ACCP Updates in Therapeutics®: Ambulatory Care Pharmacy Preparatory Review and Recertification Course

ACCP Updates in Therapeutics®:

Ambulatory Care Pharmacy Preparatory Review and Recertification Course

2016 Edition

Volume II

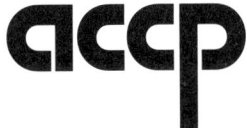

American College of Clinical Pharmacy
Lenexa, Kansas

Director of Professional Development: Nancy M. Perrin, M.A., CAE
Senior Project Manager, Education: Emma F. Webb, M.A.
Medical Editor: Kimma Sheldon, Ph.D.
Medical Editor: Anna Binda, Ph.D.
Layout Designer: Brian Rio
Layout Designer: Holly Ogden

For order information or questions, contact:
   American College of Clinical Pharmacy
   13000 W. 87th St. Parkway
   Lenexa, KS 66215-4530
   Phone: (913) 492-3311
   Fax: (913) 492-0088
   accp@accp.com
   http://www.accp.com

Printed in the United States of America.

/

To properly cite this book:

Author(s). Chapter name. In: Bainbridge JL, Cardone K, Cross LB, et al. Updates in Therapeutics®: Ambulatory Care Pharmacy Preparatory Review and Recertification Course, 2016 ed. Lenexa, KS: American College of Clinical Pharmacy, year:pages.

Note: The authors and publisher of the Ambulatory Care Pharmacy Preparatory Review and Recertification Course recognize that the development of this material offers many opportunities for error. Despite our very best efforts, some errors may persist into print. Drug dosage schedules are, we believe, accurate and in accordance with current standards. Readers are advised, however, to check other published sources to be certain that recommended dosages and contraindications are in agreement with those listed in this book. This is especially important for new, infrequently used, or highly toxic drugs.

ISBN 13: 978-1-939862-28-0
ISBN 10: 1-939862-28-0

Library of Congress Control Number: 2016931529

Continuing Pharmacy Education:

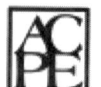

The American College of Clinical Pharmacy is accredited by the Accreditation Council for Pharmacy Education as a provider of continuing pharmacy education. The Universal Activity Numbers are: Ambulatory Care Pharmacy Preparatory Review and Recertification Course for home study, 2016 Edition:
Practice Management Issues, Activity Number: 0217-0000-16-023-H01-P; 4.0 contact hours; Biostatistics, Study Designs, and Genitourinary & Fluids/Electrolytes, Activity Number: 0217-0000-16-024-H01-P; 3.5 contact hours; Psychiatric Disorders, Neurology, and Gastrointestinal Disorders, Activity Number: 0217-0000-16-025-H01-P; 4.0 contact hours; Diabetes Mellitus, Endocrine Disorders, and Pulmonary Disorders, Activity Number: 0217-0000-16-026-H01-P; 4.5 contact hours; Cardiology and Obstetrics/Gynecology, Activity Number: 0217-0000-16-027-H01-P; 4.0 contact hours; Infectious Diseases, Renal Disorders, and Bone/Joint and Rheumatology, Activity Number: 0217-0000-16-028-H01-P; 4.5 contact hours; Health Maintenance and Public Health Activity Number: 0217-0000-16-029-H04-P; 1.5 contact hours.

All Ambulatory Care Pharmacy Preparatory Review and Recertification Course sessions are application-based activities.

To earn continuing pharmacy education credit for the home-study version of the 2016 Ambulatory Care Pharmacy Preparatory Review and Recertification Course, you must successfully complete and submit the web-based posttest associated with each program within the course no later than October 31, 2017. Statements of continuing pharmacy education credit will be available at www.accp.com/ce immediately after the submission of the successfully completed web-based posttest.

To earn BCACP recertification credit for the home-study version of the 2016 Ambulatory Care Pharmacy Preparatory Review and Recertification Course, you must successfully complete and submit the web-based posttest associated with each program within the course no later than September 1, 2016.

Errata

The authors and publisher of the Ambulatory Care Pharmacy Preparatory Review and Recertification Course recognize that the development of this material offers many opportunities for error. When possible, corrections to this publication are included in the 2016 Ambulatory Care Pharmacy Preparatory Review and Recertification Course Errata, which will be available beginning June 1, 2016, at www.accp.com/docs/products/apc16/errata.pdf.

The American College of Clinical Pharmacy (ACCP) has compiled the materials in this course book for pharmacists to use in preparing for the Board of Pharmacy Specialties (BPS) Ambulatory Care Pharmacy Specialty certification examination. There is no intent or assurance that all the knowledge on the examination will be covered in the ACCP process. Although ACCP uses the BPS Content Outline in creating the material for this course, ACCP does not know the specific content of any particular BPS examination. BPS guidelines prohibit any overlap of individuals writing the examination and developing preparatory materials.

Program Goals and Target Audience

Updates in Therapeutics®: Ambulatory Care Pharmacy Preparatory Review and Recertification Course is designed to help pharmacists who are preparing for the Board of Pharmacy Specialties certification examination in Ambulatory Care Pharmacy as well as those seeking a general review and refresher on disease states and therapeutics. The program goals are as follows:

1. To present a high-quality, up-to-date overview of disease states and therapeutics;
2. To provide a framework to help attendees prepare for the specialty certification examination in ambulatory care pharmacy; and
3. To offer participants an effective learning experience using a case-based approach with a strong focus on the thought processes needed to solve patient care problems in each therapeutic area.

FACULTY

Jacquelyn L. Bainbridge, Pharm.D., FCCP
Professor
Department of Clinical Pharmacy
Department of Neurology in the School of Medicine
University of Colorado Denver
Aurora, Colorado

Katie E. Cardone, Pharm.D., FNKF, BCACP
Associate Professor
Albany College of Pharmacy and Health Sciences
Albany, New York

L. Brian Cross, Pharm.D., BCACP, CDE
Associate Professor
Gatton School of Pharmacy
East Tennessee State University
Mountain Home, Tennessee

Alicia B. Forinash, Pharm.D., FCCP, BCPS, BCACP
Professor of Pharmacy Practice
St. Louis College of Pharmacy
St. Louis, Missouri

Shellee A. Grim, Pharm.D., BCPS
Adjunct Clinical Associate Professor
University of Illinois at Chicago
Chicago, Illinois

Adam B. Jackson, Pharm.D., BCACP
Clinical Pharmacy Specialist in Infectious Diseases
Pharmacy Department
Kaiser Permanente Colorado
Denver, Colorado

Michael P. Kane, Pharm.D., FCCP, BCPS, BCACP
Professor of Pharmacy Practice
Albany College of Pharmacy and Health Sciences;
Clinical Pharmacy Specialist
The Endocrine Group
Albany, New York

William A. Kehoe, Pharm.D., FCCP, BCPS
Professor of Clinical Pharmacy and Psychology
Chair of the Department of Pharmacy Practice
University of the Pacific
Stockton, California

Mary Ann Kliethermes, Pharm.D.
Vice Chair of the Ambulatory Care
Department of Pharmacy Practice
Associate Professor
Chicago College of Pharmacy
Midwestern University
Downers Grove, Illinois

Daniel S. Longyhore, Pharm.D., BCACP
Associate Professor
Wilkes University
Wilkes-Barre, Pennsylvania;
Ambulatory Care Pharmacist
St. Luke's Hospital & Health Network
Bethlehem, Pennsylvania

Michelle T. Martin, Pharm.D., BCPS, BCACP
Clinical Pharmacist and Assistant Professor
University of Illinois at Chicago
Chicago, Illinois

Jamie L. McConaha, Pharm.D., BCACP
Assistant Professor of Pharmacy Practice
Mylan School of Pharmacy Clinical,
Social and Administrative Sciences
Duquesne University
Pittsburgh, Pennsylvania

Emily McCoy, Pharm.D., BCACP
Associate Clinical Professor
Auburn University Harrison School of Pharmacy
Mobile, Alabama

Jean Y. Moon, Pharm.D., BCACP
Assistant Professor
North Memorial Family Medicine Residency
Program, College of Pharmacy
University of Minnesota
Minneapolis, Minnesota

Kevin M. Sowinski, Pharm.D., FCCP
Professor of Pharmacy Practice
Purdue University College of Pharmacy;
Adjunct Professor of Medicine
Indiana University School of Medicine
Indianapolis, Indiana

Jessica Tilton, Pharm.D., BCACP
Clinical Assistant Professor
Clinical Pharmacist
Medication Therapy Management Clinic;
Operations Manager
University of Illinois at Chicago
Chicago, Illinois

Joseph P. Vande Griend, Pharm.D., BCPS, CGP
Assistant Professor
University of Colorado Skaggs School of
Pharmacy and Pharmaceutical Sciences
Aurora, Colorado

Orly Vardeny, Pharm.D., BCACP
Associate Professor of Pharmacy
University of Wisconsin
School of Pharmacy
Madison, Wisconsin

Faculty Disclosures

Consultant/Member of Advisory Board: Jacquelyn L. Bainbridge (Sunovian Pharmaceuticals), Shellee A. Grimm (Astellas Pharma, Inc.), Katie E. Cardone (Fresenius Medical Care)

Grant Funding/Research Support: Jacquelyn L. Bainbridge (UCB Pharma, NIH), Michael P. Kane (AstraZeneca, Janssen Pharmaceuticals)

Speaker's Bureau: Jacquelyn L. Bainbridge (UCB Pharma)

Other: Mary Ann Kliethermes (co-owner of Clinical Pharmacy Systems, Inc.), Michelle T. Martin (owns Gilead stock)

Nothing to Disclose: L. Brian Cross, Alicia B. Forinash, Adam B. Jackson, William A. Kehoe, Daniel S. Longyhore, Jamie McConaha, Emily McCoy, Jean Y. Moon, Kevin M. Sowinski, Jessica Tilton, Joseph P. Vande Griend

Reviewer Disclosures

Consultant/Member of Advisory Board: Elizabeth Sebranek Evans (VRX)

Speaker's Bureau: Daniel M. Riche (Merck, Novo Nordisk)

Reviewers not listed above have nothing to disclose.

Acknowledgments

Jacquelyn L. Bainbridge, Pharm.D., FCCP
Professor
Department of Clinical Pharmacy
Department of Neurology in the School of Medicine
University of Colorado Denver
Aurora, Colorado

Sally Y. Barbour, Pharm.D., BCOP, CPP
Clinical Oncology Pharmacist
Duke Comprehensive Cancer Center
Duke University Medical Center
Durham, North Carolina

Ashley Branham, Pharm.D., BCACP
Director of Clinical Services
Moose Pharmacy
Concord, North Carolina

Katie E. Cardone, Pharm.D., FNKF, BCACP
Associate Professor
Albany College of Pharmacy and Health Sciences
Albany, New York

Mariann D. Churchwell, Pharm.D., BCPS
Associate Professor
University of Toledo College of Pharmacy
Toledo, Ohio

Nathan Clark, Pharm.D., FCCP, BCPS, CACP
Supervisor
Clinical Pharmacy Anticoagulation
and Anemia Services
Kaiser Permanente Colorado
Aurora, Colorado

Elizabeth A. Coyle, Pharm.D., FCCM, BCPS
Clinical Associate Professor of Infectious Diseases
University of Houston College of Pharmacy;
Director of the Infectious Diseases Pharmacy Residency
University of Texas M.D. Anderson Cancer Center
Houston, Texas

L. Brian Cross, Pharm.D., BCACP, CDE
Associate Professor
Gatton School of Pharmacy
East Tennessee State University
Mountain Home, Tennessee

Edward F. Foote, Pharm.D., FCCP, BCPS
Professor and Chair of Pharmacy Practice
Nesbitt College of Pharmacy and Nursing
Wilkes University
Wilkes-Barre, Pennsylvania

Alicia B. Forinash, Pharm.D., BCPS, BCACP
Associate Professor of Pharmacy Practice
St. Louis College of Pharmacy
St. Louis, Missouri

Wendy A. Gattis Stough, Pharm.D.
Assistant Consulting Professor in Medicine
Department of Medicine
Division of Cardiology
Duke University Medical Center
Durham, North Carolina

Shellee A. Grim, Pharm.D., BCPS
Clinical Assistant Professor
University of Illinois at Chicago
Chicago, Illinois

Ila M. Harris, Pharm.D., FCCP, BCPS
Associate Professor
Medical School
Department of Family Medicine and Community
Health, University of Minnesota
Bethesda Family Medicine
St. Paul, Minnesota

Rachel M. Heilmann, Pharm.D., BCPS
Clinical Pharmacy Specialist in Primary Care
Kaiser Permanente Colorado
Denver, Colorado

Sheryl J. Herner, Pharm.D., BCPS, CPPS
Clinical Pharmacy Specialist in Medication Safety
Kaiser Permanente Colorado
Denver, Colorado

Adam B. Jackson, Pharm.D., BCACP
Clinical Pharmacy Specialist in Infectious Diseases
Pharmacy Department
Kaiser Permanente Colorado
Denver, Colorado

Samuel G. Johnson, Pharm.D., FCCP, BCPS-AQ
Cardiology
Clinical Pharmacy Specialist – Cardiology
Kaiser Permanente Colorado Region
Denver, Colorado

Tiffany E. Kaiser, Pharm.D., FCCP, BCPS
Associate Professor of Medicine
Assistant Director of The PGY-2
Transplant Specialty Residency
University of Cincinnati Medical Center
Cincinnati, Ohio

Michael P. Kane, Pharm.D., FCCP, BCPS, BCACP
Professor of Pharmacy Practice
Albany College of Pharmacy and Health Sciences
Clinical Pharmacy Specialist
The Endocrine Group
Albany, New York

William A. Kehoe, Pharm.D., FCCP, BCPS
Professor of Clinical Pharmacy and Psychology
Chair of the Department of Pharmacy
Practice, University of the Pacific
Stockton, California

Mary Ann Kliethermes, Pharm.D.
Vice Chair of the Ambulatory Care
Department of Pharmacy Practice
Associate Professor
Chicago College of Pharmacy
Midwestern University
Downers Grove, Illinois

Sunny A. Linnebur, Pharm.D., FCCP, BCPS, CGP
Associate Professor
University of Colorado Skaggs School of
Pharmacy and Pharmaceutical Sciences
University of Colorado Anschutz Medical Campus
Aurora, Colorado

Daniel S. Longyhore, Pharm.D., BCACP
Associate Professor
Wilkes University
Wilkes-Barre, Pennsylvania;
Ambulatory Care Pharmacist
St. Luke's Hospital & Health Network
Bethlehem, Pennsylvania

Karen F. Marlowe, Pharm.D., BCPS, CPE
Assistant Dean and Associate Department Head
James T. and Anne Klein Davis Endowed Professor
Harrison School of Pharmacy
Auburn University
Mobile, Alabama

Michelle T. Martin, Pharm.D., BCPS, BCACP
Clinical Pharmacist and Assistant Professor
University of Illinois at Chicago
Chicago, Illinois

Jamie L. McConaha, Pharm.D., BCACP
Assistant Professor of Pharmacy Practice
Mylan School of Pharmacy Clinical,
Social and Administrative Sciences
Duquesne University
Pittsburgh, Pennsylvania

Karen J. McConnell, Pharm.D.,
FCCP, BCPS-AQ Cardiology
Clinical Pharmacy Specialist in Cardiology
Kaiser Permanente of Colorado;
Clinical Associate Professor
University of Colorado Skaggs School of Pharmacy and
Pharmaceutical Sciences;
Adjunct Professor of Pharmacy Practice
Regis University School of Pharmacy
Denver, Colorado

Emily McCoy, Pharm.D., BCACP
Associate Clinical Professor
Auburn University Harrison School of Pharmacy
Mobile, Alabama

Jean Y. Moon, Pharm.D., BCACP
Assistant Professor
North Memorial Family Medicine Residency
Program, College of Pharmacy
University of Minnesota
Minneapolis, Minnesota

Bruce A. Mueller, Pharm.D., FCCP
Professor of Pharmacy and Chair
Department of Clinical, Social and
Administrative Sciences
College of Pharmacy
University of Michigan;
Pharmacy Assistant Director
Department of Pharmacy Services
University Hospital
University of Michigan Health Systems
Ann Arbor, Michigan

Edith A. Nutescu, Pharm.D., FCCP
Director of the Antithrombosis Service
Associate Professor
Department of Pharmacy Practice
University of Illinois at Chicago
Chicago, Illinois

Carol A. Ott, Pharm.D., BCPP
Clinical Associate Professor of Pharmacy Practice
College of Pharmacy
Purdue University;
Clinical Pharmacy Specialist in Psychiatry
Wishard Health Services and Midtown
Community Mental Health
Indianapolis, Indiana

Ann M. Philbrick, Pharm.D., BCPS
Associate Professor
University of Minnesota;
Clinical Pharmacist
Bethesda Family Medicine
St. Paul, Minnesota

Frank Romanelli, Pharm.D., MPH, BCPS
Associate Dean
Professor of Pharmacy,
Health Sciences, and Medicine
University of Kentucky
Lexington, Kentucky

J. Mark Ruscin, Pharm.D., BCPS
Professor
Department of Pharmacy Practice
Southern Illinois University Edwardsville
Edwardsville, Illinois

Wendy L. St. Peter, Pharm.D.,
FCCP, FASN, FNKF, BCPS
Professor
College of Pharmacy
University of Minnesota;
United States Renal Data System &
Chronic Disease Research Group
Minneapolis, Minnesota

Sarah L. Scarpace, Pharm.D., BCOP
Associate Professor and Assistant Dean for
Pharmacy Professional Affairs
Albany College of Pharmacy and Health Sciences;
Clinical Pharmacy Specialist
Stratton Veterans' Affairs Medical Center
Albany, New York

Mansi Shah, Pharm.D., BCACP, CDE
Assistant Professor
University of Illinois at Chicago
College of Pharmacy
Chicago, Illinois

Kevin M. Sowinski, Pharm.D., FCCP
Professor of Pharmacy Practice
Purdue University College of Pharmacy;
Adjunct Professor of Medicine
Indiana University School of Medicine
Indianapolis, Indiana

Sarah A. Spinler, Pharm.D., FCCP, BCPS
Professor of Clinical Pharmacy
Department of Pharmacy Practice
and Pharmacy Administration
Philadelphia College of Pharmacy
University of the Sciences
Philadelphia, Pennsylvania

Michael C. Thomas, Pharm.D., BCPS
Clinical Associate Professor and Vice Chair
Department of Pharmacy Practice
Western New England University
College of Pharmacy
Springfield, Massachusetts

Jessica Tilton, Pharm.D., BCACP
Clinical Assistant Professor
Clinical Pharmacist
Medication Therapy Management Clinic;
Operations Manager
University of Illinois at Chicago
Chicago, Illinois

Andrea N. Traina, Pharm.D., BCPS, BCACP
Assistant Professor of Pharmacy Practice
St. John Fisher College
Wegmans School of Pharmacy;
Clinical Pharmacy Specialist
Endocrine-Diabetes Care and Resource Center
Rochester General Health System
Rochester, New York

Joseph P. Vande Griend, Pharm.D., BCPS, CGP
Assistant Professor
University of Colorado Skaggs School of
Pharmacy and Pharmaceutical Sciences
Aurora, Colorado

Orly Vardeny, Pharm.D., BCACP
Associate Professor of Pharmacy
University of Wisconsin
School of Pharmacy
Madison, Wisconsin

Anna Vaysman, Pharm.D., BCPS
Clinical Assistant Professor
University of Illinois at Chicago
College of Pharmacy
Chicago, Illinois

Daniel M. Witt, Pharm.D., FCCP, BCPS
Sr. Manager Clinical Pharmacy Research
& Applied Pharmacogenomics
Kaiser Permanente Central Support
Services – Pharmacy Administration
Kaiser Permanente
Aurora, Colorado

Pei Shieen Wong, Pharm.D., BCPS
Neurology Clinical Research Fellow
Department of Clinical Pharmacy
Department of Neurology in the School of Medicine
University of Colorado Denver
Aurora, Colorado

EXTERNAL REVIEWERS

The American College of Clinical Pharmacy and the authors would like to thank the following individuals for their review of Updates in Therapeutics®: Ambulatory Care Pharmacy Preparatory Review and Recertification Course.

Debra J. Barnette, Pharm.D., BCPS, BCACP
Assistant Professor
The Ohio State University
Columbus, Ohio

Julie C. Bartell, Pharm.D., BCACP, CACP
Clinical Pharmacotherapist
Pharmacy Residency Program Director
Monroe Clinic
Monroe, Wisconsin

Kevin J. Bowers, Pharm.D., BCACP
Pharmacy Manager
St. Vincent de Paul Charitable Pharmacy
Fairfield, Ohio

Benjamin Chavez, Pharm.D., BCACP, BCPP
Associate Professor
University of Colorado Denver
Denver, Colorado

Bethany S. Cross, Pharm.D., BCACP, BCPP
Clinical Pharmacy Specialist
Otsego Memorial Hospital
Gaylord, Michigan

Shawn M. Dalton, Pharm.D., BCPS, BCACP
Clinical Pharmacy Specialist
Sheridan VA Medical Center
Sheridan, Wyoming

Mary Day, Pharm.D., BCACP
Assistant Professor of Pharmacy Practice
Union University
Humboldt, Tennessee

G. Robert DeYoung, Pharm.D., BCPS
Clinical Pharmacist, Ambulatory Care
Advantage Health Physicians and St. Mary's Health Care
Grand Rapids, Michigan

Jennifer S. Dizney, Pharm.D., BCACP, BCPP, CGP
Clinical Pharmacist
St. Vincent's Medical Center - MultiSpecialty Group
Bridgeport, Connecticut

Joseph J. Fierro, Pharm.D., BCACP
Clinical Pharmacy Specialist
James A. Haley Veterans' Hospital
Spring Hill, Florida

Elisa Greene, Pharm.D., BCACP
Assistant Professor of Pharmacy Practice
Belmont University College of Pharmacy
Nashville, Tennessee

Haytham Hussein Hafez II, BScPharm, BCPS, BCACP
Senior Pharmacist
Z.M. Hospital
Abu Dhabi, United Arab Emirates

Daniel M. Hartung, Pharm.D., MPH
Assistant Professor
Oregon State University
Portland, Oregon

James D. Hicks, Pharm.D., BCACP, NCPS
LCDR
U.S. Public Health Service;
Assistant Chief Pharmacist
Winslow Indian Health Care Center
Winslow, Arizona

Libby Hinds, Pharm.D., BCACP
Clinical Pharmacy Specialist
Birmingham VAMC
Birmingham, Alabama

Emily J. Holm, Pharm.D., BCACP
Ambulatory Care Clinical Pharmacist
Mayo Clinic Health Systems
Mankato, Minnesota

Gregory J. Hughes, Pharm.D., BCPS, CGP
Assistant Clinical Professor
St. John's College of Pharmacy and
Allied Health Professions
Queens, New York

Erik C. Johnson, Pharm.D., BCACP
Clinical Pharmacist
University of Colorado Hospital
Denver, Colorado

Amber M. Kelley, Pharm.D., BCACP
Clinical Pharmacist
University of Iowa Hospitals and Clinics
Iowa City, Iowa

Craig Kimble, Pharm.D., MBA, M.S., BCACP
Director of Experiential Learning
Manager of Clinical Support Services
Assistant Professor of Pharmacy Practice
Marshall University School of Pharmacy
Huntington, West Virginia

Wichitah P. Leng, Pharm.D., BCACP
Clinical Pharmacist
Bravo Health Advanced Care Center
Philadelphia, Pennsylvania

Diane Lum, Pharm.D., BCACP
Emergency Medicine Clinical Pharmacist
Stony Brook Medicine
New York, New York

Uyen Nhi Nguyen, Pharm.D., BCACP
Clinical Pharmacy Specialist
Kaiser Permanente
Springfield, Virginia

Carol A. Ott, Pharm.D., BCPP
Clinical Associate Professor of Pharmacy Practice
College of Pharmacy
Purdue University;
Clinical Pharmacy Specialist in Psychiatry
Wishard Health Services and Midtown
Community Mental Health
Indianapolis, Indiana

Paige F. Parsons, Pharm.D., BCACP
Clinical Pharmacy Specialist
MMP Portland Family Medicine
Portland, Maine

Kayla Peeler, Pharm.D.
Pharmacist
University of Mississippi
Jackson, Mississippi

Long Pham, Pharm.D., BCPS, BCACP
Clinical Pharmacist
Exempla St. Joseph's Hospital
Frisco, Texas

Ann M. Philbrick, Pharm.D., BCPS, BCACP
Associate Professor
University of Minnesota;
Clinical Pharmacist
Bethesda Family Medicine
St. Paul, Minnesota

Darin Ramsey, Pharm.D., BCPS, BCACP
Associate Professor of Pharmacy Practice
Butler University College of
Pharmacy & Health Sciences
Indianapolis, Indiana

Holly V. Rice, Pharm.D., BCACP
Chief of Pharmacy
Indian Health Service
Sisseton, South Dakota

Daniel M. Riche, Pharm.D., FCCP, BCPS
Associate Professor
University of Mississippi
Jackson, Mississippi

Catherine S. Riggs, Pharm.D., BCACP
Primary Care Clinical Pharmacy Specialist
Kaiser Permanente Colorado
Fort Collins, Colorado

Kellie Rose, Pharm.D., BCPS, BCACP
Clinical Pharmacy Specialist-Primary Care
Staunton Community Based Outpatient Clinic
Staunton, Virginia

Annette L. Schall, Pharm.D., BCACP, CACP
Clinical Pharmacy Specialist
Providence Medical Group
Molalla, Oregon

Elizabeth Sebranek Evans, Pharm.D., BCPS, CGP
Advanced Clinical Pharmacist - Neuro
Specialty Rehabilitation
Intermountain Medical Center
Murray, Utah

Larry W. Segars, Pharm.D., DrPH, FCCP, BCPS
Chair, Department of Pharmacology & Microbiology;
Associate Professor of Pharmacology
& Preventive Medicine
Kansas City University of Medicine & Biosciences
Kansas City, Missouri

Kayce M. Shealy, Pharm.D., BCPS, BCACP
Assistant Professor of Pharmacy Practice
Presbyterian College School of Pharmacy
Clinton, South Carolina

Sneha Srivastava, Pharm.D., BCACP
Clinical Associate Professor
Chicago State University
Chicago, Illinois

Robyn M. Teply, Pharm.D., BCACP
Clinical Pharmacist
Creighton Medical Associates
Omaha, Nebraska

Tania Thomas, Pharm.D., BCACP
Clinical Pharmacy Specialist in Ambulatory Care
Parkland Health & Hospital System/
Dallas County Jail Health
Dallas, Texas

Jeremy Thoms, Pharm.D., BCACP
Geriatrics Clinical Pharmacy Specialist
Department of Veteran Affairs
Gainesville, Florida

Jeffrey M. Tingen, Pharm.D., MBA, BCPS, BCACP, CDE
Clinical Assistant Professor
PGY2 Ambulatory Care Pharmacy
Residency Program Director
University of Michigan College of Pharmacy
Ann Arbor, Michigan

Daniel B. Truelove, Pharm.D., BCPS, BCACP
Clinical Pharmacist
University of Louisville HealthCare
Louisville, Kentucky

Ryan J. Wargo, Pharm.D., BCACP
Ambulatory Care Pharmacist and Assistant Professor
Bayfront Family Medicine
Lake Erie College of Osteopathic Medicine
Bradenton, Florida

Tricia L. Watts, RPh, BCACP
Outpatient Clinical Pharmacist
VA Central Iowa
Des Moines, Iowa

Cassandra R. White, Pharm.D., BCACP, CGP
Assistant Professor
Husson University School of Pharmacy
Mount Vernon, Maine

Lori A. Wilken, Pharm.D., BCACP, TT-S, AE-C
Clinical Assistant Professor
University of Illinois at Chicago
Chicago, Illinois

Jillian N. Wilkes, Pharm.D., BCACP
Clinical Pharmacy Specialist
WJB Dorn VAMC - Florence CBOC
Scranton, South Carolina

Phillip Yamauchi, BCPS, BCACP, CDE
Clinical Pharmacist
Gila Regional Medical Center
Silver City, New Mexico

Ashley Zuppelli, Pharm.D., BCACP, AAHIVP
Assistant Professor of Pharmacy Practice
Wegmans School of Pharmacy at
St. John Fisher College
Rochester, New York

TABLE OF CONTENTS

ADDITIONAL RESOURCES

ACCP Updates in Therapeutics®: Ambulatory Care Pharmacy Preparatory Review and Recertification Course

Cardiology I

Orly Vardeny, Pharm.D., BCACP

University of Wisconsin
Madison, Wisconsin

Cardiology I

Orly Vardeny, Pharm.D., BCACP

University of Wisconsin
Madison, Wisconsin

Learning Objectives

1. Formulate appropriate oral anticoagulant treatment strategies for patients who develop venous thromboembolism (VTE) (deep venous thrombosis or pulmonary embolism) consistent with available consensus panel guidelines, recent U.S. Food and Drug Administration (FDA) approvals, and randomized clinical trials.
2. Describe key differences in onset of action, dosing, administration, absorption, effects on common coagulation tests, and drug interactions between dabigatran, rivaroxaban, apixaban, and warfarin in the management of nonvalvular atrial fibrillation (AF) and treatment and prevention of VTE.
3. Develop a comprehensive education and monitoring plan for patients receiving oral anticoagulants for treatment and prevention of VTE, stroke prevention in nonvalvular AF, and stroke prevention associated with mechanical heart valves.
4. Develop patient-specific, guideline-driven treatment, monitoring, and follow-up plans for patients with heart failure (HF).
5. Develop patient-specific, guideline-driven treatment, monitoring, and follow-up plans for rate and pharmacologic rhythm control in a patient with AF.
6. Identify patient-specific appropriate antiarrhythmic drugs for rhythm control in AF and ventricular tachycardia (VT).
7. Describe the role of catheter ablation in rhythm control management of AF and VT.
8. Develop a patient-specific monitoring plan for guideline-based medical therapies for heart failure.
9. Describe current practice standards for agent selection and duration of antithrombotic therapy for stroke prevention after transcatheter aortic valve replacement for aortic stenosis.
10. Identify treatment goals, common adverse effects, clinically important drug interactions, monitoring, and REMS (Risk Evaluation and Mitigation Strategies) requirements for oral pharmacotherapy of pulmonary arterial hypertension.

Self-Assessment Questions

Answers and explanations to these questions can be found at the end of the chapter.

1. A 55-year-old, 78-kg man with a history of hypertension (HTN) for 5 years and an acute pulmonary embolism (PE) is ready for hospital discharge. He was treated with an intravenous heparin infusion for 2 days, and his current activated partial thromboplastin time (aPTT) is 77 seconds. His only medication is losartan 50 mg orally twice daily. His serum creatinine concentration (SCr) is 0.88 mg/dL. He will initiate therapy with an oral anticoagulant now, with the heparin infusion discontinued at the time of the first dose. According to the U.S. Food and Drug Administration (FDA) approvals or favorable results in clinical trials, which option best reflects the correct treatment regimen with an intended duration of at least 6 months?

    A. Warfarin 10 mg orally daily to an international normalized ratio (INR) of 2–3.
    B. Rivaroxaban 20 mg orally daily with a meal.
    C. Apixaban 10 mg orally twice daily for 7 days; then decrease to 5 mg orally twice daily.
    D. Dabigatran 150 mg orally twice daily for 7 days; then decrease to 75 mg orally twice daily.

2. A patient with permanent atrial fibrillation (AF) taking rivaroxaban presents with acute heart failure (HF), hypotension, and a new pericardial effusion suggestive of malignancy. An urgent diagnostic and therapeutic pericardiocentesis is planned. The interventional cardiologist would like to avoid doing the procedure until the rivaroxaban dose has worn off. Which is the best laboratory test to assess whether rivaroxaban is present?

    A. International normalized ratio (INR).
    B. Activated partial thromboplastin time.
    C. Activated clotting time.
    D. Anti−factor Xa (anti-Xa) concentration.

3. Which is the preferred antithrombotic management strategy at hospital discharge for a patient with mitral stenosis in normal sinus rhythm (NSR) after placement of a bioprosthetic heart valve?

    A. Aspirin 325 mg orally daily.
    B. Dabigatran 150 mg orally twice daily.
    C. Warfarin at a goal INR of 2.0–3.0.
    D. Warfarin at a goal INR of 2.5–3.5.

4. A 78-year-old man with heart failure with reduced ejection fraction (HFrEF) and creatinine clearance (CrCl) of 45 mL/minute is initiating therapy with eplerenone 25 mg orally every other day. Which option best reflects the frequency of serum potassium and SCr monitoring recommended in the 2013 American College of Cardiology Foundation/American Heart Association (ACCF/AHA) HF guidelines?

   A. In 3 days, in 1 week, and then monthly for the first 6 months.
   B. Weekly for the first 6 months.
   C. In 2 weeks and then monthly for the first 6 months.
   D. In 1 week and then monthly for the first 6 months

5. A 68-year-old woman with HTN was recently hospitalized for heart failure with preserved ejection fraction (HFpEF) and newly diagnosed nonvalvular AF (NVAF). She is seen today in the cardiology clinic 2 weeks after hospital discharge. She is being treated with metoprolol 12.5 mg orally twice daily, enalapril 5 mg orally daily, furosemide 20 mg orally twice daily, and dabigatran 150 mg orally twice daily. She is scheduled to undergo direct current cardioversion (DCC) in 1 week. Her blood pressure (BP) is 125/80 mm Hg, heart rate (HR) is 140 beats/minute, and CrCl is 68 mL/minute. Her 12-lead electrocardiogram (ECG) shows AF and a ventricular response of 139 beats/minute. Which is the best option regarding a guideline-recommended course of action currently?

   A. No change in medications.
   B. Initiate warfarin therapy and discontinue dabigatran now.
   C. Increase enalapril to 10 mg orally daily.
   D. Increase metoprolol to 25 mg orally twice daily.

6. A 50-year-old man with nonischemic cardiomyopathy and HFrEF is admitted to the hospital for AF associated with acute HF exacerbation. He has a biventricular pacemaker (cardiac resynchronization therapy [CRT]) with an implantable defibrillator. His BP is 100/80 mm Hg, his HR is 115 beats/minute, and his laboratory test results are normal. His PR interval is 0.2 second, and his QTc is 480 milliseconds. His current medications include carvedilol 25 mg orally twice daily, lisinopril 20 mg orally daily, spironolactone 25 mg orally daily, and furosemide

40 mg orally twice daily. A decision is made to perform cardioversion after initiation of an antiarrhythmic drug. The patient is scheduled for DCC in 3 days. Which antiarrhythmic drug is the best choice, representing that recommended in the 2014 ACCF/AHA/Heart Rhythm Society (HRS) AF guidelines for maintenance of NSR, for this patient?

   A. Digoxin.
   B. Sotalol.
   C. Amiodarone.
   D. Flecainide.

7. According to the 2012 HRS consensus guidelines for the catheter ablation of AF, which option best exemplifies a patient who is not a candidate for ablation?

   A. A patient with paroxysmal AF who has signs of HF and is not maintained in NSR with dofetilide.
   B. A patient with persistent AF and palpitations with a history of amiodarone intolerance because of hyperthyroidism who is maintained in NSR with dofetilide.
   C. An asymptomatic patient with permanent AF taking no antiarrhythmic medications.
   D. A patient with paroxysmal AF with hospitalizations secondary to rapid ventricular response who is not maintained in NSR with dronedarone and sotalol.

8. A 56-year-old patient with HFrEF and a history of ventricular tachycardia (VT) is seen in the arrhythmia clinic. The patient has a biventricular implantable defibrillator that shows no firing for VT within the past 6 months. He has New York Heart Association (NYHA) class II HF symptoms, which have been stable for 6 months. His current medications include spironolactone, carvedilol, lisinopril, furosemide, and simvastatin. Amiodarone was initiated 6 months ago. In addition to a 12-lead ECG and chest radiography, which set of tests would be best to monitor for amiodarone toxicity?

   A. Slit lamp examination and lipid panel.
   B. SCr and sodium assays.
   C. Thyroid-stimulating hormone and liver function tests (LFTs).
   D. Pulmonary function tests and creatine phosphokinase assay.

9. A 68-year-old patient with HTN, AF, and HFpEF is initiating amiodarone therapy. When you review the patient's medication history, which is the best example of a concomitant medication that would require a dose adjustment currently?

   A. Warfarin.
   B. Rivaroxaban.
   C. Atorvastatin.
   D. Metoprolol.

10. An 80-year-old woman has HTN, severe aortic stenosis, HFpEF, and new-onset angina. She is currently being treated with metoprolol tartrate 75 mg orally twice daily and furosemide 20 mg orally daily. Her BP is 130/80 mm Hg, and HR is 50 beats/minute. Which is the best recommendation for treating her angina currently?

    A. Increase the metoprolol tartrate dose to 100 mg orally twice daily.
    B. Add diltiazem sustained release 120 mg orally daily.
    C. Add isosorbide mononitrate 60 mg orally daily.
    D. Add amlodipine 10 mg orally daily.

11. According to current practice standards, which is the optimal antithrombotic regimen for stroke prevention after transcatheter aortic valve replacement (TAVR) for a patient in NSR?

    A. Warfarin orally at a goal INR of 2–3 for 6 months.
    B. Warfarin orally at a goal INR of 2–3 plus aspirin 81 mg orally daily for 3 months.
    C. Prasugrel 10 mg orally daily for 6 months.
    D. Clopidogrel 75 mg orally daily plus aspirin 81 mg orally daily for 3 months.

12. In a patient being treated for pulmonary arterial hypertension (PAH), which option best represents the agent requiring LFT monitoring for early recognition of hepatotoxicity, even if the patient has no signs/symptoms of liver toxicity?

    A. Macitentan.
    B. Sildenafil.
    C. Bosentan.
    D. Riociguat.

THROMBOEMBOLISM

I. ANTITHROMBOTIC THERAPY FOR VENOUS THROMBOEMBOLISM

A. Epidemiology
1. Up to 2,000,000 symptomatic and asymptomatic cases of venous thromboembolism (VTE) occur in the United States each year, and more than 100,000 patients die of pulmonary embolism (PE).
2. Incidence of VTE doubles in each decade of life after age 50 years.
3. African American individuals are at a higher risk of VTE than are white individuals, whereas Hispanic people appear to be at a slightly lower risk.

B. Etiology *(Domain 1, Task 1)*
1. In many cases, VTE is the result of converging combinations of inherited and acquired thrombotic risk factors.
2. Many individuals with hereditary hypercoagulable conditions experience a first VTE only after being placed in situations of high risk of thrombosis such as orthopedic surgery, trauma, immobilization, use of estrogen-containing oral contraceptives, or pregnancy.

C. Risk Factors for VTE *(Domain 1, Task 2)*
1. Diagnostic workup should include a search for risk factors in the patient's medical history.
2. Cancer and prior VTE are the most significant risk factors for VTE occurrence.
3. The effects of VTE risk factors are additive. The higher the number of risk factors, the higher the likelihood of thrombosis occurring.

Table 1. Risk Factors for VTE in Hospitalized Medical Patients

Risk Factor	Points[a]
Active cancer	3
Previous VTE involving deep veins	3
Reduced mobility	3
Thrombophilia	3
Trauma or surgery within 30 days	2
Age ≥ 70 years	1
Heart and/or respiratory failure	1
Acute myocardial infarction or ischemic stroke	1
Acute infection or rheumatologic disorder	1
Obesity (BMI ≥ 30 kg/m^2)	1
Hormonal treatment	1

[a]Padua Prediction Score, high risk = 4 points or greater.

BMI = body mass index; VTE = venous thromboembolism.

Table 2. VTE Risk Stratification for Surgical Populations

AT-9 Risk Category	GI, Urologic, Vascular, Breast, and Thyroid Procedures Caprini Score[a]	Plastic and Reconstructive Surgery Caprini Score[a]	Other Populations in Risk Category	Estimated Baseline VTE Risk Without Prophylaxis, %
Very low	0	0–2	Most outpatient or same-day surgery	<0.5
Low	1–2	3–4	Spinal surgery for nonmalignant disease	1.5
Moderate	3–4	5–6	Gynecologic surgery Noncancer cardiac surgery Most thoracic surgery Spinal surgery for malignant disease	3.0
High	≥5	7–8	Bariatric surgery Gynecologic cancer surgery Pneumonectomy Craniotomy Traumatic brain injury Spinal cord injury Other major trauma Elective joint arthroplasty	6.0

[a]Caprini score: 5 points each for stroke (<30 days), elective arthroplasty, hip, pelvis, or leg fracture, or spinal cord injury (<30 days); 3 points each for age ≥ 75 years, history of VTE, family history of VTE, thrombophilia; 2 points each for age 61–74 years, arthroscopic procedure, major open surgery (>45 minutes), laparoscopic procedure (>45 minutes), malignancy, confined to bed >72 hours, plaster cast, central venous access; 1 point each for age 41–60 years, minor surgery, BMI > 25 kg/m^2, swollen legs, varicose veins, pregnant or postpartum, history of unexplained or recurrent abortion, hormone therapy, sepsis (<30 days), lung disease including pneumonia (<30 days), abnormal pulmonary function, acute myocardial infarction, congestive heart failure, history of inflammatory bowel disease, medical patient at bed rest.

AT-9 = American College of Chest Physicians (ACCP) 9th eEdition of the Chest Guidelines on Antithrombotic Therapy and Prevention of Thrombosis (AT9; BMI = body mass index; GI = gastrointestinal; VTE = venous thromboembolism.

D. Deep Venous Thrombosis (DVT) *(Domain 1, Tasks 1–, 2, 3)*
1. Clinical presentation
   a. Most thrombi begin in the lower extremities.
   b. DVTs embolize in up to 50% of cases.
   c. Superficial vein thrombi do not embolize unless they extend into a deep vein.
   d. Isolated calf DVTs are less likely to embolize than proximal DVTs.
   e. Patients often present with nonspecific symptoms; therefore, objective testing is needed to confirm the diagnosis.
   f. Many patients never develop symptoms from the acute event.
   g. Even in the absence of symptoms, patients may develop long-term consequences (e.g., postthrombotic syndrome, recurrent VTE).
   h. Most upper extremity DVTs are related to central lines.

2. Signs and symptoms of DVT
   a. Unilateral leg swelling
   b. Pain in the affected leg
   c. Calf tenderness in affected leg
   d. Increased leg warmth
   e. Erythema of affected leg
   f. A "palpable cord" may be felt in the affected leg.
3. Diagnosis
   a. D-dimer test
      i. D-dimer is a by-product of fibrin degradation.
      ii. Almost always elevated during acute VTE. (Note: Other conditions can also cause elevation such as recent surgery, trauma, pregnancy, cancer, and age older than 65 years.)
      iii. A negative D-dimer test result is effective to rule out VTE in the setting of a low pretest clinical probability.
      iv. A positive result requires further diagnostic verification.
      v. Sensitivity can be reduced if the duration of symptoms exceeds 2–3 days or if the patient received an anticoagulant.
   b. Duplex ultrasonography
      i. The most commonly used test to diagnose DVT
      ii. Preferred to venography
      iii. Can measure the rate and direction of blood flow and visualize clot formation in proximal veins of the legs
      iv. Cannot reliably detect small blood clots in distal veins
      v. Noninvasive test – Does not carry the adverse effects of venography (hypotension, cardiac arrhythmias, vessel wall irritation, and nephrotoxicity caused by the contrast medium)
      vi. A positive duplex ultrasound finding in combination with a moderate to high pretest clinical probability score or a positive D-dimer test result can be used to confirm the diagnosis.
      vii. Negative test result does not exclude DVT, particularly in calf veins.
      viii. The ability to diagnose a new DVT can be difficult in patients with a history of DVT.
   c. Venography
      i. The "gold standard" for the diagnosis of DVT
      ii. An invasive test that involves the injection of radiopaque contrast dye into a foot vein
      iii. Expensive; can cause anaphylaxis and nephrotoxicity
   d. Clinical assessment
      i. Clinical assessment significantly improves the diagnostic accuracy of noninvasive tests.
      ii. Simple assessment checklists can be used to determine whether a patient has a high, moderate, or low probability of VTE.
   e. Putting it all together
      i. Calculate pretest probability of DVT (see below).
      ii. If patient has low pretest probability, is younger than 65 years, and has a negative D-dimer test result, DVT is ruled out.
      iii. Everyone else requires duplex ultrasonography or other imaging study to confirm diagnosis.

Table 3. Wells Clinical Model for Evaluating the Pretest Probability of DVT[a,b]

Clinical Characteristic	Score
Active cancer (cancer treatment within previous 6 months or currently receivingon palliative treatment)	1
Paralysis, paresis, or recent plaster immobilization of the lower extremities	1
Recently bedridden for ≥3 days or major surgery within the previous 12 weeks requiring general or regional anesthesia	1
Localized tenderness along the distribution of the deep venous system	1
Entire leg swollen	1
Calf swelling at least 3 cm larger than that on the asymptomatic side (measured 10 cm below tibial tuberosity)	1
Pitting edema confined to the symptomatic leg	1
Collateral superficial veins (non-varicose)	1
Previously documented DVT	1
Alternative diagnosis at least as likely as DVT	−2

[a]Clinical probability of DVT: Low < 0; moderate 1–2; high > 3. In patients with symptoms in both legs, the more symptomatic leg is used.
[b]Calculator available at www.mdcalc.com/wells-criteria-for-dvt/.
DVT = deep venous thrombosis.

E. Pulmonary Embolism *(Domain 1, Tasks 1–, 2, 3)*
    1. Signs and symptoms
        a. Much like patients with DVT, patients with PE often present with atypical symptoms.
        b. Signs/symptoms are nonspecific, making diagnosis of PE challenging.
        c. Sudden death may occur before effective treatment can be initiated if symptoms are not recognized.

Table 4. Signs and Symptoms of PE

Common Signs/Symptoms	
Dyspnea	
Pleuritic chest pain with clear radiograph	
Tachypnea	
Less Common Frequent Signs/Symptoms	
Cough	Systolic murmur (tricuspid regurgitation)
Hemoptysis	
Fever	ECG findings: Right bundle branch block, S1Q3T3, and T-wave inversions in leads V1–V4
Syncope	
Diaphoresis	Wheezing
Nonpleuritic chest pain	Hypotension
Apprehension	Tachycardia
Rales	Cyanosis
Increased pulmonic component (P2) of the second heart sound	Pleural rub
	Elevated neck veins

Table 4. Signs and Symptoms of PE *(continued)*

Signs and Symptoms of Massive PE	
Hemodynamic instability	50% or more absent perfusion of the lung on angiography or ventilation/perfusion scanning
Cardiac arrest	
Cyanosis	Right ventricular strain on ECG
Hypotension	Elevated pulmonary arterial pressure
Hypoxia	Elevated B-type natriuretic peptide
Oliguria	Elevated troponin

ECG = electrocardiogram/electrocardiography; PE = pulmonary embolism.

2. Diagnosis
    a. Laboratory tests
        i. Serum concentrations of D-dimer are almost always elevated, but a negative D-dimer test result combined with a low pretest probability score in patients younger than 65 years can rule out PE.
        ii. The patient may have an elevated erythrocyte sedimentation rate and white blood cell count.
    b. Computerized tomography
        i. Most commonly used test to diagnose PE
        ii. Preferred option for PE diagnosis unless contraindications exist – Contrast dye is typically used, which can make the test unsuitable for patients with poor renal function.
        iii. Positive scan results have good specificity and generally confirm the diagnosis.
        iv. Negative scan results may require further diagnostic studies if PE seems likely because of clinical pretest probability scoring and/or D-dimer results.
        v. Both the sensitivity and specificity of the scan are improved with central clots compared with those that are more peripheral.
        vi. False positives are more common for segmental/subsegmental embolism, and follow-up testing may be needed.
    c. Ventilation/perfusion (V/Q) scanning
        i. Measures the distribution of blood flow and airflow in the lungs
        ii. When there is a large mismatch between blood flow and airflow in one area of the lung, the probability is high that the patient has a PE.
        iii. Scans with positive findings have good sensitivity and help confirm the diagnosis.
        iv. Specificity can be impaired by chronic obstructive pulmonary disease, asthma, and congestive HF.
        v. A scan with negative findings also has good specificity and generally rules out the diagnosis.
        vi. An intermediate or low radiologic probability scan lacks sensitivity and requires further diagnostic studies if PE seems likely.
        vii. V/Q scanning is often preferred in patients with renal insufficiency or with allergies to contrast dye.
    d. Pulmonary angiography
        i. The gold standard for the diagnosis of PE
        ii. An invasive test that involves the injection of radiopaque contrast dye into the pulmonary artery
        iii. Expensive and associated with a significant risk of morbidity
    e. Clinical assessment: Like in DVT, clinical assessment in PE significantly improves the diagnostic accuracy of noninvasive tests, and it should be routinely performed.

Table 5. Wells Criteria Clinical Model for Evaluating the Pretest Probability of PE[a,b]

Clinical Characteristic	Score
Cancer	+1
Hemoptysis	+1
Previous PE or DVT	+1.5
Heart rate > 100 beats/minute	+1.5
Recent surgery or immobilization	+1.5
Clinical signs of DVT	+3
Alternative diagnosis less likely than PE	+3

[a]Clinical probability of PE: Low 0–1; moderate 2–6; high ≥ 7.

[b]Calculator available at www.mdcalc.com/wells-criteria-for-pulmonary-embolism-pe/.

DVT = deep venous thrombosis; PE = pulmonary embolism.

    F.   Treatment of VTE *(Domain 1, Tasks 2, 5–, 6, 7; Domain 3, Tasks 1–, 2, 3; Domain 2, Task 5; Domain 5, Task 1)*

        1.   General treatment principles for patients with VTE (DVT and/or PE)

            a.   The diagnosis of VTE should be confirmed by objective testing.

            b.   Options for treatment are as follows:

                i.   Rapid-acting injectable anticoagulant (unfractionated heparin [UFH], low-molecular-weight heparin [LMWH], or fondaparinux) transitioned to warfarin (minimum 5 days of combined therapy)

                ii.   Rapid-acting injectable anticoagulant transitioned to dabigatran

                iii.   Sole treatment with rivaroxaban or dabigatran

            c.   If the patient's therapy is changed to warfarin, the rapid-acting anticoagulant (UFH, LMWH, or fondaparinux) should be overlapped with warfarin for at least 5 days and until the INR is greater than 2 and stable enough to allow the vitamin K antagonist sufficient time to reach its full anticoagulant effect. (Note: This is a Joint Commission VTE core measure.)

            d.   UFH is preferred for patients with severe renal insufficiency.

            e.   When intravenous UFH infusion is used, achieving a therapeutic aPTT in the first 24 hours has been linked to decreased VTE recurrence rates.

            f.   Treatment at home is recommended for patients with uncomplicated DVTs and low-risk PEs. Adequate home circumstances are required for home DVT and PE treatment, which includes well-maintained living conditions, strong support from family or friends, telephone access, and ability to return to the hospital quickly if deterioration occurs. Patient must feel well enough to be treated at home (e.g., does not have severe leg symptoms or comorbidity).

Table 6. Simplified PESI Score to Predict 30-Day Mortality After Symptomatic PE[a]

Clinical Characteristic	Score
Cancer history	+1
Age > 80 years	+1
Systolic blood pressure < 100 mm Hg	+1
Heart rate ≥ 110 beats/minute	+1
O_2 saturation < 90%	+1

[a]Clinical probability of PE: Low 0, 1% 30-day mortality, 1.5% recurrent VTE or nonfatal bleeding; high ≥ 1, 8.9% 30-day mortality.

PE = pulmonary embolism; PESI = Pulmonary Embolism Severity Index; VTE = venous thromboembolism.

From: Jiménez D, Aujesky D, Moores L, et al. Simplification of the pulmonary embolism severity index for prognostication in patients with acute symptomatic pulmonary embolism. Arch Intern Med 2010;170:1383-9.

g. Warfarin can be initiated on the first day of therapy concurrently with the parenteral anticoagulation.

h. Anticoagulants should be combined with the use of an elastic compression stocking with an ankle pressure of 30–40 mm Hg to help prevent postthrombotic syndrome, if possible; stocking use should continue for at least 2 years.

i. Upper extremity DVTs are generally treated similarly to lower extremity DVTs, but this is based on limited data.

j. Encourage early ambulation as tolerated by the patient during the initial treatment phase.

k. Target-specific oral anticoagulants (TSOACs)

    i. In the RE-COVER trial (double-blind), warfarin was compared with dabigatran 150 mg twice daily (LMWH treatment was administered for at least 5 days [median of 9 days] to both arms followed by dabigatran or warfarin with matching placebos and sham INRs in the dabigatran group) in patients with acute DVT (69%), PE (21.2%), or both (9.5%). Dabigatran was as effective as warfarin at preventing recurrent VTE or VTE-related death, with similar major bleeding at 6 months.

    ii. In the EINSTEIN trials (open-label), warfarin with enoxaparin cross-coverage at initiation was compared with rivaroxaban alone (15 mg twice daily for 21 days, followed by 20 mg once daily) for 3, 6, or 12 months in patients with acute DVT. Rivaroxaban was noninferior to enoxaparin/warfarin for prevention of recurrent symptomatic VTE as well as major bleeding. In EINSTEIN-PE, the same rivaroxaban protocol resulted in similar rates of recurrent symptomatic VTE and fewer instances of major bleeding than warfarin in patients with acute PE (1.1% vs. 2.2%).

    iii. In the AMPLIFY trial (double-blind), warfarin with enoxaparin cross-coverage at initiation was compared with apixaban alone (10 mg twice daily for 1 week then 5 mg twice daily) for 6 months in patients with either DVT (65%), PE (25.2%) or both (9.4%). Apixaban was noninferior to enoxaparin/warfarin for recurrent symptomatic VTE or VTE-related death, and major bleeding was significantly reduced (0.6% vs. 1.8%).

    iv. In the Hokusai-VTE trial (double-blind), warfarin was compared with edoxaban (both were initiated with LMWH or UFH cross-coverage for at least 5 days and for a median of 7 days in the study) in patients with acute DVT (60%) or PE (40%). The edoxaban dose was 60 mg, which was reduced to 30 mg (17% of the study population) for patients who had a CrCl of 30–50 mL/minute or weighed 60 kg or less or who were taking the concomitant P-glycoprotein (P-gp) inhibitor verapamil or quinidine at baseline. Other P-gp inhibitors, including erythromycin, azithromycin, clarithromycin, ketoconazole, and itraconazole, were prohibited at randomization but, during the study, were permitted with the dose adjusted down to 30 mg. If the P-gp inhibitor was discontinued, the edoxaban dose was increased to 60 mg again if no other reason for the lower dose existed. Edoxaban was noninferior to warfarin for preventing recurrent symptomatic VTE, with similar bleeding at a planned treatment of 3–12 months (40% of patients were treated for 12 months).

    v. Rivaroxaban and dabigatran are FDA approved for VTE treatment and prophylaxis after knee or hip replacement surgery, and edoxaban is under review by the FDA for the treatment of acute VTE but is not currently FDA approved.

    vi. All trials excluded patients with CrCl below 30 mL/minute (estimated with actual body weight).

    vii. Note that in all trials of TSOACs, the number of patients with cancer and moderate renal insufficiency was small; therefore, results may not be generalizable to these patients.

2. Considerations for the use of injectable anticoagulants in the treatment of VTE

Table 7. Injectable Options for the Treatment of Acute VTE

Unfractionated Heparin
IV administration[a]: Initial bolus and the initial rate of the continuous infusion can be either weight adjusted (80 units/kg IV bolus, followed by 18 units/kg/hour infusion) or a fixed dose (bolus 5000 units, followed by 1000 units/hour) Adjust subsequent doses to attain a goal aPTT based on the institution-specific therapeutic range or **Subcutaneous administration:** 17,500 units (250 units/kg) given every 12 hours (an initial 5000-unit IV bolus dose is recommended to attain rapid anticoagulation) Adjust subsequent doses to attain a goal aPTT based on the institution-specific therapeutic range or **Subcutaneous administration:** 333 units/kg, followed by 250 units/kg given every 12 hours (fixed-dose unmonitored dosing regimen)—Not practical for patients weighing more than 80 kg because of injection volume issues
Low-Molecular-Weight Heparins
Dalteparin: 200 units/kg subcutaneously once daily or 100 units/kg subcutaneously twice daily[b] **Enoxaparin:** 1.5 mg/kg subcutaneously once daily or 1 mg/kg subcutaneously twice daily;   if CrCl is less than 30 mL/minute: 1 mg/kg subcutaneously once daily **Tinzaparin:** 175 units/kg subcutaneously once daily
Factor Xa Inhibitor
Fondaparinux: For body weight less than 50 kg (110 lb), use 5 mg subcutaneously once daily For body weight 50–100 kg (110–220 lb), use 7.5 mg subcutaneously once daily For body weight greater than 100 kg (220 lb), use 10 mg subcutaneously once daily Contraindicated for CrCl less than 30 mL/minute

[a]IV administration preferred because of improved dosing precision.

[b]Not FDA approved for treatment of VTE in patients without cancer.

aPTT = activated partial thromboplastin time; CrCl = creatinine clearance; FDA = U.S. Food and Drug Administration; IV = intravenous; VTE = venous thromboembolism.

3. Considerations for the use of warfarin in the treatment of VTE
   a. Initial doses of 5–10 mg are preferred for otherwise healthy patients.
   b. Lower doses may be needed in some populations that are sensitive to warfarin (e.g., malnourished, drug interactions, elderly).
   c. Higher initial treatment doses (e.g., 10 mg) have been associated with obtaining a more rapid therapeutic INR in outpatients being treated for DVT.
   d. Ensure that all transitional care issues are addressed if initial therapy is given in the inpatient setting (follow-up INR scheduled, provider is aware of discharge and transition plans, therapy duration is communicated).
   e. Patients must receive complete warfarin and VTE education (Joint Commission mandates and part of the VTE core measures).
   f. Desired goal INR range is 2–3; higher INR targets have been linked to more bleeding events without greater VTE risk reduction, and lower INR targets (1.5–2) are not as effective, with no clear benefit on bleeding outcomes.

4. Considerations for the use of newer target-specific oral anticoagulants for VTE
   a. Study designs of trials differed with respect to initiation, dosing frequency, and dose-intensity modulation.
   b. Insufficient data to recommend use in patients with cancer
   c. Few patients with a CrCl less than 60 mL/minute have been studied.

Table 8. Newer Target-Specific Oral Anticoagulants for Treatment of VTE (DVT and/or PE)

Direct Thrombin Inhibitor
Dabigatran[a,b]
150 mg orally twice daily initiated after initial treatment with LMWH
Factor Xa Inhibitors
Rivaroxaban[b]
15 mg twice daily (with a meal) for 21 days, followed by 20 mg orally daily (with a meal)
Apixaban[a,b]
10 mg twice daily for 7 days followed by 5 mg twice daily
Edoxaban[a,b,c]
60 mg orally daily (for patients with estimated CrCl > 50 mL/minute and body weight > 60 kg [and not taking concomitant verapamil, quinidine, erythromycin, azithromycin, clarithromycin, ketoconazole, or itraconazole]), initiated after initial treatment with either UFH or LMWH
30 mg orally daily for patients (1) with CrCl 30–50 mL/minute, (2) with body weight of 60 kg or less, or (3) taking concomitant verapamil, quinidine, erythromycin, azithromycin, clarithromycin, ketoconazole, or itraconazole, initiated after initial treatment with either UFH or LMWH

[a]Not FDA approved for treatment of VTE as of March 1, 2014.

[b]Patients with estimated CrCl < 30 mL/minute not studied.

[c]Contraindicated for estimated CrCl < 30 mL/minute.

CrCl = creatinine clearance; DVT = deep venous thrombosis; FDA = U.S. Food and Drug Administration; LMWH = low-molecular-weight heparin; PE = pulmonary embolism; UFH = unfractionated heparin; VTE = venous thromboembolism.

   d. Patient counseling points (see Table 36)
5. Therapy duration
   a. Patients should receive 3 months of anticoagulation therapy after provoked VTE.
   b. For patients with unprovoked VTE or life-threatening PE, the long-term risks of anticoagulant use (bleeding) must be weighed against the risk of repeated thrombosis after completing a minimum of 3 months of anticoagulation therapy.
   c. The role of thrombophilia assessment to help guide the length of therapy decision is controversial. Factors associated with increased risk of VTE recurrence include hereditary thrombophilia (1.5 x x), antiphospholipid antibodies (2 x x), and residual thrombosis (1.6 x x). Normal D-dimer test result 1 month after warfarin withdrawal is protective (0.4 x x).
   d. Distal DVT (below the knee) may be managed without anticoagulation but instead by monitoring serial ultrasound findings. If the patient is very symptomatic or if the clot extends, anticoagulation should be initiated as recommended for proximal VTE.

Table 9. Duration of Anticoagulation Therapy in Patients with VTE (DVT and/or PE)

Patient Characteristic	Therapy Duration	Comments
First episode of VTE secondary to a transient (reversible) risk factor	3 months	Recommendation applies to both proximal DVT and PE
First episode of VTE and cancer	At least 3 months and consider extended duration until cancer resolves	Low-molecular-weight heparin is recommended over warfarin; warfarin is recommended over novel oral anticoagulants
First episode of unprovoked VTE	At least 3 months	Continue oral anticoagulant therapy if patient is at low risk of bleeding and adherent to therapy The risk-benefit of indefinite therapy should be reassessed at periodic intervals
First episode of VTE with inherited or acquired thrombophilia[a]	At least 3 months	Continue oral anticoagulant therapy if patient is at low risk of bleeding and adherent to therapy Several abnormalities or homozygous traits have at least additive risk The risk-benefit of indefinite therapy should be reassessed at periodic intervals
Second unprovoked VTE	Indefinite	Applies to patients at low or moderate risk of bleeding

[a]Factor V Leiden; prothrombin G20210A; antiphospholipid antibody syndrome; excess factor VIII; deficiency in protein C, protein S, or antithrombin.

DVT = deep venous thrombosis; PE = pulmonary embolism; VTE = venous thromboembolism.

Patient Cases

Questions 1–5 pertain to the following case.

R.R., a 62-year-old, overweight (weight 92 kg, height 60 inches) man, presents to the emergency department with swelling of his entire right lower extremity, erythema, and soreness of his right calf. He had knee replacement surgery 2 weeks ago. He reports no shortness of breath, cough, or chest pain. His medical history includes DVT (after plaster casting for a leg fracture) at age 24 years, diabetes mellitus, HTN, chronic kidney disease, and dyslipidemia. His estimated 10-year atherosclerotic cardiovascular disease (ASCVD) risk is 8%. His medications are metformin 500 mg orally twice daily, losartan 50 mg orally twice daily, rosuvastatin 10 mg orally daily, and aspirin 81 mg orally daily. Initial laboratory values include hematocrit 36.5% (normal 42%–52%), prothrombin time (PT) 10.8 seconds (normal 9.9–11.2 seconds), INR 1.0, aPTT 23.6 seconds (normal 24–36 seconds), platelet count 255,000/mm³ (normal 150,000–300,000/mm³), and CrCl 48 mL/minute.

1. Which risk level most accurately reflects the clinical probability of this patient's having a DVT?

    A. Low.
    B. Moderate.
    C. High.
    D. Very high.

2. Which is the best diagnostic test to objectively confirm the DVT diagnosis in this patient?

    A. D-dimer test.
    B. Duplex ultrasound scan.
    C. Venography.
    D. Computed tomography (CT) scan.

3. Which time interval best represents how long this patient should be treated with anticoagulation therapy?

    A. At least 3 months.
    B. 6 months.
    C. 12 months.
    D. Indefinitely.

4. The decision is made to initiate anticoagulation therapy in the emergency department and to discharge the patient home and treat him for DVT in the outpatient setting. Which is the best recommendation for an anticoagulant initiation regimen for this patient?

    A. Fondaparinux 5 mg subcutaneously daily and warfarin 10 mg/day orally adjusted to an INR of 2–3.
    B. Rivaroxaban 15 mg orally daily.
    C. Rivaroxaban 15 mg orally twice daily for 21 days and then 20 mg orally daily thereafter.
    D. Enoxaparin 100 mg subcutaneously daily and warfarin 5 mg/day orally adjusted to an INR of 2–3.

5. Which is the best course of action currently with respect to the patient's aspirin therapy taken for primary prevention of ASCVD?

    A. Continue aspirin 81 mg orally daily.
    B. Continue aspirin 81 mg orally daily, and revise hthe patient'sis warfarin INR target to 2.0–2.5.
    C. Increase the aspirin dose to 325 mg orally daily.
    D. Discontinue aspirin while the patient is receiving anticoagulation.

II. ANTITHROMBOTIC THERAPY IN ATRIAL FIBRILLATION

A. Stroke Prevention in Atrial Fibrillation (AF) *(Domain 1, Tasks 1–, 2, 3, 4, 5, 6, 7; Domain 3, Tasks 2, 3; Domain 2, Tasks 2, 3; Domain 5, Tasks 1, 2)*

1. AF is a major risk factor for cardiogenic embolic stroke and systemic arterial thromboembolism.
2. Around 90% of AF thromboembolic complications are stroke related, and the remaining 10% are systemic embolism.
3. Thromboembolic risks associated with AF
   a. Stasis or turbulence of blood flow within the left atrial appendage leads to thrombus formation.
   b. Dysfunction of vascular endothelium predisposes to local or systemic hypercoagulability.
   c. Conversion to normal sinus rhythm (NSR)—Spontaneous or intentional—May dislodge any existing left atrial thrombi.
4. Morbidity and mortality associated with AF
   a. 15% of all strokes occur in people with AF.
   b. The annual stroke risk in untreated patients with AF varies from 1% to greater than 10% (average is 4.5%), depending on concurrent individual risk factors.
   c. Stroke risk in AF increases with age.
      i. 1.5% in the 50- to 59-year-old age group
      ii. 23.5% in the 80- to 89-year-old age group
5. Classification of AF
   a. Acute AF: Onset within previous 48 hours
   b. Paroxysmal AF: Terminates spontaneously within 7 days (may recur)
   c. Recurrent AF: More than one episode
   d. Persistent AF: Duration of more than 7 days without spontaneous termination
   e. Permanent AF: Persistence of AF despite electrical or pharmacologic cardioversion attempts
   f. Valvular AF: Eur Heart J 2013;34:1471-4: Associated with rheumatic valvular disease, mitral stenosis, prosthetic heart valves (bioprosthetic and mechanical), or hypertrophic cardiomyopathy; 2012 European Society of Cardiology (ESC) AF guidelines: Associated with rheumatic disease and prosthetic valves
6. Tools for nonvalvular atrial fibrillation (NVAF) stroke risk stratification
   a. Various risk stratification schemes have been developed with the following goals:
      i. Identifying patients with AF having such a low stroke risk that anticoagulation-associated bleeding risk may outweigh stroke prevention benefit
      ii. Encouraging anticoagulation therapy use in patients at high risk of AF stroke when its benefit has been clearly shown
   b. $CHADS_2$ (congestive heart failure, hypertension, age at least 75 years, diabetes, previous stroke or transient ischemic attack) score – Well validated and easy to use; most popular AF stroke risk stratification tool

$CHADS_2$ Stroke Risk Factor	Points
Congestive HF	= 1
Hypertension	= 1
Age ≥ 75 years	= 1
Diabetes	= 1
Previous stroke/TIA/systemic embolus	= 2

$CHADS_2$ = congestive heart failure, hypertension, age at least 75 years, diabetes, previous stroke or transient ischemic attack; HF = heart failure; TIA = transient ischemic attack.

Table 10. CHADS$_2$ Score and Recommended Antithrombotic Therapy[a–c]

CHADS$_2$ Score	Adjusted Stroke Rate, %/Yyear (95% CI)	Recommended Therapy (2011 ASA/AHA Guidelines)
0	1.9 (1.2–3.0)	No antithrombotic therapy or aspirin for patients who choose active therapy
1	2.8 (2.0–3.8)	Warfarin (INR 2–3), apixaban, or dabigatran; for those with conditions not suitable for oral anticoagulation, aspirin or low-dose apixaban (2.5 mg bid) is suggested over no antithrombotic therapy
2	4.0 (3.1–5.1)	Warfarin (INR 2–3), apixaban, dabigatran, or rivaroxaban; for patients with conditions not suitable for oral anticoagulation, aspirin + clopidogrel is suggested over aspirin alone
3	5.9 (4.6–7.3)	
4	8.5 (6.3–11.1)	
5	12.5 (8.2–17.5)	
6	18.2 (10.5–27.4)	

[a]Interpreted to mean the "one major risk factor" equals a CHADS$_2$ point score of 1.

[b]Higher CHADS$_2$ score = higher AF stroke risk. Score of 0 = low risk; score of 1 = intermediate risk; score of ≥ 2 = high risk.

[c]CHADS$_2$ score calculator available at www.mdcalc.com/chads2-score-for-atrial-fibrillation-stroke-risk/.

AHA = American Heart Association; ASA = American Stroke Association; bid = twice daily; CHADS$_2$ = congestive heart failure, hypertension, age at least 75 years, diabetes, previous stroke or transient ischemic attack; CI = confidence interval; INR = international normalized ratio.

    c.   CHA$_2$DS$_2$-VASc (congestive heart failure, hypertension, age at least 75 years, diabetes, previous stroke or transient ischemic attack, presence of vascular disease, and age 65–74 years) score – Well validated; better than CHADS$_2$ score at identifying truly low-risk patients; primarily used for patients with a CHADS$_2$ score of 0 or 1 to assess the impact of the presence of minor risk factors on stroke risk; has been validated for patients post AF ablation

CHA$_2$DS$_2$-VASc Stroke Risk Factor[a]	Points
Congestive HF	= 1
Hypertension	= 1
Age ≥ 75 years	= 2
Diabetes	= 1
Previous stroke/TIA/systemic embolus	= 2
Vascular disease (previous MI, angina, PCI, PAD, CABG, or aortic plaque)	= 1
Age 65–74 years	= 1
Sex category (female)	= 1

[a]CHA$_2$DS$_2$-VASc score calculator is available at www.mdcalc.com/cha2ds2-vasc-score-for-atrial-fibrillation-stroke-risk/.

CABG = coronary artery bypass grafting; CHA$_2$DS$_2$-VASc = congestive heart failure, hypertension, age at least 75 years, diabetes, previous stroke or transient ischemic attack, presence of vascular disease, and age 65–74 years; HF = heart failure; MI = myocardial infarction; PAD = peripheral arterial disease; PCI = percutaneous coronary intervention; TIA = transient ischemic attack.

Table 11. CHA$_2$DS$_2$-VASc Score and Recommended Antithrombotic Therapy[a]

CHA$_2$DS$_2$-VASc Score	Adjusted Stroke Rate, %/Yyear (95% CI)	Recommended Therapy (2012 ESC Guidelines)
0	0 (0–0)	No antithrombotic therapy
1	0.6 (0–3.4)	Oral anticoagulant therapy (VKA INR 2–3, apixaban, dabigatran, or rivaroxaban)
2	1.6 (0.3–4.7)	
3	3.9 (1.7–7.6)	Consider the patient's preferences, values, and bleeding risk
4	1.9 (0.5–4.9)	
5	3.2 (0.7–9.0)	Aspirin + clopidogrel or aspirin alone may be considered in patients who refuse anticoagulation or cannot tolerate anticoagulants for any reason unrelated to bleeding
6	3.6 (0.4–12.3)	
7	8.0 (1.0–26.0)	
8	11.1 (0.3–48.3)	
9	100 (2.5–100)	

[a]In patients with a CHADS$_2$ score of 0: 1-year stroke rates in patients with a CHA$_2$DS$_2$-VASc score of 0 = 0.84%; 1 = 1.75%; 2 = 2.69%; and 3 = 3.2%.
CHA$_2$DS$_2$-VASc = congestive heart failure, hypertension, age at least 75 years, diabetes, previous stroke or transient ischemic attack, presence of vascular disease, and age 65–74 years; CI = confidence interval; ESC = European Society of Cardiology; INR = international normalized ratio; VKA = vitamin K antagonist.

    d. Risk stratification considerations
        i. No tool can incorporate all potential AF stroke risk factors. Risk stratification tools can therefore best be used only as "rough guides" to help inform clinicians.
        ii. Patient perspectives and preferences should also factor into clinical decision-making.
7. Treatment considerations
    a. Rate versus rhythm control
        i. In clinical trials, ischemic events occurred with similar frequency with either a rhythm or rate control strategy, especially when anticoagulation therapy was discontinued or was subtherapeutic.
        ii. Whether a rate or rhythm control strategy is used, patients with AF and thromboembolic risk factors should probably receive chronic therapeutic anticoagulation.
    b. Adjusted-dose warfarin versus aspirin therapy
        i. Aspirin alone provides, at best, a modest reduction in the risk of nonfatal stroke in AF and is inferior to adjusted-dose (INR 2–3) warfarin and combined therapy with clopidogrel.
        ii. A pooled analysis of trials comparing aspirin with placebo yielded a relative risk reduction estimate of 21% with a 95% confidence interval (CI) of 0%–38% compared with a relative risk reduction of 68% (95% CI, 50%–79%) with warfarin.
        iii. Compared with aspirin alone, the combination of clopidogrel and aspirin significantly reduces the rate of major vascular events (mainly stroke), but it increases the risk of serious bleeding, including intracranial hemorrhage. The American College of Chest Physicians (ACCP) 9th eEdition of the Chest Guidelines on Antithrombotic Therapy and Prevention of Thrombosis (AT-9) guidelines) state a preference for combined aspirin and clopidogrel therapy over aspirin alone.
        iv. A randomized comparison of warfarin versus clopidogrel plus aspirin was terminated early after showing the superiority of warfarin.
        v. Adding aspirin to warfarin therapy increases the risk of major bleeding and does not provide further protection against ischemic stroke in patients with AF (possible exception is patients with AF and prosthetic heart valve replacement).

c. Adjusted-dose warfarin versus newer anticoagulants
   i. Adjusted-dose warfarin has been compared with dabigatran (RE-LY trial), rivaroxaban (ROCKET AF), apixaban (ARISTOTLE), and edoxaban (ENGAGE-AF) for stroke prevention in AF.

Table 12. Major Outcomes of New Anticoagulants vs. Adjusted-Dose Warfarin[a]

Outcome (RR ± 95% CI)	RE-LY (Dabigatran 150 mg bid)	ROCKET-AF (Rivaroxaban 20 mg/day[b])	ARISTOTLE (Apixaban 5 mg bid[c])	ENGAGE-AF (Edoxaban 60 mg/day[d])
CHADS$_2$ score	2.1	3.5	2.1	2.8
Warfarin TTR	64%	55%	62.2%	68.4%
Stroke/SEE	0.65 (0.52–0.81)	0.88 (0.75–1.03)	0.79 (0.66–0.95)	0.79 (0.63–0.99)
Ischemic stroke	0.76 (0.59–0.97)	0.94 (0.75–1.17)	0.92 (0.74–1.13)	1.00 (0.83–1.19)
Hemorrhagic stroke	0.26 (0.14–0.49)	0.59 (0.37–0.93)	0.51 (0.35–0.75)	0.54 (0.38–0.77)
Major bleeding	0.93 (0.81–1.07)	1.04 (0.90–1.20)	0.69 (0.60–0.80)	0.80 (0.71–0.91)
Intracranial hemorrhage	0.40 (0.27–0.60)	0.67 (0.47–0.93)	0.42 (0.30–0.58)	0.47 (9.34–0.63)
CV mortality	0.85 (0.72–0.99)	0.89 (0.73–1.10)	0.89 (0.76–1.04)	0.92 (0.83–1.01)
All-cause mortality	0.88 (0.77–1.00)	0.85 (0.70-1.02)	0.89 (0.80–0.998)	0.86 (0.77–0.97)

[a]Patients with CrCl < 30 mL/minute were excluded from RE-LY, ROCKET-AF, and ENGAGE-AF trials; patients with CrCl < 25 mL/minute were excluded from ARISTOTLE trial. Patients with mechanical heart valves were excluded from all trials. Patients with bioprosthetic valves were excluded from RE-LY, ROCKET-AF, and ARISTOTLE trials.

[b]Dose adjusted to 15 mg/day for CrCl 30–49 mL/minute.

[c]Dose adjusted to 2.5 mg bid for two or more of the following: Age ≥ 80 years, SCr ≥ 1.5 mg/dL, body weight < 60 kg.

[d]Dose adjusted to 30 mg/day if CrCl 30–50 mL/minute, body weight ≤ 60 kg, or concomitant use of verapamil, quinidine, dronedarone; concomitant use of azithromycin, clarithromycin, ketoconazole, itraconazole, cyclosporine, and ritonavir was prohibited.

bid = twice daily; CHADS$_2$ = congestive heart failure, hypertension, age at least 75 years, diabetes, previous stroke or transient ischemic attack; CI = confidence interval; CrCl = creatinine clearance; CV = cardiovascular; RR = relative risk; SCr = serum creatinine concentration; SEE = systemic embolic event; TTR = therapeutic international normalized ratio range.

ii. The 2011 American Heart Association/American Stroke Association (AHA/ASA) guidelines recommend warfarin over newer target-specific oral anticoagulants for patients with a CrCl less than 15 mL/minute.

iii. No antidote is currently available for reversing the anticoagulant effect of any of the new anticoagulants—Management of life-threatening bleeding is unclear. Prothrombin complex concentrates (PCCs) can normalize elevated prothrombin time levels in patients treated with direct-acting factor Xa inhibitors, but their utility in bleeding patients remains to be determined.

iv. Acquisition costs for the newer target-specific oral anticoagulants are about 100 times that for warfarin.

v. Cost-effectiveness of newer target-specific oral anticoagulants compared with warfarin has been shown.

vi. Although routine laboratory monitoring is not required with the newer anticoagulants, careful monitoring and coordination of therapy for invasive procedures are still required.

vii. When deciding which oral anticoagulant to use for patients with AF, consider individual clinical features, including the ability to adhere to the requirements of therapy, the availability of the anticoagulation management program, patient preferences, and cost.

8. Transthoracic echocardiography (TTE) and transesophageal echocardiography (TEE)
   a. Can detect the presence of features associated with thromboembolism (TE), and anticoagulation therapy in patients with these features reduces stroke risk (e.g., impaired left ventricular [LV] systolic function, left atrial thrombus, dense spontaneous echo contrast [or "smoke"], or reduced velocity of blood flow in the left atrial appendage). However, the absence of these echocardiographic abnormalities has not been established as identifying a low-risk group of patients with AF who could safely forgo warfarin therapy.
   b. Valuable for detecting rheumatic mitral valve disease (there is universal agreement that these patients should receive warfarin therapy)
      i. Detection of a left atrial thrombus is a contraindication for cardioversion of AF.
      ii. TEE surpasses TTE in the evaluation of cardiogenic risk factors in patients with AF.
9. Optimal intensity of anticoagulation for AF
   a. Optimal anticoagulation intensity involves a careful balance between maximizing protection against TE while minimizing bleeding risk (intracranial hemorrhage particularly rivals ischemic stroke with respect to clinical importance).
   b. The risk of ischemic stroke is low at INR levels of 2.0 or higher.
   c. The risk of intracranial hemorrhage increases at INR levels of 3.5–4.0 and above, particularly in the elderly.
   d. An INR of less than 2.0 at admission for a new stroke substantially increases the likelihood of death and severe disability from an AF-related stroke.
   e. An INR target of 2.5 (range 2–3) should be used for most patients.
      i. The suggestion of the American College of Cardiology (ACC)/AHA/ESC 2006 guidelines that a lower target INR (1.6–2.5) may be considered in patients unable to tolerate standard-intensity warfarin therapy is not evidence based.
      ii. Narrower target ranges have been suggested in certain instances (e.g., INR 2.0–2.5 has been recommended in patients requiring warfarin, aspirin, and clopidogrel after percutaneous coronary intervention). However, such narrow ranges are not supported by good evidence, and they make achieving therapeutic INRs more difficult, usually resulting in the need for more frequent INR testing.
   f. For patients with AF and stable coronary artery disease (i.e., no acute coronary syndrome in the past year), warfarin (INR 2–3) alone without antiplatelet therapy is preferred.
10. Considerations during cardioversion
    a. Systemic embolism is the most serious complication of cardioversion, whether NSR is reestablished by electrical, pharmacologic, or spontaneous means.
    b. There is no evidence that cardioversion, followed by prolonged maintenance of NSR, effectively reduces TE in AF.
       i. At least 4 weeks of therapeutic anticoagulation is recommended after successful cardioversion.
       ii. Patients with risk factors for TE should continue anticoagulation beyond 4 weeks unless there is convincing evidence that NSR is maintained.
    c. Hemodynamically unstable patients requiring emergency cardioversion should receive therapeutic anticoagulation with either intravenous UFH or LMWH or a newer target-specific oral anticoagulant initiated as soon as possible, followed by at least 4 weeks of therapeutic anticoagulation (limited/no evidence).
    d. During the RE-LY trial, 1983 cardioversions were performed in 1270 patients: 647, 672, and 664 in the dabigatran 110-mg twice-daily, dabigatran 150-mg twice-daily, and warfarin groups, respectively. The frequencies of stroke and major bleeding within 30 days of cardioversion in patients taking the two doses of dabigatran were low and comparable with those in patients taking warfarin with or without TEE guidance.

   e. During the ROCKET-AF trial, 320 patients had a total of 460 cardioversions or AF ablations, 161 patients treated with warfarin and 160 treated with rivaroxaban. Three strokes occurred in each group.

11. Considerations during ablation procedures

   a. Patients with persistent AF who are in AF at the time of ablation should have TEE to screen for a thrombus, even if warfarin anticoagulation was used before the procedure. Usually, intraprocedural echocardiography is used to identify clot formation.

   b. The most common anticoagulation strategy is to continue therapeutic anticoagulation with warfarin and to add UFH during the procedure to inhibit activated clotting factors because warfarin just prevents the formation of active clotting factors. Most centers have abandoned LMWH bridging because it has been associated with excess bleeding risk.

   c. UFH is continued for 12–24 hours post procedure, with a brief interruption for arterial sheath pull. After the sheath pull, anticoagulation is resumed for 12–24 hours for periprocedural stroke and PE prevention.

   d. Warfarin, if selected for postablation anticoagulation, is reinitiated the evening of the procedure.

   e. If a newer oral anticoagulant is selected or dabigatran continued, the oral dose is typically restarted the morning after the procedure, once hemodynamic stability is assured and intrapericardial bleeding ruled out.

   f. Oral anticoagulation recommended in all patients for at least 2 months after an AF ablation procedure (consider prolonged therapy of at least 6 months for $CHADS_2$ score of 2 or more)

III. ANTITHROMBOTIC AGENTS: PHARMACOLOGIC AND CLINICAL CONSIDERATIONS

A. Unfractionated Heparin *(Domain 1, Tasks 2, 3, 4, 7)*

   1. Pharmacology and pharmacokinetics

      a. Rapid-acting, parenterally administered anticoagulant

      b. Heterogeneous mixture of sulfated mucopolysaccharides of variable lengths and pharmacologic properties

      c. The anticoagulant profile and clearance vary depending on chain length.

      d. UFH prevents the growth and propagation of a formed thrombus and allows the patient's own thrombolytic system to degrade the clot.

      e. Derived from bovine lung or porcine intestinal mucosa; no differences in antithrombotic activity have been shown between the two sources

      f. The subcutaneous bioavailability of UFH is dose-dependent and ranges from 30% at low doses to as much as 70% at high doses.

      g. The onset of anticoagulant effect is usually evident 1–2 hours after subcutaneous injection and peaks at 3 hours.

      h. When UFH is administered intravenously, continuous infusion is preferable.

      i. Intramuscular administration is discouraged because of erratic absorption and risk of large hematoma formation.

      j. UFH has a dose-dependent half-life of about 30–90 minutes, but it may be prolonged to as much as 150 minutes when given in high doses to some patients.

   2. Dosing and administration

      a. For prevention of VTE, UFH is given by subcutaneous injection. Typical dose for prophylaxis is 5000 units every 8–12 hours.

      b. When immediate and full anticoagulation are required, an intravenous bolus dose followed by continuous infusion is preferred (see Table 7: Initial dose of 80 units/kg followed by 18 units/kg/hour).

      c. Subcutaneous UFH (see Table 7: Initial dose of 333 units/kg, followed by 250 units/kg every 12 hours) also provides adequate therapeutic anticoagulation for the treatment of acute VTE.

3. Monitoring
   a. Administration of UFH by intravenous infusion requires close monitoring because of the unpredictable anticoagulant patient response. The utility of monitoring subcutaneously administered UFH is questionable, including at treatment doses.
   b. Tests available to monitor UFH therapy in ambulatory patients
      i. Activated partial thromboplastin time
         (a) The most widely used test to determine the degree of therapeutic anticoagulation
         (b) An institution-specific aPTT therapeutic range should be established that correlates with a plasma heparin concentration of 0.3–0.7 unit/mL by an amidolytic anti-Xa assay.
         (c) Should be measured before therapy initiation to determine the patient's baseline
         (d) When monitoring an aPTT during subcutaneous injections, the response to therapy should be measured at the mid-dosing interval two or three doses after therapy initiation or a dose change.
      ii. Anti-Xa activity (also measured at the mid-dosing interval similarly to aPTT during subcutaneous administration)
   c. Heparin resistance should be suspected in patients who require more than 35,000 units of UFH during a 24-hour period. In such cases, adjust the UFH dose according to anti-Xa concentrations.
4. Adverse effects
   a. Bleeding
      i. The presence of concomitant bleeding risks such as thrombocytopenia, the use of other antithrombotic therapy, and a preexisting source of bleeding increase the risk of UFH-induced hemorrhage.
      ii. The risk of bleeding increases with age.
      iii. Recent surgery, hemostatic defects, heavy alcohol consumption, renal failure, peptic ulcers, and neoplasms also increase the risk of major bleeding while receiving UFH.
   b. Bruising from minor trauma and at the sites of subcutaneous injections and venous access is also common.
   c. Local irritation, mild pain, erythema, histamine-like reactions, and hematoma can occur during UFH administration.
   d. Heparin-induced thrombocytopenia (HIT)
      i. A rare but serious drug-induced problem requiring immediate intervention
      ii. A baseline platelet count should be obtained before UFH therapy is initiated.
      iii. If the patient has received UFH within the previous 100 days, or if previous UFH exposure is uncertain, a repeated platelet count should be performed within 24 hours.
      iv. Monitoring platelet counts every 2–3 days from days 4 to 14 of UFH treatment or until discontinuation is recommended for patients for whom the estimated risk exceeds 1%.
      v. The incidence of HIT is greater than 1% in postoperative patients receiving prophylactic or therapeutic UFH doses. The incidence of HIT in medical patients receiving UFH ranges from less than 0.1% to 1%.
      vi. A fall in platelet count of greater than 50% from baseline but not less than 20×10^9/L is most suggestive of HIT.
   e. Long-term use of UFH has been reported to cause alopecia, priapism, and suppressed aldosterone synthesis with subsequent hyperkalemia.
   f. Use of UFH in doses of 20,000 units/day or greater for more than 3–6 months has been associated with significant bone loss and may lead to osteoporosis.

B. Low-Molecular-Weight Heparin *(Domain 1, Tasks 2, 3, 4, 7)*
1. Pharmacology and pharmacokinetics
   a. Like UFH, the LMWHs prevent the growth and propagation of formed thrombi.
   b. Both UFH and LMWH inhibit both thrombin and factor Xa. UFH inhibits both equally and LMWHs preferentially inhibit factor Xa.
   c. Three LMWH products are commercially available in the United States: Ddalteparin, enoxaparin (available as a generic), and tinzaparin.
   d. Compared with UFH, the LMWHs have a more predictable anticoagulation response.
   e. The bioavailability of the LMWHs is about 90% when administered subcutaneously.
   f. The peak anticoagulation effect is seen in 3–5 hours.
   g. The renal route is the predominant mode of elimination for the LMWHs.
   h. Their biologic half-life may be prolonged in patients with renal impairment.
2. Dosing and administration
   a. The LMWHs are given in fixed or weight-based doses according to the product and indication. See Table 7: For VTE treatment indications or as bridging in AF, enoxaparin is administered as 1 mg/kg subcutaneously twice daily or 1.5 mg/kg subcutaneously once daily. A reduced dose of 1 mg/kg once daily is recommended for patients with an estimated CrCl of less than 30 mL/minute, but published experience with this dose is lacking because patients with a CrCl of less than 30 mL/minute were excluded from clinical trials. Dalteparin is administered as 200 units/kg subcutaneously once daily.
   b. Doses should be based on actual body weight, and studies of obese patients indicate that full weight–based doses do not lead to elevated LMWH concentrations as compared with patients of normal weight.
   c. The LMWHs are generally given by subcutaneous injection in the abdominal area or the upper outer part of the thigh while the patient is in a supine position.
   d. The clinician or patient pinches a layer of skin between the thumb and forefinger and then introduces the entire length of the needle into a skinfold at a 90-degree angle. Injection sites should be alternated between right and left sides. After subcutaneous administration, the drug is absorbed slowly, resulting in sustained antithrombotic activity for several hours.
3. Therapeutic monitoring
   a. Because the LMWHs achieve a predictable anticoagulant response when given subcutaneously, routine laboratory monitoring is unnecessary to guide the dosing of these agents.
   b. Before initiating LMWH, a baseline complete blood cell count (CBC) with a platelet count and SCr measurement should be obtained.
   c. Although very limited data support the use of laboratory monitoring to guide LMWH therapy, measuring anti-Xa activity has been suggested in patients who have significant renal impairment (e.g., CrCl less than 30 mL/minute), weigh less than 50 kg, are morbidly obese, or are pregnant (because of changing pharmacokinetic variables such as volume of distribution and renal function).
      i. Anti-Xa monitoring should be used rarely because results above or below the "therapeutic range" cause difficult clinical dilemmas.
      ii. UFH is preferred for patients with a CrCl less than 30 mL/minute.

4. Adverse effects
   a. Bleeding is the most common adverse effect of the LMWHs.
      i. Major bleeding: Incidence is less than 3% and varies among the LMWH preparations, their indication for use, the patient population, and the dose administered.
      ii. Minor bleeding, particularly at the injection site, occurs often with LMWH use.
      iii. Epidural and spinal hematomas resulting in long-term or permanent paralysis have been reported with the use of LMWH during spinal and epidural anesthesia or spinal puncture. The risk of these events is higher with the use of indwelling epidural catheters and concomitant use of drugs that affect hemostasis.
   b. Heparin-induced thrombocytopenia
      i. The incidence of HIT is lower than that observed with the use of UFH in the postoperative setting. The risk of HIT in patients treated for VTE is too low to discern a difference between UFH and LMWH. Risk of HIT should not be a major determinant in selecting a parenteral anticoagulant for VTE treatment.
      ii. LMWHs have almost 100% cross-reactivity with heparin antibodies in vitro; they should be avoided in patients with an established diagnosis or history of HIT.
   c. Osteoporosis: Appears to be lower with the LMWHs than with UFH, but both agents have the potential to produce osteopenia

C. Indirect Factor Xa Inhibitor (synthetic pentasaccharide) *(Domain 1, Tasks 2, 3, 4, 7)*
   1. Fondaparinux is the only commercially available synthetic pentasaccharide.
   2. Composed of a 5 sugar moiety; the first in a class of anticoagulants that selectively inhibits factor Xa activity
   3. Pharmacology and pharmacokinetics
      a. Similar to UFH and the LMWHs, fondaparinux prevents thrombus generation and clot formation by indirectly inhibiting factor Xa activity through its interaction with antithrombin.
      b. After subcutaneous administration, bioavailability is 100%.
      c. Peak plasma concentrations are achieved in about 2 hours after a single dose and in 3 hours with repeated once-daily dosing.
      d. Fondaparinux is primarily eliminated unchanged in the urine.
      e. Contraindicated in patients with severe renal function impairment (CrCl less than 30 mL/minute); use caution in moderate renal insufficiency (CrCl 30–50 mL/minute)
      f. The terminal elimination half-life is 17–21 hours and is independent of the patient's age and sex.
      g. The anticoagulant effect of fondaparinux persists for 2–4 days after the drug is discontinued in patients with normal renal function.
   4. Dose and administration
      a. In the setting of VTE prevention, the dose of fondaparinux is 2.5 mg injected subcutaneously once daily starting 6–8 hours after surgery if hemostasis has been established. It is important to avoid initiating fondaparinux too soon because a significant relationship exists between the timing of the first dose and the risk of major bleeding complications.
      b. Patients who weigh less than 50 kg should not be given fondaparinux for VTE prophylaxis.
      c. For the treatment of DVT or PE, the dose of fondaparinux is 7.5 mg given subcutaneously once daily. Patients who weigh more than 100 kg should be given 10 mg once daily, and those who weigh less than 50 kg should receive 5 mg/day.
      d. Similar to the LMWHs, fondaparinux is administered to the fatty tissue of the abdominal wall. Patients should be instructed to pinch a fold of skin at the injection site and hold it throughout the injection. The needle should be inserted at a 90-degree angle. Injection sites should be alternated from side to side.

5. Therapeutic monitoring
   a. A CBC and SCr should be measured at baseline.
   b. Kidney function should be monitored closely in patients at risk of developing renal failure.
   c. Fondaparinux should be discontinued if the CrCl drops below 30 mL/minute.
   d. Signs and symptoms of bleeding should be monitored daily, particularly in patients with a baseline CrCl between 30 and 50 mL/minute. If neuraxial anesthesia has been used, patients should be closely monitored for signs and symptoms of neurologic impairment.
   e. Fondaparinux does not alter coagulation tests such as the aPTT and PT. The role of anti-Xa monitoring during fondaparinux is not well defined. Patients receiving fondaparinux therapy do not require routine coagulation testing.
6. Adverse effects
   a. Bleeding is the primary adverse effect associated with fondaparinux therapy.
   b. The rate of major bleeding in the VTE prophylaxis trials was around 2%–3%.
   c. Similar to UFH and the LMWHs, fondaparinux should be used with extreme caution in patients with neuraxial anesthesia or after a spinal puncture because of the risk of spinal or epidural hematoma formation.
   d. Unlike UFH and the LMWHs, fondaparinux has not been associated with HIT and does not produce cross-sensitivity in vitro. Fondaparinux has been used in the treatment of HIT.

Table 13. Comparison of UFH, LMWHs, and Fondaparinux

Property	UFH	LMWH	Fondaparinux
Molecular weight range[a]	3000–30,000	1000–10,000	1728
Average molecular weight[a]	12,000–15,000	4000–5000	1728
Anti−factor Xa/anti−factor IIa activity	1:1	2:1–4:1	>100:1
aPTT monitoring required	Yes	No	No
Inactivation by platelet factor 4	Yes	No	No
Capable of inactivating platelet-bound factor Xa	No	Yes	Yes
Inhibition of platelet function	++++	++	No
Increases vascular permeability	Yes	No	No
Protein binding	++++	+	No
Endothelial cell binding	+++	+	No
Dose-dependent clearance	Yes	No	No
Primary route of elimination	1. Saturable binding processes and depolymerization 2. Renal	Renal	Renal
Elimination half-life	30–150 minutes	2–6 hours	17 hours

[a]Measured in daltons.

aPTT = activated partial thromboplastin time; LMWH = low-molecular-weight heparin; UFH = unfractionated heparin.

D. Warfarin *(Domain 1, Tasks 2, 3, 4, 5, 6, 7)*
   1. Currently, the most commonly used anticoagulant when long-term or extended anticoagulation is indicated
   2. Warfarin is FDA approved for the prevention and treatment of VTE, as well as for the prevention of thromboembolic complications associated with AF, heart valve replacement, and myocardial infarction (MI).
   3. Because of its narrow therapeutic index, predisposition to drug and food interactions, and propensity to cause hemorrhage, warfarin requires continuous patient monitoring and education to achieve optimal outcomes.
   4. Pharmacology and pharmacokinetics
      a. Warfarin exerts its anticoagulation effect by inhibiting vitamin K epoxide reductase, the enzyme responsible for the cyclic interconversion of vitamin K in the liver.
      b. Reduced vitamin K is a cofactor required for the carboxylation of the vitamin K–dependent coagulation proteins; factors II (prothrombin), VII, IX, and X; and the endogenous anticoagulant proteins C and S.
      c. Warfarin has no direct effect on previously circulating clotting factors or previously formed thrombi.
      d. The time required for warfarin to achieve its pharmacologic effect depends on the elimination half-lives of the coagulation proteins.
      e. Given that prothrombin has a 2- to 3-day half-life, the full antithrombotic effect is not achieved for 7–15 days after warfarin initiation.
      f. By suppressing the production of active clotting factors, warfarin prevents the initial formation and propagation of a thrombus.

Table 14. Elimination Half-lives of Vitamin K–Dependent Clotting Factors

Clotting Factor	Half-life, hours
II	42–72
VII	4–6
IX	21–30
X	27–48
Protein C	9
Protein S	60

      g. Warfarin is a racemic mixture of R- and S-enantiomers that differ with respect to elimination half-life, metabolism, pathways of oxidative metabolism, and potency.

Table 15. Comparison of R- and S-Warfarin

	R-Warfarin	*S*-Warfarin
Elimination half-life	45 hr (20–70 hr)	29 hr (18–52 hr)
Metabolism	40% reduction 60% oxidation	10% reduction 90% oxidation
Oxidative metabolism	1A2 > 3A4 > 2C19	2C9 > 3A4
Potency	1.0 (reference)	2.7–3.8 times R-warfarin

hr = hours.

    h. Warfarin is 99% bound to plasma proteins (mostly albumin).

    i. Undergoes stereoselective metabolism by cytochrome P450 (CYP) 1A2, 2C9, 2C19, 2C8, 2C18, and 3A4 isoenzymes in the liver, with CYP2C9 being the main enzyme to modulate in vivo anticoagulant activity

    j. Pharmacokinetic variables of warfarin, particularly hepatic metabolism, vary substantially between individuals, leading to large interpatient differences in dose requirements.

    k. Genetic variations in the gene that codes for the CYP2C9 isoenzyme, vitamin K epoxide reductase complex 1 (VKORC1), correlate with warfarin dose requirements.

    l. Warfarin dosing algorithms that incorporate pharmacogenetic information are being evaluated, but they have yet to show improved clinical outcomes (e.g., reduced bleeding).

    m. Clinical utility and cost-effectiveness of using pharmacogenetic information to guide warfarin initiation remain unproven.

5. Dosing and administration

    a. The dose of warfarin is patient-specific depending on the desired intensity of anticoagulation and the patient's individual response.

    b. Because of tremendous interpatient and intrapatient variability in dose response, the warfarin dose must be based on continual clinical and laboratory monitoring.

    c. Although the average weekly warfarin dose is between 25 and 55 mg, some patient-related variables are associated with lower-than-usual dose requirements.

    d. For most patients, initiating therapy with 5–10 mg/day and adjusting the dose according to the INR response will produce therapeutic INRs in 5–7 days.

6. Initiation dosing of warfarin therapy. Outpatients: Warfarin initiation using the average daily dosing method

    a. This nomogram is useful in outpatients for whom INR cannot be checked on a daily basis.

    b. The response to therapy should be measured every 1–3 days until stabilized.

    c. Factors that increase sensitivity to warfarin

        i. Age older than 75 years

        ii. Clinical congestive HF

        iii. Clinical hyperthyroidism

        iv. Decreased oral intake

        v. Diarrhea

        vi. Drug-drug interactions

        vii. Elevated baseline INR

        viii. End-stage renal disease

        ix. Fever

        x. Hepatic disease

        xi. Hypoalbuminemia

        xii. Known CYP2C9 variant

        xiii. Malignancy

        xiv. Malnutrition

        xv. Postoperative status

Table 16. Warfarin Initiation in Outpatients

	Nonsensitive Patients	**Sensitive Patients**[a]
Initial dose	5 mg/day	2.5 mg/day
First INR	3 days	3 days
<1.5	7.5–10 mg/day	5–7.5 mg/day
1.5–1.9	5 mg/day	2.5 mg/day
2.0–3.0	2.5 mg/day	1.25 mg/day
3.1–4.0	1.25 mg/day	0.5 mg/day
>4.0	Hold	Hold
Next INR	2–3 days	2–3 days
Subsequent dosing and monitoring	Continue dose escalation and frequent monitoring until lower limit of therapeutic range is reached	

[a]See earlier section for factors that influence sensitivity to warfarin.

INR = international normalized ratio.

7. Maintenance dosing of warfarin therapy
   a. When adjusting the warfarin dose, the clinician should allow sufficient time for changes in the INR to occur.
   b. In general, maintenance dose changes should not be made more often than every 3 days.
   c. Doses should be adjusted by calculating the weekly dose and reducing or increasing the weekly dose by 5%–20%.
   d. Use of dosing algorithms (computerized or paper-based) is strongly encouraged. See www.warfarindosing.org.
   e. The effect of dose changes may not become evident for 7 days or greater if alternate-day dosing is used.

Table 17. Consideration for Adjustments of Warfarin Maintenance Dose for Goal INR of 2–3 (after at least 7 days of continuous dosing)[a]

INR	Suggested Change in Total "Weekly" Dosage
<1.5	Give extra daily dose once and increase weekly dose by 10%–20%
1.5–1.9	Increase weekly dose by 5%–15% (may give extra daily dose x 1)[b]
2.0–3.0	Maintain same dose
3.1–4.0	Hold zero to one daily dose and decrease weekly dose by 5%–20%[b]
4.1–5.0	Hold up to two daily doses and decrease weekly dose by 10%–20%[b]
≥5	Hold dose, consider administration of vitamin K

[a]Assumes no active bleeding.

[b]If transient cause is identified or if previously stable and INR ≤ 0.5 unit is out of range, may not need to increase/decrease weekly dose.

INR = international normalized ratio.

8. Therapeutic monitoring
   a. Warfarin requires frequent laboratory monitoring to ensure optimal therapeutic outcomes and to minimize bleeding complications.
   b. The PT is used to monitor the anticoagulation effects of warfarin.
   c. The PT measures the biologic activity of factor II, VII, and X activity and correlates well with warfarin's anticoagulation effect.
   d. The INR corrects for differences in thromboplastin reagents.
   e. Although the INR system has several potential problems, it is currently the best means available to interpret the PT and is the preferred method for monitoring oral anticoagulation therapy.
   f. The recommended target INR and associated goal range are based on the therapeutic indication.
   g. For most indications, the target INR is 2.5 with an acceptable range of 2.0–3.0.
   h. The target INR is higher for some patients with mechanical prosthetic heart valves (target INR 3.0, range 2.5–3.5).
   i. A baseline PT and CBC should be obtained before initiating warfarin therapy.
   j. In patients with an acute thromboembolic event, an INR should be measured minimally every 3 days during the first week of therapy (daily INRs are optimal to minimize need for cross-coverage with injectable anticoagulants during outpatient DVT treatment).
   k. Once the patient's dose response is established, an INR should be determined every 7–14 days until it stabilizes and, optimally, every 4–6 weeks thereafter.
   l. Recent evidence indicates INR recall intervals as long as 12 weeks may be used in patients with very stable conditions.
   m. When the warfarin dose is adjusted for significantly out-of-range INRs (e.g., greater than 4.0 or less than 1.5), an INR should be rechecked within 7 days. For INRs less severely out of range, a 14-day recall interval is acceptable.
   n. For patients with previously stable INR control, avoid changing the warfarin dose for mildly out-of-range INR (e.g., 1.5–3.5); instead, increase INR monitoring frequency.
9. Patient assessment and management: With each INR, the patient should also be assessed for other factors that can influence the anticoagulant effect of warfarin.
   a. Verification of the warfarin dose administered or taken
   b. Changes in current medications (prescription, over-the-counter, herbal)
   c. Acute illnesses (nausea, vomiting, diarrhea)
   d. Changes in diet (especially foods rich in vitamin K or decreased oral intake)
   e. Binge alcohol use
   f. Assess patient for signs and symptoms of TE.
   g. Assess patient for signs and symptoms of bleeding.
10. Adverse effects
    a. Bleeding
       i. As with the other anticoagulants, bleeding is the most common adverse effect.
       ii. The gastrointestinal (GI) tract and the nose are the most frequent sites of bleeding. Intracranial hemorrhage is the most serious and feared complication related to warfarin therapy, often resulting in permanent disability or death.
       iii. The annual incidence of major bleeding ranges from 1% in highly selected patient populations who are carefully managed to greater than 10% in patients who are medically managed in less structured environments.
       iv. Few studies have prospectively evaluated the incidence of minor bleeding, but it is likely to be greater than 15% annually, even in the most expertly treated patients.
       v. Several risk factors for bleeding while taking anticoagulation therapy have been identified.

Table 18. Risk Factors for Major Bleeding While Taking Anticoagulation Therapy

Anticoagulation intensity (e.g., INR > 4.0)
Therapy initiation (first few weeks)
Unstable anticoagulation response (INR control)
Age > 65 years
Concurrent antiplatelet drug use
Concurrent nonsteroidal anti-inflammatory drug use
History of gastrointestinal bleeding
Recent surgery or trauma
High risk of fall/trauma
Heavy alcohol use
Renal failure
Cerebrovascular disease
Malignancy

INR = international normalized ratio.

Reprinted from: Talbert RL, DiPiro JT, Matzke GR, et al., eds. Pharmacotherapy: A Pathophysiological Approach, 8th ed. New York: McGraw-Hill, 2011. With permission from The McGraw-Hill Companies.

vi. Intensity of anticoagulation therapy appears to be the most powerful risk factor for bleeding.

vii. Patients whose target INR is greater than 3.0 have twice the incidence of major bleeding than those having a target of 2.5.

viii. Unstable INR control also appears to be associated with an increased risk of bleeding.

ix. The risk of hemorrhage is greatest during the first few weeks of therapy.

x. However, bleeding can occur at any time, and the cumulative incidence steadily increases over time.

xi. Scoring systems have been developed to assess the risk of major bleeding in patients taking warfarin. To date, no bleeding prediction rule has shown sufficient predictive accuracy or had sufficient validation to be recommended for routine use in practice.

Table 19. Scoring Systems to Assess the Risk of Major Bleeding in Patients Taking Warfarin (validated only in patients with AF—Note also that CHADS$_2$ scores correlate with bleeding risk [i.e., higher scores = higher bleeding risk])

Scoring System	Criteria	Point Scores	Risk of Major Bleeding
Outpatient Bleeding Risk Index	Age > 65 years	1	<u>Score MB/pt-yr</u>
	History of GI bleed	1	Low (0) 3%
	History of stroke	1	Intermediate (1–2) 8%
	One or more of diabetes, hematocrit < 30%, SCr > 1.5 mg/dL, or recent MI	1	High (3–4) 30%
HEMORR$_2$HAGES scoring system	Hepatic or renal disease	1	<u>Score MB/pt-yr</u>
	Ethanol abuse	1	Low (0–1) 1.9%–2.5%
	Malignancy	1	Intermediate (2–3)
	Older (age > 75 years)	1	5.3%–8.4%
	Reduced platelet count or function	1	High (≥4) 10.4%–12.3%
	Rebleeding risk	2	
	Hypertension (uncontrolled)	1	
	Anemia	1	
	Genetic factors (CYP2C9 polymorphism)	1	
	Excessive fall risk	1	
	Stroke	1	
HAS-BLED[a]	Uncontrolled hypertension (SBP > 160 mm Hg)	1	<u>Score MB/pt-yr</u>
	Renal disease (SCr > 2.6 mg/dL, dialysis, transplant)	1	Low (0) 0.9%
	Hepatic disease (cirrhosis, bilirubin > 2 x ULN, AST/ALT > 3 x ULN)	1	Intermediate (1–2) 3.7%
	Stroke		High (≥3) 6.7%
	Prior major bleeding or predisposition	1	
	Labile INR (<60% time in range)	1	
	Elderly (age > 75 years)	1	
	Drugs/alcohol concomitantly	1 (1 each)	
ATRIA	Anemia	3	<u>Score MB/pt-yr</u>
	Severe renal disease	3	Low (0–3) 0.76%
	Age ≥ 75 years	2	Intermediate (4) 2.62%
	Any prior hemorrhage diagnosis	1	High (5–10) 5.76%
	Diagnosed hypertension	1	

[a]HAS-BLED calculator available at www.mdcalc.com/has-bled-score-for-major-bleeding-risk/.

AF = atrial fibrillation; AST/ALT = aspartate aminotransferase/alanine aminotransferase; CHADS$_2$ = congestive heart failure, hypertension, age at least 75 years, diabetes, previous stroke or transient ischemic attack; CYP = cytochrome P450; GI = gastrointestinal; INR = international normalized ratio; MB = major bleeding; MI = myocardial infarction; pt-yr = patient-year; SBP = systolic blood pressure; SCr = serum creatinine; ULN = upper limit of normal.

> xii. Serious bleeding, such as intracranial hemorrhage, necessitates holding warfarin and administering of 10 mg of vitamin K by slow intravenous infusion for 1 hour and PCC administration. Only the four-factor PCC (Kcentra) is FDA approved for warfarin reversal. The dose of Kcentra is based on the patient's INR, body weight, and factor IX concentration of the vial.

    b.   The "purple toe syndrome"

        i.   Manifested as a purplish discoloration of the toes

        ii. An extremely rare event reported in a small percentage of patients

        iii. The etiology of this unusual phenomenon is unknown, but it is thought to be the result of cholesterol microembolization into the arterial circulation of the toes.

    c.   Warfarin-induced skin necrosis

        i.   An uncommon but very serious dermatologic reaction

        ii. Manifested by a painful maculopapular rash and ecchymosis or purpura that subsequently progresses to necrotic gangrene

        iii. Usually appears in areas of the body rich in subcutaneous fat, such as the breasts, thighs, buttocks, and abdomen

        iv. Incidence is less than 0.1%.

        v.   Usually occurs in middle-aged women being treated for acute VTE

        vi. Although symptoms generally appear during the first week of therapy, symptoms have been reported in a few patients who had taken warfarin for months and even years.

        vii. Patients with protein C or S deficiency appear to be at greater risk. Patients who receive large "loading" doses of warfarin may also be at greater risk.

        viii. Overlapping warfarin and injectable anticoagulants is especially important in any patient thought to have a hypercoagulable state or with a strong family history of VTE. Warfarin-induced skin necrosis can occur despite concomitant parenteral anticoagulation.

        ix. If skin necrosis is suspected, warfarin therapy should be immediately discontinued, fresh frozen plasma and vitamin K administered, and full-dose UFH or LMWH therapy initiated.

        x.   Warfarin therapy should be reinitiated with extreme caution in patients having a history of skin necrosis, using small doses and gradual titration until a therapeutic INR has been achieved, if at all.

11. Drug and dietary interactions

    a.   The pharmacokinetic and pharmacodynamic properties of warfarin, together with its narrow therapeutic index, predispose this agent to numerous clinically important drug and food interactions.

    b.   Drug interactions

        i.   Pharmacokinetic drug interactions with warfarin are primarily a result of alterations in hepatic metabolism or binding to plasma proteins.

        ii. Drugs that inhibit or induce the CYP2C9, CYP1A2, and CYP3A4 isoenzymes have the greatest potential to significantly alter the response to warfarin therapy.

        iii. Protein-binding displacement interactions can also occur. However, in the absence of hepatic disease or a diminished capacity to metabolize warfarin (e.g., concurrent CYP enzyme inhibition), changes in protein binding should result in only transient changes in the INR.

        iv. Drugs that alter hemostasis, platelet function, or the clearance of clotting factors (e.g., thyroid hormone replacement) can alter the response to warfarin therapy or increase the risk of bleeding by pharmacodynamic mechanisms.

        v.   In most cases, increasing the frequency of INR monitoring and adjusting the warfarin dose as needed are preferable to preemptive empiric warfarin dose adjustment.

Table 20. Clinically Important Warfarin Drug Interactions

Medications That Increase INR	Proposed Mechanism	Medications That Decrease INR	Proposed Mechanism
Amiodarone	CYP3A4, CYP1A2, and CYP2C9 inhibitor	Carbamazepine	Induces CYP3A4
Cimetidine	CYP3A4 and CYP1A2 inhibitor	Methimazole	Unknown
Ciprofloxacin	CYP1A2 inhibitor	Nelfinavir	Unknown
Clarithromycin	CYP3A4 inhibitor	Nevirapine	CYP3A4 inducer
Cyclosporine	CYP3A4 substrate	Phenobarbital	Induces CYP3A4
Efavirenz	CYP2C9 inhibitor	Phenytoin	Induces CYP3A4
Erythromycin	CYP3A4 inhibitor	Rifampin	Induces CYP3A4 and CYP2C9
Fenofibric acid	CYP2C9 inhibitor	Ritonavir, Ritonavir/ Lopinavir	CYP3A4 and CYP2C9 inducer
Fluconazole	CYP3A4 and CYP2C9 inhibitor		
Fluorouracil	CYP2C9 inhibitor		
Fluvastatin	CYP2C9 inhibitor		
Fluvoxamine	CYP1A2 inhibitor		
Itraconazole	CYP3A4 inhibitor		
Ketoconazole	CYP3A4 inhibitor		
Levofloxacin	CYP1A2 inhibitor		
Lovastatin	CYP3A4 substrate		
Metronidazole	CYP3A4 inhibitor		
Miconazole	CYP3A4 inhibitor		
Nelfinavir	CYP3A4 inhibitor		
Phenytoin	CYP2C9 substrate		
Prednisone	CYP3A4 inhibitor		
Rosuvastatin	Unknown		
Saquinavir	CYP3A4 substrate and inhibitor		
Simvastatin	CYP3A4 substrate		
Sulfamethoxazole	CYP3A4 substrate		
Tamoxifen	CYP2C9 substrate		
Voriconazole	CYP3A4 and CYP2C9 inhibitor		

CYP = cytochrome P450; INR = international normalized ratio.

Reprinted from: Levine GN. Cardiology Secrets, 4th ed. Philadelphia: Saunders, 2013. With permission from Elsevier.

c. Dietary interactions
   i. Vitamin K
      (a) Vitamin K can reverse warfarin's pharmacologic activity, and many foods contain sufficient vitamin K to reduce the anticoagulation effect of warfarin if a patient consumes them in unusually large portions or repetitively within a short period.
      (b) Patients should be given a list of vitamin K–rich foods and instructed to maintain a relatively consistent intake. Patients with consistently higher intake of dietary vitamin K have less variable INR response and warfarin dosing requirements; therefore, it is important to stress consistency and moderation rather than abstinence.
      (c) Abrupt changes in vitamin K intake should be considered when unexplained changes in the INR occur.
      (d) Alternative sources of vitamin K, such as multivitamins and nutritional supplements (e.g., Sustacal and Ensure), should also be considered.
      (e) Patients who require parenteral nutrition should not receive a weekly bolus dose of vitamin K if they are receiving warfarin therapy.

Table 21. Vitamin K Content of Select Foods[a]

Very High (>200 mcg)	High (100–200 mcg)	Medium (50–100 mcg)	Low (<50 mcg)
Brussel sprouts	Basil	Apple, green	Apple, red
Chickpea	Broccoli	Asparagus	Avocado
Collard greens	Chive	Cabbage	Beans
Coriander	Coleslaw	Cauliflower	Breads, grains
Endive	Cucumber (with peel)	Mayonnaise	Carrot
Kale	Canola oil	Nuts, pistachio	Cereal
Lettuce, red leaf	Green onion/scallion	Squash, summer	Celery
Parsley	Lettuce, butterhead		Coffee
Spinach	Mustard greens		Corn
Swiss chard	Soybean oil		Cucumber (without peel)
Tea, green			Dairy products
Tea, black			Eggs
Turnip greens			Fruit (varies)
Watercress			Lettuce, iceberg
			Meats, fish, poultry
			Pasta
			Peanuts
			Peas
			Potato
			Rice
			Tomato

[a]Approximate amount of vitamin K per 100-g (3.5 oz.) serving.

Reprinted from: Talbert RL, DiPiro JT, Matzke GR, et al., eds. Pharmacotherapy: A Pathophysiological Approach, 8th ed. New York: McGraw-Hill, 2011. With permission from The McGraw-Hill Companies.

ii. Other dietary and herbal supplements

    (a) All patients receiving warfarin therapy should be questioned regarding the use of herbal drugs and dietary supplements.

    (b) Clinicians should advise patients receiving warfarin therapy to seek information about potential interactions with warfarin whenever they start to take a new drug product, whether it is prescribed or purchased over the counter.

    (c) If there is a known drug interaction or doubt about its potential to alter the response to warfarin, more frequent INR testing after the new agent is initiated is prudent.

Table 22. Warfarin Drug Interactions with Dietary Supplements

Mechanism	Effect	Supplement
Inhibition of warfarin metabolism	Increased INR	Chinese wolfberry Cranberry juice Grapefruit juice
Contain coumarin derivatives	Increased INR	Dan shen Dong quai Fenugreek
Unknown	Increased INR	Curbicin Devil's claw Glucosamine-chondroitin Melatonin Papaya extract Guilinggao
Inhibition of platelet aggregation	Increased bleeding	Garlic Ginger Ginkgo
Contain vitamin K/derivatives	Decreased INR	Coenzyme Q_{10}Green tea Some multivitamins
Induction of CYP3A4	Decreased INR	St. John's wort
Unknown	Decreased INR	Ginseng Melatonin

CYP = cytochrome P450; INR = international normalized ratio.

Table 23. Warfarin Drug-Disease State Interactions

Clinical Condition	Effect on Warfarin Therapy
Advanced age	Increased sensitivity to warfarin because of reduced vitamin K stores and/or lower plasma concentrations of vitamin K–dependent clotting factors
Pregnancy	Teratogenic; avoid exposure during pregnancy
Lactation	Not excreted in breast milk; can be used postpartum by nursing mothers
Alcoholism	Acute ingestion: Inhibits warfarin metabolism, with acute elevation in INR Chronic ingestion: Induces warfarin metabolism, with higher dose requirements

Table 23. Warfarin Drug-Disease State Interactions *(continued)*

Clinical Condition	Effect on Warfarin Therapy
Liver disease	May induce coagulopathy by decreased production of clotting factors, with baseline elevation in INR May reduce clearance of warfarin
Renal disease	Reduced activity of CYP2C9, with lower warfarin dose requirements
Heart failure	Reduced warfarin metabolism because of hepatic congestion
Cardiac valve replacement	Enhanced sensitivity to warfarin postoperatively because of hypoalbuminemia, lower oral intake, decreased physical activity, and reduced clotting factor concentrations after cardiopulmonary bypass
Nutritional status	Changes in dietary vitamin K intake (intentional or because of disease, surgery, etc.) alter response to warfarin, especially in patients with lower-than-average baseline dietary vitamin K intake
Use of tube feedings	Decreased sensitivity to warfarin, possibly caused by changes in absorption or vitamin K content of nutritional supplements
Thyroid disease	Hypothyroidism: Decreased catabolism of clotting factors requiring increased dosing requirements Hyperthyroidism: Increased catabolism of clotting factors causing increased sensitivity to warfarin
Smoking and tobacco use	Smoking: May induce CYP1A2, increasing warfarin dosing requirements Chewing tobacco: May contain vitamin K, increasing warfarin dosing requirements
Fever	Increased catabolism of clotting factors, causing acute increase in INR
Diarrhea	Reduction in secretion of vitamin K by gut flora, causing acute increase in INR
Acute infection/ inflammation	Increased sensitivity to warfarin
Malignancy	Increased sensitivity to warfarin by many factors; increased bleeding risk

CYP = cytochrome P450; INR = international normalized ratio.

E. Newer Target-Specific Oral Anticoagulants: Dabigatran *(Domain 1, Tasks 2, 3, 4, 5, 6, 7; Domain 3, Tasks 2, 3)*

Table 24. Dabigatran Characteristics

Characteristic	Dabigatran
Protein binding	35%
Volume of distribution	50–70 L
Time to maximal serum concentrations	1 (fasted) to 2 (fed) hours
Elimination half-life	CrCl ≥ 80 mL/minute = 13 hours CrCl 50–80 mL/minute = 15 hours CrCl 30–50 mL/minute = 18 hours CrCl 15–30 mL/minute = 27 hours
Activation	Prodrug dabigatran etexilate converted to active drug dabigatran by esterase hydrolysis
Metabolism	Conjugation
Renal excretion of unchanged drug	80% (of the absorbed dose, <7% of dabigatran etexilate absorbed)
Dialyzable	Yes

CrCl = creatinine clearance.

Table 25. Dabigatran – Considerations for Use

Dosage availability	75- and 150-mg oral capsules Do not chew, break, or open capsules; this can substantially increase the bioavailability (once open, the bottle expires in 4 months)
Dosage form	Capsules contain many drug pellets with a tartaric acid core (coated with dabigatran etexilate) that creates an acidic microenvironment to improve dissolution and absorption independently of gastric pH
Dosing	Nonvalvular atrial fibrillation CrCl > 30 mL/minute: 150 mg orally twice daily CrCl 15–30 mL/minute: 75 mg orally twice daily CrCl < 15 mL/minute or receiving dialysis: Not recommended
Hemodialysis	Removes a substantial amount of dabigatran (62% at 2 hours, 68% at 4 hours); may be considered if overdose
Instructions if missed dose	Take on the same day as soon as possible; skip the missed dose if it cannot be taken at least 6 hours before the next scheduled dose; dosing should not be doubled to make up for a missed dose
Hepatic impairment	No adjustment required
Elderly	No significant pharmacokinetic differences in healthy elderly individuals, but the elderly may be at higher bleeding risk from dabigatran
Reversal	Activated charcoal may decrease absorption if used within 1–2 hours of ingestion Hemodialysis (see above) One case report of FEIBA and two with rFVIIa (vitamin K, FFP, PCCs, protamine, and aminocaproic acid are not expected to have any effect)
Converting dabigatran to warfarin	Adjust the starting time of warfarin based on CrCl CrCl > 50 mL/minute: InitiateStart warfarin 3 days before discontinuing dabigatran CrCl 31–50 mL/minute: InitiateStart warfarin 2 days before discontinuing dabigatran CrCl 15–30 mL/minute: InitiateStart warfarin 1 day before discontinuing dabigatran CrCl < 15 mL/minute: Not recommended Note: Dabigatran can elevate the INR; the INR will better reflect warfarin's effect after dabigatran has been discontinued for at least 2 days
Converting warfarin to dabigatran	Discontinue warfarin and initiatestart dabigatran when the INR is below 2
Converting to or from a parenteral anticoagulant	When a parenteral anticoagulant is in use, initiatestart dabigatran 0–2 hours before the next subcutaneous dose of parenteral drug was to have been administered or when a continuously administered IV parenteral drug is discontinued For patients currently taking dabigatran, wait 12 hours (CrCl ≥ 30 mL/minute) or 24 hours (CrCl < 30 mL/minute) after the last dabigatran dose before initiating the parenteral (subcutaneous or IV) anticoagulant

Table 25. Dabigatran – Considerations for Use *(continued)*

Surgery or invasive procedures	Discontinue dabigatran 2 days (CrCl ≥ 50 mL/minute) or 2 days (CrCl 30-49 mL/minute) or 4 days (<30 mL/minute) before invasive or surgical procedures, if possible, to reduce the risk of bleeding
	Note: Depending on the risk of bleeding, urgency of the procedure, and thrombosis risk, holding for a shorter period may be considered
	Longer holding periods to establish complete hemostasis may be considered for major surgery, spinal puncture, or placement of a spinal or epidural catheter or port
	If a delay in surgery is not possible, the increased risk of bleeding should be weighed against the urgency of intervention
Contraindications	Active bleeding
	History of serious hypersensitivity reaction to dabigatran
	CrCl < 15 mL/minute
	Mechanical heart valve
	Avoid dabigatran in patients taking P-gp inhibitors with CrCl 15–30 mL/minute
Warnings and precautions	Risk of bleeding: Dabigatran can cause serious and sometimes fatal bleeding; promptly evaluate signs and symptoms of blood loss
	Temporary discontinuation: Avoid lapses in therapy to minimize stroke risk
	Discontinuation puts the patient at increased thrombosis risk
Adverse reactions	GI adverse effects are the most common: Dyspepsia, nausea, vomiting, constipation

CrCl = creatinine clearance; FEIBA = factor eight inhibitor bypass activity; FFP = fresh frozen plasma; GI = gastrointestinal; INR = international normalized ratio; IV = intravenous(ly); PCC = prothrombin complex concentrate; P-gp = P-glycoprotein; rFVIIa = recombinant factor VIIa.

Table 26. Dabigatran Drug Interactions

↑ **Dabigatran serum concentration**
• Amiodarone
• Dronedarone (reduce dose to 75 mg bid if CrCl 30–50 mL/minute)
• Quinidine
• Ketoconazole (reduce dose to 75 mg bid if CrCl 30–50 mL/minute)
• Verapamil
Avoid dabigatran if patient taking P-gp inhibitor and CrCl 15–30 mL/minute
↓ **Dabigatran serum concentration**
• Rifampin (significant interaction to avoid)
↑ **Anticoagulation effect**
• Other anticoagulants
• Antiplatelet agents
• Salicylates
• SSRIs
• SNRIs

bid = twice daily; CrCl = creatinine clearance; P-gp = P-glycoprotein; SNRI = serotonin-norepinephrine reuptake inhibitor; SSRI = selective serotonin reuptake inhibitor.

F. Direct Xa Inhibitors; Oral Xa Inhibitors: Rivaroxaban, Apixaban, Edoxaban
   (Domain 1, Tasks 2–, 3, 4, 5, 6, 7; Domain 3, Tasks 2, 3)
   1. Rivaroxaban

Table 27. Rivaroxaban Characteristics

Characteristic	**Rivaroxaban**
Protein binding	92%–95%
Volume of distribution	50 L
Time to maximal serum concentrations	2–4 hours
Elimination half-life	5–9 hours
Metabolism	Oxidative metabolism by CYP3A4/5
Renal excretion of unchanged drug	66% of the total dose/33% of the absorbed dose
Dialyzable	Unlikely (because of high plasma protein binding)

CYP = cytochrome P450.

Table 28. Rivaroxaban – Considerations for Use

Dosage availability	10-, 15-, and 20-mg oral film-coated tablets
Dosing	Nonvalvular atrial fibrillation CrCl > 50 mL/minute: 20 mg orally once daily with evening meal CrCl 15–50 mL/minute: 15 mg once daily with evening meal CrCl < 15 mL/minute or receiving dialysis: Avoid use VTE treatment CrCl ≥ 30 mL/minute: 15 mg once daily orally twice daily with a meal for 21 days; then 20 mg orally once daily with a meal thereafter CrCl < 30 mL/minute: Avoid use VTE prophylaxis CrCl ≥ 30 mL/minute: 10 mg once daily orally once daily with evening meal CrCl < 30 mL/minute: Avoid use
Hemodialysis	Because of high plasma protein binding, not expected to be dialyzable
Instructions if missed dose	If a dose is not taken at the scheduled time, administer the dose as soon as possible on the same day
Hepatic impairment	Avoid use in patients with moderate (Child-Pugh B) and severe (Child-Pugh C) hepatic impairment or with any hepatic disease associated with coagulopathy
Elderly	No significant pharmacokinetic differences in healthy elderly individuals, but elderly may be at higher bleeding risk from rivaroxaban
Reversal	Use of activated charcoal to reduce absorption in case of overdose may be considered No specific antidote is available Benefits of rFVIIa is unknown, limited evidence indicates four-factor PCCs (Kcentra) may reverse anticoagulant effect (vitamin K, FFP, protamine, and aminocaproic acid are not expected to have any effect)

Table 28. Rivaroxaban – Considerations for Use *(continued)*

Converting rivaroxaban to warfarin	No clinical trial data are available to guide converting patients' therapy from rivaroxaban to warfarin
	Rivaroxaban affects INR, so INR measurements made during coadministration with warfarin may not be useful for determining the appropriate dose of warfarin
	One (unproven) approach is to discontinue rivaroxaban and begin both a parenteral anticoagulant and warfarin when the next dose of rivaroxaban would have been taken (an increased rate of stroke was observed during the transition from rivaroxaban to warfarin in clinical trials of patients with atrial fibrillation)
	Another (unproven) approach is based on CrCl:
	CrCl > 50 mL/minute: InitiateStart warfarin 4 days before discontinuing rivaroxaban
	CrCl 31–50 mL/minute: InitiateStart warfarin 3 days before discontinuing rivaroxaban
	CrCl 15–30 mL/minute: InitiateStart warfarin 2 days before discontinuing rivaroxaban
Converting warfarin to rivaroxaban	Discontinue warfarin and initiate rivaroxaban as soon as the INR is below 3.0 to avoid periods of inadequate anticoagulation
Converting to or from anticoagulants other than warfarin	Initiate rivaroxaban 0–2 hours before the next scheduled evening administration of the drug (e.g., LMWH or non-warfarin oral anticoagulant) and omit administration of the other anticoagulant
	For UFH being administered by continuous infusion, discontinue the infusion and initiate rivaroxaban at the same time
	For patients currently taking rivaroxaban and transitioning to an anticoagulant with rapid onset, discontinue rivaroxaban and give the first dose of the other anticoagulant (oral or parenteral) when the next rivaroxaban dose would have been taken
Surgery or invasive procedures	Discontinue at least 24 hours before the procedure; in deciding whether a procedure should be delayed until 24 hours after the last dose of rivaroxaban, weigh the increased risk of bleeding against the urgency of intervention; reinitiate after the surgical or other procedures as soon as adequate hemostasis has been established; if oral medication cannot be taken after surgical intervention, consider administering a parenteral anticoagulant
Contraindications	Active bleeding
	History of serious hypersensitivity reaction to rivaroxaban
Warnings and precautions	Risk of bleeding: Rivaroxaban can cause serious and sometimes fatal bleeding; promptly evaluate signs and symptoms of blood loss
	Temporary discontinuation: Avoid lapses in therapy to minimize stroke risk
Adverse reactions	Low incidence of adverse reactions other than bleeding

CrCl = creatinine clearance; FFP = fresh frozen plasma; INR = international normalized ratio; LMWH = low-molecular-weight heparin; PCC = prothrombin complex concentrate; rFVIIa = recombinant factor VIIa; UFH = unfractionated heparin; VTE = venous thromboembolism.

Table 29. Rivaroxaban Drug Interactions

↑ **Rivaroxaban serum concentration**
• Combined P-gp and strong CYP3A4 inhibitors (avoid use)
• Ketoconazole
• Itraconazole
• Lopinavir/ritonavir
• Ritonavir
• Indinavir/ritonavir
• Conivaptan
↓ **Rivaroxaban serum concentration**
• Combined P-gp and strong CYP3A4 inducers (avoid use)
• Carbamazepine
• Phenytoin
• Rifampin
• St. John's wort
Weigh risk vs. benefit in patients with CrCl 15–50 mL/minute taking concomitant P-gp and weak or moderate CYP3A4 inhibitors
↑ **Anticoagulation effect**
• Other anticoagulants
• Antiplatelet agents
• NSAIDs
• SSRIs
• SNRIs

CrCl = creatinine clearance; CYP = cytochrome P450; NSAID = nonsteroidal anti-inflammatory drug; P-gp = P-glycoprotein; SNRI = serotonin-norepinephrine receptor inhibitor; SSRI = selective serotonin receptor inhibitor.

2. Apixaban

Table 30. Apixaban Characteristics

Characteristic	Apixaban
Protein binding	87%
Volume of distribution	21 L
Time to maximal serum concentrations	3–4 hours
Elimination half-life	12 hours
Metabolism	Oxidative metabolism primarily by CYP3A4
Renal excretion of unchanged drug	27% of total dose
Dialyzable	Yes

CYP = cytochrome P450.

Table 31. Apixaban – Considerations for Use

Dosage availability	2.5- and 5-mg film-coated oral tablets
Dosing	Nonvalvular atrial fibrillation 5 mg orally bid for CrCl ≥ 15 mL/minute Reduce dose to 2.5 mg orally bid if two of the following are present: Age > 80 years, body weight ≤ 60 kg, SCr ≥ 1.5 mg/dL Patients receiving hemodialysis (excluded from trials): Prescribing information recommends a dose of 5 mg bid unless one of the following is present: Age > 80 years, body weight ≤ 60 kg; then reduce dose to 2.5 mg orally bid VTE and PE treatment 10 mg orally bid for days 1–7, then 5 mg orally bid VTE prophylaxis 2.5 mg orally bid
Hemodialysis	Dialysis clearance 18 mL/minute (compared with renal clearance in healthy normal volunteers of 11 mL/minute), representing a 14% decrease in exposure compared with an off-dialysis period; 7% of dose removed by hemodialysis
Instructions if missed dose	If a dose is not taken at the scheduled time, administer the dose as soon as possible on the same day, and twice-daily administration should be resumed
Hepatic impairment	No dosage adjustment in mild hepatic impairment; avoid use in patients with severe hepatic impairment
Reversal	Use of activated charcoal to reduce absorption in case of overdose may be considered No specific antidote is available Benefits of rFVIIa are unknown; limited evidence indicates four-factor PCCs (not available in the United States) may reverse anticoagulant effect (vitamin K, FFP, protamine, and aminocaproic acid are not expected to have any effect)
Converting apixaban to warfarin	Apixaban affects INR, so INR measurements made during coadministration with warfarin may not be useful for determining the appropriate dose of warfarin One (unproven) approach is to discontinue apixaban and begin both a parenteral anticoagulant and warfarin when the next dose of apixaban would have been taken (an increased rate of stroke was observed during the transition from apixaban to warfarin in clinical trials of patients with atrial fibrillation)
Converting warfarin to apixaban	Discontinue warfarin and initiate apixaban as soon as the INR is below 2.0 to avoid periods of inadequate anticoagulation
Converting to or from anticoagulants other than warfarin	Initiate apixaban at the same time as the next scheduled dose and omit administration of the other anticoagulant For UFH being administered by continuous infusion, discontinue the infusion and initiate apixaban at the same time For patients currently taking apixaban and transitioning to an anticoagulant with rapid onset, discontinue apixaban and give the first dose of the other anticoagulant (oral or parenteral) when the next rivaroxaban dose would have been taken

Table 31. Apixaban – Considerations for Use *(continued)*

Surgery or invasive procedures	Discontinue at least 24 hours before a procedure with a low bleeding risk and at least 48 hours before a procedure with a moderate or high bleeding risk; reinitiate after the surgical or other procedures as soon as adequate hemostasis has been established; if oral medication cannot be taken after surgical intervention, consider administering a parenteral anticoagulant
Contraindications	Active bleeding History of serious hypersensitivity reaction to apixaban
Warnings and precautions	Risk of bleeding: Apixaban can cause serious and sometimes fatal bleeding; promptly evaluate signs and symptoms of blood loss Temporary discontinuation: Avoid lapses in therapy to minimize stroke risk
Adverse reactions	Low incidence of adverse reactions other than bleeding

bid = twice daily; CrCl = creatinine clearance; FFP = fresh frozen plasma; INR = international normalized ratio; PCC = prothrombin complex concentrate; PE = pulmonary embolism; rFVIIa = recombinant factor VIIa; SCr = serum creatinine concentration; UFH = unfractionated heparin; VTE = venous thromboembolism.

Table 32. Apixaban Drug Interactions

↑ **Rivaroxaban serum concentration** • Combined P-gp and strong CYP3A4 inhibitors (reduce 5-mg dose bid to 2.5 mg bid, and if 2.5 mg bid, avoid use) • Ketoconazole • Itraconazole • Lopinavir/ritonavir • Ritonavir • Indinavir/ritonavir • Clarithromycin
↓ **Rivaroxaban serum concentration** • Combined P-gp and strong CYP3A4 inducers (avoid use) • Carbamazepine • Phenytoin • Rifampin • St. John's wort
↑ **Anticoagulation effect** • Other anticoagulants • Antiplatelet agents • NSAIDs • SSRIs • SNRIs

bid = twice daily; CYP = cytochrome P450; NSAID = nonsteroidal anti-inflammatory drug; P-gp = P-glycoprotein; SNRI = serotonin-norepinephrine receptor inhibitor; SSRI = selective serotonin receptor inhibitor.

3. Edoxaban

Table 33. Edoxaban Characteristics

Characteristic	Edoxaban
Protein binding	55%
Volume of distribution	21 L
Time to maximal serum concentrations	2 hours
Elimination half-life	12 hours
Metabolism	Oxidative metabolism primarily by CYP3A4, conjugation
Renal excretion of unchanged drug	50% of total dose
Dialyzable	No

CYP = cytochrome P450.

Table 34. Edoxaban – Considerations for Use

Dosage availability	30- and 60-mg film-coated oral tablets
Dosing	Nonvalvular atrial fibrillation 60 mg orally daily for CrCl ≥ 50 mL/minute Reduce dose to 30 mg orally daily if CrCl between 15 and -50 mL/minute Patients receiving hemodialysis (excluded from trials): Not recommended VTE and PE treatment 60 mg taken orally once daily after following 5 to 10 days of initial therapy with a parenteral anticoagulant
Hemodialysis	A 4- hour hemodialysis session reduced total edoxaban exposure by less than 7%
Instructions if missed dose	If a dose is not taken at the scheduled time, administer the dose as soon as possible on the same day, and once-daily administration should be resumed the next day
Hepatic impairment	No dosage adjustment in mild hepatic impairment; avoid use in patients with moderate to severe hepatic impairment
Reversal	Use of activated charcoal to reduce absorption in case of overdose may be considered No specific antidote is available Benefits of rFVIIa are unknown; limited evidence indicates four-factor PCCs (not available in the United States) may reverse anticoagulant effect (vitamin K, FFP, protamine, and aminocaproic acid are not expected to have any effect)
Converting edoxaban to warfarin	Decrease edoxaban to 30 mg daily and initiatestart warfarin; continue edoxaban until INR ≥ 2.0 OR, discontinue edoxaban and initiatestart warfarin (recommend parenteral anticoagulation until INR > 2)
Converting warfarin to edoxaban	InitiateStart edoxaban when INR is ≤ 2.5

Table 34. Edoxaban – Considerations for Use *(continued)*

Converting to or from anticoagulants other than warfarin	Initiate edoxaban at the same time as the next scheduled dose and omit administration of the other anticoagulant
	For UFH being administered by continuous infusion, discontinue the infusion and initiate edoxaban 4 hours later
	For patients currently taking edoxaban and transitioning to an anticoagulant with rapid onset, discontinue edoxaban and give the first dose of the other anticoagulant (oral or parenteral) when the next edoxaban dose would have been taken
Surgery or invasive procedures	Discontinue at least 24 hours before invasive or surgical procedures; reinitiate after the surgical or other procedures as soon as adequate hemostasis has been established; if oral medication cannot be taken after surgical intervention, consider administering a parenteral anticoagulant
Contraindications	Active bleeding History of serious hypersensitivity reaction to edoxaban
Warnings and precautions	Risk of bleeding: Eedoxaban can cause serious and sometimes fatal bleeding; promptly evaluate signs and symptoms of blood loss Temporary discontinuation: Avoid lapses in therapy to minimize stroke risk
Adverse reactions	Low incidence of adverse reactions other than bleeding

bid = twice daily; CrCl = creatinine clearance; FFP = fresh frozen plasma; INR = international normalized ratio; PCC = prothrombin complex concentrate; PE = pulmonary embolism; rFVIIa = recombinant factor VIIa; SCr = serum creatinine concentration; UFH = unfractionated heparin; VTE = venous thromboembolism.

Table 35. Edoxaban Drug Interactions

↓ **Edoxaban serum concentration** • Combined P-gp and strong CYP3A4 inducers (avoid use) • Carbamazepine • Phenytoin • Rifampin • St. John's wort
Verapamil: Ffor VTE, reduce dose to 30 mg daily
↑ **Anticoagulation effect** • Other anticoagulants • Antiplatelet agents • NSAIDs • SSRIs •SNRIs

bid = twice daily; CYP = cytochrome P450; NSAID = nonsteroidal anti-inflammatory drug; P-gp = P-glycoprotein; SNRI = serotonin-norepinephrine receptor inhibitor; SSRI = selective serotonin receptor inhibitor; VTE = venous thromboembolism..

Patient Cases

Questions 6–8 pertain to the following case.

S.K. is a 78-year-old, 58-kg woman with a history of uncontrolled HTN, diabetes mellitus, GI bleeding, chronic kidney disease, and chronic NVAF. Her current medications include metformin, carvedilol, digoxin, aspirin, and lansoprazole; her SCr is 0.94 mg/dL; and her calculated CrCl is 45 mL/minute.

6. Which is the best choice for S.K.'s CHADS$_2$ score and classification for stroke risk?

   A. 0 (Low).
   B. 1 (Moderate).
   C. 2 (High).
   D. 3 (High).

7. Which is the best choice for S.K.'s HAS-BLED score and classification of bleeding risk?

   A. 1 (Intermediate).
   B. 2 (Intermediate).
   C. 3 (High).
   D. 4 (High).

8. A decision is made to administer anticoagulants to S.K. Which represents the most appropriate choice?

   A. Apixaban 5 mg orally twice daily.
   B. Rivaroxaban 20 mg orally daily.
   C. Dabigatran 75 mg orally twice daily.
   D. Aspirin 81 mg plus clopidogrel 75 mg orally daily.

IV. THERAPY PRECAUTIONS AND MANAGEMENT OF ADVERSE EVENTS *(Domain 1, Tasks 2, 3, 4)*

Table 36. General Contraindications to Anticoagulation Therapy

Active major bleeding
Hemophilia or other hemorrhagic tendencies
Severe liver disease with elevated baseline PT
Severe thrombocytopenia (platelet count < 20,000/mm³)
Malignant hypertension
Inability to meticulously supervise and monitor treatment

PT = prothrombin time.

Table 37. Reversal Considerations for LMWH or Fondaparinux

LMWHs	Fondaparinux
Protamine can be used as a "partial" reversal agent for the effects of LMWH Protamine neutralizes around 60% of the anti–factor Xa activity If LMWH was given in the previous 8 hours, then 1 mg of protamine should be administered for every 100 IU (or 1 mg) of the LMWH If the LMWH dose is given in the previous 8–12 hours, a 0.5-mg dose of protamine should be given for every 100 anti–factor Xa units Use of protamine sulfate is not recommended if the LMWH was administered more than 12 hours earlier	No specific antidote exists

LMWH = low-molecular-weight heparin.

Table 38. Guidelines for Reversal of an Elevated INR in a Patient Taking Warfarin

INR	Recommendation
<5	Lower or hold dose
5–10	Hold one or two doses
≥10	Hold warfarin and give vitamin K (2.5 mg orally); use additional vitamin K, if necessary
Serious bleeding with high INR	Hold warfarin and give vitamin K (10-mg slow IV infusion) supplemented with fresh frozen plasma, prothrombin complex concentrate, or recombinant factor VIIa; may repeat vitamin K every 12 hours, if necessary
Life-threatening bleeding	Hold warfarin and give prothrombin complex concentrates or recombinant factor VIIa supplemented with vitamin K (10-mg slow IV infusion); repeat as necessary

INR = international normalized ratio; IV = intravenous.

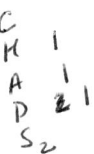

V. PATIENT EDUCATION CONSIDERATIONS

A. Oral Anticoagulants *(Domain 2, Task 5)*

Table 39. Key Elements of Patient Education Regarding Warfarin, Apixaban, Dabigatran, Rivaroxaban, and Edoxaban

Identification of generic and brand names
Purpose of therapy
Expected therapy duration
Dosing and administration
Visual recognition of drug and tablet or capsule dosage strength
Importance of taking exactly as prescribed
What to do if a dose is missed
Importance of prothrombin time/INR monitoring (warfarin only)
Importance of kidney function monitoring (apixaban, dabigatran, and rivaroxaban only)
Recognition of signs and symptoms of bleeding
Recognition of signs and symptoms of TE
What to do if bleeding or TE occurs
Potential for interactions with prescription and over-the-counter medications and natural/herbal products
Dietary considerations (warfarin only) and use of alcohol
MustNeed to take with food (rivaroxaban only)
Expiration of tablets (dabigatran only)
Importance of not crushing or breaking capsule (dabigatran only)
Avoidance of pregnancy
Significance of informing other health care providers that anticoagulant has been prescribed
When, where, and with whom follow-up will be provided
Ensure that the patient can pay for the drug before a final decision on treatment is made

INR = international normalized ratio; TE = thromboembolism.

B. LMWH/Fondaparinux for Home Use *(Domain 2, Tasks 3, 5)*

Table 40. Use of LMWH/Fondaparinux at Home

Ensure that the patient/caregiver is fully educated on administering the injection and is willing to adhere
Ensure that the follow-up appointments have been made for anticoagulation monitoring
Ensure that the outpatient provider clearly understands the treatment plan and the importance of making sure the patient follows up
Ensure that the patient can pay for the drug before a final decision on treatment is made
Ensure that the pharmacy where the patient will obtain the drug has it in stock
Ensure that the patient has telephone numbers to call if he or she has any questions/concerns about therapy when at home and that the care providers have the patient's contact information, if needed

C. Periprocedural Anticoagulation Bridging *(Domain 1, Tasks 2, 3, 4, 7)*

Table 41. Risk Stratification for Determining the Need for Bridge Therapy

Risk Stratum	Indication for VKA Therapy		
	Mechanical Heart Valve	**Atrial Fibrillation**	**Venous Thromboembolism**
High	Any mitral valve prosthesis Older (caged-ball or tilting disk) aortic valve prosthesis Recent (within 6 months) stroke or transient ischemic attack	$CHADS_2$ score of 5 or 6 Recent (within 3 months) stroke or transient ischemic attack Rheumatic valvular heart disease	Recent (within 3 months) VTE Severe thrombophilia (e.g., deficiency of protein C, protein S, or antithrombin; antiphospholipid antibodies; many abnormalities)
Moderate	Bileaflet aortic valve prosthesis and one of the following: Atrial fibrillation, previous stroke or transient ischemic attack, hypertension, diabetes, congestive heart failure, age > 75 years	$CHADS_2$ score of 3 or 4	VTE within the past 3–12 months (Consider VTE prophylaxis rather than full-intensity bridge therapy) Nonsevere thrombophilic conditions (e.g., heterozygous factor V Leiden mutation, heterozygous factor II mutation) Recurrent VTE Active cancer (treated within 6 months or palliative)
Low	Bileaflet aortic valve prosthesis without atrial fibrillation and no other risk factors for stroke	$CHADS_2$ score of 0–2 (no previous stroke or transient ischemic attack)	Single VTE occurred greater than 12 months ago and no other risk factors

$CHADS_2$ = congestive heart failure, hypertension, age at least 75 years, diabetes, previous stroke or transient ischemic attack; VKA = vitamin K antagonist; VTE = venous thromboembolism.

Table 42. Warfarin to Parenteral Anticoagulant Bridge Therapy Guidelines for Invasive Procedures

Thromboembolic Risk[a]	Renal Function	Bridge Therapy
Low	All patients	Last dose of warfarin on day −6 pre procedure Hold warfarin day from day −5 through day −1 Consider vitamin K 2.5 mg PO on day −2 or day −1 if INR ≥ 1.5 Resume warfarin 12–48 hours post procedure at usual maintenance dose (decision based on postoperative assessment of bleeding risk)
High	CrCl > 30 mLl/minute	Last dose of warfarin on day −6 pre procedure Hold warfarin day −5 through day −1 Start LMWH on day −3 (or when INR < lower limit of range) Consider vitamin K 2.5 mg PO on day 2 or day 1 if INR ≥ 1.5 Last dose of LMWH 24 hours pre procedure (On day −1, give one-half dose of LMWH if patient is receiving once-daily LMWH) Resume warfarin 12–24 hours post procedure at usual maintenance dose (decision predicated on postprocedure assessment of bleeding risk) Resume LMWH 24 hours post procedure (or 48–72 hours for major surgery or high bleeding risk procedure) and continue until INR > lower limit of therapeutic range
	CrCl ≤ 30 mLl/minute	Last dose of warfarin on day −6 pre procedure Hold warfarin day −5 through day −1 Consider vitamin K 2.5 mg PO or 1 mg IV x on day −2 or day −1 pre procedure if INR ≥ 1.5 Admit on day −1 pre procedure and begin IV UFH (70 units/kg bolus, 15 units/kg/hour infusion and adjust per inpatient protocol) Discontinue IV UFH 6 hours pre procedure Resume warfarin 12–24 hours post procedure at the usual maintenance dose (decision based on postoperative assessment of bleeding risk) Resume IV UFH 24 hours post procedure (or 48–72 hours for major surgery or high-bleeding-risk procedure) and continue until INR > lower limit of therapeutic range

[a]The decision to bridge patients with a moderate risk of thromboembolism should be based on surgery and patient-related factors.

CrCl = creatinine clearance; INR = international normalized ratio; IV = intravenous; LMWH = low-molecular-weight heparin; PO = orally; UFH = unfractionated heparin.

VI. CONSIDERATIONS FOR PATIENT SAFETY AND DELIVERY OF QUALITY PATIENT CARE

A. Systematic Management *(Domain 4, Task 1)*
   1. Anticoagulation therapy management services can improve the care of patients who take warfarin therapy.
   2. Provides structured and comprehensive patient education and evaluation
   3. Improves the safety and effectiveness of warfarin therapy compared with "usual" medical care
   4. Lowers the overall cost of care by reducing the frequency of major bleeding and recurrent thromboembolic events
   5. However, the benefit of anticoagulation management services is not supported by high-quality evidence.

B. Home Management of Warfarin Oral Anticoagulation: Portable Fingerstick INR Devices Are Available for Monitoring Warfarin Therapy. *(Domain 1, Task 5)*
   1. Self-monitoring at home: Requires that the patient report his or her test results to a health care professional. The clinician continues to make warfarin dosing decisions.
   2. Self-management at home: Highly motivated patients can be trained to manage dosing themselves, independently altering the warfarin therapy dose according to their INR results.
   3. Patients who engage in INR self-monitoring and warfarin self-management report high levels of satisfaction with care, with modest improvement in percentage time in therapeutic INR range, compared with those who are medically managed by "usual care."
   4. Home INR testing and self-management require careful patient selection and considerable education.
   5. Most benefit is seen in the reduction of thromboembolic complication risk in patients with mechanical valves who self-manage INRs. Minimal benefit has been shown with self-testing in patients with AF (e.g., the THINRS [The Home INR Study] trial did not show any benefit of self-testing).
   6. Patients with very stable conditions probably do not need the frequent testing usually used with self-testing and self-management.

C. National Quality Initiatives *(Domain 5, Tasks 1, 2)*
   1. The recent national focus on quality health care has been emphasized by the call to accountability through the Joint Commission's Agenda for Change; the Institute of Medicine's report on medical errors; the endorsed safe practices of the National Quality Forum (NQF); the Leapfrog Group's recommendations; and the demand for value by health care consumers.

Table 43. Organizations Monitoring Quality of Venous Thromboembolism Care

The Joint Commission - www.jointcommission.org
A not-for-profit health care accreditation organization that issues performance-based standards and assesses organizational compliance with improved patient safety and quality of care
Leapfrog Group - www.leapfroggroup.org
An initiative of health care–purchasing organizations seeking improvements in safety, quality, and affordability of health care, with funding from the Business Roundtable, Robert Wood Johnson Foundation, and member organizations
National Quality Forum - www.qualityforum.org
A not-for-profit organization that develops and implements national strategies for health care quality measurement and reporting

   2. The NQF has developed national consensus standards for VTE prevention and treatment that will apply to a variety of health care settings.
      a. The outcomes of this effort will provide a framework for measuring the effective screening, prevention, and treatment of VTE.
      b. The NQF's recommendations include developing organizational policies that address staff education, treatment protocols, and compliance measurements to improve VTE prevention in the hospital.
      c. The ultimate goal of the NQF consensus standards is to facilitate the early promulgation of VTE policies, risk assessment, prophylaxis, diagnosis, and treatment services as well as patient education and organizational accountability.
      d. To that end, the Joint Commission has developed performance measures to enforce the NQF's recommendations.

Table 44. The Joint Commission's Proposed Performance Measures for the Prevention and Treatment of Venous Thrombosis

Number	Description of Proposed Performance Measure
1	Documentation of Venous Thromboembolism Risk Assessment/Prophylaxis Within 24 Hours of Hospital Admission
2	Documentation of Venous Thromboembolism Risk Assessment/Prophylaxis Within 24 Hours of Transfer to ICU
3	Venous Thromboembolism Patients with Overlap of Parenteral and Warfarin Anticoagulation Therapy
4	Venous Thromboembolism Patients Receiving Unfractionated Heparin by Nomogram/Protocol with Platelet Count Monitoring
5	Venous Thromboembolism Discharge Instructions
6	Incidence of Potentially Preventable Hospital-Acquired Venous Thromboembolism

ICU = intensive care unit.

Table 45. The Joint Commission National Patient Safety Goals on Anticoagulation Therapy Elements of Performance

Use only oral unit-dose products, prefilled syringes, or premixed infusion bags when these types of products are available – Note: For pediatric patients, prefilled syringe products should be used only if specifically designed for children

Use approved protocols for the initiation and maintenance of anticoagulant therapy

Before initiating warfarin therapy for a patient, assess the patient's baseline coagulation status; for all patients receiving warfarin therapy, use a current INR to adjust this therapy; the baseline status and current INR are documented in the medical record

Use authoritative resources to manage potential food and drug interactions for patients receiving warfarin

When heparin is administered both intravenously and continuously, use programmable pumps to provide consistent and accurate dosing

A written policy addresses baseline and ongoing laboratory tests that are required for anticoagulants

Provide education regarding anticoagulant therapy to prescribers, staff, patients, and families; patient/family education includes the following:

- The importance of follow-up monitoring
- Adherence
- Drug-food interactions
- The potential for adverse drug reactions and interactions

Evaluate anticoagulation safety practices, take action to improve practices, and measure the effectiveness of those actions in a period determined by the organization

INR = international normalized ratio.

Table 46. Useful Resources Involving Anticoagulation Therapy

Reference	Web Site	Comment
American College of Chest Physicians guidelines	http://journal. publications.chestnet. org/ss/guidelines.aspx	The oldest and most established evidence-based guideline involving antithrombotic therapy
Anticoagulation Forum	www.acforum.org/	Multidisciplinary professional organization for those who manage anticoagulation therapy; helpful clinical resources are posted on the site as well as professional guidelines that describe best practice for outpatient (2008) and inpatient (2013) anticoagulation services
ClotCare	www.clotcare.com/ clotcare/index.aspx	Regularly updated site mainly focused on keeping professionals abreast of cutting-edge information involving antithrombotic therapy; site also contains helpful information for patients

HEART FAILURE

VII. DIAGNOSIS

A. Symptoms Suggestive of HF *(Domain 1, Task 2)*
   1. Dyspnea at rest or on exertion
   2. Reduced exercise capacity, unexplained fatigue, or weakness
   3. Orthopnea
   4. Paroxysmal nocturnal dyspnea or nocturnal cough
   5. Early satiety, nausea and vomiting, abdominal discomfort, or constipation
   6. Wheezing or cough
   7. Confusion, delirium, or depression

B. Physical Examination Findings *(Domain 1, Task 2)*
   1. Elevated jugular venous pressure or hepatojugular reflux
   2. S3 gallop
   3. Rales
   4. Displaced apical pulse, or PMI ("point of maximum impulse")
   5. Ascites
   6. Edema
   7. Cardiac enlargement
   8. Cardiac murmurs suggesting valvular dysfunction
   9. Narrow pulse pressure
   10. Cool extremities

C. Other Pertinent Diagnostic and Laboratory Findings *(Domain 1, Tasks 2, 3)*
   1. Assessment of B-type natriuretic peptide (BNP) or N-terminal proBNP (NT-proBNP) concentration is recommended by guidelines, especially when the diagnosis is uncertain.
   2. BNP greater than 100 pg/mL: May be used to monitor the success of goal-directed medical therapy (GDMT)

3. NT-proBNP cut points of more than 450 pg/mL for patients younger than 50 years, more than 900 pg/mL for patients 50–74 years of age, and more than 1800 pg/mL for patients 75 years and older are predictive of HF. May be used to monitor the success of GDMT

4. Left ventricular ejection fraction (LVEF) less than 40% as determined by echocardiography, radionuclide angiography (MUGA [multiple gated acquisition] blood scan, considered the gold standard for LVEF measurement), or coronary angiography. Even though a MUGA scan provides the most accurate assessment of ejection fraction (EF), it is seldom used because of its higher cost and invasiveness.

5. Models that can be used in ambulatory patients to predict mortality
   a. Seattle Heart Failure Model (http://SeattleHeartFailureModel.org)
   b. Heart Failure Survival Score (http://handheld.softpedia.com/dyn-search.php)

D. Definitions *(Domain 1, Task 2)*
   1. HFrEF is HF with reduced LVEF (historically called systolic HF): A clinical syndrome characterized by signs and symptoms of HF and reduced LVEF defined as 40% or less. Usually associated with LV chamber dilation
   2. HFpEF is HF with preserved LVEF (historically called diastolic HF): A clinical syndrome characterized by signs and symptoms of HF with preserved LVEF defined as 50% or greater. Usually associated with a nondilated LV chamber
   3. NYHA classes I–IV and ACC/AHA stages A–D (Table 474)

Table 47. Clinical Classifications of Heart Failure Severity

NYHA Functional Classification		ACC/AHA Stages of Heart Failure	
		Stage A	At high risk of heart failure; no identified structural or functional abnormality; no signs or symptoms
Class I	No limitation of physical activity; ordinary physical activity does not cause undue fatigue, palpitation, or dyspnea	Stage B	Developed structural heart disease that is strongly associated with the development of heart failure but without signs or symptoms
Class II	Slight limitation of physical activity; comfortable at rest, but ordinary physical activity results in fatigue, palpitation, or dyspnea	Stage C	Symptomatic heart failure associated with underlying structural heart disease
Class III	Marked limitation of physical activity; comfortable at rest, but less than ordinary activity results in fatigue, palpitation, or dyspnea		
Class IV	Unable to carry on any physical activity without discomfort; symptoms present at rest; if any physical activity is undertaken, discomfort is increased	Stage D	Advanced structural heart disease and marked symptoms of heart failure at rest despite maximal medical therapy

ACC/AHA = American College of Cardiology/American Heart Association; NYHA = New York Heart Association.

Reprinted with permission from: McMurray JJV. Systolic heart failure. N Engl J Med 2010;362:228-38.

VIII. STANDARD PHARMACOLOGIC MANAGEMENT STRATEGIES FOR HEART FAILURE WITH REDUCED LEFT VENTRICULAR EJECTION FRACTION

A. Angiotensin-Converting Enzyme (ACE) Inhibitors *(Domain 1, Tasks 2, 3, 5, 6, 7; Domain 3, Tasks 2, 3)*
   1. ACE inhibitors are recommended in all patients with symptomatic HFrEF, unless contraindicated. Randomized controlled trials with ACE inhibitors in HF have shown the following:
      a. Improved survival
      b. Reduced rate of HF hospitalizations, even among patients with asymptomatic HFrEF
   2. In general, ACE inhibitor therapy is widely tolerated; however, ACE inhibitors should be avoided in patients with the following:
      a. History of angioedema
      b. Bilateral renal artery stenosis
      c. Severe aortic stenosis
      d. Labile BP and hypotension, which increases risk of cardiogenic shock
      e. Pregnancy
   3. In general, ACE inhibitors should be used cautiously and with close monitoring in patients with a serum potassium concentration greater than 5.5 mmol/L because of the potential for hyperkalemia.
   4. Early worsening renal function (decrease in estimated glomerular filtration rate of 20% or greater) after ACE inhibitor initiation is not predictive of smaller mortality benefit (compared with placebo in the Studies of Left Ventricular Dysfunction [SOLVD] trial). Therefore, in practice, increases in SCr of 30%–50% are tolerated.
   5. In patients admitted with acute HF and significant worsening of renal dysfunction, ACE inhibitors, angiotensin receptor blockers (ARBs), and mineralocorticoid receptor antagonists (MRAs) may be temporarily discontinued until renal function improves. Every effort should be made to reinitiate an ACE inhibitor or ARB and an MRA before hospital discharge.
   6. Table 485 lists specific ACE inhibitors and recommended doses. In general, the benefits of ACE inhibitors are considered to be a class effect, and doses should be titrated to doses proven effective in randomized trials. In the ATLAS (Assessment of Treatment with Lisinopril and Survival) trial, patients randomly assigned to receive high-dose lisinopril (32.5–35 mg/day) had a significantly lower risk of all-cause death or all-cause hospitalization, as well as a lower risk of HF-specific hospitalization, than did patients randomly assigned to receive low-dose lisinopril (2.5–5 mg/day); all-cause mortality alone was not significantly different between the high- and low-dose groups.

Table 48. ACE Inhibitors and Doses

Generic Name	Trade Name	Initial Daily Dose	Target Dose	Mean Dose Achieved in Clinical Trials
Captopril	Capoten	6.25 mg tid	50 mg tid	122.7 mg/day
Enalapril	Vasotec	2.5 mg bid	10 mg bid	16.6 mg/day
Fosinopril	Monopril	5–10 mg daily	80 mg daily	N/A
Lisinopril	Zestril, Prinivil	2.5–5 mg daily	20 mg daily	[a]4.5 mg/day (low-dose ATLAS) 33.2 mg/day (high-dose ATLAS)
Quinapril	Accupril	5 mg bid	80 mg daily	N/A
Ramipril	Altace	1.25–2.5 mg daily	10 mg daily	N/A
Trandolapril	Mavik	1 mg daily	4 mg daily	N/A

[a]No difference in mortality between high- and low-dose groups, but a 12% lower risk of death or hospitalization in high- versuss. low-dose group.

ACE = angiotensin-converting enzyme; ATLAS = Assessment of Treatment with Lisinopril and Survival; bid = twice daily; N/A = not applicable; tid = three times daily.

Reprinted with permission from: Lindenfeld J, Albert NM, Boehmer JP, et al. HFSA 2010 comprehensive heart failure practice guideline. J Card Fail 2010;16:e1-194.

7. Monitoring
   a. SCr assessed within 1–2 weeks after initiation and periodically thereafter
   b. Serum potassium concentration assessed within 1–2 weeks after initiation and periodically thereafter

8. Major adverse effects
   a. Angioedema
   b. Hyperkalemia
   c. Hypotension (potentiated by diuretics)
   d. Worsening renal function (e.g., rapid increase of SCr by 30%–50% over baseline)
   e. Persistent nonproductive cough

B. Angiotensin Receptor Blockers *(Domain 1, Tasks 2, 3, 5, 6, 7; Domain 3, Tasks 2, 3)*
   1. ARBs for ACE inhibitor–intolerant patients
      a. An ARB is a useful alternative to an ACE inhibitor because of intolerance.
         i. Data from the ELITE II (Losartan Heart Failure Survival Study) trial showed no differences in all-cause mortality for patients randomly assigned to the ARB losartan arm versus captopril.
         ii. In the Candesartan in Heart Failure Assessment of Reduction in Morbidity and Mortality (CHARM) Alternative study, candesartan was associated with a 23% reduction (hazard ratio 0.77; 95% CI, 0.67–0.89, p=0.0004) compared with placebo for the primary end point of cardiovascular (CV) death or HF hospitalization among patients who were intolerant of ACE inhibitors.
      b. In general, ARBs are routinely recommended for patients intolerant of ACE inhibitors because of cough. However, ACE inhibitors are still considered the <u>first-line</u> vasodilator therapy in heart failure because of stronger mortality data.
      c. Patients intolerant of ACE inhibitors because of worsening renal function, hyperkalemia, or hypotension are likely to experience similar effects with ARBs; thus, ARBs should also be used cautiously and with close monitoring in those situations.

Table 49. Angiotensin Receptor Blockers and Recommended Doses

Generic Name	Trade Name	Initial Daily Dose	Target Dose	Mean Dose Achieved in Clinical Trials
Candesartan	Atacand	4–8 mg daily	32 mg daily	24 mg/day
Losartan	Cozaar	12.5–25 mg daily	150 mg daily	129 mg/day
Valsartan	Diovan	40 mg bid	160 mg bid	254 mg/day

bid = twice daily.

Reprinted with permission from: Lindenfeld J, Albert NM, Boehmer JP, et al. HFSA 2010 comprehensive heart failure practice guideline. J Card Fail 2010;16:e1-194.

   2. Addition of an ARB to ACE inhibitor therapy
      a. Adding an ARB may be recommended for patients with HF who remain symptomatic despite optimal treatment with ACE inhibitors and β-blockers (unless contraindications are present) and for whom an MRA is not indicated or not tolerated.
      b. Several studies have evaluated the addition of an ARB to background ACE inhibitor therapy
         i. The Valsartan Heart Failure Trial (Val-HeFT) showed a 13% reduction (relative risk [RR] 0.87; 97.5% CI, 0.77–0.97; p=0.009) in the combined end point of mortality and morbidity for patients randomly assigned to receive valsartan versus placebo. Mortality was similar between groups. Around 93% of the patients studied received background ACE inhibitor therapy.

ii. In the CHARM-Added trial, the addition of candesartan for patients with HF receiving background ACE inhibitor therapy provided a 15% reduction (hazard ratio 0.85; 95% CI, 0.75–0.96; p=0.011) in the primary end point of CV death or HF hospitalization, compared with placebo.

iii. Of note, combination therapy is associated with a higher risk of hyperkalemia and increase in SCr; thus, patients should be carefully selected and closely monitored while receiving combined ARB and ACE inhibitor therapy. In general, combination of ACE inhibitor and ARB has fallen out of favor clinically.

3. ARBs for patients with evidence of LV systolic dysfunction post MI with or without HF symptoms

a. Valsartan showed noninferiority to captopril for the end points of mortality alone and fatal and nonfatal CV events in the Valsartan in Acute Myocardial Infarction (VALIANT) trial; thus, either ARB or ACE inhibitors are appropriate in this setting.

b. Combining valsartan with captopril was not associated with improvements in clinical outcomes; however, adverse event rates were higher in this group. Thus, there is no advantage to using combination therapy for these patients.

c. Use of ARBs in post-MI patients with reduced EF or HF symptoms who are intolerant of ACE inhibitors is recommended by the ACC/AHA acute coronary syndrome guidelines (class I recommendation).

C. Angiotensin Rreceptor Nneprilysin Iinhibitor *(Domain 1, Tasks 2, 3, 5, 6, 7; Domain 3, Tasks 2, 3)*

1. Natriuretic peptides, or NPs (atrial natriuretic peptide [ANP], B-type natriuretic peptide [BNP], and c-type natriuretic peptides [CNPs]), are responsible for natriuresis, and help maintain sodium and fluid balance. NPs are released in the setting of excess plasma volume and elevated left ventricular filling pressures. Other benefits include cGMP-mediated vasodilation, and reduction in renin-angiotensin-aldosterone (RAAS) activation.

a. NPs are cleared through the natriuretic receptor, and through peptide-mediated breakdown byvia neprilysin. Because neprilysin also breaks down angiotensin II, an inhibitor of this enzyme must needs to be combined with RAAS blockade.

b. A new drug, sacubitril/valsartan (formerly known as LCZ696), is an angiotensin receptor neprilysin inhibitor, which is a fixed- dose combination of the ARB valsartan and the neprilysin inhibitor sacubitril.

2. In the Prospective Comparison of ARNI wWith ACEI to Determine Impact on Global Mortality and Morbidity in Heart Failure (PARADIGM-HF) trial, patients with NYHA functional classFC II–-IV and reduced LVEF of less than <40% (, later changed to ≤35% or less) were randomly assignedized to receive enalapril 10 mg twice daily or sacubitril/valsartan 200 mg twice daily. Compared to enalapril, sacubitril/valsartan reduced the primary composite end point of cardiovascular death or HF heart failure hospitalization by 20% (hazard ratio [HR]: 0.80; 95% confidence interval [CI],: 0.73– to 0.87; p < 0.0000004), and reduced all-cause mortality by 16% (hazard ratioHR: 0,86XX; 95% CI,: 0.76– to 0.93; p < 0.0002).

3. In July 2015, sacubitril/valsartan was FDA approved to reduce the risk of cardiovascular death and hospitalization for HF in patients with chronic HF heart failure (NYHA class II–IV) and reduced EF ejection fraction, to be used in place of an ACE inhibitor or ARB. Updated HF heart failure treatment guidelines will incorporate this new drug and provide recommendations on its place in therapy in the setting of chronic HFheart failure.

4. Adverse effects of sacuibtril/valsartan include hyperkalemia, hypotension, and renal dysfunction.

5. Three doses of sacubitril/valsartan are available: 24/26 mg, 49/51 mg, and 97/103 mg. The starting dose is 49/50 mg twice daily, titrated to a goal dose of 97/103 mg twice daily.

D. β-Adrenergic Blockers *(Domain 1, Tasks 2, 3, 5, 6, 7; Domain 3, Tasks 2, 3)*
   1. β-Blockers, in conjunction with ACE inhibitors, are the cornerstone of HF pharmacotherapy.
   2. Use of specific β-blockers (e.g., bisoprolol, carvedilol, or metoprolol succinate) is recommended for all patients with HFrEF or without current symptoms and without contraindications because of compelling evidence from randomized controlled trials.
   3. Use of immediate-release metoprolol (metoprolol tartrate) is not recommended for patients with HF because of the lack of compelling evidence in these patients.
   4. These recommendations are based on four landmark studies (three that were placebo controlled and one that compared carvedilol with metoprolol tartrate) evaluating β-blockers in HF: The Cardiac Insufficiency Bisoprolol Study (CIBIS II), the Carvedilol Prospective Randomized Cumulative Survival trial (COPERNICUS), the Metoprolol Randomized Intervention Trial in Congestive Heart Failure (MERIT-HF), and the Carvedilol Or Metoprolol European Trial (COMET).
   5. Data from the aforementioned trials consistently show a 34%–35% reduction in the primary end point of all-cause mortality. All patients in these studies received background ACE inhibitor therapy.
   6. β-Blockers inhibit the deleterious effects of the sympathetic nervous system (i.e., norepinephrine) on HF progression, prevent/reverse cardiac remodeling, and reduce the risk of sudden cardiac death (SCD).
   7. β-Blockers are generally well tolerated, but they should be newly initiated only in patients who are currently clinically stable and euvolemic. Initiation at the lowest possible dose with uptitration at 2-week intervals (and potentially longer for older adults) is recommended to reduce the risk of short-term worsening of HF symptoms.
   8. Every effort should be made to up-titrate β-blocker doses to the concentration achieved in clinical trials to promote reverse remodeling and improve LVEF. Studies consistently show that benefits of therapy increase with higher doses.
   9. During hospitalization for acute HF, every effort should be made to continue the β-blocker, and a temporary dose reduction or discontinuation should be considered only for patients who have recently initiated β-blocker therapy and who have marked volume overload or low cardiac output with hemodynamic instability. The β-blocker should be reinitiated before hospital discharge.
   10. In practice, metoprolol succinate is often used in patients who need HR control, such as those with concomitant AF or post MI, whereas carvedilol is selected for patients needing additional vasodilating effects, such as those with HTN.

Table 50. β-Blockers and Recommended Doses

Generic Name	Trade Name	Initial Daily Dose	Target Dose	Mean Dose Achieved in Clinical Trials
Bisoprolol	Zebeta	1.25 mg daily	10 mg daily	8.6 mg/day
Carvedilol	Coreg	3.125 mg bid	25 mg bid[a]	37 mg/day
Carvedilol	Coreg CR	10 mg daily	80 mg daily	N/A
Metoprolol succinate	Toprol XL	12.5–25 mg daily	200 mg daily	159 mg/day

[a]A dose of 50 mg twice daily has been used in patients weighing more than 85 kg if lower doses have been tolerated.

bid = twice daily; CR = controlled release; N/A = not applicable; XL = extended release.

Reprinted with permission from: Lindenfeld J, Albert NM, Boe hmer JP, et al. HFSA 2010 comprehensive heart failure practice guideline. J Card Fail 2010;16:e1-194.

E. Mineralocorticoid Receptor Antagonists *(Domain 1, Tasks 2, 3, 5, 6, 7; Domain 3, Tasks 2, 3)*
1. Treatment with an MRA is recommended for patients with symptomatic HFrEF (NYHA class II– IV) and LVEF of 35% or less. In NYHA class II, patients should also have a history of prior cardiovascular hospitalization or elevated natriuretic peptide values.
2. Treatment with an MRA is recommended for patients post MI with an LVEF of 40% or less and either HF symptoms or diabetes mellitus according to the results of the Eplerenone Post–Acute Myocardial Infarction Heart Failure Efficacy and Survival Study (EPHESUS).
3. The 2013 ACCF (American College of Cardiology Foundation)/AHA guideline wording removed the stipulation that patients must be treated with an optimized ACE inhibitor/ARB and β-blocker before MRA initiation.
4. In the Randomized Aldactone Evaluation Study (RALES), spironolactone reduced the risk of all-cause mortality by 30%, compared with standard therapy (RR 0.69; 95% CI, 0.58–0.82; p<0.001).
5. The Eplerenone in Patients with Systolic Heart Failure and Mild Symptoms (EMPHASIS-HF) study showed a reduced risk of death and hospitalization (hazard ratio 0.63; 95% CI, 0.54–0.74; p<0.001) among patients with systolic HF and mild symptoms (NYHA class II). Patients underwent randomization if they were 55 years or older, had NYHA class II symptoms, had EF of 30% or less, and were receiving treatment with an ACE inhibitor or an ARB and a β-blocker (at maximally tolerated doses). Eplerenone was initiated at 25 mg orally daily for the first 4 weeks and then titrated to 50 mg orally daily thereafter, depending on the patient's renal function.
6. In EPHESUS, eplerenone reduced all-cause mortality by 15% (RR 0.85; 95% CI, 0.75–0.96; p=0.008) and CV death or CV hospitalization by 13% (RR 0.87; 95% CI, 0.72–0.94; p=0.005), compared with placebo.
7. Treatment with an MRA is not indicated in the following instances:
   a. Patients with CrCl less than 30 mL/minute
   b. SCr greater than 2.5 mg/dL in male individuals or greater than 2.0 mg/dL in female individuals
   c. Serum potassium concentration greater than 5.0 mEq/L
   d. Patients already receiving combination therapy with an ACE inhibitor plus an ARB (a combination of an ACE inhibitor and an ARB already not preferred because of hyperkalemia risk)

Table 51. Other Evidence-Based Therapies and Recommended Doses

Generic Name	Trade Name	Initial Daily Dose	Target Dose	Mean Dose Achieved in Clinical Trials
Aldosterone receptor antagonists				
Spironolactone	Aldactone	12.5–25 mg/day	25 mg/day	26 mg/day
Eplerenone	Inspra	25 mg/day	50 mg/day	42.6 mg/day
Other vasodilators				
Fixed-dose hydralazine/ isosorbide dinitrate	BiDil	37.5 mg hydralazine/20 mg isosorbide dinitrate tid	75 mg hydralazine/ 40 mg isosorbide dinitrate tid	143 mg hydralazine/76 mg isosorbide dinitrate/day
Hydralazine	Apresoline	37.5 mg tid	100 mg tid	N/A
Isosorbide dinitrate	Isordil	20 mg tid	40 mg tid	N/A
Loop diuretics				
Furosemide	Lasix	20–40 mg/day or bid		
Bumetanide	Bumex	0.5–1.0 mg/day or bid		
Torsemide	Demadex	10–20 mg/day		

bid = twice daily; N/A = not applicable; tid = three times daily.

Adapted from: Lindenfeld J, Albert NM, Boehmer JP, et al. HFSA 2010 comprehensive heart failure practice guideline. J Card Fail 2010;16:e1-194.

8. Hyperkalemia is a significant complication of MRA therapy. In the RALES trial, the incidence of hyperkalemia was only 2%, but it was 12% in EMPHASIS-HF. However, outside the rigorous follow-up of a clinical trial, much higher rates of hyperkalemia have been reported (11 hyperkalemia-associated hospitalizations per 100 patients treated).

9. The incidence of gynecomastia with spironolactone in the RALES trial was 10% and does not occur with eplerenone.

10. Careful patient selection and close laboratory monitoring help minimize hyperkalemia-related complications in these patients.

Table 52. Guidelines for Minimizing the Risk of Hyperkalemia in Patients Treated with MRAs

1. Serum potassium concentrations should be monitored at 3 days, 1 week, and monthly for at least 3 months after initiation of an MRA
2. Discontinue or reduce dose if serum potassium concentration > 5.5 mEq/L
3. Initiate an MRA at a dose appropriate for the patient's renal function, and increase it at appropriate intervals
4. The risk of hyperkalemia is increased with the concomitant use of MRAs with higher doses of ACEIs (captopril ≥ 75 mg/daily; enalapril or lisinopril ≥ 10 mg/daily)
5. Potassium supplements should be discontinued or reduced
6. Diarrhea or other causes of dehydration should be addressed emergently

ACEI = angiotensin-converting enzyme inhibitor; MRA = mineralocorticoid receptor antagonist.

Table 53. Dosing and Titration of MRAs

Estimated CrCl	30–49 mL/minute		≥50 mL/minute	
MRA	Eplerenone	Spironolactone	Eplerenone	Spironolactone
Initial dose (only if K^+ ≤ 5.0 mEq/L)	25 mg every other day	12.5 mg daily or every other day	25 mg daily	12.5–25.0 mg daily
Maintenance dose (after 4 wk for serum K^+ ≤ 5.0 mEq/L)[a]	25 mg once daily	12.5–25.0 mg daily	50 mg daily	25 mg daily or bid

[a]After dose initiation, if potassium concentration increases to ≤6.0 mEq/L or worsening renal function, hold until potassium concentration < 5.0 mEq/L. Consider reinitiating reduced dose after confirming the resolution of hyperkalemia/renal insufficiency for at least 72 hours.

bid = twice daily; CrCl = creatinine clearance; K^+ = potassium; MRA = mineralocorticoid receptor antagonist; wk = weeks.

Adapted from: Yancy CW, Jessup M, Bozkurt B, et al. 2013 ACCF/AHA guideline for the management of heart failure: a report of the American College of Cardiology Foundation/American Heart Association Task Force on Practice Guidelines. J Am Coll Cardiol 2013;62:e147-239.

11. Both eplerenone and spironolactone are MRAs, but eplerenone is a selective MRA that has a lower incidence of endocrine-related adverse effects (i.e., gynecomastia) because of its reduced affinity for glucocorticoid, androgen, and progesterone receptors.

F. Hydralazine and Isosorbide Dinitrate *(Domain 1, Tasks 2, 3, 5, 6, 7; Domain 3, Tasks 2, 3)*
   1. The combination of hydralazine and nitrate is recommended for African American patients with NYHA class III and IV HFrEF added to ACE inhibitor and β-blocker (and MRA) therapy unless contraindicated.
   2. The combination of hydralazine and nitrate is recommended for symptomatic patients with HFrEF who are intolerant of ACE inhibitors or ARBs because of renal insufficiency, hyperkalemia, or, in some cases, angioedema, regardless of race.

3. The African American Heart Failure Trial (A-HeFT) showed a 43% reduction in all-cause mortality (hazard ratio 0.57; p=0.01) for patients randomly assigned to receive hydralazine plus isosorbide dinitrate compared with placebo.

4. The 2013 ACCF/AHA HF guidelines removed the specification that the product be a "fixed-dose" combination. It is jJust stated that hydralazine and nitrates may be given in two pills three times daily.

G. Diuretics *(Domain 1, Tasks 2, 3, 5, 6, 7; Domain 3, Tasks 2, 3)*

1. In general, loop diuretics are preferred for patients with HF and symptoms related to hypervolemia owing to their potency.

2. The lowest dose needed to achieve euvolemia should be prescribed.
    a. Some patients with HF can be educated to "self-manage" diuretic dosing, using a dosing approach dictated by the patient's weight.
    b. This approach requires careful patient education and access to a health care provider, should problems or questions arise.

3. Not all patients with HF will require loop diuretic therapy, particularly in the early stages of HFrEF when symptoms may be adequately managed with other evidence-based therapies; loop diuretics provide only symptomatic relief, and they do not demonstrably affect mortality. Some retrospective analyses have linked diuretics, particularly high doses, with harm.

4. Patients with HFpEF may be especially sensitive to the BP-lowering effects of diuretics.

5. Special attention should be paid to pharmacodynamic drug interactions. Diuretics may increase the hypotensive response to ACE inhibitors. If hypotension or increases in SCr occur, it may be reasonable to decrease the diuretic first (depending on whether the patient shows signs or symptoms of congestion). This action may allow the ACE inhibitor to be maintained and/or the dose titrated.

6. Diuretic resistance is a clinical scenario whereby some patients have an inadequate response to conventionally dosed loop diuretic regimens. In such cases, the following options should be considered. (1) Emphasize sodium and fluid restriction. (2) Increase the loop diuretic dose. (3) If the patient is taking furosemide, change to bumetanide or torsemide for improved oral absorption. (4) Switch from oral dosing to parenteral dosing. (5) Consider adding a second diuretic agent (e.g., distal tubular diuretics metolazone or chlorthalidone) given 30 minutes before loop diuretic administration to augment diuretic effects. Use of ultrafiltration (discussed in further detail in the Ultrafiltration section) may be an alternative strategy.

7. Routine laboratory studies (e.g., blood urea nitrogen, SCr, potassium) should be performed to monitor patients for the development of renal impairment or electrolyte abnormalities. In addition, orthostasis (sitting, standing BP, and HR) should be checked routinely to assess for volume depletion.

H. Digoxin *(Domain 1, Tasks 2, 3, 5, 6, 7; Domain 3, Tasks 2, 3)*

1. Digoxin continues to be used in patients with symptomatic HF after standard therapy. The optimal therapeutic range is 0.5–0.9 ng/mL according to a post hoc analysis of the Digitalis Investigative Group (DIG) trial (although the 2013 ACCF/AHA guidelines state 0.4–0.9 ng/mL).

2. In the DIG trial, digoxin was associated with a lower risk of HF hospitalization, compared with placebo. Of note, the DIG trial was conducted before β-blockers were adopted as evidence-based therapy; thus, the impact of adding digoxin to regimens including an ACE inhibitor and a β-blocker is unknown. Digoxin had no mortality benefit in this trial.
    a. Digoxin may be particularly useful in the subset of patients with AF and HFrEF.
    b. There are no apparent differences in the effectiveness of digoxin in men and women, and there is no evidence that women are at increased risk of mortality from digoxin.

    c.   Signs and symptoms of digoxin toxicity include the following:
        i.   Arrhythmias, including ventricular ectopy, atrioventricular (AV) conduction block of any degree (although rarely Mobitz type II), paroxysmal atrial tachycardia with block, accelerated junctional rhythm, and bidirectional VT (rare)
        ii.   GI disturbances (usually observed first)
        iii.   Central nervous system disturbances
        iv.   Visual changes
    d.   Significant drug interactions with digoxin include the following (not all-inclusive):
        i.   Amiodarone
        ii.   Dronedarone
        iii.   Verapamil
        iv.   Erythromycin
        v.   Clarithromycin
        vi.   Telaprevir
        vii.   Quinidine
        viii.   Saquinavir

I. Ivabradine *(Domain 1, Tasks 2, 3, 5, 6, 7; Domain 3, Tasks 2, 3)*
    1.   Mechanism of action: Bblockade of hyperpolarization-activated cyclic nucleotide–-gated channel, resulting in reduction of the spontaneous pacemaker activity of the cardiac sinus node by selectively inhibiting the If current (If)
    2.   In the Systolic Heart failure treatment with the If inhibitor ivabradine Trial (SHIFT) study, ivabradine was found to reduce the primary composite end point of cardiovascular death or hospitalization for HF heart failure by 18%, compared to placebo, in patients with symptomatic HFrEF. The results were mainly driven by a reduction in heart failure hospitalizations for HF.
    3.   Ivabradine was approved in April 2015 to reduce the risk of hospitalization for worsening HF in patients with stable, symptomatic chronic HF with an whose and LVEF of $\leq$ is 35% or less and whose heart rate of $\geq$ is 70 beats/minute or above.
        a.   Patients should be receiving either on maximally tolerated doses of β-blockers or have a contraindication to βbeta-blocker use.
        b.   Avoid use in patients with atrial fibrillation, in those who have third-3rd degree heart block, BP below< 90/50mmHg, acute 90/50 mm Hg, acute HFheart failure, severe hepatic impairment, pacemaker dependencyt, resting heart rate below< 60 beats/minute, or in combination with strong cytochrome CYP3A4 inhibitors (diltiazem, verapamil, and grapefruit juice), or CYP3A4 inducers (St. John's wort, rifampicin, barbiturates, and phenytoin).
    4.   Adverse eEffects:
        a.   Bradycardia
        b.   Hypertension
        c.   Atrial fFibrillation
        d.   Phosphenes: Ttransiently enhanced brightness in a limited area of the visual field, halos, image decomposition (stroboscopic or kaleidoscopic effects), colored bright lights, or several multiple images (retinal persistency).
    5.   Dose: 5 mg twice daily, increase to 7.5 mg twice daily after 2 weeks.
        a.   In patients with conduction defects or in whom bradycardia could lead to hemodynamic compromise, initiate dosing at 2.5 mg twice daily.

Patient Cases

Questions 9 and 10 pertain to the following case.

R.R., a 68-year-old African American woman with HF, presents to your clinic. Comorbidities include HTN and type 2 diabetes mellitus. During the past year, she has had two hospitalizations for decompensated HF and significant volume overload with each hospitalization. Her current symptoms are shortness of breath with minimal exertion and 2+ peripheral edema bilaterally. Other pertinent findings include BP 120/72 mm Hg, HR 58 beats/minute, SCr 1.60 mg/dL (estimated CrCl 36 mL/minute), BUN 25 mg/dL, potassium 5.1 mEq/L, sodium 140 mEq/L, hemoglobin A1C 7.1%, digoxin 0.5 ng/mL, and LVEF 28%. Current medications include enalapril 10 mg twice daily, metoprolol XL (extended release) 150 mg once daily, metformin 500 mg twice daily, digoxin 0.125 mg daily, and furosemide 40 mg twice daily.

9. Which of the following best describes R.R.'s current HF type, stage, and classification?

    A. HFpEF, stage B, NYHA class II.
    B. HFpEF, stage C, NYHA class III.
    C. HFrEF, stage B, NYHA class II.
    D. HFrEF, stage C, NYHA class III.

    [handwritten: class III]

10. Which is the best recommendation for R.R.?

    A. Increase the digoxin dose to 0.25 mg daily.
    B. Add spironolactone 25 mg orally daily.
    C. Add hydralazine 50 mg orally three times daily and isosorbide dinitrate 20 mg orally three times daily.
    D. Add eplerenone 50 mg orally daily.

11. P.N. is a 60-year-old, 78-kg, white man with ischemic cardiomyopathy and LVEF 25%. He was recently hospitalized with acute MI and acute HF. He underwent percutaneous coronary intervention with bare metal stent placement to his right coronary artery. He is currently treated with enalapril 10 mg orally twice daily, carvedilol 25 mg twice daily, furosemide 40 mg/day, aspirin 81 mg/day, clopidogrel 75 mg/day, and atorvastatin 80 mg/day. He has stable NYHA class II HF symptoms. Other pertinent clinical findings include BP 114/70 mm Hg, HR 67 beats/minute, 1+ edema bilaterally, SCr 1.0 mg/dL, and potassium 4.0 mEq/L. Other laboratory values are within normal limits. Which is the best recommendation for this patient currently?

    A. Add valsartan 80 mg orally daily.
    B. Add spironolactone 25 orally daily.
    C. Add hydralazine 50 mg orally three times daily and isosorbide dinitrate 20 mg orally three times daily.
    D. Increase enalapril dose to 20 mg orally twice daily.

IX. STANDARD PHARMACOLOGIC MANAGEMENT STRATEGIES FOR HEART FAILURE WITH PRESERVED EJECTION FRACTION

A. Pathophysiology *(Domain 1, Task 1)*
   1. Characterized by LV hypertrophy, concentric remodeling, increased extracellular matrix, abnormal relaxation and filling, and decreased diastolic distensibility
   2. Activation of the renin-angiotensin-aldosterone system and the sympathetic nervous system is common.

B. Diagnostic Criteria *(Domain 1, Tasks 2, 3)*
   1. Clinical signs and symptoms of HF
   2. Evidence of preserved or normal LVEF
   3. Evidence of LV diastolic dysfunction on echocardiography or LV angiography
   4. Excludes other noncardiac causes of HF

C. Treatment *(Domain 1, Tasks 2, 3, 5, 6, 7; Domain 3, Tasks 2, 3)*
   1. No therapy was shown to decrease morbidity and mortality in this population in an adequately powered randomized controlled clinical trial.
   2. In patients with HTN, BP should be monitored and optimally controlled.
   3. Patients with HTN should be counseled to follow a low-sodium diet.
   4. Diuretics are recommended for patients with volume overload.
   5. ACE inhibitors or ARBs may be used for patients with HFpEF; however, there is no evidence that these agents reduce morbidity or mortality.
      a. The ARB irbesartan was studied in the Irbesartan in Heart Failure with Preserved Ejection Fraction (I-PRESERVE) study, but irbesartan failed to show a clinical effect in this population. In the irbesartan group, 36% died or experienced a CV hospitalization, compared with 37% in the placebo group (hazard ratio 0.95; 95% CI, 0.86–1.05; p=0.35). No between-group differences were detected in any of the secondary end points.
      b. In the CHARM-Preserved study, there was no difference in the composite end point of CV death or HF hospitalization for patients randomly assigned to receive candesartan versus placebo. Fewer patients randomly assigned to receive candesartan were hospitalized for HF (p=0.017).
   6. β-Blocker therapy is recommended in guidelines for patients with HFpEF, particularly if they are post MI, or have AF requiring rate control.
   7. TOPCAT (Treatment of Preserved Cardiac Function Heart Failure with an Aldosterone AnTagonist): Spironolactone (15, 30, and 45 mg daily) versus placebo in patients with symptomatic HF, LVEF of 45% or greater, and either prior hospitalization for HF or elevated BNP or NT-proBNP concentration. Excluded patients with a CrCl less than 30 mL/minute, serum potassium concentration greater than 5 mEq/L, AF and HR greater than 90 beats/minute, recent acute coronary syndrome, or uncontrolled HTN. There was no significant difference in the 3-year primary composite outcome of CV mortality, aborted cardiac arrest, or hospitalization for HF. High rate of study drug discontinuation (spironolactone 34.3% and placebo 31.4%). Spironolactone (mean dose at 8 months of 25 mg/day) reduced the secondary end point of hospitalization for HF by 15% (12.0% vs. 14.2%, p=0.042; 2.8/100 patient-years vs. 4.6/100 patient-years). Rates of hyperkalemia, defined as serum potassium concentration of 5.5 mEq/L or greater, were higher with spironolactone than placebo (18.7% vs. 9.1%, p<0.001). Post-hoc analyses revealed substantial regional differences in response to spironolactone, such that participants from the Americas (USA, Canada, South America) had higher event rates and observed benefits with spironolactone versus placebo, compared to patients in Russia and the Republic of Georgia. Therefore, clinicians may find it reasonable to use spironolactone in the setting of HFpEF as long as appropriate monitoring is in place for hyperkalemia.

Patient Cases

Questions 12 and 13 pertain to the following case.

J.J. is a 62-year-old, 88-kg white man with a history of HTN and intolerance of ACE inhibitors secondary to cough. He was recently discharged from an HF-related hospitalization and presents to the clinic for follow-up 1 week after hospital discharge. Before hospitalization, his medication regimen included valsartan 80 mg twice daily, metoprolol XL 100 mg/day, and furosemide 40 mg twice daily. The patient's condition is now stable, with no symptoms at rest and some shortness of breath when walking around his home. Other pertinent diagnostic and laboratory findings include BUN 30 mg/dL, SCr 1.4 mg/dL, potassium 4 mEq/L, LVEF 65%, BP 154/70 mm Hg, and HR 77 beats/minute.

12. Which of the following best describes J.J.'s HF type and classification?
    A. HFpEF, NYHA class III.
    B. HFpEF, NYHA class IV.
    C. HFrEF, NYHA class III.
    D. HFrEF, NYHA class IV.

13. Given J.J.'s persistent symptoms, which is the best recommendation for him?
    A. Increase the furosemide dose to 80 mg orally twice daily.
    B. Increase metoprolol succinate to 150 mg orally daily.
    C. Add eplerenone 25 mg orally daily.
    D. Add hydralazine 50 mg orally three times daily plus isosorbide dinitrate 20 mg orally three times daily.

X. STANDARD DEVICE MANAGEMENT STRATEGIES

A. Implantable Cardioverter Defibrillator (ICD) *(Domain 3, Tasks 2, 3)*
   1. SCD accounts for about half of all HF-related deaths, particularly in patients with less severe symptoms.
   2. ICD therapy is indicated for primary prevention of SCD and to reduce mortality for patients with LVEF of 35% or less, receiving GDMT, and with NYHA class II or III symptoms who have either nonischemic dilated cardiomyopathy or ischemic heart disease and who are at least 40 days post MI.
   3. In the SCD-HeFT trial, an ICD reduced all-cause mortality by 23% (hazard ratio 0.77; 97.5% CI, 0.62–0.96; p=0.007).
   4. In the Multicenter Automatic Defibrillator Implantation Trial II (MADIT II), an ICD reduced the risk of all-cause mortality by 31% (hazard ratio 0.69; 95% CI, 0.51–0.93; p=0.016) compared with conventional therapy among patients with a prior MI and LVEF 30% or less.
   5. Antiarrhythmic therapies may be used as adjunctive therapies for the management of arrhythmia-prone patients under special circumstances. Amiodarone, dofetilide, and sotalol reduce the frequency of ICD shock therapy, thus increasing ICD generator battery life and reducing patient morbidity (namely posttraumatic stress disorder). Amiodarone is the preferred agent for patients with significant renal impairment.

B. Cardiac Resynchronization Therapy (CRT) *(Domain 3, Tasks 2, 3)*
   1. It is estimated that cardiac dyssynchrony affects 15%–30% of patients with HF, resulting in decreased systolic function and increased systolic volumes.
   2. By applying biventricular stimulation, CRT aims to restore appropriate activation of the intraventricular septum and LV free wall.

3. CRT therapy is indicated for patients with LVEF of 35% or less and NYHA class II, III, or ambulatory class IV symptoms who are receiving GDMT and who fulfill the following criteria:
   a. Have sinus rhythm or left bundle branch block (LBBB) with a QRS of 150 milliseconds or greater on 12-lead ECG or
   b. Have non-LBBB pattern with a QRS of 150 milliseconds or greater on 12-lead ECG or
   c. Have LBBB with a QRS of 120–149 milliseconds on 12-lead ECG
   d. Are undergoing new or replacement device implantation with anticipated ventricular pacing (greater than 40%)
4. Initial studies observed improvements in NYHA functional class, quality of life, 6-minute walk distance, exercise test duration, and EF for patients randomly assigned to CRT.
5. In the Comparison of Medical Therapy, Pacing, and Defibrillation in Heart Failure (COMPANION) trial, CRT was associated with a 19% reduction (hazard ratio 0.81; 95% CI, 0.69–0.96; p=0.014) in the primary end point of all-cause death or all-cause hospitalization among patients with NYHA class III–IV HF, LVEF of 35% or less, and QRS of 120 milliseconds or more. The effect of CRT on all-cause mortality alone did not reach statistical significance (hazard ratio 0.76; 95% CI, 0.58–1.01; p=0.059). Patients randomly assigned to CRT plus an ICD showed a 20% reduction (hazard ratio 0.8; 95% CI, 0.68–0.95; p=0.01) in all-cause death or hospitalization and a 36% reduction (hazard ratio 0.64; 95% CI, 0.48–0.86; p=0.003) in all-cause mortality.
6. The Cardiac Resynchronization Heart Failure (CARE-HF) study evaluated CRT alone (without an ICD) in 813 patients with NYHA class III–IV symptoms, LVEF of 35% or less, LV end-diastolic dimension of at least 30 mm, and QRS duration of 120 milliseconds or more. CRT reduced the primary end point of all-cause mortality or CV hospitalization by 37% (hazard ratio 0.63; 95% CI, 0.51–0.77; p<0.001). CRT was also associated with a 36% reduction in all-cause mortality (hazard ratio 0.64; 95% CI, 0.48–0.85; p<0.002).
7. Echocardiographic measurements also improved for the CRT group compared with placebo, including higher EF, lower end-systolic volume index, smaller area of mitral regurgitation, and shorter interventricular mechanical delay, suggesting CRT exerted favorable effects on remodeling.
8. The 2012 device guideline update from ACCF/AHA/HRS increased the QRS requirement from 120 milliseconds, which was used in the trials described above, to 150 milliseconds according to additional data from subgroup analyses and meta-analyses from the (five) trials reporting that patients who benefited were those with a QRS of 150 milliseconds or greater and that a QRS of less than 150 milliseconds was a predictor of failure to respond to CRT.

C. LV Assist Device (LVAD) *(Domain 3, Tasks 2, 3)*
   1. The application of LVADs is largely limited to use as a bridge to transplantation and to treating patients with acute, severe myocarditis; however, some centers use LVADS as destination therapy. Such use is typically reserved for selected patients with refractory end-stage HF and estimated 1-year mortality greater than 50% with medical therapy.
   2. 2011 data from the International Society for Heart & Lung Transplantation (ISHLT) mechanical circulatory support device database show that 75% of patients survive for at least 1 year when devices are implanted as a bridge to transplantation.
   3. LVAD devices may also be used as permanent or destination therapy in selected patients with refractory HF and an estimated 1-year mortality exceeding 50%.
   4. Guidelines: The 2013 ISHLT data describe candidate selection.
      a. Evaluate a candidate's suitability for transplantation because current outcomes with transplants are superior to those with LV assist devices.
      b. An LVAD candidate has ventricular function that has been deemed unlikely to recover without support or who cannot be weaned from inotropes.

    c. An LVAD candidate should have the capacity for meaningful recovery of end-organ function and quality of life.

    d. An LVAD candidate should have no irreversible end-organ damage.

5. The 2013 ISHLT guidelines recommend antithrombotic therapy for mechanical circulatory support devices consisting of the following: Warfarin at a goal INR of 2–3 and aspirin 81–325 mg/day for the HeartMate II device and the HeartWare HVAD; warfarin at a goal INR of 2.5–3.5 and aspirin 81–325 mg/day for the pulsatile mechanical circulatory support devices (e.g., the Thoratec PVAD [paracorporeal ventricular assist device]/IVAD [implantable ventricular assist device]), and warfarin at a goal INR of 2.5–2.5 and aspirin 81–325 mg/day and dipyridamole 75 mg three times daily for the CardioWest temporary total artificial heart.

6. Recent data indicate that the HeartMate II device (Thoratec Corp.) thrombosis rates started to increase in March 2011 and that they have continued to do so.

D. Ultrafiltration *(Domain 3, Tasks 2, 3)*

1. Ultrafiltration carries a class IIb recommendation for patients with volume overload and congestion symptoms (level of evidence B) and for patients unresponsive to GDMT.

2. The Ultrafiltration Versus Intravenous Diuretics for Patients Hospitalised for Acute Decompensated Heart Failure (UNLOAD) study (n=200) showed a greater degree of weight loss at 48 hours among patients randomly assigned to ultrafiltration compared with those treated with standard-care intravenous diuretics. At 90 days, patients receiving ultrafiltration had fewer HF hospitalizations, rehospitalization days, and unscheduled visits than did patients receiving intravenous diuretics alone. No adverse safety signals were detected.

3. Typically, ultrafiltration is used in hospitalized patients whose condition is unresponsive to high-dose diuretics.

E. Disease Management and the Role of the Pharmacist *(Domain 1, Tasks 5, 6; Domain 2, Tasks 2, 3, 4; Domain 4, Tasks 1, 4, 6, 7)*

1. Pharmacists play a key role in HF management (Pharmacotherapy 2013;33:529-48; J Card Fail 2013;19:354-69).

2. Pharmacist involvement in care has been associated with a decreased HF readmission, all-cause readmission, and emergency department visits.

3. Ensure use of GDMT.

4. Ensure use of target doses of evidence-based therapy.

5. Avoid/minimize drug-drug and drug-disease interactions.

6. Prevention of adverse reactions and medication errors

7. Medication reconciliation: Assist with patient follow-up, identify signs of worsening HF so that appropriate therapeutic interventions can be implemented, and prevent the need for hospitalization/rehospitalization.

8. Resources for health care providers to assist in preventing hospital readmissions for HF: Hospital to Home (H2H) sponsored by the ACC and Institute for Healthcare Improvement (www.h2hquality.org/): Patient appointment within 7 days of hospital discharge (See You in 7)

9. Provide patient education/adherence reinforcement (Pharmacotherapy 2013;33:558-80).

10. Dietary counseling

    a. Fluid restriction

    b. Sodium restriction (1500 mg/day or less)

    c. Potassium-containing foods/salt substitutes for patients receiving MRAs

11. Disease education

12. End-of-life discussions when appropriate

13. Ensure medication access: Assist patients in identifying patient assistance programs.
    a. Several Web sites: www.rxassist.org, www.pparx.org, www.patientassistance.com
    b Many local communities have programs/resources.
    c. Suggest contacting individual companies as well – Some have programs that are not advertised – Policies/procedures/requirements change often.

F. Quality of Care
    1. Several studies have shown that a treatment gap exists between HF guideline–recommended therapies and the actual treatments received by patients with HF in both the inpatient and outpatient settings.
        a. OPTIMIZE (inpatient)
        b. IMPROVE (outpatient)
        c. AHA Get With The Guidelines-Heart Failure
    2. Performance improvement interventions are quite successful at improving the use of evidence-based therapies both in the inpatient and outpatient settings: Improvements in use of β-blockers, MRAs, CRT, ICDs, and delivery of HF education
    3. Interventions include the following:
        a. Clinical decision support tools (e.g., algorithms, pathways)
        b. Structured improvement strategies
        c. Chart audits with feedback

G. Resources for Patients with HF *(Domain 5, Task 2)*
    1. American Heart Association: www.heart.org/HEARTORG/Conditions/HeartFailure/Heart-Failure_UCM_002019_SubHomePage.jsp
    2. Get With The Guidelines-Heart Failure (sponsored by AHA): www.heart.org/HEARTORG/HealthcareResearch/GetWithTheGuidelinesHFStrokeResus/GetWithTheGuidelinesHeartFailureHomePage/Get-With-The-Guidelines-Heart-Failure-Clinical-Tools-Library_UCM_305817_Article.jsp
    3. Heart Failure Society of America: www.hfsa.org/heart_failure_education_modules.asp
    4. National Heart Lung and Blood Institute: www.nhlbi.nih.gov/health/dci/Diseases/Hf/HF_WhatIs.html

ARRHYTHMIAS

XI. ATRIAL FIBRILLATION AND ATRIAL FLUTTER

A. Atrial Fibrillation *(Domain 1, Tasks 1, 2, 5, 6, 7; Domain 3, Tasks 2, 3)*
    1. Classification
        a. Paroxysmal AF: Spontaneously self-terminates in fewer than 7 days; recurrent if two or more episodes
        b. Persistent AF
            i.   Continues for greater than 7 days
            ii. Does not self-terminate, requires chemical or electrical cardioversion
        c. Permanent AF: Does not convert with chemical or electrical cardioversion
        d. Lone AF
            i.   Established or paroxysmal AF
            ii. Patient is younger than 60 years and without heart disease.
        e. Postoperative AF
            i.   AF that occurs 3–5 days after surgery
            ii. Usually self-terminating

2. Epidemiology
   a. The most common arrhythmia found in clinical practice
   b. Accounts for about one-third of hospitalizations from arrhythmias
   c. Affects 1.5%–2% of the general population
   d. Average age is 75–85 years.
   e. Sixty percent of those 75 years and older are women.
   f. The 3-year incidence in patients with HF is 10%.
   g. Mortality rate is double that of patients in NSR and is linked to the severity of the underlying heart disease.
   h. Presentation: 400–600 atrial beats/minute with varying ventricular response (irregularly irregular rhythm)
   i. Symptoms
      i. Dizziness
      ii. Shortness of breath or exacerbation of HF
      iii. Fatigue
      iv. Palpitations
      v. Syncope
3. Pathophysiologic mechanisms
   a. Enhanced automaticity in several rapidly depolarizing foci or reentry involving several circuits
   b. Foci usually originate in the pulmonary veins.
   c. Foci can also occur in the right atrium.
   d. Foci infrequently occur in the superior vena cava or coronary sinus.
   e. Longer episodes (greater than 24 hours) are more difficult to terminate because AF causes mechanical and electrical remodeling of the atrial tissue.
   f. Causes
      i. Organic heart disease that activates the renin-angiotensin-aldosterone system through atrial stretch
         (a) Ischemia/infarction
         (b) Hypertensive heart disease
         (c) Valvular disorders
         (d) Dilated or hypertrophic cardiomyopathy
         (e) In addition, there are disease states that cause right atrial stretch.
            (1) Pulmonary embolism
            (2) Pulmonary hypertension
      ii. Associated with a high degree of adrenergic tone
         (a) Surgery/anesthesia induction
         (b) Thyrotoxicosis
         (c) Alcohol withdrawal
         (d) Sepsis
         (e) Excessive physical exertion
      iii. Perpetuated by high cholinergic tone
         (a) After meals
         (b) During sleep
      iv. Idiopathic
4. Complications
   a. Thromboembolic risk
      i. Thrombi located in the left atrium; usually found in the left atrial appendage because of blood stasis, endothelial dysfunction, and systemic hypercoagulability
      ii. There is a 5-fold increase in risk of stroke in patients with NVAF compared with patients without AF.

iii. Risk increases with advanced age.
    (a) 1.5% annual risk among 50- to 59-year-old individuals
    (b) 23.5% annual risk among 80- to 89-year-old individuals
    (c) Lone AF is at a lower risk of stroke.
b. Heart failure (3-fold incidence)
    i. Tachycardia-induced cardiomyopathy
    ii. Impaired diastolic filling
    iii. Loss of atrial kick
c. Rapid ventricular response
    i. AF conducted over an accessory pathway, potentially leading to lethal ventricular fibrillation
    ii. Can exacerbate ischemia, HF, or tachycardia-induced cardiomyopathy
5. Treatment: Rate versus rhythm control strategy
a. Rate control
    i. Indications
        (a) No symptoms to minimal symptoms
        (b) Treatment of choice for persistent or permanent AF
    ii. Goal is an HR less than 110 beats/minute with persistent AF in the following instances:
        (a) Stable LV function (LVEF greater than 40%)
        (b) Asymptomatic or acceptable symptoms
        (c) Of note: Might be associated with reversible decline in ventricular performance over time (called tachycardia-associated cardiomyopathy)
    iii. Treatment options

Table 54. Nonacute Setting and Chronic Maintenance Rate Control Therapy of AF

Drug	Loading Dose (Oral)	Onset	Maintenance Dose (Oral)	Major Adverse Effects
Rate Control				
Metoprolol	Same as maintenance	4–6 hours	25–100 mg twice daily	Hypotension, bradycardia, heart failure and asthma exacerbation, heart block
Propranolol (for thyrotoxicosis-associated AF)	Same as maintenance	60–90 minutes	80–240 mg in divided doses	Hypotension, bradycardia, heart failure and asthma exacerbation, heart block
Diltiazem	Same as maintenance	2–4 hours	120–360 mg/day in divided doses; slow release available	Hypotension, heart failure exacerbation, heart block
Verapamil	Same as maintenance	1–2 hours	120–360 mg/day in divided doses; slow release available	Hypotension, heart failure exacerbation, heart block, digoxin interaction

Table 54. Nonacute Setting and Chronic Maintenance Rate Control Therapy of AF *(continued)*

Drug	Loading Dose (Oral)	Onset	Maintenance Dose (Oral)	Major Adverse Effects
Rate control in patients with heart failure and without accessory pathway				
Digoxin	0.5 mg/day	2 days	0.125–0.375 mg/day	Digoxin toxicity; GI, neurologic and electrophysiologic changes. Goal concentrations for AF are higher (typically, 1–2 ng/mL) than for HFrEF
Amiodarone	800 mg/day for 1 week 600 mg for 1 week 400 mg for 4–6 weeks	1–3 weeks	200 mg/day	See Table 574

AF = atrial fibrillation; GI = gastrointestinal; HFrEF = heart failure with reduced ejection fraction.

Originally published in: Fuster V, Rydén LE, Cannom DS, et al. ACC/AHA/ESC 2006 guidelines for the management of patients with atrial fibrillation—executive summary: a report of the American College of Cardiology/American Heart Association Task Force on Practice Guidelines and the European Society of Cardiology Committee for Practice Guidelines (Writing Committee to Revise the 2001 Guidelines for the Management of Patients With Atrial Fibrillation). Circulation 2006;114:700-52. Published online before print August 2, 2006.

- (a) β-Blockers (above is not a complete list of options)
    - (1) Added mortality benefit in post-MI and LV systolic dysfunction
    - (2) Younger patients may not tolerate because they are unable to quickly increase HR during exercise.
- (b) Nondihydropyridine calcium channel blockers: Avoid in LV dysfunction.
- (c) Digoxin
    - (1) Not usually used as monotherapy
    - (2) Controls rate only at rest with increased vagal tone
    - (3) Consider in patients with HF.
- (d) Amiodarone:
    - (1) Can be used as rate control when not responding to AV node blockers. Decreases number of AF episodes; therefore, more tolerable to the patient
    - (2) Note: Can cause conversion to normal sinus rhythm, so need to ensure no clot is present before use or patient has to receive anticoagulation therapy
- (e) AV nodal ablation with pacemaker pacing
- (f) Suggested reference: RACE II (Rate Control Efficacy in Permanent Atrial Fibrillation II) study
    - (1) Noninferiority trial of lenient rate control (resting HR less than 110 beats/minute) versus strict rate control (resting HR less than 80 beats/minute with moderate exercise) in patients with permanent AF
    - (2) No statistically significant difference for CV death or hospitalization for HF, stroke, systemic embolism, bleeding, and life-threatening arrhythmic events
    - (3) Lenient rate control is more convenient; fewer outpatient visits and examinations are needed.
    - (4) Of note, only 67% of patients obtained strict rate control, and the mean resting HR at the end was 93 ± 9 beats/minute in the lenient control group.

   b. Rhythm control
- i. Prevention of AF may stop the progression to persistent or permanent AF.
- ii. Indication
    - (a) Symptomatic patients despite adequate rate control
    - (b) Hemodynamically unstable condition
    - (c) Patients with HF
    - (d) AF secondary to a trigger or substrate (e.g., ischemia, hyperthyroidism) that has been corrected
    - (e) Not an option for permanent AF
- iii. Pharmacologic cardioversion
    - (a) Class Ic
        - (1) Flecainide
        - (2) Propafenone
        - (3) Note: Avoid in patients with structural heart disease.
    - (b) Class III
        - (1) Sotalol—Not efficacious for conversion to sinus rhythm, but beneficial in prevention of recurrence
        - (2) Amiodarone—More effective than other agents; 61%–86% success rate
        - (3) Dofetilide
        - (4) Dronedarone – Although included in the guidelines, adverse effects and black box warnings have all but eliminated this agent as a therapeutic option: Increased risk of HF and death in patients with recent symptomatic HF), liver toxicity, interstitial lung pneumonitis, pulmonary fibrosis
    - (c) "Pill-in-the-pocket" cardioversion for hemodynamically stable, recurrent symptomatic paroxysmal AF
        - (1) Single oral loading dose of propafenone or flecainide may terminate AF in ambulatory outpatients already taking a β-blocker, diltiazem, or verapamil (to prevent rapid AV conduction if atrial flutter occurs).
        - (2) Prior safety of the agent should have been shown for the patient in-hospital.
        - (3) Patients may not have sinus or AV node dysfunction, bundle-branch block, QT-interval prolongation, Brugada syndrome, or structural heart disease.
- iv. Maintenance of sinus rhythm: When comparing rate control with rhythm control, there was no difference in mortality, stroke, or quality of life (NEJM 2002;347:1825-33), and study confirmed that chronic anticoagulation therapy is needed in either rate or rhythm control. Moreover, rhythm control had a statistically significant increase in hospitalizations and adverse drug effects.

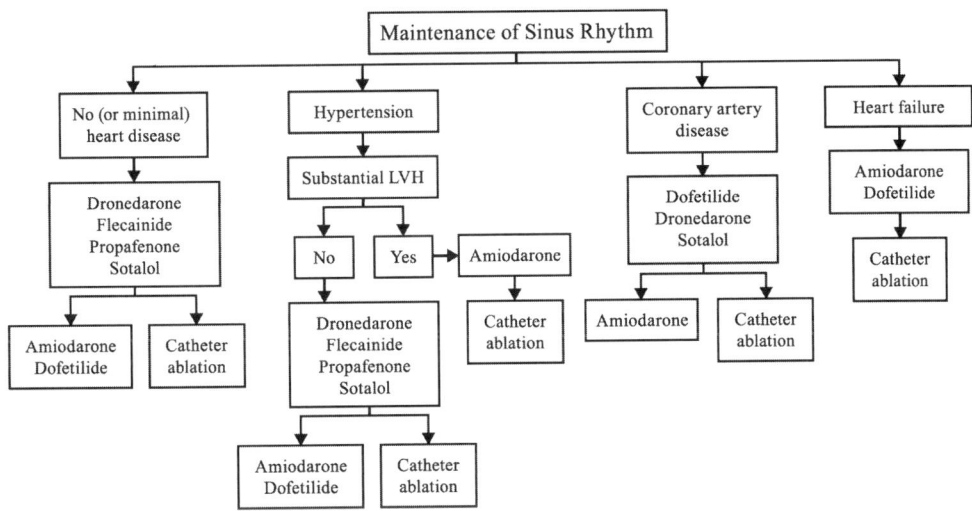

Figure 1. Rhythm control for recurrent paroxysmal or persistent atrial fibrillation.

Drugs listed in alphabetic order, not in order of suggested use.

LVH = left ventricular hypertrophy.

Originally published in: Wann LS, Curtis AB, January CT, et al.; writing on behalf of the 2006 ACC/AHA/ESC Guidelines for the Management of Patients With Atrial Fibrillation Writing Committee. 2011 ACCF/AHA/HRS focused update on the management of patients with atrial fibrillation (updating the 2006 guideline): a report of the American College of Cardiology Foundation./American Heart Association Task Force on Practice Guidelines. Circulation 2011;123:104-23.

   (2) ANDROMEDA
      (A) Dronedarone versus placebo in patients hospitalized with severe HF (NYHA class III or IV) and severe LV systolic dysfunction (LVEF around 35% or less)
      (B) Patients given dronedarone had a 2-fold increase in mortality related to worsening of HF.
   (3) ATHENA
      (A) Dronedarone decreased the incidence of hospitalization caused by CV events.
      (B) Dronedarone reduced the incidence of death in patients with AF.
   (4) DIONYSOS
      (A) Patients taking dronedarone for the prevention of recurrent AF were half as likely to remain in sinus rhythm as patients taking amiodarone.
      (B) However, these patients were less likely to discontinue antiarrhythmic therapy because of adverse effects.
   (5) PALLAS
      (A) Evaluated the use of dronedarone compared to placebo in patients with permanent AF and at least one other ASCVD risk factor
      (B) Study was discontinued early because of the significant excess of CV events in the dronedarone group compared to placebo.
   c. Direct current cardioversion (DCC)
      i. Indication
         (a) When rapid ventricular response does not respond to pharmacologic measures
         (b) When patient is hemodynamically unstable
         (c) When patient finds symptoms unacceptable
         (d) Contraindicated with digitalis toxicity and hypokalemia

      ii. DCC alone

     iii. DCC with pharmacologic enhancement; pretreatment with amiodarone, flecainide, propafenone, sotalol, or dronedarone and continue. Useful to prevent recurrence of AF

d. Ablation for AF or surgical Cox maze III ("maze") procedure

      i. Two types of ablation: Ablation of focal triggers in and around pulmonary veins (called pulmonary vein isolation) and ablation at the site of origin of trigger (preferred, because the patient is left in NSR) versus ablation of the AV node with implant of pacemaker (controls only the HR and the patient remains in AF)

      ii. Maze procedure is done only if patient has AF and is undergoing cardiothoracic surgery for another reason such as coronary artery bypass grafting surgery or valve repair/replacement.

     iii. Ablation is currently first-line therapy or an alternative to antiarrhythmic therapy to prevent recurrent AF.

     iv. Good option for patients who are symptomatic with little or no left atrial enlargement

      v. Ablation is indicated for the following:

        (a) Symptomatic paroxysmal (class I recommendation) or persistent AF (class IIa recommendation) intolerant of at least one antiarrhythmic drug or

        (b) Symptomatic paroxysmal AF (class IIa recommendation) before the initiation of antiarrhythmic drugs (first line)

      vi. Risk of AF recurrence is highest 6–12 months post ablation.

     vii. Patients are at risk of TE (stroke or PE) during and for at least 6 weeks after ablation because of damaged left atrial endothelium and placement of transseptal sheaths and electrode catheters during the procedure, as well as left atrial stunning.

    viii. Suggested reference

        Heart Rhythm 2012;9:632-96: A report of the Heart Rhythm Society (HRS) Task Force on Catheter and Surgical Ablation of Atrial Fibrillation. Developed in partnership with the European Heart Rhythm Association (EHRA), a registered branch of the European Society of Cardiology (ESC) and the European Cardiac Arrhythmia Society (ECAS); and in collaboration with the ACC, AHA, the Asia Pacific Heart Rhythm Society (APHRS), and the Society of Thoracic Surgeons (STS). Endorsed by the governing bodies of the ACCF, the AHA, the ECAS, the EHRA, the STS, the APHRS, and the HRS

e. Preventing thromboembolism in AF

      i. See Thromboembolism chapter for stroke prevention in AF.

      ii. Antithrombotic therapy after AF ablation

        (a) Therapeutic warfarin anticoagulation maintained pre, during, and post ablation

        (b) Newer oral anticoagulant switched to warfarin about 1 month before ablation, and therapeutic warfarin anticoagulation maintained pre and during ablation; then patient's medication switched back to newer oral anticoagulant once INR is less than 2

        (c) Limited experience with maintaining newer oral anticoagulant until 24 or 48 hours before procedure or maintaining during procedure and no warfarin or LMWH bridge

        (d) LMWH bridging has been abandoned secondary to excessive bleeding risk.

        (e) Consensus recommendation from 2012 HRS AF ablation guidelines is that all patients undergoing AF ablation receive therapeutic anticoagulation with warfarin or a newer oral direct thrombin inhibitor or factor Xa inhibitor for at least 2 months post procedure, regardless of $CHADS_2$ score. A longer duration of anticoagulation for high-risk patients is strongly encouraged, with discontinuation done in the setting of ambulatory continuous rhythm monitoring for AF recurrence.

f. Prevention of thromboembolism when undergoing cardioversion
    i. Patients in stable condition in AF for less than 48 hours
        (a) Sinus rhythm obtained and no risk factors for AF: Anticoagulation unnecessary
        (b) Sinus rhythm obtained and risk factors for AF
            (1) Oral anticoagulation after cardioversion; duration of 4 weeks
            (2) Consider long-term anticoagulation after cardioversion if stroke risk factors and/or risk of AF recurrence/presence of thrombus
    ii. Patients in stable condition in AF for 48 hours or more
        (a) Anticoagulation at least 3 weeks before (prevents new thrombi and permits any potential thrombi to organize and adhere to the atrial wall, where they will likely not embolize before sinus rhythm is restored) and 4 weeks after (normal atrial contraction may not return for 2 weeks, and any newly formed thrombi may embolize) electric or pharmacologic cardioversion
        (b) Alternatively, cardioversion can be performed immediately after a TEE revealing no left atrial/left atrial appendage clot in the setting of current therapeutic anticoagulation with UFH/LMWH/warfarin or, more recently, at least 2–4 hours after the first dose of a newer oral anticoagulant (see Thromboembolism chapter for time to Cmax).
    iii. Hemodynamically unstable, immediate cardioversion required, and in AF 48 hours or more
        (a) A TEE can be used to evaluate for thrombus in the left atrium or left atrial appendage.
        (b) Intravenous heparin (fully anticoagulated) or LMWH before cardioversion
        (c) Oral anticoagulation after cardioversion; duration of 4 weeks
    iv. Hemodynamically unstable, immediate cardioversion required, and in AF less than 48 hours: Cardioversion administered without delay for anticoagulation

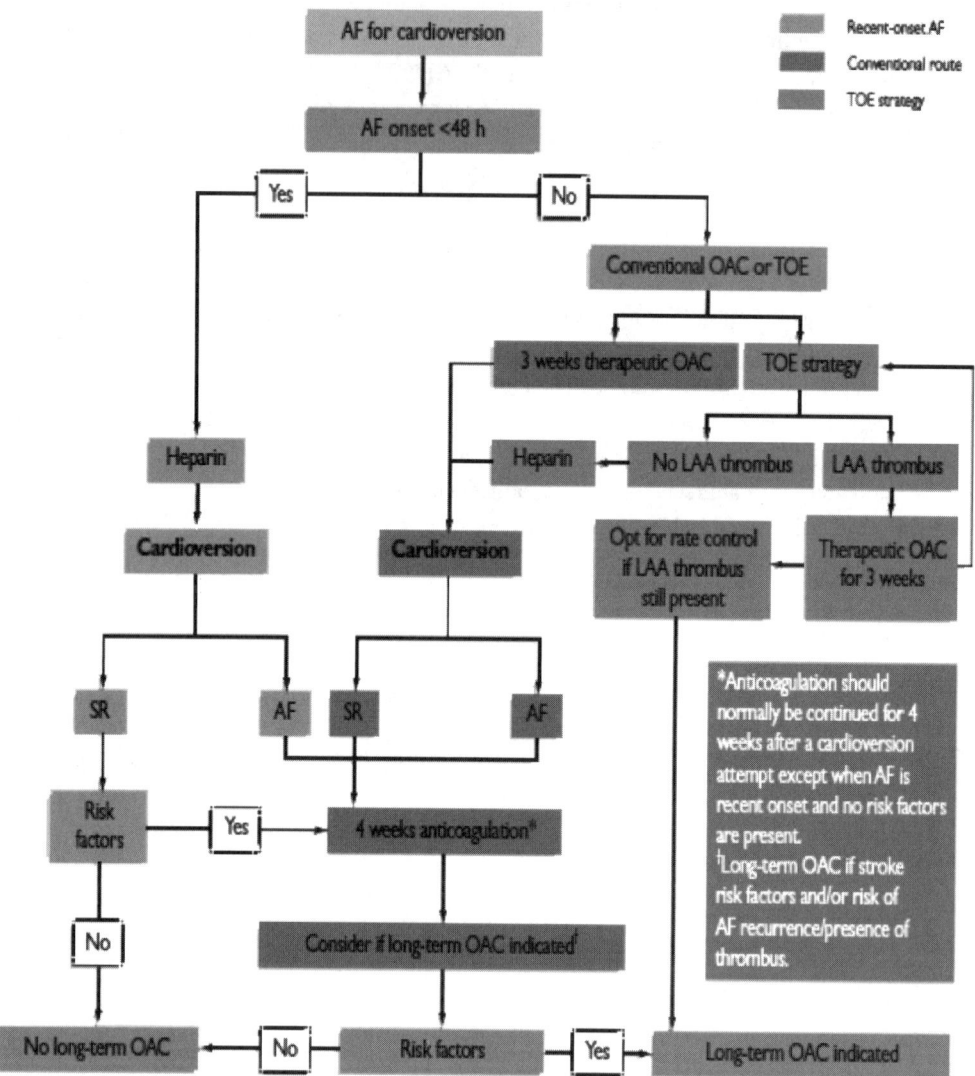

Figure 2. Cardioversion of hemodynamically stable AF, the role of TEE, and subsequent anticoagulation strategy.

AF = atrial fibrillation; DCC = direct current cardioversion; LA = left atrium; LAA = left atrial appendage; OAC = oral anticoagulant; SR = sinus rhythm; TEE = transesophageal echocardiogram.

Reprinted with permission from the European Society of Cardiology. Originally published in: Camm AJ, Kirchhof P, Lip GYH, et al. Guidelines for the management of atrial fibrillation: the Task Force for the Management of Atrial Fibrillation of the European Society of Cardiology (ESC). Eur Heart J 2010;31:2369-429.

Patient Cases

Questions 14 and 15 pertain to the following case.

T.T. is a 55-year-old-man with a medical history significant for coronary artery disease, NYHA class III HF, LVEF 35%, two cardioembolic strokes, and diabetes mellitus who presents to the clinic today with new palpitations, fatigue, shortness of breath, and dizziness for the past 3 weeks. A 12-lead ECG shows AF with an HR of 101 beats/minute and a QTc of 420 milliseconds. The patient is currently taking carvedilol 12.5 mg twice daily, lisinopril 20 mg/day, aspirin 81 mg/day, and insulin glargine 20 units at bedtime. His blood pressure is 120/80 mm Hg. Laboratory testing shows the following: SCr 0.80 mg/dL, hemoglobin 14.0 g/dL, and INR 1.0.

14. Which option best reflects the HR goal for T.T.?

    A. Less than 150 beats/minute.

    B. Less than 110 beats/minute.

    C. Less than 80 beats/minute.

    D. Not specified in a practice guideline.

15. Which is the best course of action to treat T.T. currently?

    A. Perform DCC to obtain NSR.

    B. Increase carvedilol dose to 25 mg orally twice daily, and add rivaroxaban 20 mg orally daily with food.

    C. Add dofetilide 250 mcg orally twice daily and rivaroxaban 20 mg orally daily with food.

    D. Increase carvedilol dose to 25 mg orally twice daily, add dofetilide 250 mcg orally twice daily, and add rivaroxaban 20 mg orally daily with food.

Questions 16 and 17 pertain to the following case.

H.W. is a 50-year-old man with symptomatic paroxysmal AF and HTN. He is seen in the arrhythmia clinic, where he is refusing ablation. His current medications include apixaban 5 mg orally twice daily, enalapril 10 mg orally twice daily, hydrochlorothiazide 25 mg orally daily, and metoprolol tartrate 50 mg orally twice daily. His laboratory test results are normal (with apixaban coagulation effects), BP 120/70 mm Hg, and HR 75 beats/minute. He has no LV hypertrophy on ECG, and his QTc is 400 milliseconds. His LVEF is 65% on echocardiography, and he has no evidence of clot. He attests to high medication adherence.

16. Which option best reflects the HR goal for H.W.?

    A. Less than 150 beats/minute.

    B. Less than 110 beats/minute.

    C. Less than 80 beats/minute.

    D. Not specified in a practice guideline.

17. A decision is made to start rhythm control for H.W. Which would be the best antiarrhythmic drug to treat H.W. currently?

    A. Amiodarone.

    B. Dofetilide.

    C. Dronedarone.

    D. Flecainide.

B. Atrial Flutter *(Domain 1, Tasks 1, 2, 5, 6, 7; Domain 3, Tasks 2, 3)*
1. Classifications
   a. Type I flutter: Classic form ("saw-tooth" P waves in inferior leads)
   b. Type II flutter: Atypical atrial flutter circuits, often faster
2. Epidemiology
   a. Less common than AF; however, there are many similarities
   b. Occurs in 25%–35% of patients with AF
   c. Presentation (type I flutter): 250–350 atrial beats/minute
   d. Symptoms
      i. Dyspnea
      ii. Fatigue
      iii. Palpitations
      iv. Chest discomfort
      v. Exercise-induced fatigue
      vi. Worsening HF
3. Pathophysiologic mechanisms
   a. Reentry within the atrial wall
      i. Type I flutter: Macroreentrant circuit depends on the cavotricuspid isthmus.
      ii. Type II flutter: Less common lesion-related macroreentrant (surgical scar)
   b. Causes: Can be precipitated by forms of organic heart disease that cause atrial stretch
      i. Hypertension
      ii. Chronic obstructive pulmonary disease
      iii. Valvular disorders
      iv. Dilated or hypertrophic cardiomyopathy
      v. Cardiac disease
      vi. Surgery
      vii. Ischemia/infarction
4. Complications: Embolic risk. The risk of stroke is lower than with AF.
5. Treatment (treated similarly to AF)
   a. Preventing thromboembolism
      i. Risk of embolism is lower.
      ii. No appropriate trials to evaluate anticoagulation; therefore, AF guidelines extend to atrial flutter (see above Atrial Fibrillation and Thromboembolism sections)
   b. Direct current cardioversion
   c. Ablation: First-line treatment because it most effectively increases quality of life
   d. Pharmacologic (limited data to evaluate antiarrhythmic medications)
      i. AV nodal–blocking agents; more difficult-to-control rate
      ii. Class Ia and Ic drugs
      iii. Class III drugs

Table 55. Recommendations for Long-term Management of Atrial Flutter

Clinical Status/Proposed Therapy	Recommendation[a]
First-episode and well-tolerated atrial flutter	1. Cardioversion 2. Catheter ablation
Recurrent and well-tolerated atrial flutter	1. Catheter ablation 2. Dofetilide 3. Amiodarone, sotalol, flecainide, quinidine, propafenone
Poorly tolerated atrial flutter	1. Catheter ablation
Atrial flutter appearing after use of class Ic agents or amiodarone for treatment of atrial fibrillation	1. Catheter ablation
Symptomatic non–cavotricuspid isthmus-dependent flutter after failed antiarrhythmic drug therapy	1. Catheter ablation

[a]Recommendations are numbered by classification of supporting evidence.

Originally published in: Blomstrom-Lundqvist C, Scheinman MM, Aliot EM, et al. ACC/AHA/ESC guidelines for the management of patients with supraventricular arrhythmias – executive summary: a report of the American College of Cardiology/American Heart Association Task Force on Practice Guidelines, and the European Society of Cardiology Committee for Practice Guidelines (Writing Committee to Develop Guidelines for the Management of Patients With Supraventricular Arrhythmias.). J Am Coll Cardiol 2003;42:1493-531.

XII. VENTRICULAR ARRHYTHMIAS

A. VT with Pulse *(Domain 1, Tasks 1, 2)*
1. Classification
   a. ECG morphology (monomorphic or polymorphic)
   b. Duration (sustained or nonsustained)
   c. Location
   d. Hemodynamic significance (stable, unstable, pulseless)
   e. Mechanism (reentrant, automatic)
2. Epidemiology
   a. ECG: Typically wide QRS
   b. Rate: Greater than 100 beats/minute
   c. The mortality risk correlates with the degree of structural heart disease.
   d. Symptoms
      i. Dyspnea
      ii. Syncope
      iii. Palpitations
3. Pathophysiologic mechanism
   a. Impulse is generated from increased automaticity of a single point in either the left or the right ventricle or is caused by a reentry circuit within the ventricle.
   b. Nonsustained VT—Three or more consecutive premature ventricular contractions (PVCs) lasting less than 30 seconds and terminating spontaneously
   c. Sustained VT—Three or more consecutive PVCs at a rate greater than 100 beats/minute lasting more than 30 seconds and/or lasting less than 30 seconds but requiring termination because of hemodynamic compromise
   d. Causes
      i. Idiopathic
      ii. Sleep apnea
      iii. Myocardial scarring from previous MI: Scar cannot conduct electrical activity, causing a potential circuit around it.

     iv. Coronary artery disease

     v. Hypertrophic cardiomyopathy

     vi. Nonischemic cardiomyopathies

     vii. Electrolyte abnormalities

     viii. Right ventricular dysplasia

B. Chronic Treatment *(Domain 1, Tasks 3, 4, 5, 6)*
1. Nonsustained VT
   a. EF greater than 40% and asymptomatic; usually does not require therapy
   b. Symptomatic; β-blockers or amiodarone
   c. EF less than 40%; amiodarone
2. Sustained VT
   a. Implantable cardioverter defibrillator
   b. If VT reoccurs after ICD placement or if ICD is not an option
     i. Ablation
     ii. Sotalol
     iii. β-Blocker plus amiodarone
     iv. Amiodarone
     v Correct underlying cause.

XIII. PHARMACIST ROLE IN ARRHYTHMIA MANAGEMENT *(Domain 2, Tasks 1, 5)*

A. Medication Reconciliation

B. Patient Education (medications, signs and symptoms of stroke)
Available resources: www.hrsonline.org/Patient-Resources/Patient-Information-Sheets#axzz2qrUgkpeG

C. Anticoagulation Management for AF/Atrial Flutter

D. Evaluate for Drug Interactions.

E. Ensure that 12-lead ECG is obtained and QTc interval determined for appropriate antiarrhythmic agents causing torsades de pointes.

F. Prevent adverse drug events by ensuring the drug's appropriateness according to the patient's comorbidities and medication profile.

G. Identify Adverse Drug Events with Frequent Monitoring.
1. Subjective questioning
2. Laboratory draws

H. Historian: Identify the Medications the Patient Has Taken in the Past to Treat the Arrhythmia. Make recommendations according to the patient's past treatments and current disease states.

I. Ensure Continuity of Care.

J. Keep Nurses and Physicians Up to Date on Current Cardiac Medication Literature and Ongoing Trials.

K. Ensure Medications Can Be Obtained by the Patient According to Cost and/or Formulary.

L. Facilitate Prior Authorizations from Insurance Company.

M. Create Collaborative Agreements or Standing Orders.

XIV. ANTIARRHYTHMIC MEDICATIONS *(Domain 1, Tasks 2, 3)*

Table 56. Oral Antiarrhythmic Medications (classification, mechanism, drugs, and indication)

Vaughan-Williams Classification	Indications[a]	Drugs	Mechanism of Action
Ia	AF, atrial flutter, paroxysmal supraventricular tachycardia, ventricular arrhythmias [a]Disopyramide – Only paroxysmal supraventricular tachycardia	Quinidine	Channel blocked: Na (intermediate association and dissociation), K, Ach, α ECG manifestations: May ↑ sinus rate; ↑ QT (not dose related); ↑ QRS high dose
		Disopyramide	Channel blocked: Na (intermediate association and dissociation), K, Ach ECG manifestations: May ↑ sinus rate; ↑ QT (not dose related); ↑ QRS high dose
Ib	Ventricular arrhythmias [a]Used most commonly as add-on to amiodarone and not as sole agent	Mexiletine	Channel blocked: Na (fast association and dissociation) ECG manifestations: May ↓ sinus rate, generally do not affect QRS or QT
Ic	AF and atrial flutter, paroxysmal supraventricular tachycardia, ventricular arrhythmias [a]May precipitate atrial flutter in patients with AF if no rate-controlling agent coadministered	Propafenone	Channel blocked: Na (slow association and dissociation), β ECG manifestations: May ↓ sinus rate; ↑ PR, ↑ QRS
		Flecainide	Channel blocked: Na (slow association and dissociation) ECG manifestations: May ↓ sinus rate; ↑ PR, ↑ QRS
II	AF, atrial flutter, paroxysmal supraventricular tachycardia, ventricular arrhythmias	ß-Blockers (i.e., metoprolol)	Channel blocked: β, indirect CaECG manifestations: ↓ Sinus rate

Table 56. Oral Antiarrhythmic Medications (classification, mechanism, drugs, and indication) *(continiued)*

Vaughan-Williams Classification	Indications[a]	Drugs	Mechanism of Action
III	Amiodarone: Supraventricular and ventricular arrhythmias Dronedarone: Paroxysmal or persistent atrial fibrillation and atrial flutter Sotalol: Ventricular arrhythmias; maintenance of AF and flutter Dofetilide: Supraventricular arrhythmias; atrial flutter and fibrillation conversion	Amiodarone	Channel blocked: K, Na, Ca, β, α, Ach ECG manifestations: ↓ Sinus rate, ↑ PR, ↑ QRS, ↑ QT
		Dronedarone	Channel blocked: K, Na, Ca, β, α, Ach ECG manifestations: ↓ Sinus rate, ↑ PR
		Sotalol	Channel blocked: K, β ECG manifestations: ↓ Sinus rate, may ↑ PR, ↑ QT (dose related)
		Dofetilide	Channel blocked: K ECG manifestations: ↑ QT (dose related)
IV	AF, atrial flutter, paroxysmal supraventricular tachycardia	Diltiazem Verapamil	Channel blocked: CaECG manifestations: ↓ Sinus rate
Additional agents	AF	Digoxin	Channel blocked: Positive inotropic effect, enhanced vagal tone, and decreased ventricular rate to fast atrial arrhythmias ECG manifestations: ↓ Sinus rate

[a]Including off-label uses.

Ach = acetylcholine; AF = atrial fibrillation; Ca = calcium; ECG =, electrocardiographic; K = potassium; Na = sodium.

Table 57. Antiarrhythmic Medications (oral class I and III agents only) Properties and Dosing

Drug	Mechanism of Action, Pharmacokinetics, Contraindications, Adverse Effects, Drug Interactions	Dosing
Class Ia – Na⁺ channel blockers		
Quinidine (Quinidex, Quinaglute)	MOA: Strong vagolytic and anticholinergic properties, Na⁺ and K⁺ channel blockage	Sulfate (extended release): 300 mg PO every 8–12 hours Gluconate (extended release): 324–648 mg PO every 8–12 hours
	PK: Half-life 5–9 hours Substrate CYP3A4 Inhibitor CYP2D6	
	AEs: Nausea/vomiting/diarrhea (30%) TdP (first 72 hours, not dose related) "Cinchonism": CNS symptoms, tinnitus Thrombocytopenia, rash, pruritus	
	DIs: Warfarin, digoxin	
Disopyramide (Norpace, Norpace CR, Rythmodan, Rythmodan-LA)	MOA: Potent Na⁺ and M2 blockade, Ach; strong negative inotrope	Initial dose 400–800 mg/day in divided doses; IR every 6 hours, CR every 12 hours Maximum 1200–1600 mg/day Dose adjustment required for renal insufficiency
	PK: Half-life 4–8 hours Substrate CYP3A4	
	CIs: Glaucoma	
	AEs: Anticholinergic adverse effects TdP ADHF	
Class Ib – Na⁺ channel blockers		
Mexiletine (Mexitil)	MOA: Inactive Na⁺ channel blocker	VT maintenance: 200–300 mg every 8 hours Maximum of 1200 mg/day
	PK: Half-life 12–20 hours Substrate CYP2D6, CYP1A2 Inhibitor CYP1A2	
	CIs: Third-degree AV heart block	
	AEs: GI upset (administer with food); CNS: Tremor, dizziness, ataxia, nystagmus	
Class Ic – Na⁺ channel blockers (*avoid with HF or post MI)**		
Propafenone (Rythmol)	MOA: Na⁺ and Ca²⁺ channel blocker; ß-blocker	AF conversion: 600 mg (IR) PO × 1 (efficacy 45% in 3 hours) AF maintenance: IR: 150–300 mg PO every 8 hours SR: 225–425 mg PO every 12 hours
	PK: Half-life 10–25 hours Substrate CYP2D6, CYP1A2 Inhibitor CYP2D6	
	CIs: HF NYHA III–IV, liver disease, valvular disease (TdP), CAD, VT	
	AEs: Metallic taste, dizziness	
	DIs: Propafenone may ↑ digoxin concentrations, may decrease warfarin metabolism, has β-blocker properties and pharmacokinetic interaction increasing β-blocker concentrations – Need to monitor HR and reduce β-blocker dose if necessary to prevent symptoms/heart block	

Table 57. Antiarrhythmic Medications (oral class I and III agents only) Properties and Dosing *(continued)*

Drug	Mechanism of Action, Pharmacokinetics, Contraindications, Adverse Effects, Drug Interactions	Dosing
Class Ic – Na$^+$ channel blockers (***avoid with HF or post MI) *(continued)*		
Flecainide (Tambocor)	MOA: Strong Na$^+$ channel blockade; vagolytic, anticholinergic, and negative inotrope	AF conversion: 300 mg PO × 1 (efficacy 50% in 3 hours) AF maintenance: 50–200 mg PO bid
	PK: Half-life 10–20 hours Substrate CYP2D6 Inhibitor CYP2D6	
	CIs: HF, CAD, valvular/LV hypertrophy (TdP)	
	AEs: Dizziness, tremor, HF exacerbation, VT, atrial flutter (in patients with AF)	
	DI: May increase digoxin concentrations; flecainide concentrations increased by haloperidol, cimetidine, and fluoxetine	
Class III – K$^+$ channel blockers		
Amiodarone (Cordarone, Pacerone)	MOA: K$^+$, Na$^+$, Ca^{2+} channel blocker, ß-blocker	AF/VT conversion/maintenance: 600–800 mg/day in divided doses until 10 g total; then 100–400 mg/day maintenance *** Maintenance doses are often started before the patient completes the 10-g loading dose.
	PK: Half-life 26–107 days (chronic oral dosing), large volume of distribution (high affinity for adipose tissue) Substrate CYP3A4, CYP1A2, CYP2C9 Inhibitor CYP3A4, CYP2D6, CYP2C9, CYP1A2, CYP2C19, intestinal P-glycoprotein	
	CIs: Iodine hypersensitivity, hyperthyroidism, third-degree AV heart block	
	AEs: Pulmonary fibrosis (1.7% in outpatient setting), thyroid dysfunction (2%–23%), hepatotoxicity (3%–20%), neurologic toxicity (4%–9%), TdP (< 1%), AV block (14%), photosensitivity (3%–10%), visual disturbances (4%–9%), sinus bradycardia ***The 2007 HRS amiodarone guidelines and prescribing information recommend the following: Baseline thyroid panel and liver function tests repeated every 6 months; chest radiography and physical examination at baseline and repeated every 3 to 6 months with a high-resolution CT scan if new symptoms of pulmonary toxicity appear such as dyspnea, cough, or chest radiograph changes	

Table 57. Antiarrhythmic Medications (oral class I and III agents only) Properties and Dosing *(continued)*

Drug	Mechanism of Action, Pharmacokinetics, Contraindications, Adverse Effects, Drug Interactions	Dosing
Class III – K⁺ channel blockers *(continued)*		
Amiodarone (Cordarone, Pacerone)	Since the 2007 guidelines were published, new AEs of optic neuritis and neuritis leading to blindness were added to prescribing information and require regular ophthalmologic examinations (including funduscopy and slit lamp examination) ***Most AEs are dose-dependent; reduce to lowest effective dose ***Does not increase mortality in HF	AF/VT conversion/maintenance: 600–800 mg/day in divided doses until 10 g total; then 100–400 mg/day maintenance *** Maintenance doses are often started before the patient completes the 10-g loading dose.
	DIs: Warfarin (reduce dose by 25%–50%, recheck INR accordingly), digoxin (reduce dose by 50%), statins (simvastatin 20 mg maximal dose) Dabigatran effects increased but not clinically relevant,dabigatran	
Sotalol (Betapace)	MOA: K⁺ channels, blocks ß₁- and ß₂-receptors	AF conversion: No effect!
	PK: Renally eliminated Half-life 30–40 hours	AF maintenance: Dose 80–160 mg Twice daily; CrCl > 60 mL/minute
	CIs: Baseline QTc > 0.45 seconds or CrCl < 40 mL/minute in atrial arrhythmias only	Daily; CrCl 40–60 mL/minute Contraindicated; CrCl < 40 mL/minute
	AEs: HF exacerbation, bradycardia, AV heart block, bronchospasm, TdP 3%–8% within 3 days of initiation ***Ideally initiated in hospital, because of proarrhythmia	VT maintenance: Dose 80–160 mg Twice daily; CrCl > 60 mL/minute Daily; CrCl 30–60 mL/minute Every 48 hours; CrCl 10–30 mL/minute
	DIs: Has β-blocker properties, so the dose of concomitant β-blockers may need tapering after sotalol initiation; monitor HR	Every 72 hours; CrCl > 10 mL/minute
Dofetilide (Tikosyn)	MOA: K⁺ channel blocker only	AF conversion/maintenance: (CrCl > 60 mL/minute) 500 mcg PO twice daily
	PK: Renal and hepatic elimination Half-life 6–10 hours Substrate CYP3A4	(CrCl 40–60 mL/minute) 250 mcg PO twice daily (CrCl 20–40 mL/minute) 125 mcg PO twice daily
	CIs: Baseline QTc > 0.44 seconds or CrCl < 20 mL/minute	Contraindicated CrCl < 20 mL/minute *If initiated after amiodarone failure, need a 3-month washout period

Table 57. Antiarrhythmic Medications (oral class I and III agents only) Properties and Dosing *(continued)*

Drug	Mechanism of Action, Pharmacokinetics, Contraindications, Adverse Effects, Drug Interactions	Dosing
Class III – K⁺ channel blockers *(continued)*		
Dofetilide (Tikosyn)	AEs: TdP (0.8%; 4% if not renally dosed), dizziness, diarrhea ***Does not increase mortality in HF DIs: CYP3A4 inhibitors or cation drug transport system inhibitor drugs secreted by the kidney (ketoconazole, verapamil, trimethoprim, megestrol, dolutegravir, prochlorperazine), HCTZ (should be discontinued as concentrations of dofetilide increase)	REMS: ***Ensuring dofetilide is prescribed only by certified prescribers, dispensed only by certified dispensers (retail pharmacy must be enrolled in TIPS), and dispensed for use only with documentation of safe use conditions ***Educating health care providers about the risks and the need to initiate and reinitiate therapy in a hospital (at least a 72-hour stay) that can provide calculations of CrCl, continuous ECG monitoring, and cardiac resuscitation; do not initiate if QTc is > 0.44 second or 0.5 second in patients with baseline conduction abnormalities; obtain QTc 2–3 hours after first five doses, reduce by 50% if QTc ↑ > 15% (QTc should never exceed 0.5 second or 0.55 second in patients with baseline conduction system abnormality); if QTc prolongs by more than 15% or 0.5 second in patients with baseline conduction abnormalities of baseline after any dosage adjustment, dofetilide must be discontinued and deemed treatment failure; before the patient is discharged, the health care facility must either provide a free 7-day supply of dofetilide and the medication guide to patients or ensure the patient's take-home prescription is filled ***Inform the patient about the serious risks associated with dofetilide therapy (medication guide mandated) ***Mandates K⁺, Mg, SCr, and 12-lead ECG monitoring at least every 3 months

Ach = acetylcholine; ADHF = acute decompensated heart failure; AE = adverse effect; AF = atrial fibrillation; AV = atrioventricular; bid = twice daily; Ca²⁺ = calcium; CAD = coronary artery disease; CI = contraindicationt; CNS = central nervous system; CR = controlled release; CrCl = creatinine clearance; CT = computed tomography; CYP = cytochrome P450; DI = drug interaction; ECG = electrocardiogram; GI = gastrointestinal; HCTZ = hydrochlorothiazide; HF = heart failure; HR = heart rate; HRS = Heart Rhythm Society; INR = international normalized ratio; IR = immediate release; IV = intravenously; K⁺ = potassium; LA = long acting; LV = left ventricular; LVEF = left ventricular ejection fraction; Mg = magnesium; MI = myocardial infarction; MOA = mechanism of action; Na⁺ = sodium; NYHA = New York Heart Association; PK = pharmacokinetics; PO = orally; QTc = corrected QT interval; REMS = Risk Evaluation and Mitigation Strategies; SCr = serum creatinine; SR = sustained release; TdP = torsades de pointes; TIPS = Tikosyn In Pharmacy Systems; VF = ventricular fibrillation; VT = ventricular tachycardia.

Patient Case

18. A 75-year-old man with a history of MI, AF, and stage C HFrEF presents to the clinic 2 weeks after hospitalization for VT ablation. His current medications include amiodarone 400 mg/day (after a 5-g loading dose administered during his recent hospitalization), aspirin 81 mg orally daily, warfarin 5 mg orally daily (INR 2.4), simvastatin 40 mg orally daily, lisinopril 20 mg orally daily, spironolactone 25 mg orally daily, metoprolol succinate 100 mg orally twice daily, and digoxin 0.25 mg orally daily. His estimated CrCl is 55 mL/minute, and other chemistry test and LFT results are normal. Serum digoxin concentration is 1.5 ng/mL. His BP is 120/70 mm Hg, and HR is 59 beats/minute. Which is the best course of action currently?

   A. Decrease his warfarin dose to 2.5 mg orally daily, and decrease his amiodarone dose to 200 mg orally daily.
   B. Decrease his simvastatin dose to 20 mg orally daily, and decrease his amiodarone dose to 200 mg orally daily.
   C. Decrease his warfarin dose to 2.5 mg orally daily, and decrease his digoxin dose to 0.125 mg orally daily.
   D. Decrease his simvastatin dose to 20 mg orally daily, and decrease his digoxin dose to 0.125 mg orally daily.

VALVULAR HEART DISEASE

XV. THROMBOEMBOLISM PREVENTION

A. Prevention of TE in Patients with Valvular Heart Disease or Prosthetic Heart Valves *(Domain 1, Tasks 2, 3)*
   1. Patients with valvular AF are considered at "high risk" of cardioembolic stroke and should receive anticoagulation and, in some cases, added aspirin.
   2. Patients with mechanical valve prosthesis without AF are at high risk of thromboembolic complications (mainly cardioembolic stroke and valve thrombosis) and require lifelong antithrombotic prophylaxis.
   3. Prosthetic valves are made of various materials that differ in thrombogenicity.
      a. Newer materials reduce thrombogenicity, and future materials such as polymerics may reduce thrombogenicity even more.
      b. Bioprosthetic valves are less thrombogenic, but they are not as durable as mechanical valve prosthesis and are thus more prone to failure, requiring replacement.
      c. Because valve position, type, and materials affect thrombogenicity, correct use of anticoagulation therapy requires a determination of exactly which valve(s) has(have) been replaced and the type of prosthesis used so that mistakes in anticoagulation are avoided.
   4. Risk factors for thrombosis
      a. Annual risk of TE ranges from 4% to 23% without prophylaxis.
      b. Prophylaxis reduces the risk of TE to less than 2% a year.
      c. Risk of TE is highest in the early postsurgical period because of exposed valvular components (e.g., suturing ring, valve surfaces). After about 3 months, endothelialization occurs, and TE risk decreases.

5. Types of valves
   a. Mechanical prosthetic valves
      i. Three basic types of mechanical valves: Caged-ball/disk, tilting disk, and bileaflet

Table 58. Types of Mechanical Heart Valves

Valve Type	Model
Caged-ball	Starr-Edwards
Tilting disk	Björk-Shiley Monostrut Medtronic-Hall Omniscience Omnicarbon Ultracor
Bileaflet	St. Jude On-X Carbomedics Baxter TEKNA Duromedics Sorin Bicarbon

      ii. Older caged-ball and tilting disk valves are more thrombogenic than bileaflet valves.
      iii. Annual TE event rate in patients who receive anticoagulation treatment to an INR of 2.5–4.9
         (a) Bileaflet 0.5% a year
         (b) Tilting disk 0.7% a year
   b. Bioprosthetic valves
      i. Bioprosthetic valves use a ring of material from an animal source (e.g., porcine, bovine).
      ii. Porcine valves use the tissue valve from pig hearts (usually aortic valves).
      iii. Pericardial valves use tissue from the bovine pericardium to make the valve leaflets, which are supported by a synthetic frame.
      iv. Less thrombogenic and less durable than mechanical valves

Table 59. Bioprosthetic Valve Types

Valve Type	Model
Porcine	Hancock I Hancock II Intact Carpentier-Edwards Freestyle Bicor
Pericardial (bovine)	Carpentier-Edwards Perimount Ionescu-Shiley Mitroflow

6. Position of valves: Valve position influences thrombogenicity. Mechanical mitral valves are more thrombogenic than mechanical aortic valves.

7. Antithrombotic prophylaxis

   a. Intravenous adjusted-dose UFH or subcutaneous LMWH can be used postoperatively after valve insertion as a transition to warfarin and continued until INR is therapeutic and stable.

   b. A recent observational study suggests that discontinuation of warfarin after placement of a bioprosthetic aortic valve is associated with an increased risk of thromboembolism and CV death; therefore, future guidelines may suggest anticoagulation after aortic bioprosthetic surgery, as they now do for mitral bioprosthetic valve placement (JAMA 2012;308:2118-25).

   c. In the only study reported with mechanical heart valves and a target-specific oral anticoagulant (phase II, open-label, RE-ALIGN trial), patients treated with dabigatran had increased thrombotic and bleeding risk, compared with patients treated with warfarin, and the trial was terminated prematurely. Dabigatran is the only newer oral agent that specifically carries a contraindication for use in patients with mechanical heart valves.

   d. All patients with a mechanical valve should receive lifelong warfarin therapy adjusted to the recommended INR range.

   e. Patients with bioprosthetic valves and AF should receive lifelong anticoagulation therapy. Although not contraindicated in current (January 1, 2014) product labeling of dabigatran, rivaroxaban, and apixaban, these agents have not been studied in this group of patients.

   f. Patients with either mitral stenosis or a bioprosthetic heart valve were enrolled in the ENGAGE-AF trial comparing edoxaban and warfarin, but results in this important subgroup have not yet been presented or published.

Table 60. Chest Guideline Recommendations for Antithrombotic Prophylaxis

Valve Position	Bioprosthetic	Mechanical[a]
Aortic	Aspirin[b]	Warfarin (INR 2–3)[c]
Mitral	Warfarin (INR 2–3) x 3 months; then aspirin[b]	Warfarin (INR 2.5–3.5)

[a]Recommend adding low-dose aspirin 50–100 mg orally daily for all patients with mechanical valves and low risk of bleeding.

[b]Aspirin 50–100 mg/day. Recommend against giving aspirin to patients at high risk of bleeding (e.g., history of GI bleed, age > 80 years).

[c]ACC/AHA recommends INR 2.5–3.5 for all caged-ball and tilting disk valves.

GI = gastrointestinal; INR = international normalized ratio.

8. Patients who develop systemic embolism despite a therapeutic INR

   a. If patient was not previously taking aspirin, add aspirin 50–100 mg/day.

   b. Titrate warfarin to a higher INR range.

Previous INR Range	Postsystemic Embolism INR Range
2–3	2.5–3.5
2.5–3.5	3.5–4.5

INR = international normalized ratio.

Patient Cases

19. A 78-year-old woman with a history of permanent AF, dyslipidemia, HTN, and prior GI bleed is hospitalized with planned St. Jude mechanical aortic valve surgery for aortic stenosis. Diagnostic angiography before surgery revealed no significant coronary artery disease. Her CrCl is 55 mL/minute, and her medications at the time of admission for surgery were enalapril 10 mg orally twice daily and atorvastatin 40 mg orally daily. Which is the best antithrombotic regimen for stroke prevention for this patient after surgery?

    A. Aspirin 325 mg orally plus warfarin orally at a goal INR of 2–3.
    B. Dabigatran 150 mg orally twice daily.
    C. Warfarin at a goal INR of 2.5–3.5.
    D. Warfarin orally at a goal INR of 2–3.

20. A 68-year-old patient with a medical history of HTN and bicuspid aortic stenosis and bioprosthetic valve replacement 2 years ago presents with AF. Current medications are metoprolol succinate 100 mg orally twice daily and aspirin 325 mg orally daily. The patient has a HAS-BLED score of 2 and a CrCl of 80 mL/minute. Which is the best antithrombotic strategy for stroke prevention for this patient currently?

    A. Add clopidogrel 75 mg orally daily.
    B. Add warfarin at a goal INR of 2.5–3.5.
    C. Dabigatran 150 mg twice daily.
    D. Discontinue aspirin and add warfarin at a goal INR of 2–3.

XVI. AORTIC STENOSIS (Domain 1, Tasks 2, 3; Domain 3, Task 2)

A. Epidemiology
   1. Most common type of valvular heart disease
   2. Affects up to 5% of the elderly older than 75 years
   3. High risk of SCD in symptomatic patients
   4. Most common cause is calcific aortic stenosis.

B. Diagnosis Is Usually Made by Heart Murmur on Physical Examination by Auscultation: Typically, crescendo-decrescendo systolic ejection murmur radiating to the neck and confirmed by echocardiography

C. Severe Aortic Stenosis: Defined by Doppler echocardiography as a maximum aortic jet velocity greater than 4 m/second, mean transvalvular pressure gradient greater than 40 mm Hg, and continuity equation valve area less than 1.0 cm^2 or valve area index less than 0.6 cm^2

D. Pathophysiology: Pressure Overload Hypertrophy

E. Signs and Symptoms
   1. Three classic signs and symptoms: HF, syncope, and angina
   2. HF is caused by hypertrophy and the failure to eject blood effectively from the ventricles, leading to fluid overload; syncope secondary to diminished carotid blood flow and angina secondary to diminished coronary flow to the hypertrophied heart
   3. Typically, symptom-free until late in the disease course
   4. Interval from the onset of symptoms to the time of death is around 2 years in patients with HF, 3 years in those with syncope, and 5 years in those with angina.

F. Treatment of Severe Aortic Stenosis
    1. Medical management of severe aortic stenosis has a mortality rate of 50% at 1 year.
    2. Mechanical or bioprosthetic valve replacement surgery provides symptom relief and mortality reduction in appropriate candidates.
    3. Candidates are screened for surgical acceptability by using the STS (Society of Thoracic Surgeons) score, which predicts operative and short-term postoperative survival, using a model of 24 variables. See http://riskcalc.sts.org/STSWebRiskCalc273/de.aspx.
    4. Transcatheter aortic valve replacement (TAVR) (nonsurgical placement of a porcine or bovine aortic valve)
    5. Aortic balloon valvuloplasty (now used primarily as a bridge to TAVR or as palliation because durability is short). Two valves are FDA approved: SAPIEN (Edwards) and CoreValve system (Medtronic).

G. TAVR with SAPIEN Valve (Edwards): Placed primarily by using a transfemoral approach and, less preferably, a transapical approach. FDA approved according to the PARTNER trial
    1. PARTNER (Placement of AoRtic TraNscathetER Valve) trial was a prospective, unblinded, multicenter randomized trial that compared medical management with TAVR in patients who were not considered surgical candidates (cohort B) and with aortic valve replacement (AVR) in patients deemed high-risk operable (cohort A).
    2. Cohort B results: Compared with medical management of TAVR
        a. Reduced all-cause mortality by 38% at 1 year (p<0.001)
        b. Reduced the composite of all-cause mortality and rehospitalization at 1 year by 38% (p<0.001)
        c. 2-fold increased risk of major bleeding (p<0.001)
        d. 2-fold increased risk of stroke (p=0.03)
        e. Improved quality of life
    3. Cohort A results: Compared with AVR
        a. Noninferior for 1-year mortality (24.2% vs. 26.8%; hazard ratio 0.93; 95% CI, 0.71–1.22, p=0.001 for noninferiority)
        b. Increased risk of stroke at 1 year (8.3%–4.3%; p=0.04)
        c. Reduced bleeding risk at 1 year (14.7% compared with 25.7%; p<0.01)
        d. Two-year outcomes showed similar mortality and stroke risk between TAVR and AVR.
        e. PARTNER II trial comparing TAVR and AVR in patients at intermediate surgical risk is ongoing, with expected completion in 2015.

H. Antithrombotic Therapy for Stroke Prevention After TAVR
    1. Around 32% of patients undergoing TAVR develop AF within 48 hours of the procedure.
    2. Completed randomized trials comparing aspirin alone or with aspirin plus clopidogrel for stroke prevention after TAVR have been underpowered.
    3. 2012 ACCP guidelines recommend aspirin 50–100 mg plus clopidogrel 75 mg daily for at least the first 3 months after TAVR.
    4. PARTNER trial regimen was aspirin 75–100 mg plus clopidogrel 300 mg pre procedure and aspirin 75–100 mg indefinitely plus clopidogrel 75 mg daily for 6 months.
    5. No information with newer $P2Y_{12}$ agents such as prasugrel or ticagrelor
    6. Variable practice if patients require anticoagulation for another reason, such as AF. Some centers use triple antithrombotic therapy, whereas others use anticoagulation plus one antiplatelet.

I. Medical Therapy for the Inoperable Patient or the Symptomatic Patient Awaiting Surgery/TAVR
    1. Maintain sinus rhythm if the patient develops AF (administer an antiarrhythmic agent).

2. Avoid hypotension.
3. Digoxin for HF and depressed LVEF
4. Angina
   a. First-line therapy: β-Blocker
   b. Second-line therapy: Calcium channel blocker
   c. Avoid long-acting nitrates because reduction in preload may lead to worsening symptoms.
5. Heart failure
   a. Cautious use of diuretics (avoid dehydration)
   b. First-line β-blocker and ACE inhibitor or ARB (monitor for hypotension and worsening symptoms with addition of vasodilator)
6. Hypertension
   a. First-line β-blocker
   b. Second-line ACE inhibitor or ARB

Patient Case

21. A 78-year-old woman who underwent TAVR 1 month ago presents for follow-up at surgical clinic. She developed postoperative AF and received a 1-week course of amiodarone while hospitalized and aspirin 81 mg orally daily with warfarin anticoagulation since hospital discharge. She has maintained sinus rhythm since hospital discharge. Her surgeon wants to discontinue her oral anticoagulation nowcurrently. Which is the best strategy for stroke prevention currently?

   A. Aspirin 325 mg orally daily indefinitely.
   B. Aspirin 81 mg orally daily indefinitely.
   C. Clopidogrel 75 mg orally daily for 3 months.
   D. Aspirin 81 mg orally daily plus clopidogrel 75 mg orally daily for at least 2 months.

PULMOPNARY ARTERIAL HYPERTENSION

XVII. DEFINITION, DIAGNOSIS, AND TREATMENT GOALS (5TH WORLD SYMPOSIUM 2013)

A. Pulmonary Arterial Hypertension (PAH) *(Domain 1, Task 1)*
   1. Pulmonary hypertension (PH) is defined by a mean pulmonary arterial pressure (mPAP) of 25 mm Hg or greater at rest as measured at right heart catheterization (RHC).
   2. PAH is a subpopulation of PH hypertension that includes an end-expiratory pulmonary artery wedge pressure or LV end-diastolic pressure of 15 mm Hg or less and a pulmonary vascular resistance greater than 3 Wood units at RHC.

B. Classification *(Domain 1, Task 2)*
   1. Group 1: PAH (includes idiopathic, heritable, drug/toxin induced, connective tissue disease such as scleroderma, portal HTN, congenital, and human immunodeficiency virus [HIV] infection) (4.2%)
   2. Group 2: PH caused by left heart disease (78.7%)
   3. Group 3: PH caused by chronic lung disease and/or hypoxia (9.7%)
   4. Group 4: Chronic thromboembolic PH (0.6%)
   5. Group 5: PH caused by multifactorial mechanisms (6.8%)

C. Symptoms *(Domain 1, Task 2)*
1. Dyspnea with exertion (60% of patients), fatigue, chest pain, syncope, weakness (40%) – Caused by impaired oxygen delivery to tissues and diminished cardiac output
2. Orthopnea, peripheral edema, liver congestion, abdominal bloating, and other signs of right ventricular hypertrophy and failure occur when disease progresses to involve the heart.

D. Diagnosis and Classification *(Domain 1, Task 2)*

Table 61. Diagnostic Findings of Pulmonary Arterial Hypertension

Hemodynamic alterations	mPAP ≥ 25 mm Hg, PCWP ≤ 15 mm Hg, and PVR > 3 Wood units on RHC
Electrocardiogram	Signs of RV hypertrophy, right-axis deviation, and anterior ST- and T-wave abnormalities consistent with RV strain pattern
Echocardiography	Estimated RV systolic pressure elevation, enlarged RV, RV dysfunction
Chest radiography	Enlarged pulmonary arteries and diminished peripheral pulmonary vascular markings, RV enlargement
Physical examination	Cool and/or cyanotic extremities, jugular venous distension, pulsatile hepatomegaly, peripheral edema, ascites
Laboratory testing	Elevated BNP concentration

BNP = B-type natriuretic peptide; mPAP = mean pulmonary arterial pressure; PA = pulmonary artery; PCWP = pulmonary capillary wedge pressure; PVR = pulmonary vascular resistance; RHC = right heart catheterization; RV = right ventricle/ventricular.

Table 62. Classification of Pulmonary Arterial Hypertension Symptoms
WHO/Modified NYHA Classification

Class	Definition
I	No symptoms (dyspnea, fatigue, syncope, chest pain) with normal daily activities
II	Symptoms with strenuous normal daily activities that slightly limit functional status and activity level
III	Symptoms of dyspnea, fatigue, syncope, and chest pain with normal daily activities that severely limit functional status and activity level
IV	Symptoms at rest; cannot perform normal daily activities without symptoms

NYHA = New York Heart Association; WHO = World Health Organization.

E. Treatment Goals *(Domain 1, Task 3)*
1. Relieve acute dyspnea symptoms: Functional class I or II.
2. Improve exercise capacity: 6-minute walk test of at least 380 (to 440) m.
3. Normalization of right ventricular function: Right atrial pressure less than 8 mm Hg and cardiac index greater than 2.5 L/minute/m^{2}4.   Cardiopulmonary exercise testing: Peak oxygen consumption greater than 15 mL/minute/kg and ventilatory equivalent for carbon dioxide less than 45 L/minute
5. BNP concentration normal

F. For Acute Vasodilator Response Testing *(Domain 1, Task 2)*
1. Use intravenous epoprostenol, inhaled nitric oxide, or intravenous adenosine.
2. Positive response: Reduction in mPAP of at least 10 mm Hg to an absolute mPAP of less than 40 mm Hg
3. Positive response predicts mortality reduction with long-term calcium channel blocker or vasodilator use.

XVIII. TREATMENT OF PULMONARY HYPERTENSION *(Domain 1, Tasks 3, 4, 5, 6)*

A. Reassessment – Should include functional class determination and a 6-minute walk test every 3–6 months, with RHC less often

B. Satisfactory Condition – Functional classes I and II, ambulated 380 m or greater (or 1250 ft) during 6-minute walk test, with a cardiac index of 2.2 L/minute/m^2 or greater and an mPAP less than 12 mm Hg

Table 63. Initial PAH Treatment Algorithm

Supportive Care: Treat corrective causes of hypoxemia, and avoid dehydration, pain, fatigue, high altitude, smoking, pregnancy, iron deficiency, etc.
Oxygen to maintain O_2 saturation > 90%, diuretic if peripheral edema or ascites
Supervised exercise activity (avoid strenuous exercise)
Oral anticoagulation, warfarin (INR 1.5–2.5) if IPAH, heritable PAH, or PAH caused by anorexigens, or associated PAH;   ± diuretics ± digoxin   (anticoagulation to prevent catheter thrombosis [IV prostaglandin use] and venous thromboembolism)
Immunizations for influenza and Pneumococcus
Avoid pregnancy: Discuss effective methods of birth control with women of childbearing potential
Positive response to acute vasoreactivity testing
Initiate oral CCB   - If sustained response, continue CCB   - If no sustained response, initiate one or more agents below based on the WHO FC

CCB = calcium channel blocker; INR = international normalized ratio; IPAH = idiopathic pulmonary arterial hypertension; IV = intravenous; PAH = pulmonary arterial hypertension; WHO FC = World Health Organization functional class.

C. Therapy Options
   1. Initial therapy with one agent from the endothelin pathway, prostacyclin pathway, or nitric oxide pathway (most common in practice), followed by sequential combination therapy; or
   2. Initial therapy with combination therapy of two agents from different classes/having differing actions

Recommendation Grade[a]	WHO FC II	WHO FC III	WHO FC IV
I	Ambrisentan Bosentan Macitentan[b]Riociguat Sildenafil Tadalafil	Ambrisentan Bosentan Macitentan[b]Riociguat Sildenafil Tadalafil Epoprostenol IV[b]Iloprost inhaled Treprostinil subcutaneous or inhaled	Epoprostenol IV[b]
IIa		Iloprost IV Treprostinil IV	Ambrisentan Bosentan Macitentan[b]Riociguat Sildenafil Tadalafil Iloprost inhaled and IV Treprostinil Subcutaneous, IV, or inhaled
IIb	Initial combination therapy	Initial combination therapy	Initial combination therapy

[a]Grade I recommendation is one with strong evidence that is recommended or indicated. Grade IIa recommendation is one where evidence favors use, and treatment should be considered. Grade IIb recommendation is one where usefulness/efficacy is less well established or is based on opinion: May be recommended.

[b]Morbidity or mortality as a primary end point in a randomized controlled study or a reduction in all-cause mortality (prospectively defined).

IV = intravenous; WHO FC = World Health Organization functional class.

From: 5th World Symposium on Pulmonary Hypertension (sponsored by the European Respiratory Society), 2013; Nice, France. If refractory/unresponsive, reassess: Consider combination therapy, investigational protocols, atrial septostomy, lung transplantation.

Table 64. Overview of PAH Treatment Options (5th World Symposium)

Drug/Mechanism/ Indication	Dose	Adverse Effects	Considerations
Calcium channel blockers Class II PAH	Varies by agent and patient tolerance	Hypotension, headache, dizziness, peripheral edema, cardiac conduction delay (diltiazem)	Should not be used empirically without positive response to acute vasodilatory response testing Diltiazem, amlodipine, nifedipine most commonly used Select agent on the basis of HR at baseline If tachycardia, choose diltiazem If bradycardia, choose amlodipine, nifedipine
Epoprostenol (Flolan, Veletri) Prostanoid Class III–IV PAH	2–40 ng/kg/ minute IV	Jaw pain, nausea, vomiting, flushing, headache, muscle aches and pain, catheter-related thrombosis, and IV line infections; rebound worsening of symptoms if abruptly discontinued	Continuous IV infusion by pump Flolan: Unstable at acidic pH and room temperature (refrigerate or use ice packs before and during infusion) Veletri: Stable at room temperature Drug requires reconstitution in sterile environment Medical emergency if infusion interrupted (half-life – 6 minutes) – Spare drug cassette and infusion pump should be kept available
Treprostinil (Remodulin, Tyvaso) Prostanoid Class III–IV PAH	1.25- to 40-ng/ kg/minute subcutaneous infusion, IV Inhaled	Severe erythema and induration (83%) and injection site pain (85%) limits use; also headache, nausea, diarrhea, rash	Longer half-life (half-life – 3 hours) – Longer to seek medical attention Premixed, prefilled syringe easier to administer Local treatments (hot/cold packs or topical analgesics) can be used to minimize infusion site discomfort Moving infusion site every 3 days minimizes irritation
Inhaled iloprost (Ventavis) Prostanoid Class III–IV PAH	2.5 × 1; then 5 mcg/inhalation by nebulizer six to nine times daily while awake	Mild, transient cough, flushing, headache, syncope	Requires 6–9 inhalations daily (15 minutes each with jet nebulizer) Prodose AAD nebulization system required Inhaled form has fewer systemic adverse reactions Use no more than every 2 hours

Table 64. Overview of PAH Treatment Options (5th World Symposium) *(continued)*

Drug/Mechanism/ Indication	Dose	Adverse Effects	Considerations
Bosentan (Tracleer) Nonselective endothelin receptor antagonist (ET_A and ET_B) Class II–IV PAH	62.5–125 mg PO twice daily Initiate at 62.5 mg orally twice daily for 4 weeks; then increase to 125 mg twice daily Patients weighing <40 kg should receive 62.5 mg twice daily	Peripheral edema 5%–14%, hypotension 7%, increased LFTs 11%, flushing 7%–14%, palpitations 5%, anemia 3%	Severe drug interactions with glyburide (increased LFT results) and cyclosporine (decreased efficacy of both cyclosporine and bosentan) Monitor LFTs monthly (repeat if >3 times baseline to confirm; if >5 x baseline, discontinue; if >3 and ≤5 x baseline, reduce dose to 62.5 mg daily; repeat LFTs every 2 weeks if >3 x baseline Monitor hemoglobin/hematocrit at initiation, 1 month, 3 months, and every 3 months thereafter Potential teratogen; if childbearing age, use two contraceptive methods (reduced efficacy of hormonal contraceptives); monthly pregnancy test required; decreases concentrations of norethindrone and ethinyl estradiol Bosentan is a substrate of CYP2C9 and CYP3A Bosentan is an inducer of CYP3A and CYP2C9 Bosentan is a substrate of OATP Efficacy decreased with inducers, and toxicity increased with inhibitors of CYP 2C9 and 3A4 Concomitant cyclosporine contraindicated (bosentan concentrations increased 4-fold and cyclosporine concentrations decreased by 50), glyburide contraindicated (increased LFT values, bosentan concentrations decreased 30% and glyburide increased 40%) May decrease the concentrations/efficacy of simvastatin, lovastatin, atorvastatin Animal data indicate increased concentrations of bosentan when tacrolimus coadministered Warfarin coadministration showed no significant INR changes Coadministration with sildenafil reduces sildenafil concentrations by 63% and increases bosentan concentrations by 50% (no dose change recommended) Discontinue bosentan 36 hours before initiating ritonavir; then initiate bosentan at 62.5 mg daily or every other day

Table 64. Overview of PAH Treatment Options (5th World Symposium) *(continued)*

Drug/Mechanism/ Indication	Dose	Adverse Effects	Considerations
Ambrisentan (Letairis) Selective endothelin receptor antagonist (ET$_A$ only) Class II–II PAH	5–10 mg PO once daily	Peripheral edema 17%, hypotension 0%, increased LFT results 0%–2.8%, flushing 4%, palpitations 5%, fluid retention, anemia (decreases in Hgb of 0.9–1.2 g/dL observed within first few weeks of initiation)	Caution with cyclosporine – Maximal dose is 5 mg daily Contraindicated in patients with idiopathic pulmonary fibrosis Potential teratogen (see above comments) Measure Hgb at initiation, 1 month, and periodically thereafter Coadministration with cyclosporine resulted in 2-fold increases in ambrisentan concentrations – Limit ambrisentan dose to 5 mg orally daily
Macetentan[a] (Opsumit) Nonselective endothelin receptor antagonist (ET$_A$ and ET$_B$)	10 mg PO once daily	Anemia (13%), nasopharyngitis/ pharyngitis (20%), bronchitis (12%), headache (14%), influenza (6%), and urinary tract infection (9%)	REMS: Potential teratogen; if childbearing age, use two contraceptive methods (reduced efficacy of hormonal contraceptives); monthly pregnancy test required Periodic Hgb/Hct monitoring (recommended at initiation and as clinically indicated; studies required laboratory tests at baseline, 3 months, 6 months, and every 6 months thereafter) Baseline LFTs and, if clinically indicated, signs of liver failure such as nausea, vomiting, right upper quadrant pain, anorexia, vomiting, etc. (trials did not show increased risk of hepatotoxicity) Active metabolite contributes 40% of activity Half-life of parent drug is 16 hours and active metabolite 48 hours CYP3A4 and CYP2C19 (lesser) substrate Avoid strong CYP3A4 inducers (e.g., rifampin) and strong CYP3A4 inhibitors (e.g., ritonavir, ketoconazole stated in labeling but also clarithromycin, itraconazole, posaconazole, voriconazole)
Sildenafil (Revatio) Phosphodiesterase inhibitor Class II–IV PAH	20 mg PO three times daily (doses as high as 80 mg three times daily have been used in some trials)	Headache, epistaxis, facial flushing, bluish or blurry vision, light sensitivity, dyspepsia, insomnia	Half-life 4–5 hours May augment effects of other vasodilators when used in combination (especially prostacyclin, α-blockers, amlodipine, other antihypertensives, and alcohol) Contraindicated in patients receiving nitrates Sildenafil is a CYP3A4 substrate Avoid combined use with strong CYP3A4 inhibitors (e.g., ritonavir, cimetidine, erythromycin) and inducers (rifampin) (The FDA lists cimetidine as a weak inhibitor and erythromycin as a moderate inhibitor)

Table 64. Overview of PAH Treatment Options (5th World Symposium) *(continued)*

Drug/Mechanism/ Indication	Dose	Adverse Effects	Considerations
Tadalafil (Adcirca) Phosphodiesterase inhibitor Class II–IV PAH	40 mg PO once daily; initiate 20 mg PO once daily if concomitant ritonavir	Headache, flushing, indigestion, nausea, backache, myalgia, nasopharyngitis, respiratory tract infection	Half-life 17.5 hours May augment effects of other vasodilators when used in combination (especially prostacyclin, α-blockers, antihypertensives, alcohol) Contraindicated in patients receiving nitrates If CrCl = 31–80 mL/minute, initiate 20 mg PO once daily and titrate as tolerated If CrCl < 30 mL/minute or hemodialysis, avoid use If Child-Pugh class A or B, initiate 20 mg PO once daily and titrate as tolerated If Child-Pugh class C, avoid use Tadalafil is a CYP3A substrate Avoid use with potent CYP3A4 inhibitors (erythromycin, ketoconazole, itraconazole, grapefruit juice)/inducers (rifampin, carbamazepine, phenytoin, phenobarbital) When initiating ritonavir, discontinue tadalafil at least 24 hours before starting ritonavir; then reinitiate tadalafil at 20 mg daily after at least 1 week of ritonavir
Riociguat (Adempas) sGC stimulator[b] For chronic thromboembolic PH and class II–IV PAH	1 mg PO three times daily up to 2.5 mg PO three times daily (can be tapered to 0.5 mg PO three times daily if intolerance)	Headache, dyspepsia, GERD, gastritis, nausea, vomiting, dizziness, hypotension, bleeding, anemia, diarrhea, constipation	P-gp and BCRP substrate (consider lower dose for patients receiving concomitant strong inhibitors; cyclosporine is an inhibitor of BCRP) No experience with CrCl < 15 mL/minute Contraindicated with nitrates and NO donors including specific PDE-5 inhibitors (sildenafil, tadalafil, vardenafil) or nonspecific PDE-5 inhibitors (dipyridamole, theophylline) Potential teratogen; if childbearing age, use two contraceptive methods (reduced efficacy of hormonal contraceptives); monthly pregnancy test required Black box warning regarding embryo/fetal toxicity: REMS for female patients regardless of childbearing potential; pharmacies must register and dispense only to authorized users

[a]SERAPHIN study results: Macitentan 10 mg daily reduced the risk of the primary composite end point - Death, atrial septostomy, lung transplantation, initiation of treatment with intravenous or subcutaneous prostanoids, or worsening of PAH - By 45% compared with placebo with hazard ratioHR 0.55 (97.5% CI, 0.39–0.76; p<0.001). Other results included a significant increase in 6-minute walk of 12.5 m and a reduction in hospitalizations.

[b]sGC is an enzyme in the cardiopulmonary vasculature that serves as the receptor for NO. Activation of sGC by NO causes synthesis of cGMP, regulating vascular tone, proliferation, fibrosis, and inflammatory processes. Riociguat has a dual mechanism of action: (1) Sensitizes sGC to endogenous NO through stabilization of the sGC-NO complex and (2) direct agonist of sGC (not NO-dependent). Riociguat induces vasodilation through stimulation of the NO-sGC-cGMP pathway by increasing concentrations of cGMP.

AAD = antiarrhythmic drug; BCRP = human breast cancer resistance protein; cGMP = cyclic guanosine monophosphate; CI = confidence interval; CrCl = creatinine clearance; CYP = cytochrome P450; ET antagonists = endothelin antagonists; FDA = U.S. Food and Drug Administration; GERD = gastroesophageal reflux disease; Hct = hematocrit; Hgb = hemoglobin; HR = heart rate; INR = international normalized ratio; IV = intravenous; LFT = liver function test; NO = nitric oxide; OATP = organic anion transport protein; PAH = pulmonary arterial hypertension; PDE-5 = phosphodiesterase type-5; P-gp = P-glycoprotein; PO = orally; REMS = Risk Evaluation and Mitigation Strategies; sGC = soluble guanylate cyclase.

Reference: Galie N, Corris PA, Frost A, et al. Updated treatment algorithm of pulmonary arterial hypertension. J Am Coll Cardiol 2013;62(25 suppl):D60-72.

Table 65. Cost Comparison of Oral Agents Used to Treat PAH in Nonresponders to CCB Therapy

Drug	AWP Unit Price	30-Day Supply
Riociguat (Adempas, Bayer AG) 2.5-mg tablets	$100.00/tablet tid	$9000.00
Bosentan (Tracleer, Actelion) 125-mg tablets	$136.80/tablet bid	$8208.00
Macitentan (Opsumit, Actelion) 10-mg tablets	$273.60/tablet daily	$8208.00
Ambrisentan (Letairis, Gilead) 10-mg tablets	$257.93/tablet daily	$7737.90
Sildenafil (Revatio, Pfizer) 20-mg tablets	$25.72/tablet tid	$2314.80
Tadalafil (Adcirca, Lilly) 20-mg tablets	$34.85/tablet x 2 tablets daily	$2091.00

AWP = average wholesale price; bid = twice daily; CCB = calcium channel blocker; PAH = pulmonary arterial hypertension; tid = three times daily.

From: Red Book Online [Internet]. Greenwood Village, CO: Truven Health Analytics, 2014. Available at http://www.redbook.com/redbook/online/. Accessed January 20, 2014

Patient Cases

Questions 22 and 23 pertain to the following case.

P.L. is a 35-year-old woman with PAH associated with HIV infection who has dyspnea and fatigue with activities of daily living but not at rest. Her LFT results are normal, hemoglobin concentration is 13.5 g/dL, and CrCl is 90 mL/minute.

22. Which option best represents the World Health Organization (WHO) functional class in which her PAH symptoms fall?

   A. I.
   B. II.
   C. III.
   D. IV.

23. P.L. is unresponsive to vasodilator testing. Concomitant medications include ritonavir-boosted atazanavir and tenofovir disoproxil fumarate/emtricitabine. Atazanavir is a CYP3A4 inhibitor. Which is the best first-line therapy for treatment of PAH in P.L.?

   A. Sildenafil.
   B. Ambrisentan.
   C. Bosentan.
   D. Macitentan.

REFERENCES

Thromboembolism

1. Ageno W, Gallus AS, Wittkowsky A, et al. Oral anticoagulant therapy: Antithrombotic Therapy and Prevention, 9th ed: American College of Chest Physicians Evidence-Based Clinical Practice Guidelines. Chest 2012;141:e44s-88s.

2. Agnelli G, Buller HR, Cohen A, et al. Apixaban for extended treatment of venous thromboembolism. N Engl J Med 2013;368:699-708.

3. Agnelli G, Buller HR, Cohen A, et al. Oral apixaban for the treatment of acute venous thromboembolism. N Engl J Med 2013;369:799-808.

4. Barrett YC, Wang Z, Frost C, et al. Clinical laboratory measurement of direct factor Xa inhibitors: anti-Xa assay is preferable to prothrombin time assay. Thromb Haemost 2010;104:1263-71.

5. Camm AJ, Kirchhof P, De Caterina R, et al. 2012 focused update of the ESC Guidelines for the management of atrial fibrillation: an update of the 2010 ESC Guidelines for the management of atrial fibrillation: developed with the special contribution of the European Heart Rhythm Association. Eur Heart J 2012;33:2719-47.

6. Connolly G, Spyropoulos AC. Practical issues, limitations, and periprocedural management of the NOAC's. J Thromb Thrombolysis 2013;36:212-22.

7. Connolly SJ, Ezekowitz MD, Yusuf S, et al. Dabigatran versus warfarin in patients with atrial fibrillation. N Engl J Med 2009;361:1139-51.

8. Connolly SJ, Ezekowitz MD, Yusuf S, et al. Newly identified events in the RE-LY trial. N Engl J Med 2010;363:1875-6.

9. Douketis JD, Spyropoulos AC, Spencer FA, et al. Perioperative management of antithrombotic therapy: Antithrombotic Therapy and Prevention, 9th ed: American College of Chest Physicians Evidence-Based Clinical Practice Guidelines. Chest 2012;141:e326s-50s.

10. Eikelboom JW, Connolly SJ, Bruecmann M, et al. Dabigatran versus warfarin in patients with mechanical heart valves. N Engl J Med 2013;369:1206-14.

11. The EINSTEIN-DVT Investigators. Oral rivaroxaban for symptomatic venous thromboembolism. N Engl J Med 2010;363:2499-510.

12. The EINSTEIN-PE Investigators. Oral rivaroxaban for the treatment of symptomatic pulmonary embolism. N Engl J Med 2012;366:127-97.

13. Fang MC, Go AS, Borowsky LH, et al. A new risk scheme to predict warfarin-associated hemorrhage: the ATRIA (Anticoagulation and Risk Factors in Atrial Fibrillation) Study. J Am Coll Cardiol 2011;58:395-401.

14. Friberg L, Rosenqvist M, Lip GY. Evaluation of risk stratification schemes for ischaemic stroke and bleeding in 182,678 patients with atrial fibrillation: the Swedish Atrial Fibrillation cohort study. Eur Heart J 2012;33:1500-10.

15. Furie KL, Goldstein LB, Albers GW, et al. Oral antithrombotic agents for the prevention of stroke in nonvalvular atrial fibrillation: a science advisory for healthcare professionals from the American Heart Association/American Stroke Association. Stroke 2012;43:3442-53.

16. Fuster V, Ryden LE, Cannom DS, et al. ACC/AHA/ESC 2006 guidelines for the management of patients with atrial fibrillation: a report of the American College of Cardiology/American Heart Association Task Force on Practice Guidelines and the European Society of Cardiology Committee for Practice Guidelines (Writing Committee to Revise the 2001 Guidelines for the Management of Patients With Atrial Fibrillation): developed in collaboration with the European Heart Rhythm Association and the Heart Rhythm Society. Circulation 2006;114:e257-354.

17. Gage BF, Waterman AD, Shannon W, et al. Validation of clinical classification schemes for predicting stroke: results from the National Registry of Atrial Fibrillation. JAMA 2001;285:2864-70.

18. Garcia DA, Baglin TP, Weitz JI, et al. Parental anticoagulants: Antithrombotic Therapy and Prevention, 9th ed: American College of Chest Physicians Evidence-Based Clinical Practice Guidelines. Chest 2012;141:e24s-43s.

19. Giugliano RP, Ruff CT, Braunwald E, et al. Edoxaban versus warfarin in patients with atrial fibrillation. N Engl J Med 2013;369:2093-104.

20. Gould MK, Garcia DA, Wren SM, et al. Prevention of VTE in nonorthopedic surgical patients: Antithrombotic Therapy and Prevention, 9th ed: American College of Chest Physicians Evidence-Based Clinical Practice Guidelines. Chest 2012;141:e227s-77s.

21. Granger CB, Alexander JH, McMurray JJ, et al. Apixaban versus warfarin in patients with atrial fibrillation. N Engl J Med 2011;365:981-92.

22. Heneghan C, Ward A, Perera R; The Self-Monitoring Trialist Collaboration. Self-monitoring of oral anticoagulation: systematic review and meta-analysis of individual patient data. Lancet 2012;379:322-34.

23. The Hokusai-VTE Investigators. Edoxaban versus warfarin for the treatment of symptomatic venous thromboembolism. N Engl J Med 2013;369:1406-15.

24. Holbrook A, Schulman S, Witt DM, et al. Evidence-based management of anticoagulant therapy: Antithrombotic Therapy and Prevention, 9th ed: American College of Chest Physicians Evidence-Based Clinical Practice Guidelines. Chest 2012;141:e152s-84s.

25. Kahn SR, Lim W, Dunn AS, et al. Prevention of VTE in nonsurgical patients: Antithrombotic Therapy and Prevention, 9th ed: American College of Chest Physicians Evidence-Based Clinical Practice Guidelines. Chest 2012;141:e195S-226s.

26. Kearon C, Akl EA, Comerota AJ, et al. Antithrombotic therapy for VTE disease: Antithrombotic Therapy and Prevention, 9th ed: American College of Chest Physicians Evidence-Based Clinical Practice Guidelines. Chest 2012;141:e419s-94s.

27. Lip GYH, Nieuwlaat R, Pisters R, et al. Refining clinical risk stratification for predicting stroke and thromboembolism in atrial fibrillation using a novel risk factor-based approach: the Euro Heart Survey on Atrial Fibrillation. Chest 2010;137:263-72.

28. Nutescu EA, Dager WE, Kalus JS, et al. Management of bleeding and reversal strategies for oral anticoagulants: clinical practice considerations. Am J Health Syst Pharm 2013;70:1914-29.

29. Nutescu EA, Shapiro NL, Ibrahim S, et al. Warfarin and its interactions with foods, herbs and other dietary supplements. Expert Opin Drug Saf 2006;5:433-51.

30. Patel MR, Mahaffey KW, Garg J, et al. Rivaroxaban versus warfarin in nonvalvular atrial fibrillation. N Engl J Med 2011;365:883-91.

31. Schulman S, Kearon C, Kakkar AK, et al. Extended use of dabigatran, warfarin or placebo in venous thromboembolism. N Engl J Med 2013;368:709-18.

32. Siegal DM, Cuker A. Reversal of novel oral anticoagulants in patients with major bleeding. J Thromb Thrombolysis 2013;35:391-8.

33. Wann LS, Curtis AB, Ellenbogen KA, et al. 2011 ACCF/AHA/HRS focused update on the management of patients with atrial fibrillation (update on dabigatran). Circulation 2011;123:104-23.

34. Wells PS, Owen C, Doucette S, et al. Does this patient have deep vein thrombosis? JAMA 2006;295:199-207.

35. Whitlock RP, Sun JC, Fremes SE, et al. Antithrombotic and thrombolytic therapy for valvular heart disease: Antithrombotic Therapy and Prevention, 9th ed: American College of Chest Physicians Evidence-Based Clinical Practice Guidelines. Chest 2012;141:e576s-600s.

36. You JJ, Singer DE, Howard DA, et al. Antithrombotic therapy for atrial fibrillation: Antithrombotic Therapy and Prevention, 9th ed: American College of Chest Physicians Evidence-Based Clinical Practice Guidelines. Chest 2012;141:e531s-75s.

Heart Failure

1. Abraham WT, Fisher WG, Smith AL, et al. Cardiac resynchronization in chronic heart failure. N Engl J Med 2002;346:1845-53.

2. Ahmed A, Rich MW, Love TE, Lloyd-Jones DM, et al. Digoxin and reduction in mortality and hospitalization in heart failure: a comprehensive post hoc analysis of the DIG trial. Eur Heart J 2006;27:178-86.

3. Bristow MR, Saxon LA, Boehmer J, et al. Cardiac-resynchronization therapy with or without an implantable defibrillator in advanced chronic heart failure. N Engl J Med 2004;350:2140-50.

4. CIBIS II Investigators. The Cardiac Insufficiency Bisoprolol Study II (CIBIS-II): a randomised trial. Lancet 1999;353:9-13.

5. Cleland JG, Daubert JC, Erdmann E, et al. The effect of cardiac resynchronization on morbidity and mortality in heart failure. N Engl J Med 2005;352:1539-49.

6. Cohn JN, Tognoni G; Valsartan Heart Failure Trial Investigators. A randomized trial of the angiotensin-receptor blocker valsartan in chronic heart failure. N Engl J Med 2001;345:1667-75.

7. Feldman D, Pamboukian SV, Teuteberg JJ, et al. The 2013 International Society for Heart and Lung Transplantation guidelines for mechanical circulatory support: executive summary. J Heart Lung Transplant 2013;32:157-87.

8. Fonarow GC, Abraham WT, Albert NM, et al. Influence of a performance-improvement initiative on quality of care for patients hospitalized with heart failure: results of the Organized Program to Initiate Lifesaving Treatment in Hospitalized Patients with Heart Failure (OPTIMIZE-HF). Arch Intern Med 2007;167:1493-502.

9. Granger CB, Ertl G, Kuch J, et al. Randomized trial of candesartan cilexetil in the treatment of patients with congestive heart failure and a history of intolerance to angiotensin-converting enzyme inhibitors. Am Heart J 2000;139:609-17.

10. Koshman SL, Charrois TL, Simpson SH, et al. Pharmacist care of patients with heart failure: a systematic review of randomized trials. Arch Intern Med 2008;168:687-94.

11. Long JW, Kfoury AG, Slaughter MS, et al. Long-term destination therapy with the HeartMate XVE left ventricular assist device: improved outcomes since the REMATCH study. Congest Heart Fail 2005;11:133-8.

12. Massie BM, Carson PE, McMurray JJ, et al. Irbesartan in patients with heart failure and preserved ejection fraction. N Engl J Med 2008;359:2456-67.

13. McMurray JJ, Ostergren J, Swedberg K, et al. Effects of candesartan in patients with chronic heart failure and reduced left-ventricular systolic function taking angiotensin-converting-enzyme inhibitors: the CHARM-Added trial. Lancet 2003;362:767-71.

14. McMurray JJ, Packer M, Desai AS, et al. Angiotensin-neprilysin inhibition versus enalapril in heart failure. N Engl J Med. 2014;371(11):993-1004

15. MERIT-HF Investigators. Effect of metoprolol CR/XL in chronic heart failure: Metoprolol CR/XL Randomised Intervention Trial in Congestive Heart Failure (MERIT-HF). Lancet 1999;353:2001-7.

16. Milfred-LaForest SK, Chow SL, DiDomenico RJ, et al. Clinical pharmacy services in heart failure: an opinion paper from the Heart Failure Society of America and American College of Clinical Pharmacy Cardiology Practice and Research Network. Pharmacotherapy 2013;33:529-48.

17. Moss AJ, Hall WJ, Cannom DS, et al. Cardiac-resynchronization therapy for the prevention of heart-failure events. N Engl J Med 2009;361:1329-38.

18. Packer M, Coats AJ, Fowler MB, et al. Effect of carvedilol on survival in severe chronic heart failure. N Engl J Med 2001;344:1651-8.

19. Pfeffer MA, McMurray JJ, Velazquez EJ, et al. Valsartan, captopril, or both in myocardial infarction complicated by heart failure, left ventricular dysfunction, or both. N Engl J Med 2003;349:1893-906.

20. Pitt B, Remme W, Zannad F, et al. Eplerenone, a selective mineralocorticoid receptor blocker, in patients with left ventricular dysfunction after myocardial infarction. N Engl J Med 2003;348:1309-21.

21. Pitt B, Zannad F, Remme WJ, et al. The effect of spironolactone on morbidity and mortality in patients with severe heart failure: Randomized Aldactone Evaluation Study Investigators. N Engl J Med 1999;341:709-17.

22. Poole-Wilson PA, Swedberg K, Cleland JG, et al. Comparison of carvedilol and metoprolol on clinical outcomes in patients with chronic heart failure in the Carvedilol Or Metoprolol European Trial (COMET): randomised controlled trial. Lancet 2003;362:7-13.

23. Pruett AE, Lee AK, Patterson JH, et al. Biomarker guided therapy for heart failure: focus on natriuretic peptides [published online ahead of print November 17, 2013]. Curr Cardiol Rev.

24. Starling RC, Moazami N, Silvestry SC, et al. Unexpected abrupt increase in left ventricular assist device thrombosis. N Engl J Med 2014;370:33-40.

25. Swedberg K, Komajda M, Böhm M, et al. Ivabradine and outcomes in chronic heart failure (SHIFT): a randomised placebo-controlled study. Lancet. 2010;376(9744):875-85

26. Taylor AL, Ziesche S, Yancy C, et al. Combination of isosorbide dinitrate and hydralazine in blacks with heart failure. N Engl J Med 2004;351:2049-57.

27. The Digitalis Investigation Group. The effect of digoxin on mortality and morbidity in patients with heart failure. N Engl J Med 1997;336:525-33.

28. Yancy CW, Jessup M, Bozkurt B, et al. 2013 ACCF/AHA guideline for the management of heart failure: a report of the American College of Cardiology Foundation/American Heart Association Task Force on Practice Guidelines. J Am Coll Cardiol 2013;62:e147-239.

29. Zannad F, McMurray JJ, Krum H, et al. Eplerenone in patients with systolic heart failure and mild symptoms. N Engl J Med 2011;364:11-21.

Arrhythmias

1. Anderson JL, Halperin JL, Albert JM, et al. Management of patients with atrial fibrillation (compilation of 2006 ACCF/AHA/ESC and 2011 ACCF/AHA/HRS recommendations): a report of the American College of Cardiology/American Heart Association Task Force on Practice Guidelines. J Am Coll Cardiol 2013;61:1935-44.

2. January CT, Wann S, Alpert JS, et al. 2014 AHA/ACC/HRS Guideline for the Management of Patients With Atrial Fibrillation: executive summary. J Am Coll Cardiol 2014. doi: 10.1016/j.jacc.2014.03.021. Blomstrom-Lundqvist C, Scheinman MM, Aliot EM, et al. ACC/AHA/ESC 2003 guidelines for the management of patients with supraventricular arrhythmias – executive summary: a report of the American College of Cardiology/American Heart Association Task Force on Practice Guidelines and the European Society of Cardiology Committee for Practice Guidelines. J Am Coll Cardiol 2003;42:1493-531.

3. Calkins H, Kuck KH, Cappato R, et al. 2012 HRS/EHRA/ECAS expert consensus statement on catheter and surgical ablation of atrial fibrillation: recommendations for patient selection, procedural techniques, patient management and follow-up, definitions, endpoints, and research trial design: a report of the Heart Rhythm Society (HRS) Task Force on Catheter and Surgical Ablation of Atrial Fibrillation. Developed in partnership with the European Heart Rhythm Association (EHRA), a registered branch of the European Society of Cardiology (ESC) and the European Cardiac Arrhythmia Society (ECAS); and in collaboration with the American College of Cardiology (ACC), American Heart Association (AHA), the Asia Pacific Heart Rhythm Society (APHRS), and the Society of Thoracic Surgeons (STS): endorsed by the governing bodies of the American College of Cardiology Foundation, the American Heart Association, the European Cardiac Arrhythmia Society, the European Heart Rhythm Association, the Society of Thoracic Surgeons, the Asia Pacific Heart Rhythm Society, and the Heart Rhythm Society. Heart Rhythm 2012;9:632-96.

4. Camm AJ, Lip G, De Caterina R, et al. 2012 focused update of the ESC guidelines for the management of atrial fibrillation: an update of the 2012 ESC guidelines for the management of atrial fibrillation: developed with the special contribution of the European Heart Rhythm Association. Eur Heart J 2012;33:2719-47.

5. Goldschlager N, Epstein AE, Naccarelli GV, et al. A practical guide for clinicians who treat patients with amiodarone: 2007. Heart Rhythm 2007;4:1250-9.

6. January CT, Wann S, Alpert JS, et al. 2014 AHA/ACC/HRS Guideline for the Management of Patients With Atrial Fibrillation: executive summary. J Am Coll Cardiol 2014. doi: 10.1016/j.jacc.2014.03.021.

7. Sanoski CA, Bauman JL. The arrhythmias. In: Talbert RL, DiPiro JT, Matzke GR, et al., eds. Pharmacotherapy: A Pathophysiologic Approach, 8th ed. New York: McGraw-Hill, 2011:XXX-XXX273-309.

8. Wann LS, Curtis AB, January CT, et al. 2011 ACCF/AHA/HRS focused update on the management of patients with atrial fibrillation (updating the 2006 guidelines): a report of the American College of Cardiology Foundation/American Heart Association Task Force on Practice Guidelines. Circulation 2011;123:104-23.

9. Zimetbaum P. Antiarrhythmic drug therapy for atrial fibrillation. Circulation 2012;125:381-9.

10. Zipes DP, Camm AJ, Borggrefe M, et al. ACC/AHA/ESC 2006 guidelines for the management of patients with ventricular arrhythmias and the prevention of sudden cardiac death – executive summary: a report of the American College of Cardiology/American Heart Association Task Force on Practice Guidelines and the European Society of Cardiology Committee for Practice Guidelines. J Am Coll Cardiol 2006;48:1064-108.

Pulmonary Arterial Hypertension

1. Bishop BM, Mauro VF, Skouri SJ. Practical considerations for the pharmacotherapy of pulmonary arterial hypertension. Pharmacotherapy 2012;32:838-55.

2. Galie N, Corris PA, Frost A, et al. Updated treatment algorithm of pulmonary arterial hypertension. J Am Coll Cardiol 2013;62(suppl):D60-72.

3. Galie N, Hoeper MM, Humbert M, et al. Guidelines for the diagnosis and treatment of pulmonary hypertension: the Task Force for the Diagnosis and Treatment of Pulmonary Hypertension of the European Society of Cardiology (ESC) and the European Respiratory Society (ERS), endorsed by the International Society of Heart and Lung Transplantation (ISHLT). Eur Heart J 2009;30:2493-537.

4. Ghofrani HA, D'Armini AM, Grimminger, F, et al. Riociguat for the treatment of chronic thromboembolic pulmonary hypertension. N Engl J Med 2013;369:319-29.

5. Ghofrani HA, Galié N, Grimminger F, et al. Riociguat for the treatment of pulmonary arterial hypertension. N Engl J Med 2013;369:330-40.

6. Hoeper MM, Bogaard HJ, Condliffe R, et al. Definitions and diagnosis of pulmonary hypertension. J Am Coll Cardiol 2013;62(suppl):D42-50.

7. McLaughlin VV, Gaine SP, Howard LS, et al. Treatment goals of pulmonary hypertension. J Am Coll Cardiol 2013;62(suppl):D73-81.

8. Pulido T, Adzerikho I, Channick RN, et al. Macitentan and morbidity and mortality in pulmonary arterial hypertension. N Engl J Med 2013;369:809-18.

9. Simonneau G, Gatzoulis MA, Adatia I, et al. Updated clinical classification of pulmonary hypertension. J Am Coll Cardiol 2013;62(suppl):D34-41.

10. Tackett KL, Stajich GV. Combination pharmacotherapy in the treatment of pulmonary arterial hypertension: continuing education article. J Pharm Pract 2013;26:18-28.

11. Tackett KL, Stajich GV. Combination pharmacotherapy in the treatment of pulmonary arterial hypertension: continuing education article. J Pharm Pract 2013;26:18-28.

12. Yao AY. Recent advances and future perspectives in therapeutic strategies for pulmonary arterial hypertension. J Cardiol 2012;60:344-9.

ANSWERS AND EXPLANATIONS TO PATIENT CASES

1. Answer C

The clinical probability score for this patient is 4; thus, he has a high probability of experiencing a DVT (see Table 3). He presents with swelling of his entire right lower extremity (1 point), erythema, and soreness of his right calf (1 point); he was recently bedridden because he underwent knee replacement surgery 2 weeks ago (1 point), and he has a history of DVT (1 point). There is no "very high" risk category.

2. Answer B

Use of D-dimer testing is effective to rule out VTE in the setting of a low pretest clinical probability; however, it is not as useful in cases of high pretest clinical probability. The diagnosis of DVT should be confirmed by objective testing before anticoagulation therapy is initiated. Although venography is the gold standard for diagnosis of DVT, it is rarely used in clinical practice because of technical difficulty and risk of adverse effects. A CT scan of the chest is used in the diagnosis of PE and not DVT. Duplex ultrasonography is considered a noninvasive test, has very good sensitivity and specificity for DVT, and is therefore considered the diagnostic test of choice.

3. Answer A

Although this is a recurrent DVT for this patient, indefinite treatment is not necessary. The previous DVT episode was secondary to a reversible risk factor (as is the current DVT) and occurred more than 25 years ago. Treatment for at least 3 months is an evidence-based recommendation. Longer treatment durations could be considered after 3 months, depending on the patient's preference and whether the patient tolerates the treatment well.

4. Answer C

Answer C (rivaroxaban 15 mg orally twice daily for 21 days, followed by 20 mg orally daily thereafter) is correct. OptionAnswers A, B, and D have either incorrect doses or frequencies. See Tables 7 and 8 for dosing guidelines.

5. Answer D

Many patients do not have an indication for dual antithrombotic therapy. In this case, whether the patient should even receive aspirin for primary prevention is controversial, with the U.S. Preventive Services Task Force recommending no aspirin at all because this patient's 10-year ASCVD risk is less than 10%, whereas the AHA/American Diabetes Association(ADA) recommends "optional" aspirin for a 10-year risk of 5%–10%. Only the Chest guidelines recommend aspirin because the patient is older than 50 years. Dual antithrombotic therapy significantly increases bleeding risk. Therefore, with unsure benefit and increased risk, aspirin therapy should at least be temporarily interrupted while the patient is receiving anticoagulation.

6. Answer D

The patient's $CHADS_2$ score is 3: age 75 years or older (1 point), uncontrolled HTN (1 point), and diabetes mellitus (1 point). A score of 0 is low risk, 1 is intermediate risk, and 2 or greater is high risk.

7. Answer: D

The patient's HAS-BLED score is 4: uncontrolled HTN (1 point), age older than 75 years (1 point), and prior bleeding (1 point, concomitant aspirin 1 point). Patients with scores of 3 or higher are at a high risk of bleeding.

8. Answer A

OptionAnswer B is incorrect because the patient's CrCl is less than 50 mL/minute, and the correct dose of rivaroxaban is 15 mg orally daily. OptionAnswer C is incorrect because a dabigatran dose of 150 mg twice daily is appropriate for a CrCl of 48 mL/minute. Aspirin plus clopidogrel is not an anticoagulant therapy, making OptionAnswer D incorrect. The patient has only one of the factors to dose-adjust apixaban (low body weight); therefore, the usual dose of apixaban 5 mg twice daily orally is correct. Apixaban is also an appropriate choice because it is the only agent among the answers to show lower bleeding risk than warfarin.

9. Answer: D

The patient's EF is less than 40%; therefore, she has HFrEF, not HFpEF (LVEF greater than 50%), making OptionAnswer A and OptionAnswer B incorrect. The patient has symptoms with minimal activity and is therefore in NYHA class III rather than II, making OptionAnswer A and OptionAnswer C incorrect. The patient has structural heart disease, as evidenced by her reduced LVEF, and has symptoms; therefore, she does not have stage-B HF, making OptionAnswer A and OptionAnswer C incorrect. The patient has stage-C HF (structural heart disease and symptoms) and reduced EF, making Answer D correct.

10. Answer: C

The patient's serum digoxin concentration is within the target desired for HF (0.4–0.9 ng/mL), making OptionAnswer A incorrect. The patient's serum potassium concentration is above 5 mEq/L; thus, an MRA should not be initiated currently, making OptionAnswer B and OptionAnswer D incorrect. The initial spironolactone dose for a patient with a CrCl of 36 mL/minute is 12.5 mg daily or every other day, making OptionAnswer B incorrect. The initial eplerenone dose for a patient with a CrCl of 36 mL/minute is 25 mg every other day, making OptionAnswer D incorrect. The combination of hydralazine and a nitrate was shown to reduce mortality in the AHeFT trial, and it is recommended by the 2013 ACCF/AHA HF guideline to be added to a β-blocker and ACE inhibitor for cases of persistent symptomatic NYHA class III or IV HF in an African American patient, making Answer C correct.

11. Answer: B

The patient, who has HFrEF, is receiving a target dose of an ACE inhibitor. Therefore, adding an ARB is not recommended, and Option Answer A is incorrect. The patient is not African American and is not receiving an MRA, and the patient has no contraindication to an MRA (renal function or potassium); therefore, an MRA is preferred to adding hydralazine plus nitrates currently, making Option Answer C incorrect. The estimated CrCl of this patient is 87 mL/minute; therefore, the initial eplerenone dose recommended is 25 mg/day, making Option Answer D incorrect. The correct spironolactone dose for a patient with a CrCl of 87 mL/minute is 12.5–25 mg/day, making Answer B correct.

12. Answer: A

The patient has HF symptoms and an EF greater than 50%; therefore, the patient has HFpEF, making Option Answer C and Option Answer D incorrect. The patient has no HF symptoms at rest and therefore does not have NYHA class IV symptoms, making Option Answer B and Option Answer D incorrect. Answer A is correct because the patient has HFpEF and symptoms with minimal activity.

13. Answer: B

Because the patient has HFpEF and HTN, the goal is to control BP according to established guidelines. He has no jugular venous distension or peripheral edema, so the diuretic dose should not be increased, making OptionAnswer A incorrect. The MRAs are indicated for HFrEF or as a fourth-line antihypertensive agent, making OptionAnswer C incorrect. The JNC 8 (Eighth Joint National Committee) recommends a goal BP of less than 140/90 mm Hg. His current HR is high enough to increase the metoprolol dose, making Answer B correct.

14. Answer: D

This patient has HFrEF. Patients with unstable HF were excluded from the RACE II trial comparing strict with lenient rate control; current AF practice guidelines describing the goal HR in AF exclude patients with an LVEF less than 40%, making Answer D correct and OptionAnswers A, B, and C incorrect.

15. Answer: B

OptionAnswer A is incorrect because the patient is not receiving anticoagulation and has not had a TEE showing no left atrial clot. OptionAnswer C and OptionAnswer D are incorrect because dofetilide is initiated only in hospitalized patients (and after serum, potassium, and magnesium concentrations are shown to be normal). Answer B is correct because anticoagulation is indicated for at least 3 weeks before cardioversion in the absence of a TEE. Rate control can be enhanced with an increased carvedilol dose, which may also be titrated to a target dose (25 mg orally twice daily) according to the patient's diagnosis of HFrEF.

16. Answer: B

This patient has an EF greater than 40%; therefore, the target HR, as specified in the 2011 ACCF/AHA/HRS AF guidelines, is less than 110 beats/minute (lenient rate control), making Answer B correct and OptionAnswers A, C, and D incorrect.

17. Answer: D

This patient has a structurally normal heart. Amiodarone is reserved for patients with structurally abnormal hearts (e.g., reduced LVEF) because of its toxicities with chronic use, making OptionAnswer A incorrect. The patient is currently taking hydrochlorothiazide, which is contra-indicated with dofetilide; therefore, OptionAnswer B is incorrect. Dronedarone has toxicities similar to those of amiodarone and is therefore reserved for patients whose other agents fail and who are intolerant of amiodarone; thus, OptionAnswer C is incorrect. According to the 2011 ACCF/AHA/HRS AF guidelines, flecainide is a first-line choice for patients with structurally normal hearts without QT prolongation, making Answer D correct.

18. Answer: D

The patient has been receiving amiodarone for weeks; therefore, drug interactions are already manifest. The patient's INR is within goal so the warfarin dose should not be changed, making OptionAnswer A and OptionAnswer C incorrect. The patient has not yet received a 10-g loading dose of amiodarone; therefore, the current dose of 400 mg should not be reduced, making OptionAnswer B incorrect. The serum digoxin concentration is above the goal range for a patient with HF (less than 1.0 ng/mL), and the patient's HR is low; therefore, the digoxin dose should be reduced. The maximal simvastatin dose that should be coadministered with amiodarone is 20 mg (see Table 574). Therefore, Answer D is correct.

19. Answer: D

This patient has a history of GI bleeding and therefore has a higher risk of bleeding. Anticoagulation is indicated because this is a mechanical heart valve. OptionAnswer B is incorrect because dabigatran is contraindicated in a patient with a mechanical heart valve. For mechanical valves in the aortic position, the intensity of warfarin recommended is an INR of 2–3; therefore, OptionAnswer C is incorrect and Answer D is correct. Aspirin is indicated at a dose of 81 mg for stroke prevention in all patients who are at low risk of bleeding; therefore, OptionAnswer A is incorrect.

20. Answer: D

Dabigatran should be avoided in patients with bioprosthetic valves, making OptionAnswer C incorrect. This patient is at high risk of stroke because the patient has a bioprosthetic valve plus AF; thus, anticoagulation is indicated, making OptionAnswer A, dual antiplatelet therapy, incorrect. The Chest guidelines recommend an INR of 2–3 for patients with a bioprosthetic valve and AF; therefore, Answer D is correct and OptionAnswer B is incorrect.

21. Answer: D

Guidelines recommend that in the absence of a requirement for anticoagulation (e.g., AF in this patient), dual antiplatelet therapy with low-dose aspirin and clopidogrel be given for 3 months after TAVR. This patient received 1 month of anticoagulation therapy; therefore, an additional 2 months of dual antiplatelet therapy with low-dose aspirin in indicated, making Answer D correct. OptionAnswer A is incorrect because it is single antiplatelet therapy, and the dose of aspirin is too high. OptionAnswer B and OptionAnswer C are incorrect because they represent single antiplatelet therapy.

22. Answer: C

This patient has symptoms with ordinary daily activity, but not at rest, making Answer C correct and OptionAnswer A (no symptoms), OptionAnswer B (symptoms only at moderate activity), and OptionAnswer D (symptoms at rest) incorrect.

23. Answer: B

Sildenafil (OptionAnswer A), bosentan (OptionAnswer C), and macitentan (OptionAnswer D) should be avoided in patients taking CYP3A4 inducers or strong CYP3A4 inhibitors and are not preferred in patients taking any inhibitors or substrates for CYP3A4. Ambrisentan has only one clinically significant drug interaction with cyclosporine; thus, ambrisentan would be preferred for this patient, for whom the HIV medications must need to be maintained, making Answer B correct.

ANSWERS AND EXPLANATIONS TO SELF-ASSESSMENT QUESTIONS

1. Answer: C

Warfarin should be overlapped with heparin for at least 5 days, making Option Answer A incorrect. The FDA-approved rivaroxaban dose for treatment of a PE is 15 mg twice daily, followed by 20 mg daily; thus, Option Answer B is incorrect. The dabigatran dose tested in the RE-MEDY and RE-SONATE trials was 150 mg twice daily, and parenteral anticoagulation is required for 5–10 days before starting dabigatran; therefore, Option Answer D is incorrect. The apixaban dose studied in the AMPLIFY trial was 10 mg twice daily for 7 days, followed by 5 mg twice daily for 6 months; therefore, Answer C is correct.

2. Answer: D

Rivaroxaban is a direct-acting factor Xa inhibitor. The sensitivity to a change in INR with PT, as well as aPTT and activated clotting times, is variable; therefore, Option Answer A is incorrect. The best measure of effect of a factor Xa concentration is an anti-Xa concentration; thus, Answer D is correct.

3. Answer: C

The patient has valvular heart disease and a bioprosthetic valve; therefore, newer oral anticoagulants should be avoided, making Option Answer B incorrect. The American College of Chest Physicians recommends warfarin for the first 3 months, followed by low-dose aspirin for stroke prevention after bioprosthetic mitral valve placement; therefore, Option Answer A, aspirin alone at the time of hospital discharge, is incorrect. The target INR therapeutic range for a patient with a bioprosthetic valve and requiring anticoagulation is 2–3, making Answer C correct.

4. Answer: A

Because of the increased risk of hyperkalemia when a mineralocorticoid receptor antagonist is added to an ACE inhibitor, frequent monitoring of potassium—within 3 days, at 1 week, and then monthly for the first 6 months—is recommended by the 2013 ACCF/AHA HF guidelines, making Answer A correct and OptionAnswers B, C, and D incorrect.

5. Answer: D

β-Blockers are the first-line rate control medication recommended by the ACCF/AHA/HRS AF guidelines; therefore, Answer D is correct. The patient requires additional rate control because the goal HR is less than 110 beats/minute for a patient with HFpEF, and the patient's current HR is 140 beats/minute; therefore, Option Answer A is incorrect. The patient's BP is high enough to tolerate an increased β-blocker dose. Enalapril does not lower HR, and the patient is at goal BP; therefore, Option Answer C is incorrect. Because warfarin is not effective immediately, it would require overlap with warfarin for at least 2–3 days before warfarin would become effective, making Option Answer B incorrect.

6. Answer: C

Digoxin is not effective for converting or maintaining NSR, making Option Answer A incorrect. The guidelines recommend that patients with structural heart disease (e.g., HFrEF) avoid sotalol and flecainide, making Option Answer B and Option Answer D incorrect.

7. Answer: C

The 2012 HRS guidelines recommend catheter ablation only for symptomatic patients with persistent or paroxysmal AF who have not responded to or had an arrhythmia recurrence while receiving one or more antiarrhythmic medications. Therefore, the patients in Options Answers A, B, and D have indications for catheter ablation of AF and these answers are incorrect. The patient in Answer C has permanent AF and therefore is not a candidate for ablation.

8. Answer: C

Liver function tests and a thyroid-stimulating hormone test are recommended to be done every 6 months, making Answer C correct. A lipid panel, SCr, and serum sodium are not a recommended component of amiodarone monitoring, making Option Answer A and Option Answer B incorrect. Pulmonary function testing is recommended only if the patient has symptoms; therefore, Option Answer D is incorrect.

9. Answer: A

The dose of warfarin should be reduced by 33%–50% when amiodarone is added; therefore, Answer A is correct. No dosing adjustments are required with rivaroxaban or atorvastatin when amiodarone is added; therefore, Option Answer B and Option Answer C are incorrect. Although amiodarone has β-blocking activity, the metoprolol dose need not be reduced proactively, but the HR should be monitored during the early phase of therapy in patients who do not have a pacemaker. Therefore, Option Answer D is incorrect.

10. Answer: D

The patient has sinus bradycardia and an HR of 50 beats/minute. Therefore, increasing the metoprolol dose (OptionAnswer A) and adding diltiazem (Option Answer B) are incorrect because this would increase the risk of heart block. Nitrates are contraindicated in severe aortic stenosis because they are venodilators, reducing preload and then LV volume, which may lead to worsening myocardial ischemia and hypotension because of reduced cardiac output, making Option Answer C incorrect. Answer D, amlodipine, is a second-line antianginal agent for a patient with severe aortic stenosis. Amlodipine does not lower HR but may increase coronary artery blood flow; it would therefore be preferred in a patient unable to tolerate other agents secondary to bradycardia.

11. Answer: D

For a patient in sinus rhythm, combination therapy with low-dose aspirin and clopidogrel is recommended for at least 3 months in patients undergoing TAVR, making Answer D correct. There is no published experience with prasugrel and TAVR, making Option Answer C incorrect. Anticoagulation would be indicated only for a patient with another reason for anticoagulation, such as AF, and in those situations, there are no specific guideline recommendations regarding triple therapy with anticoagulation plus dual antiplatelet therapy or anticoagulation with a single antiplatelet agent. Option Answer A and Option Answer B contain anticoagulation and are incorrect because the patient is in sinus rhythm.

12. Answer: C

The only agent that requires LFT monitoring is bosentan, a selective endothelin antagonist. Therefore, Answer C is correct, and OptionAnswers A, B, and D are incorrect.

Cardiology II

Emily K. McCoy, Pharm.D., BCACP

Auburn University
Harrison School of Pharmacy
Mobile, Alabama

Karen J. McConnell, Pharm.D., BCPS-AQ Cardiology, FCCP

Kaiser Permanente of Colorado
University of Colorado Skaggs School of Pharmacy
and Pharmaceutical Sciences
Denver, Colorado

Anne M. Denham, Pharm.D., BCPS-AQ Cardiology

Kaiser Permanente of Colorado
University of Colorado Skaggs School of Pharmacy
and Pharmaceutical Sciences
Denver, Colorado

Cardiology II

Emily K. McCoy, Pharm.D., BCACP

Auburn University
Harrison School of Pharmacy
Mobile, Alabama

Karen J. McConnell, Pharm.D., BCPS-AQ Cardiology, FCCP

Kaiser Permanente of Colorado
University of Colorado Skaggs School of Pharmacy
and Pharmaceutical Sciences
Denver, Colorado

Anne M. Denham, Pharm.D., BCPS-AQ Cardiology

Kaiser Permanente of Colorado
University of Colorado Skaggs School of Pharmacy
and Pharmaceutical Sciences
Denver, Colorado

Learning Objectives

1. Recommend regimens for primary and secondary prevention of coronary heart disease (CHD) events according to current guidelines and performance measures.
2. Calculate a patient's 10-year risk of CHD events by using the 2013 Pooled Cohort Equation.
3. Recommend an appropriate antiplatelet regimen after percutaneous coronary intervention according to current guidelines and product labeling for P2Y12 inhibitors and protease-activated receptor (PAR-1) antagonists.
4. Apply an understanding of the mechanism of action and effects of antihypertensive medications to construct an appropriate pharmacologic and therapeutic monitoring plan for a patient with hypertension (HTN).
5. Design an evidence-based HTN medication regimen according to comorbid conditions (e.g., chronic kidney disease [CKD], diabetes mellitus, CHD).
6. Develop a treatment strategy for patients who require combination antihypertensive therapy to achieve their blood pressure goals.
7. Integrate an understanding of the mechanism of action and effects of lipid medications to select appropriate pharmacologic therapy and develop a monitoring plan.
8. Create an evidence-based lipid-lowering medication regimen for primary and secondary prevention.
9. Formulate an appropriate pharmacotherapeutic regimen for patients with dyslipidemia and comorbid conditions (e.g., CKD, potential drug interactions, chronic elevation in creatine kinase).
10. Develop a treatment strategy for patients with peripheral arterial disease.
11. Recommend an evidence-based medication regimen for secondary prevention of stroke and transient ischemic attack (TIA).

Self-Assessment Questions

Answers and explanations to these questions can be found at the end of the chapter.

1. A 56-year-old white man with type 2 diabetes mellitus (DM) who is a nonsmoker is concerned about his risk of CHD. His vital signs include blood pressure (BP) 145/98 mm Hg, heart rate (HR) 70 beats/minute, and body mass index (BMI) 26.5 kg/m². His fasting laboratory test results today include serum creatinine (SCr) 0.8 mg/dL, total cholesterol (TC) 188 mg/dL, low-density lipoprotein cholesterol (LDL-C) 130 mg/dL, high-density lipoprotein cholesterol (HDL-C) 40 mg/dL, and triglycerides (TG) 90 mg/dL. Which is the best strategy for primary prevention of CHD for this patient?

   A. Ramipril 5 mg orally.
   B. Aspirin 81 mg/day orally.
   C. Simvastatin 80 mg/day orally plus lisinopril 10 mg/day orally.
   D. Aspirin 81 mg/day orally plus atorvastatin 40 mg/day orally plus lisinopril 10 mg/day orally.

2. A 56-year-old female nonsmoker presents to your clinic for her annual physical examination. Her vital signs include BP 130/88 mm Hg, HR 65 beats/minute, and BMI 30 kg/m². Her fasting laboratory values today are SCr 0.7 mg/dL, glucose 75 mg/dL, TC 190 mg/dL, HDL-C 46 mg/dL, and TG 80 mg/dL. Which is the best recommendation to make regarding aspirin therapy for this patient currently for primary prevention of stroke according to the U.S. Preventive Services Task Force (USPSTF) guidelines?

   A. Because the patient is 56 years old, aspirin is indicated for primary prevention of stroke.
   B. Because the patient is 56 years old and her 10-year risk of CHD is greater than 5%, aspirin is indicated for primary prevention of myocardial infarction (MI).
   C. Because the patient's 10-year risk of CHD is greater than 5%, aspirin is indicated for primary prevention of both stroke and MI.
   D. Because the patient's 10-year risk of stroke is less than 10%, aspirin is not indicated for primary prevention of stroke.

3. A 55-year-old, 66-kg Hispanic man with HTN and an MI 9 months ago, leading to placement of a bare metal stent (BMS), presents to the primary care clinic. His current medications include aspirin 325 mg/day orally, clopidogrel 75 mg/day orally, atorvastatin 40 mg/day orally, and metoprolol succinate 50 mg/day orally. His vital signs are BP 145/88 mm Hg and HR 52 beats/minute. His laboratory test results show LDL-C 68 mg/dL and SCr 1.0 mg/dL. Which recommendation is best for secondary prevention of CHD currently?

A. Decrease aspirin dose to 81 mg/day, and add lisinopril to 5 mg/day orally.

B. Increase atorvastatin to 80 mg/day orally, and increase metoprolol succinate to 100 mg/day orally.

C. Decrease aspirin dose to 81 mg/day, and increase metoprolol succinate to 100 mg/daily orally.

D. Discontinue clopidogrel, and increase atorvastatin to 80 mg/day orally.

4. A patient is being discharged from the hospital after admission for non–ST-segment elevation MI (NSTEMI). The patient received a percutaneous coronary intervention (PCI) with a drug-eluting stent (DES) and is at low risk of bleeding. Which is the best recommendation for aspirin and P2Y$_{12}$ inhibitor therapy according to the 2011 American Heart Association/American College of Cardiology Foundation (AHA/ACCF) PCI guidelines?

A. Aspirin 325 mg indefinitely and ticagrelor for at least 1 year.

B. Aspirin 325 mg for 1 month; then 81 mg indefinitely and clopidogrel for 6 months.

C. Aspirin 81 mg indefinitely and clopidogrel for 1 month.

D. Aspirin 81 mg indefinitely and prasugrel for at least 1 year.

5. A patient with a medical history of NSTEMI, peripheral arterial disease (PAD), HTN, and dyslipidemia (DLD) presents to the primary care clinic. He was discharged 2 weeks ago for a recurrent NTEMI, for which he received PCI without stenting. At the time of discharge, the patient was taking quinapril 40 mg/day orally, atenolol 100 mg/day orally, atorvastatin 80 mg/day orally, aspirin 81 mg/day orally, and clopidogrel 75 mg daily. The patient is considered to be at low risk of bleeding. Owing to the patient's risk of recurrent cardiovascular (CV) events, the decision is made to try vorapaxar. Which of the following is the most appropriate use of vorapaxar in this patient?

A. Initiate vorapaxar 2.08 mg/day orally and discontinue clopidogrel 75 mg.

B. Initiate vorapaxar 2.08 mg/day orally and discontinue aspirin 81 mg.

C. Initiate vorapaxar 2.08 mg/day orally and continue both aspirin 81 mg and clopidogrel 75 mg.

D. Initiate vorapaxar 2.08 mg/day orally, discontinue clopidogrel 75 mg, and initiate ticagrelor 90 mg twice daily orally.

6. A patient with a medical history of everolimus drug-eluting coronary artery stent placement and acute coronary syndrome (ACS) 5 months ago is scheduled to undergo radical prostatectomy for prostate cancer. He underwent a noninvasive stress test, with findings negative for myocardial ischemia. His current medications include aspirin 81 mg/day orally and clopidogrel 75 mg/day orally. Which is the best recommendation regarding the management of the patient's dual antiplatelet therapy (DAPT)?

A. Discontinue both aspirin and clopidogrel at least 7 days before the procedure.

B. Continue clopidogrel, but discontinue aspirin at least 5 days before the procedure.

C. Continue aspirin, but discontinue clopidogrel at least 7 days before the procedure.

D. Continue both aspirin and clopidogrel without interruption.

7. B.L. is a 52-year-old white man with type 2 DM for the past 15 years. He is upset because his physician is now telling him he has high BP, and the physician wants to initiate therapy with "another medicine." His vital signs today include BP 147/78 mm Hg, repeated BP 144/77 mm Hg; HR 58 beats/minute; weight 82 kg (182 lb); and height 69 inches. His laboratory test results show SCr 1.3 mg/dL and potassium (K) 4.4 mEq/L. Which option is the best therapeutic plan, given B.L.'s history?

A. Initiate ramipril 5 mg/day.

B. Initiate terazosin 1 mg/day.

C. Initiate atenolol 25 mg/day.

D. No medication changes are needed.

8. T.R. is a 50-year-old African American woman with PAD. She has been unable to tolerate angiotensin-converting enzyme (ACE) inhibitors and angiotensin receptor blockers (ARBs) because of hyperkalemia. Her current medication regimen is amlodipine 10 mg/day, metoprolol succinate 25 mg/day, simvastatin 20 mg/day, and aspirin 81 mg/day. Her vital signs today include BP 146/82 mm Hg, repeated BP 148/85 mm Hg; HR 60 beats/minute; weight 69 kg (154 lb); and height 64 inches. Her laboratory tests reveal K 4.9 mEq/L and creatinine clearance (CrCl) 65 mL/minute. Which option is the best therapeutic plan for T.R.?

   A. No medication changes are warranted.

   B. Initiate terazosin 1 mg at bedtime.

   C. Increase metoprolol XR (extended release) to 50 mg/day.

   D. Initiate hydrochlorothiazide 12.5 mg/day.

Questions 9 and 10 pertain to the following case.
A.M. is a 32-year-old woman with type 1 DM and HTN. Her current medication regimen is as follows: ramipril 10 mg/day, chlorthalidone 25 mg/day, amlodipine 10 mg/day, ethinyl estradiol 20 mcg/norethindrone 1 mg (for the past 2 years), and insulin as directed. Her vital signs today include BP 145/83 mm Hg, repeated BP 145/81 mm Hg; HR 82 beats/minute; height 66 inches; weight 70 kg (155 lb); and BMI 24.5 kg/m². A.M. would prefer not to take any more drugs, if possible.

9. Which option is the best clinical plan for A.M.?

   A. No change in therapy is warranted currently.

   B. Advise weight loss, and recheck her BP in 3 months.

   C. Change chlorthalidone to hydrochlorothiazide.

   D. Discuss changing her contraceptive method.

10. A.M. and her husband have decided they are ready to have children. Which is the best medication option for A.M.?

   A. No change in therapy is warranted currently.

   B. Discontinue ramipril and replace with labetalol.

   C. Increase chlorthalidone to 50 mg/day.

   D. Discontinue all antihypertensive therapy.

11. P.T. is a 75-year-old Asian woman with a history of coronary artery disease (CAD) (stent placement 5 years ago) and osteoarthritis. She has adhered to her medication regimen since her stent placement without problems. She has been checking her BP at home, and it has been steadily increasing (range during the past 2 weeks: 150s–160s/80s–90s mm Hg). Her medication regimen includes carvedilol 25 mg twice daily, ramipril 5 mg/day, atorvastatin 40 mg/day, and aspirin 81 mg/day. She started taking ibuprofen 600 mg twice daily 1 month ago after a fall. Her laboratory test results are as follows: creatinine (Cr) 1.7 mg/dL (CrCl [ideal body weight {IBW}] 24.7 mL/minute), BMI 22.4 kg/m², K 4.9 mEq/L, sodium (Na) 143 mEq/L, and thyroid-stimulating hormone (TSH) 1.56 μIU/mL. Which option is the most likely cause of her increasing BP?

   A. Medication nonadherence.

   B. Poor diet and lack of exercise.

   C. Nonsteroidal anti-inflammatory drug (NSAID) use and renal function.

   D. Thyroid disorder.

12. A.D. is a 45-year-old woman with CKD and worsening HTN. Her home BP readings have ranged from the 130s to the 140s/70s mm Hg for the past month. Her current antihypertensive regimen includes lisinopril 40 mg/day, felodipine 10 mg/day, and atenolol 25 mg/day. Her vital signs today include BP 139/75 mm Hg, repeated BP 138/72 mm Hg; HR 58 beats/minute; weight 56 kg (125 lb); and height 62 inches. Her laboratory values are as follows: Cr 1.9 mg/dL (CrCl [IBW] 29.6 mL/minute), K 4.9 mEq/L, Na 145 mEq/L, fasting blood glucose (FBG) 97 mg/dL, TSH 2.65 μIU/mL, and albumin/Cr ratio 66. Her nephrologist would like you to use the recent KDIGO (Kidney Disease: Improving Global Outcomes) guidelines to set her BP goal. Which is the next best step to control her BP?

   A. Add hydrochlorothiazide 12.5 mg/day.

   B. Add furosemide 20 mg twice daily.

   C. Change lisinopril to losartan 100 mg/day.

   D. Increase atenolol dose to 50 mg/day.

13. B.L. is a 62-year-old white man who has had type 2 DM for the past 25 years. He is a moderate alcohol consumer (three drinks per night, with occasional binges) and is obese (BMI 40.1 kg/m^2). In the past year, he had an MI and five-vessel coronary artery bypass grafting (CABG). He has well-controlled BP (125/70 mm Hg). He currently takes metformin 1 g twice daily, glipizide 10 mg twice daily, aspirin 81 mg/day, simvastatin 40 mg/day, metoprolol 25 mg twice daily, lisinopril 40 mg/day, and nitroglycerin sublingually as needed. Fasting laboratory test results show TC 148 mg/dL, TG 220 mg/dL, HDL-C 32 mg/dL, LDL-C 72 mg/dL, non–HDL-C 116 mg/dL, SCr 1.3 mg/dL, Na 142 mEq/L, K 4.5 mEq/L, hemoglobin A1C (A1C) 6.8%, and alanine aminotransferase (ALT) 75 IU/L (history of ALT readings between 56 and 92 IU/L during the past 3 years). His primary care physician asks you about his chronically elevated ALT concentration and about continuing his statin therapy. Which is the best response?

    A. Discontinue simvastatin because of elevated ALT values and alcohol use.

    B. Change simvastatin to ezetimibe 10 mg/day.

    C. Lower simvastatin dose to 10 mg/day because of elevated ALT values and alcohol use.

    D. Change simvastatin to atorvastatin 40 mg/day.

14. A.M. is a 45-year-old African American woman with PAD and atrial fibrillation whose metoprolol was switched to verapamil today for better rate control. Today, her BP is 135/81 mm Hg. She has been taking simvastatin 80 mg/day for cholesterol for the past 4 years. Fasting laboratory test results show TC 196 mg/dL, TG 85 mg/dL, HDL-C 50 mg/dL, LDL-C 129 mg/dL, non–HDL-C 146 mg/dL, SCr 1.3 mg/dL, Na 141 mEq/L, and K 4.0 mEq/L. Which is the best way to address her lipid values?

    A. No change in therapy is warranted currently.

    B. Change simvastatin to rosuvastatin 20 mg/day.

    C. Change simvastatin to lovastatin 40 mg twice daily.

    D. Lower simvastatin dose to 40 mg/day.

15. P.T. is a 73-year-old Asian woman with a history of CAD (with stent placement 5 years ago). She has adhered to her medication regimen since her stent placement without any problem. Her primary care physician checked her creatine kinase (CK) concentration because she was prescribed chronic statin therapy. She has no muscle symptoms. Her medication regimen includes atorvastatin 40 mg/day, aspirin 81 mg/day, carvedilol 6.25 mg twice daily, and omeprazole 20 mg as needed. Fasting laboratory test results show TC 135 mg/dL, TG 85 mg/dL, HDL-C 50 mg/dL, LDL-C 68 mg/dL, non–HDL-C 85 mg/dL, SCr 1.2 mg/dL (CrCl [IBW] 32 mL/minute), Na 141 mEq/L, K 4.0 mEq/L, and CK 303 U/L (normal limits 20–200 U/L). Which is the next best step for P.T.?

    A. Continue atorvastatin.

    B. Discontinue atorvastatin; statin therapy is contraindicated for this patient.

    C. Discontinue atorvastatin and initiate lovastatin 40 mg every evening.

    D. Lower atorvastatin dose to 20 mg every evening.

16. M.Z. is a 55-year-old woman with CKD. Two months ago, therapy with simvastatin 40 mg/day was initiated, to which she has been adherent. She exercises 5 days/week and eats a heart-healthy diet. Fasting laboratory test results show TC 176 mg/dL, TG 100 mg/dL, HDL-C 41 mg/dL, LDL-C 115 mg/dL, non–HDL-C 135 mg/dL, and SCr 2.3 mg/dL (CrCl [IBW] 28.9 mL/minute). Which is the best way to address her elevated LDL-C and non–HDL-C values?

    A. No change in therapy is warranted currently.

    B. Increase simvastatin to 80 mg/day.

    C. Change simvastatin to atorvastatin 40 mg/day.

    D. Lower simvastatin to 20 mg/day.

17. J.M. is a 41-year-old African American man who presents to the clinic for a follow-up. Three months ago, he was told for the first time that his cholesterol concentration was high and that he had to work on his diet and exercise. He is otherwise healthy, does not smoke, and is taking no prescription medications. His BP today is 121/68 mm Hg. Fasting laboratory test results today show TC 262 mg/dL (down from 273 mg/dL), TG 145 mg/dL (down from 160 mg/dL), HDL-C 42 mg/dL (no change), LDL-C 191 mg/dL (down from 199 mg/dL), non–HDL-C 220 mg/dL (down from 231 mg/dL), and SCr 1.0 mg/dL. Which is the best way to treat his cholesterol?

    A. Continue to work on diet and exercise; no medications needed.

    B. Continue to work on diet and exercise, and initiate atorvastatin 80 mg/day.

    C. Continue to work on diet and exercise, and initiate lovastatin 20 mg/day.

    D. Continue to work on diet and exercise, and initiate simvastatin 40 mg every evening.

18. J.T. is a 36-year-old man with heterozygous familial hypercholesterolemia (HeFH) who presents to the primary care clinic for a follow-up. His current medications include atorvastatin 80 mg/day orally and ezetimibe 10 mg/day orally. J.T. reports adherence to all medications and states he follows a low-fat diet and exercises 40 minutes/day 4 days/week. Fasting laboratory test results today show TC 275 mg/dL (baseline 320 mg/dL), TG 204 mg/dL (baseline 265 mg/dL), HDL-C 75 mg/dL (increased from 50 mg/dL), LDL-C 160 mg/dL (down from 217 mg/dL), and non–HDL-C 200 mg/dL (down from 270 mg/dL). Which of the following would be the best way to treat his cholesterol?

    A. Initiate alirocumab 75 mg subcutaneously every 2 weeks.

    B. Initiate evolocumab 140 mg subcutaneously every 2 weeks.

    C. Initiate fenofibrate 54 mg/day orally.

    D. Initiate colesevelam 3750 mg/day orally.

I. CARDIOVASCULAR DISEASE (CVD)

A. Leading Cause of Death in the United States (1 in every 2.9 deaths) in Both Men and Women

B. Components
   1. Hypertension (HTN)
   2. Coronary heart disease (CHD)
      a. Myocardial infarction (MI)
      b. Angina pectoris
      c. Asymptomatic atherosclerotic coronary artery disease (CAD)
   3. Stroke and transient ischemic attack (TIA)
   4. Arrhythmias
   5. Cardiomyopathy and heart failure (HF)
   6. Congenital heart disease

II. CORONARY HEART DISEASE

A. CHD Events Make Up More than Half of All CVD Events.

B. Lifetime Risk is 49% in Men and 32% in Women After Age 40 Years.

C. About 1 in Every 6 Deaths (more than 370,000 people annually) in the United States

D. From 1998 to 2008, the Annual CHD Death Rate Declined by 30.6%. About 40% of this reduction was attributable to lifestyle and diet risk factor modifications and 50% attributable to treatments.

E. Fifty Percent of Men and 69% of Women Who Die of CHD Have No Prior Symptoms. Hospital mortality for MI in both men and women who present without chest pain is higher than in patients presenting with chest pain.

F. A Total of 1.36 Million ACS (unstable angina [UA], NSTEMI, and ST-segment elevation MI [STEMI]) Hospital Discharges Annually

III. PRIMARY PREVENTION OF CHD EVENTS

A. Definition of Primary Prevention: Prevention of the First Occurrence of CHD *(Domain 1)*

B. 2009 ACCF/AHA Primary Prevention Performance Measures *(Domains 1, 2, 5)*
   1. Measure quality of care and identify areas for improvement.
   2. Accountability and public reporting versus internal quality improvement

Table 1. 2009 ACCF/AHA Primary Prevention Performance Measures

Performance Measure	Description	A/PR vs. IQI Designation
Global risk assessment	Estimation of a patient's absolute risk of CHD by using a multivariate risk score	IQI
Lifestyle and risk factor screening	Assessment of a patient's lifestyle and physical activity risk factors for developing CHD	A/PR, IQI
Dietary intake counseling	Counseling to eat a healthy diet	A/PR
Physical activity counseling	Counseling to engage in regular physical activity	A/PR
Smoking and tobacco use screening	Risk assessment for current smoking and tobacco use behaviors	A/PR, IQI
Smoking cessation counseling	Cessation intervention for active smoking	A/PR
Weight assessment	Measurement of weight and body mass index and/or waist circumference	A/PR, IQI
Weight management	Counseling to achieve and maintain ideal body weight	A/PR, IQI
Blood pressure measurement	Measurement of blood pressure	A/PR
Blood pressure control	Effective blood pressure control or combination drug therapy	A/PR, IQI
Lipid profile measurement	Fasting lipid profile performed	A/PR, IQI
Lipid-lowering therapy and control	LDL-C at target or prescribed	A/PR
Aspirin use	Aspirin use in patients without clinical evidence of atherosclerotic disease but at high risk of events	IQI

ACCF = American College of Cardiology Foundation; AHA = American Heart Association; A/PR = accountability/public reporting; CHD = coronary heart disease; IQI = internal quality improvement; LDL-C = low-density lipoprotein cholesterol.

Patient Case

1. A 69-year-old Hispanic man with a medical history of HTN for 5 years, type 2 DM for 4 years, and dyslipidemia for 8 years presents to his primary care physician for an annual physical examination. He is a nonsmoker. His current medications include losartan 50 mg orally once daily and metformin 500 mg orally twice daily. His BP is 148/89 mm Hg, and HR is 78 beats/minute. Results of today's fasting laboratory tests are as follows: SCr 0.8 mg/dL, TC 240 mg/dL, LDL-C 158 mg/dL, HDL-C 35 mg/dL, TG 110 mg/dL, and FBG 108 mg/dL. Using the Pooled Cohort Equation for CHD risk assessment (http://my.americanheart.org/cvriskcalculator), which percentage best estimates the risk of 10-year atherosclerotic cardiovascular disease (ASCVD) events for this patient?

    A. 17%.
    B. 30%.
    C. 46%.
    D. 51%.

C. ASCVD Risk Assessment *(Domain 1)*
1. Assess risk for adults 20–79 years of age at least once every 4–6 years.
    a. Age 20–39 years
        i. Assess risk factors
        ii. Risk factors include age, sex, total and HDL-C, systolic BP, use of antihypertensive therapy, diabetes, current smoking.
    b. Age 40–79 years – Use Pooled Cohort Equations.
2. Non-Hispanic African American and white individuals have sex- and race-specific Pooled Cohort Equations to predict 10-year risk of ASCVD.
3. Other patient populations
    a. Consider using the non-Hispanic Caucasian Pooled Cohort Equation for other populations.
    b. Important to remember that the estimated risks may be overestimates, particularly for Hispanics and Asian-Americans
4. If, after using the Pooled Cohort Equations, risk-based treatment decisions remain unclear, may consider factoring in family history, high-sensitivity C-reactive protein (hs-CRP), coronary artery calcium score, or ankle brachial index (ABI)

D. Pooled Cohort Equation (http://my.americanheart.org/cvriskcalculator). Risk assessment based on:
1. Age
2. Sex
3. Race
4. TC concentration
5. LDL-C concentration
6. Systolic blood pressure (SBP)
7. Treatment for HTN
8. Presence of diabetes
9. Current (day of assessment) smoker status

Patient Case

2. A 58-year-old male smoker with no significant medical history presents to the wellness clinic at your hospital for BP, diabetes, and cholesterol screening. You perform the fasting screening tests, which show BP 135/85 mm Hg, LDL-C 110 mg/dL, HDL-C 50 mg/dL, TG 80 mg/dL, and FBG 80 mg/dL. He asks you whether he should take a baby aspirin daily for the prevention of CVD. According to current practice guidelines, which is the best response to his question?

A. Yes, a daily aspirin will help prevent stroke.
B. Yes, a daily aspirin will help prevent heart attack.
C. No, his risk of intracranial bleeding is higher than his risk of heart attack.
D. No, his risk of gastrointestinal (GI) bleeding is higher than his risk of stroke.

E. Lifestyle Counseling: Diet and Physical Activity *(Domains 1–3)*
1. Recommend 40 minutes of moderate to vigorous intensity aerobic activity on 3 or 4 days of the week.
2. Diet recommendations
    a. 2013 AHA scientific statement on lifestyle management to reduce CV risk
        i. Consume vegetables, fruit, whole grains, low-fat dairy, poultry, fish, legumes, nontropical vegetable oils, and nuts.
        ii. Limit sweets, sugar-sweetened beverages, and red meat.
        iii. Consume appropriate calorie requirements.
        iv. Modify to meet personal and cultural food preferences and nutritional needs for concomitant diseases.

v. Limit intake of saturated fats to less than 5%–6% of calories, and reduce percentage of calories from trans fat.

vi. For BP lowering, lower Na intake.

    (a) Consume no more than Na 2400 mg/day.

    (b) Consuming less than 1500 mg/day Na can further lower BP.

    (c) Reduce Na intake by at least 1000 mg/day if unable to achieve daily Na recommendations.

b. AHA Healthy People 2020 diet score. Desire a score of 4 of 5 of the following:

i. Fruits and vegetables: 4½ cups or more a day

ii. Fish: Two or more 3½-oz servings a week (preferably oily fish)

iii. Fiber-rich whole grains (1.1 g of fiber per 10 g of carbohydrate): Three or more 1-oz-equivalent servings a day

iv. Sodium: Less than 1500 mg/day

v. Sugar-sweetened beverages: 450 kcal (36 oz) or less a week

F. Smoking Status Assessment and Cessation Counseling (USPSTF 2015 recommendation) (Ann Int Med 2015;163:622-34. doi:10.7326/M15-2023) *(Domains 1, 2, 5)*

1. Assess tobacco use at least once every 2 years and preferably at every visit for active smokers.

2. Ask about secondhand smoke exposure.

3. Common approaches

a. The 5 A's (Ask, Advise, Assess, Assist, Arrange follow-up and support)

b. Ask, Advise, Refer.

i. Refer to telephone quit lines and/or other evidence-based cessation interventions.

4. Nonpregnant adults 18 years or older: Provide pharmacotherapy and behavioral interventions for cessation.

5. Pregnant adults 18 years or older: Provide behavioral interventions for cessation.

6. Behavioral interventions

a. In-person behavioral support and counseling

b. Telephone counseling

c. Self-help materials

7. Pharmacologic therapy for smoking cessation

a. Nicotine replacement therapy (NRT)

i. Products

    (a) Over the counter (OTC): Patch, gum, lozenge

    (b) Prescription: Oral inhaler, nasal spray

ii. Superior to placebo, increases quit rates by about 2-fold

iii. In a 2012 Cochrane systematic review, combination nicotine replacement (patch plus gum, spray, or inhaler) was more effective than any treatment alone (relative risk [RR] 1.34; 95% confidence interval [CI], 1.18–1.51).

iv. A 2014 systematic review of more than 11,000 patients found that NRT was associated with a higher rate of all CV events (RR 1.81; 95% CI, 1.35–2.43), which was driven by minor events such as tachycardia and arrhythmia; no increase in major CV events was found.

b. Bupropion sustained release (SR) 150 mg twice daily

i. Almost doubles quit rate compared with placebo

ii. In a 2014 systematic review on the use of antidepressants for smoking cessation, bupropion SR was associated with higher rates of smoking cessation at 6 months than placebo or no bupropion SR (RR 1.62; 95% CI, 1.4–1.76).

        iii. Combination therapy with nicotine replacement with bupropion may be beneficial in treatment-refractory patients.

        iv. No significant difference found between bupropion and placebo in all CV events

        v. No significant increase in serious psychiatric events with bupropion SR

           (a) Label does include boxed warning about serious neuropsychiatric events.

    c. Varenicline

        i. Increases quit rate by 3 times compared with placebo

        ii. Dosing

           (a) 0.5 mg at bedtime, days 1–3; then

           (b) 0.5 mg twice daily, days 4–7; then

           (c) 1 mg twice daily, weeks 2–12

        iii. Warning regarding worsening depression and risk of suicide

        iv. In 2014 meta-analysis, no significant increase in all CV adverse events (RR 1.24; 95% CI, 0.85–1.81).

    d. Electronic nicotine delivery systems (ENDS):

        i. Insufficient evidence on the benefit, and the balance of benefits and harms cannot be determined.

        ii. No ENDS manufacturer has applied for/received U.S. Food and Drug Administration (FDA) approval for smoking cessation.

G. Weight Assessment and Counseling *(Domains 1, 2)*

  1. Assess BMI and/or weight and waist circumference at least once annually.

  2. When BMI is 25 kg/m² or greater, patients may be at increased risk of CVD. The higher the BMI, the greater the risk of CVD, DM, and all-cause mortality.

  3. For overweight and obese individuals, a sustained body weight reduction of 3%–5% can produce clinically meaningful results (reduction in lipids and blood glucose).

H. Aspirin Use *(Domain 1)*

  1. Dose 75–162 mg orally daily; doses higher than 81 mg/day are no more effective and are associated with increased risk of GI bleeding (JAMA 2007;297:2018-24).

    a. Risk factors associated with bleeding include dose of aspirin used, history of GI ulcers or upper GI pain, bleeding disorders, renal failure, severe liver disease, thrombocytopenia, concurrent anticoagulation therapy, NSAID use, uncontrolled HTN, male sex, and older age.

    b. Increased risk of hemorrhagic stroke in men.

  2. Clopidogrel is an alternative if true aspirin allergy.

  3. All patients with CAD, stroke, and PAD are at high risk of CVD events.

  4. 2012 American College of Chest Physicians (ACCP) guidelines recommend low-dose aspirin (75–100 mg orally daily) for patients older than 50 years without symptomatic CVD (Chest 2012;141:e637S-68S).

Table 2. Benefits and Risks of Aspirin for Primary Prevention of Cardiovascular Disease

Risk Group	MIs Prevented per 1000 Patients Treated	Strokes Prevented per 1000 Patients Treated	Total Mortality Reduction per 1000 Patients Treated	Major Bleeds per 1000 Patients Treated
Lower risk (5% 10-year CHD risk)	6	–	–	4
Moderate risk (15% 10-year CHD risk)	19	–	–	16
High risk (25% 10-year CHD risk)	31	–	6	22

CHD = coronary heart disease; MI = myocardial infarction.

From: Vandvik PO, Lincoff AM, Gore LM, et al.; American College of Chest Physicians. Primary and secondary prevention of cardiovascular disease: Antithrombotic Therapy and Prevention of Thrombosis, 9th ed: American College of Chest Physicians Evidence-Based Clinical Practice Guidelines. Chest 2012;141(2 suppl):e637S-68S.

5. In 2014, the FDA issued a public health advisory stating that the evidence to use aspirin for primary prevention was lacking.
   a. Aspirin provides modest benefit in preventing MI, has no effect on total mortality or CV mortality.
   b. In women, benefit was limited to stroke prevention.
   c. Aspirin can increase risk of bleeding.
6. 2009 Primary Prevention Performance Measure: Advise patients without overt CVD to use aspirin if global risk assessment for 10-year CHD risk is 20% or more.
7. 2009 USPSTF Aspirin for the Prevention of Cardiovascular Disease recommendations are available at www.uspreventiveservicestaskforce.org/uspstf/uspsasmi.htm.
   a. Inconclusive evidence to recommend aspirin to men or women 80 years or older, men younger than 45 years, and women younger than 55 years
8. 2015 USPSTF Aspirin for the Prevention of Cardiovascular Disease and Cancer recommendations are currently under review and open for comment.
   a. Low-dose aspirin is recommended in adults aged 50–59 years who have a 10% or greater 10-year CVD risk, are not at increased risk of bleeding, have a life expectancy of at least 10 years, and are willing to take low-dose aspirin daily for at least 10 years.
   b. The decision to use low-dose aspirin in adults aged 60–69 years who have a 10-year risk that is greater than 10% is an individual one. Those who are not at an increased risk of bleeding, have a life expectancy of 10 years or more, and are willing to take aspirin daily for 10 years are more likely to benefit.
   c. Inconclusive evidence to recommend aspirin to men or women 70 years and older or younger than 50 years

Table 3. 2009 USPSTF Recommendations for Aspirin Use in Men 45–79 Years of Age

The shaded areas indicate the estimates where the risk of harm from aspirin (GI bleeding and intracranial hemorrhage) equals or exceeds the benefit in reduction of 10-year risk of MI.			
Variable	**Estimated MIs Prevented (per 1000 men treated), N**		
10-Year CHD Risk, %	**Age 45–59 Years**	**Age 60–69 Years**	**Age 70–79 Years**
1	3.2	3.2	3.2
2	6.4	6.4	6.4
3	9.6	9.6	9.6
4	12.8	12.8	12.8
5	16	16	16
6	19.2	19.2	19.2
7	22.4	22.4	22.4
8	25.6	25.6	25.6
9	28.8	28.8	28.8
10	32	32	32
11	35.2	35.2	35.2
12	38.4	38.4	38.4
13	41.6	41.6	41.6
14	44.8	44.8	44.8
15	48	48	48
16	51.2	51.2	51.2
17	54.4	54.4	54.4
18	57.6	57.6	57.6
19	60.8	60.8	60.8
20	64	64	64

Type of event	**Estimated Harm (per 1000 men treated), N**		
GI bleeding	8	24	36
Hemorrhagic stroke	1	1	1

CHD = coronary heart disease; GI = gastrointestinal; MI = myocardial infarction; USPSTF = U.S. Preventive Services Task Force.

Reproduced with permission from: US Preventive Services Task Force. Aspirin for the prevention of cardiovascular disease: US Preventive Services Task Force recommendation statement. Ann Intern Med 2009;150:396-404.

Table 4. 2009 USPSTF Recommendations for Aspirin Use in Women 55–79 Years of Age

The shaded areas indicate the estimates where the risk of harm from aspirin (GI bleeding and intracranial hemorrhage) equals or exceeds the benefit in reduction of 10-year risk of ischemic stroke.		
Variable	**Estimated Strokes Prevented (per 1000 women treated), N**		
10-Year Stroke Risk, %	**55–59 Years of Age**	**60–69 Years of Age**	**70–79 Years of Age**
1	1.7	1.7	1.7
2	3.4	3.4	3.4
3	5.1	5.1	5.1
4	6.8	6.8	6.8
5	8.5	8.5	8.5
6	10.2	10.2	10.2
7	11.9	11.9	11.9
8	13.6	13.6	13.6
9	15.3	15.3	15.3
10	17	17	17
11	18.7	18.7	18.7
12	20.4	20.4	20.4
13	22.1	22.1	22.1
14	23.8	23.8	23.8
15	25.5	25.5	25.5
16	27.2	27.2	27.2
17	28.9	28.9	28.9
18	30.6	30.6	30.6
19	32.3	32.3	32.3
20	34	34	34
Type of event	**Estimated Harm (per 1000 women treated), N**		
GI bleeding	4	12	18

GI = gastrointestinal; N = number; USPSTF = U.S. Preventive Services Task Force.

I. Aspirin Use in Patients with DM (The reader is also referred to the Diabetes Mellitus chapter.) *(Domains 1, 3)*
1. American Diabetes Association (ADA) 2016 Standards of Medical Care in Diabetes
    a. Estimate CVD risk (see global risk assessment above; suggest 2008 modified Framingham risk score, even in women with DM).
        i. Various risk tools are currently available.
        ii. 2010 Consensus Statement risk tools included the UKPDS (UK Prospective Diabetes Study) Risk Engine and ARIC (Atherosclerosis Risk in Communities) CHD Risk Calculator (J Am Coll Cardiol 2010;55:2878-88).

    b. Aspirin 75–162 mg/day indicated if 10-year CVD risk greater than 10%

        i. Per 2016 Scientific Statement, low-dose aspirin is reasonable in adults with intermediate (5%–10%) risk (Diabetes Care 2016;39 Suppl 1:S1-S112).

        ii. Clinical judgment should be used until further research is available.

    c. If no risk assessment

        i. Men and women older 50 years and older who have at least one other risk factor for CHD and are not at increased risk for bleeding

        ii. Risk factors for CHD

            (a) Family history of premature ASCVD

            (b) Hypertension

            (c) Smoking

            (d) Dyslipidemia

                (1) Low HDL-C values

                (2) Elevated LDL-C values

                (3) Elevated TG values

            (e) Albuminuria defined as urinary albumin excretion of 30 mg or more every 24 hours.

2. Meta-analysis of nine randomized controlled trials (RCTs) of 11,787 patients (J Am Coll Cardiol 2010;55:2878-78)

    a. No overall benefit in CHD events or stroke

    b. Aspirin resistance is higher in patients with DM, but data on recommending a higher dose to overcome effects and reduce outcomes are lacking.

3. 2009 Cochrane meta-analysis of six randomized placebo-controlled trials of 10,117 patients (BMJ 2009;339:b4531)

    a. No overall benefit in CVD events, stroke, CVD death, or all-cause mortality

    b. Forty-three percent reduction in MI in men (RR 0.57; 95% CI, 0.34–0.94; p=0.03)

4. Meta-analysis of six RCTs (five of six were placebo controlled) (Expert Opin Pharmacother 2010;11:1459-66)

    a. n=7374 patients with DM

    b. No difference in total mortality (RR 0.96; 95% CI, 0.78–1.18); the composite of CV death, MI, or stroke (RR 0.90; 95% CI, 0.78–1.05); or MI (RR 0.95, 95% CI, 0.76–1.18)

    c. No difference in major bleeding (RR 2.49; 95% CI, 0.70–8.84)

J. Aspirin Use in Patients with CKD *(Domains 1, 3)*

  1. KDIGO 2012 Clinical Practice Guideline for the Evaluation and Management of CKD states that aspirin is not indicated for primary prevention for patients (only secondary prevention).

  2. Post hoc analysis of the Hypertension Optimal Treatment (HOT) study

    a. Patients with estimated glomerular filtration rate (eGFR) less than 45 mL/minute/m^2: 95% did not have CVD at baseline, and less than 10% had DM.

    b. Lower all-cause mortality (11.03% vs. 5.68%; hazard ratio 0.51; 95% CI, 0.27–0.94), CV mortality (6.25% vs. 2.27%; hazard ratio 0.35; 95% CI, 0.14–0.90), and strokes (5.15% vs. 1.14%; hazard ratio 0.06–0.75) for patients taking aspirin 75 mg/day compared with placebo

    c. Major bleeding similar to placebo in patients with eGFR less than 45 mL/minute/m^2. Per every 1000 individuals treated with aspirin for 3.8 years, an excess 27 major bleeds occurred.

    d. The authors concluded that the increased risk of major bleeding appears to be outweighed by the benefits.

Patient Cases

Questions 3 and 4 pertain to the following case.

R.R., a 56-year-old African American woman with a medical history of type 2 DM for 2 years and a family history of a father with an MI at 45 years of age, presents to her primary care physician for an annual physical examination. She is a nonsmoker and has no known drug allergies. Her current medications include metformin 500 mg orally twice daily. Her BP is 145/89 mm Hg, and her HR is 80 beats/minute—values similar to the office results obtained 6 months ago. Results of the past week's fasting laboratory tests are as follows: SCr 0.9 mg/dL, TC 181 mg/dL, LDL-C 110 mg/dL, HDL-C 51 mg/dL, TG 100 mg/dL, A1C 7.2%, and FBG 180 mg/dL. Her 10-year ASCVD risk is 11.9%.

3. Which is the best recommendation to make regarding aspirin therapy for primary prevention of CHD events for R.R. according to the ADA 2015 guidelines?

   A. Aspirin 81 mg/day orally.
   B. Aspirin 325 mg/day orally.
   C. Aspirin 650 mg/day orally.
   D. No aspirin indicated.

4. Which is the best recommendation currently for initiating additional pharmacotherapy for R.R. to prevent a CHD event?

   A. Enalapril 5 mg/day and atorvastatin 40 mg/day.
   B. Atenolol 50 mg/day and simvastatin 40 mg/day.
   C. Ramipril 2.5 mg/day and rosuvastatin 5 mg/day.
   D. Hydrochlorothiazide 12.5 mg/day.

V. SECONDARY PREVENTION OF MYOCARDIAL INFARCTION

   A. Lifestyle Counseling: Diet and Physical Activity: Encourage consumption of fish. *(Domains 1, 2)*
      1. Same counseling as primary prevention patient, except exercise as tolerated
      2. Encourage consumption of fish.

   B. Smoking Cessation *(Domains 1, 5)*

   C. Referral to a Cardiac Rehabilitation Program *(Domains 1, 2)*
      1. American Association of Cardiovascular and Pulmonary Rehabilitation (AACVPR): www.aacvpr.org/
      2. 2010 AACVPR/ACCF/AHA Performance Measures for Cardiac Rehabilitation and Secondary Prevention Services
         a. All patients hospitalized for MI, PCI, or cardiac surgery should be referred before discharge.
         b. All outpatients who did not participate in a program within the past 12 months after hospitalization should be referred.
      3. Core Components of a Cardiac Rehabilitation Program for Secondary Prevention of CHD (2007 AHA/AACVPR)
         a. Patient assessment
         b. Nutritional counseling
         c. Lipid management
         d. BP management

    e. Smoking cessation
    f. Weight management
    g. Diabetes management
    h. Psychosocial management
    i. Physical activity counseling
    j. Exercise training

  D. AHA 2008 Performance Measures for MI *(Domains 1,2)*

Table 5. ACC/AHA 2008 Quality Performance Measures for MI

Aspirin at arrival
Aspirin prescribed at discharge
β-Blocker prescribed at hospital discharge
Statin prescribed at hospital discharge (for patients with LDL-C > 100 mg/dL)
ACE inhibitor or ARB for LVD prescribed at discharge
Evaluation of LV function
Time to fibrinolytic therapy for patients with STEMI or LBBB
Time to PCI for patient with STEMI
Time from ED arrival to ED discharge when transferring for STEMI PCI to another hospital
Time from ED arrival at STEMI referral facility to PCI at receiving facility
Percentage of eligible patients with STEMI or LBBB receiving reperfusion therapy
Smoking cessation counseling
Cardiac rehabilitation referral

ACC = American College of Cardiology; ACE = angiotensin-converting enzyme; AHA = American Heart Association; ARB = angiotensin receptor blocker; ED = emergency department; LBBB = left bundle branch block; LDL-C = low-density lipoprotein cholesterol; LV = left ventricular; LVD = left ventricular dysfunction; MI = myocardial infarction; PCI = percutaneous coronary intervention; STEMI = ST-segment elevation myocardial infarction.

  E. Antiplatelets for Patients Not Undergoing PCI *(Domains 1, 3)*
    1. Guideline recommendations

Table 6. Aspirin Therapy for Secondary Prevention in Patients Not Undergoing Percutaneous Coronary Intervention (ACCF/AHA guideline recommendations)

ACS	Initial Dose	Subsequent Doses Starting on Day 2 and Therapy Duration
NSTE ACS medical management	162–325 mg of nonenteric-coated formulation either oral or chewed	75–100 mg/day indefinitely
STEMI medical management (including fibrinolysis)	162–325 mg of nonenteric-coated formulation either oral or chewed	75–100 mg/day indefinitely

ACCF/AHA = American College of Cardiology Foundation/American Heart Association; ACS = acute coronary syndrome; NSTE = non–ST-segment elevation; STEMI = ST-segment elevation myocardial infarction.

Table 7. P2Y$_{12}$ Inhibitor Therapy for Secondary Prevention in Patients Not Undergoing Percutaneous Coronary Intervention (ACCF/AHA guideline recommendations)

ACS	Initial Dose	Subsequent Doses Starting on Day 2 and Therapy Duration
NSTE ACS medical management	Clopidogrel 300-600 mg Ticagrelor 180 mg[a]	Clopidogrel 75 mg/day for at least 12 months[b]Ticagrelor 90 mg twice daily for at least 12 months[b,c]
STEMI medical management (including fibrinolysis)	For patients >75 years: Clopidogrel 75 mg	Clopidogrel 75 mg/day on days 2–14 post MI
	For patients ≤75 years: Clopidogrel 75 mg or 300 mg (including fibrinolysis)	Clopidogrel 75 mg/day on days 2–14 post MI

[a]Concomitant aspirin dose must be 81 mg daily.

[b]Unless bleeding risk outweighs anticipated benefit. Duration after ACS is the same regardless of stent type.

[c]It is reasonable to use ticagrelor in preference to clopidogrel for P$_2$Y$_{12}$ treatment in patients with NSTE-ACS who undergo and early ichemia-guided strategy per 2014 ACCF/AHA NSTEMI guidelines (IIa).

ACCF/AHA = American College of Cardiology Foundation/American Heart Association; ACS = acute coronary syndrome; MI = myocardial infarction; NSTE = non–ST-segment elevation; STEMI = ST-segment elevation myocardial infarction.

2. Efficacy and treatment goals
   a. Non–ST-segment elevation (NSTE) ACS
      i. Aspirin reduced the risk of death or MI by 49% in a meta-analysis of four placebo-controlled unstable angina trials.
      ii. Clopidogrel reduced the risk of death, MI, or stroke (composite end point) by 20% (similar to patients undergoing PCI according to the subgroup analysis of the Clopidogrel in Unstable Angina to Prevent Recurrent Events [CURE] trial).
      iii. Ticagrelor reduced the risk of CV death, MI, or stroke by 15% in a subgroup of the Platelet Inhibition and Outcomes (PLATO) trial.
   b. ST-segment elevation MI
      i. Aspirin reduced CV mortality by 20% compared with placebo in the Second International Study of Infarct Survival (ISIS-2) trial.
      ii. Clopidogrel reduced mortality by 7%, and death, reinfarction, or stroke by 9% compared with placebo when added to aspirin and standard therapy in the Clopidogrel and Metoprolol in Myocardial Infarction Trial (COMMIT).
      iii. Ticagrelor reduced the risk of CV death, MI, or stroke by 15% in a subgroup of the PLATO trial.
   c. When aspirin, clopidogrel, and warfarin are combined, use aspirin 81 mg and warfarin target international normalized ratio (INR) 2.0–2.5 (2012 ACCF/AHA/SCAI [Society for Cardiovascular Angiography and Intervention STEMI guidelines]) (e.g., patients with atrial fibrillation, venous thromboembolism, or left ventricular thrombus). Please see Anticoagulation section in Cardiology I chapter for more details.
      i. Ticagrelor and prasugrel should not be used owing to risk of bleeding and lack of evidence in this setting.

F. Dual Antiplatelet Therapy (DAPT) for Patients Undergoing PCI *(Domains 1, 3)*
   1. Guideline recommendations (2011 ACCF/AHA PCI guidelines, 2013 ACCF/AHA STEMI guidelines, 2014 AHA/ACC NSTE-ACS guidelines)

Table 8. Aspirin in PCI

NSTE-ACS and STEMI	Initial Dose	Subsequent Doses Starting on Day 2 and Therapy Duration
Bare metal stent	325 mg before PCI	81 mg/day orally indefinitely
Drug-eluting stent	325 mg before PCI	81 mg/day orally indefinitely

ACS = acute coronary syndrome; NSTE = non–ST-segment elevation; PCI = percutaneous coronary intervention; STEMI = ST-segment elevation myocardial infarction.

Table 9. Concomitant $P2Y_{12}$ Inhibitor Therapy in PCI

ACS	Initial Dose	Subsequent Doses Starting Day 2 and Therapy Duration (Class Recommendation[a])
Bare metal stent (STEMI primary PCI, UA, and NSTEMI)	Clopidogrel 600 mg orally	Clopidogrel 75 mg orally daily for at least 12 months (I)[b]
	Prasugrel 60 mg orally	Prasugrel 10 mg/day orally for at least 12 months (I)[b,d]; consider dose reduction to 5 mg/day orally for patients weighing <60 kg or >75 years; contraindicated for patients with prior stroke/TIA (III)
	Ticagrelor 180 mg orally	90 mg twice daily orally ideally for at least 12 months (I)[b,d]
Drug-eluting stent (STEMI primary PCI, UA, and NSTEMI)	Clopidogrel 300–600 mg orally	Clopidogrel 75 mg/day orally for at least 12 months (I)[b,c]
	Prasugrel 60 mg orally	Prasugrel 10 mg/day orally for at least 12 months (I)[b,c,d]; consider dose reduction to 5 mg/day orally for patients weighing <60 kg[b] (I); in general, not recommended for patients 75 years or older (I); contraindicated in patients with prior stroke or TIA (III)
	Ticagrelor 180 mg orally	90 mg twice daily orally for at least 12 months (I)[b,c,d]
STEMI nonprimary PCI	If fibrinolytic administered, continue clopidogrel if already initiated; otherwise, administer 300–600 mg	Same as above as indicated by stent type
	If fibrinolytic not administered, initiate clopidogrel, prasugrel, or ticagrelor as above for primary PCI	

[a]Class recommendations refer to the 2011 ACCF/AHA PCI guidelines.

[b]Option to discontinue sooner if risk of bleeding outweighs the anticipated benefit (I).

[c]Option to continue beyond 12 months for DES (IIb).

[d] Prasugrel or ticagrelor may be reasonable to choose over clopidogrel per 2014 ACCF/AHA NSTEMI guidelines(IIa)

ACS = acute coronary syndrome; DES = drug-eluting stent; MI = myocardial infarction; NSTEMI = non–ST-segment elevation myocardial infarction; PCI = percutaneous coronary intervention; STEMI = ST-segment elevation myocardial infarction; TIA = transient ischemic attack; UA = unstable angina.

2. Efficacy and treatment goals
   a. Weak data to support the benefit of aspirin 325 mg versus 81 mg orally daily
      i. Clopidogrel and Aspirin Optimal Dose Usage to Reduce Recurrent Events – Seventh Organization to Assess Strategies in Ischemic Symptoms (CURRENT OASIS-7) trial, PCI subgroup analysis
         (a) A total of 17,263 patients randomly assigned in a 2 x 2 fashion to low-dose (75–100 mg/day) or high-dose (300–325 mg/day) aspirin and either clopidogrel 300 mg followed by 75 mg/day or 600 mg followed by 150 mg/day on days 2–7; then 75 mg/day through day 30.
         (b) The rates of the primary end point of CV death, MI, or stroke, as well as a secondary end point of stent thrombosis, at 30 days were not different between low- and high-dose aspirin.
         (c) Occurrence of major bleeding at 30 days was not different between low- and high-dose aspirin.
      ii. Individual stent labels recommend low-dose aspirin.
      iii. Xience stent (everolimus) product labeling states that 75 mg of aspirin daily was administered in clinical trials.
      iv. 2011 PCI guidelines state that aspirin 81 mg is "preferable" to higher doses (class IIa recommendation).
   b. Prasugrel versus clopidogrel – Trial to Assess Improvement in Therapeutic Outcomes by Optimizing Platelet Inhibition with Prasugrel–Thrombolysis in Myocardial Infarction (TRITON-TIMI) 38.
      i. Studied only in patients undergoing PCI (NSTE-ACS and STEMI)
      ii. Prasugrel reduced the risk of the primary end point of CV death, MI, or stroke at 30 days and 15 months, compared with clopidogrel.
      iii. Increased risk of bleeding, including life-threatening bleeding, with prasugrel in overall study (2.4% vs. 1.8%) at 15 months
      iv. Increased risk of bleeding in patients with low body weight (less than 60 kg)
      v. Contraindicated in patients with prior stroke or TIA
      vi. Subgroups in which benefit was found without increased bleeding risk
         (a) ST-segment elevation MI
         (b) Diabetes mellitus
      vii. Core cohort of patients without history of stroke or TIA, weighing 60 kg or more, and younger than 75 years
         (a) Twenty-six percent reduction in CV death, MI, or stroke
         (b) No increased bleeding risk
   c. Ticagrelor versus clopidogrel – PLATO
      i. Studied in both NSTE-ACS and STEMI in patients with intended medical management (results described above) and those with intended early coronary angiography/ revascularization
      ii. Ticagrelor reduced CV death, MI, or stroke as composite end point, as well as individual end points of CV death, MI, and all-cause mortality, compared with clopidogrel.
      iii. No difference in study-defined bleeding, but non–coronary artery bypass grafting (CABG)-related major bleeding was higher with ticagrelor.
   d. Extended duration of DAPT
      i. Twelve or 30 Months of Dual Antiplatelet Therapy After Drug-Eluting Stents (DAPT study)
         (a) A total of 9961 patients were enrolled after drug-eluting stent (DES) placement. After 12 months of treatment with either clopidogrel or prasugrel plus aspirin, patients were randomly assigned to continue either DAPT or aspirin monotherapy for an additional 18 months.

(b) Coprimary efficacy end points: Stent thrombosis and major adverse CV and cerebrovascular events occurring between 12 to 30 months

(c) Primary safety end point: Moderate or severe bleeding

(d) Patients in the DAPT group had a reduced rate of stent thrombosis (hazard ratio 0.29; 95% CI, 0.17–0.48; p<0.001) and major adverse CV and cerebrovascular events (4.3% vs. 5.9%; hazard ratio 0.71; 95% CI, 0.59–0.85; p<0.001).

(e) Moderate or severe bleeding was higher in the DAPT group (2.5% vs. 1.6%, p=0.001).

(d) All-cause mortality was 2.0% in the DAPT group versus 1.5% in the aspirin monotherapy group (hazard ratio 1.36; 95% CI, 1.00–1.85; p=0.05).

   ii. Long-term use of ticagrelor in patients with prior myocardial infarction (PEGASUS-TIMI 54)

(a) Evaluation of prolonged use of ticagrelor in patients older than 50 years who had a prior MI 1 to

3 years before enrollment plus at least one additional risk factor (65 years of age or older, diabetes mellitus requiring medication, second prior spontaneous MI, multivessel CAD, chronic renal dysfunction)

(b) Patients were randomly assigned to one of two doses of ticagrelor (90 mg twice daily or 60 mg twice daily) or placebo; all patients received aspirin.

(c) Primary efficacy end point: CV death, MI, and stroke

(d) Primary safety end point: TIMI major bleeding

(e) The primary efficacy end point was significantly reduced in both ticagrelor groups compared to placebo.

    (1) Ticagrelor 90 mg twice daily versus placebo: 7.85% versus 9.04% (hazard ratio 0.85; 95% CI, 0.75–0.96, p=0.008)

    (2) Ticagrelor 60 mg twice daily versus placebo: 7.77% versus 9.04% (hazard ratio 0.84; 95% CI, 0.75-.095, p=0.004)

(f) TIMI major bleeding events were higher with ticagrelor (2.60% with 90 mg twice daily vs. 2.30% with 60 mg twice daily vs. 1.06% with placebo; p<0.001 for each ticagrelor dose vs. placebo).

  e. Triple antiplatelet therapy

   i. Vorapaxar: Competitive inhibitor of platelet protease-activated receptor (PAR-1) receptor on platelet surface; blocks thrombin-mediated platelet activation.

(a) TRACER trial: Vorapaxar 40-mg loading dose and 2.5-mg daily maintenance dose compared to placebo in addition to standard therapy (91.1% taking clopidogrel) in 12,944 patients with NSTE-ACS

    (1) Vorapaxar did not achieve primary efficacy end point (CV death, MI, stroke, recurrent ischemia with rehospitalization, or urgent coronary revascularization), compared to placebo (hazard ratio 0.92, p=0.07).

    (2) Prespecified secondary end point (CV death, MI, stroke) reduced with vorapaxar (hazard ratio 0.89, p=0.02), which was mostly driven by reduction in MI.

    (3) GUSTO trail: Moderate or severe bleeding at 2 years significantly increased in the vorapaxar group (7.2% vs. 5.2%; hazard ratio 1.35; 95% CI, 1.16–1.58; p<0.01).

(b) TRA 2P=TIMI 50 trial: Vorapaxar 2.5 mg daily added to aspirin and/or thienopyridine (majority received clopidogrel; only 0.7% received prasugrel) as part of standard care, compared to placebo in 26,449 patients with a history of atherosclerotic CVD, including MI, stroke, or PAD, within 2 weeks to 12 months of enrollment. Mean follow-up was 30 months.

    (1) Vorapaxar reduced primary combined end point of CV death, MI, and stroke (9.3% vs. 10.5%; hazard ratio 0.87; 95% CI, 0.80–0.94; p<0.001).

    (2) GUSTO trial: Moderate or severe bleeding significantly increased with vorapaxar (4.2% vs. 2.5%; hazard ratio 1.66; 95% CI, 1.43–1.93; p<0.001).

> (3) Net clinical benefit was found in patients with MI (reduction in primary end point) and PAD (reduction in hospitalization for limb ischemia and peripheral artery revascularization).
>
> (4) Stroke arm of the trial was discontinued early owing to increased risk of intracranial hemorrhage.

    (c) FDA approval: Patients with a history of MI or PAD in adjunct to aspirin, clopidogrel, or both. Contraindicated in patients with history of stroke, TIA, intracranial hemorrhage, or active bleeding

> (1) Approved dose is 2.08 mg daily
>
> (2) This dose is equivalent to 2.5 mg of vorapaxar sulfate.

Patient Case

5. A 66-year-old man with a medical history of HTN, and an MI with coronary stent placement 8 months ago, presents to the primary care clinic. Current medications include aspirin 81 mg/day orally, prasugrel 10 mg/day orally, nitroglycerin 0.4-mg tablets sublingually as needed for chest pain, metoprolol succinate 75 mg/day orally, ramipril 10 mg/day orally, and atorvastatin 20 mg/day orally. He asks you how long he will need to take prasugrel. Which is the best answer?

    A. If you have a bare metal stent (BMS), call your physician because you should be able to stop prasugrel now.

    B. If you have a DES, call your physician because you should be able to stop prasugrel now.

    C. You will need to take prasugrel indefinitely.

    D. You will need to take prasugrel for at least 1 year after your MI and stent placement.

G. Monitoring Antiplatelet Therapy for Adverse Effects *(Domain 1)*
1. Aspirin: GI bleeding and bruising. Major bleeding about 2%–3% in first year
2. Clopidogrel: Bleeding, diarrhea, rash – An additional absolute risk of 1% major (severe or life-threatening) bleeding when added to aspirin (3%–4% per year in combination with aspirin) in first year. Similar to aspirin alone after the first year in patients able to tolerate DAPT in the first year in a post hoc substudy of the Clopidogrel for High Atherothrombotic Risk and Ischemic Stabilization, Management, and Avoidance (CHARISMA) trial
3. Prasugrel: Bleeding, diarrhea, rash: An additional absolute risk of 0.6% major and 0.5% life-threatening bleeding, compared with clopidogrel
4. Ticagrelor: Bleeding, bradycardia, heart block, dyspnea
5. Vorapaxar: Bleeding, anemia, depression, rashes, skin eruptions, exanthemata
6. Reduction of Atherothrombosis for Continued Health (REACH) bleeding risk score
    a. Nine clinical factors
    b. High risk of bleeding with score greater than 10

H. Limitations of Therapy *(Domain 1)*
1. Clopidogrel
    a. Nonuniform platelet activity, and only about 50% of patients achieve greater than 50% platelet inhibition with clopidogrel after a 600-mg loading dose. It is estimated that about 30% of patients have inadequate response

   b. Reduced effectiveness shown in carriers of reduced-function alleles, particularly CYP2C19*2
      i. TRITON-TIMI 38: Carriers had lower levels of active metabolite, diminished platelet inhibition, and increased rates of major CV events and stent thrombosis. However, this has not been confirmed in other studies.
      ii. Clinical trials have failed to demonstrate ability to modulate clinical outcomes with genetic-based therapy.
   c. Proton-pump inhibitors, specifically omeprazole, can interfere with metabolism and result in diminished in vitro platelet activity, but this does not appear to correlate to worse clinical outcomes.
2. Prasugrel should not be used in patients with history of stroke or TIA and was not shown to be beneficial in patients 75 years or older or weighing less than 60 kg in the TRITON-TIMI 38 trial.
3. Ticagrelor should only be used with low-dose aspirin, with doses not to exceed 81 mg, on the basis of the PLATO trial, which demonstrated a smaller effect in North America. In addition, in this trial the number of patients with prior strokes was small, which limited the ability to detect differences in rates of intracranial hemorrhage in this population.
4. Vorapaxar should not be used in patients with severe hepatic dysfunction owing to bleeding risk and is contraindicated in patients with a history of stroke, TIA, or intracranial hemorrhage (ICH) owing to the increased risk of ICH in this patient population.
   a. Vorapaxar should only be used with clopidogrel because it has not been studied with prasugrel or ticagrelor.

Table 10. REACH Bleeding Risk Score

Factor	Value	Point(s)
Age, years	45–54	0
	55–64	2
	65–74	4
	≥75	6
Peripheral arterial disease	Yes	1
	No	0
Heart failure	Yes	2
	No	0
Diabetes mellitus	Yes	1
	No	0
Hypercholesterolemia	No	1
	Yes	0
Hypertension	Yes	2
	No	0
Smoking	Current	2
	Former	1
	Never	0
Antiplatelets prescribed	Two or more	4
	Nonaspirin antiplatelet alone	2
	Aspirin alone	1
	None	0
Oral anticoagulant prescribed	Yes	4
	No	0

REACH = Reduction of Atherothrombosis for Continued Health.

Table 11. REACH Scoring (sum the score associated with each of the nine factors)

Score	2-Year Risk of Serious Bleeding, %
0–6	0.46
7–8	0.95
9–10	1.25
11–21	2.76

REACH = Reduction of Atherothrombosis for Continued Health.

I. Management of DAPT in Patients Undergoing a Surgical Procedure *(Domain 1)*
1. For patients with past ACS and no stent who are transitioning to nonurgent CABG surgery (ACCF/AHA 2013 guideline recommendation)
    a. Continue low-dose aspirin.
    b. Discontinue clopidogrel or ticagrelor at least 5 days before surgery.
    c. Discontinue prasugrel at least 7 days before surgery.
2. For patients with a coronary stent (2011 ACCF/AHA/SCAI PCI guidelines)
    a. Select BMS over DES for patients likely to undergo invasive procedures.
    b. Avoid elective surgery within 4–6 weeks of BMS placement or 12 months of DES placement.
3. For urgent surgical procedures (either BMS or DES) (2013 ACCF/AHA STEMI guidelines)
    a. Continue aspirin.
    b. Discontinue clopidogrel or ticagrelor at least 5 days before surgery and prasugrel at least 7 days before surgery, if possible.
    c. Discontinue clopidogrel or ticagrelor at least 24 hours before on-pump CABG surgery.
    d. Urgent off-pump CABG surgery may be considered earlier than 24 hours after discontinuing clopidogrel or ticagrelor.
    e. Reinitiate the P2Y12 inhibitor as soon as possible postoperatively.
4. 2012 ACCP Chest Guidelines
    a. No prior stent: Continue aspirin for patients undergoing noncardiac or CABG surgery unless low risk of events, in which case, discontinue.
    b. Prior stent
        i. Aspirin should be continued.
        ii. Elective surgery should be deferred, if possible, for at least 6 weeks after BMS placement and for at least 6 months after DES placement.
        iii. Patients with a BMS who require surgery within 6 weeks of placement should continue clopidogrel/prasugrel.
        iv. Patients with a DES who require surgery within 12 months of placement should continue clopidogrel/prasugrel.
        v. For surgery more than 6 weeks after placement of a BMS or 6 months after placement of a DES, continue aspirin and discontinue clopidogrel/prasugrel at least 5 days before surgery.
5. Transition to urgent noncardiac surgery (J Am Coll Cardiol 2012;60:2005-16).
    a. High bleed risk: Aspirin or no antiplatelet therapy
    b. High cardiac event risk and not a high bleed risk
        i. If less than 4 weeks after stent placement, continue DAPT or discontinue the $P2Y_{12}$ inhibitor and continue aspirin.
        ii. If more than 4 weeks after stent placement, continue DAPT.
    c. Not a high cardiac event risk and not a high bleed risk
        i. If less than 4 weeks after stent placement, continue DAPT.
        ii. If more than 4 weeks after stent placement, continue DAPT or discontinue $P2Y_{12}$ inhibitor and continue aspirin.

6. 2012 Society of Thoracic Surgeons Guideline on Use of Antiplatelet Drugs in Patients Having Cardiac and Noncardiac Operations (Ann Thorac Surg 2012;94:1761-81)
   a. Elective cardiac surgery without ACS and no prior stent: Discontinuing aspirin for a few days before surgery is "reasonable."
   b. Noncardiac surgery and no prior stent: Continue antiplatelet monotherapy (either aspirin or clopidogrel).
   c. Noncardiac surgery and prior stent: Continue DAPT unless bleeding risk is prohibitive.
   d. Urgent surgery while undergoing DAPT
      i. Continue aspirin.
      ii. Delay surgery for 1–2 days after discontinuing the $P2Y_{12}$ inhibitor, if possible.
      iii. If DES was placed less than 1 year ago, surgery should be performed less than 5 days after discontinuing the $P2Y_{12}$ inhibitor.
   e. Consider platelet aggregation testing, but the target level of platelet aggregation inhibition when surgery can commence safely has not been established.

J. Statins – See Dyslipidemia Section for Additional Details. Initiation Recommendations *(Domain 1)*
   1. 2013 ACCF/AHA/SCAI STEMI guidelines – A high-intensity statin is recommended before hospital discharge for all patients without contraindications, regardless of baseline LDL-C concentration (atorvastatin 80 mg specifically mentioned).
   2. 2013 AHA/ACC dyslipidemia guidelines - for patients with clinical ASCVD, a high-intensity statin is recommended for patients 75 years and younger, and a moderate-intensity statin is recommended for patients older than 75 years or if not a candidate for high-intensity statin therapy.

K. β-Blockers *(Domain 1)*
   1. Guideline recommendations
      a. Initiate an oral β-blocker within 24 hours for patients without contraindications.
      b. Reevaluate patients with initial contraindication(s) for possible initiation before discharge.
      c. Class I recommendation
         i. Use for all patients with left ventricular systolic dysfunction (LVSD, ejection fraction less than 40%) with HF or prior MI, unless contraindicated.
         ii. Start therapy and continue for 3 years for all patients with history of MI or ACS.
      d. Class IIa recommendation
         i. Reasonable to continue as chronic therapy after 3 years in all patients with history of MI or ACS
         ii. Reasonable for patients with LVSD without HF or prior MI
      e. Class IIb recommendation
         i. Consider as chronic therapy for all other patients with coronary or other vascular disease.
   2. Efficacy and treatment goals
      a. No effect on mortality, but reduced risk of ventricular arrhythmias in COMMIT
      b. Worsened mortality if initiated at higher doses with fixed titration in patients with signs of HF presenting with an acute MI

L. ACE Inhibitors *(Domains 1, 3)*
   1. Guideline recommendations
      a. Initiate within 24 hours in patients with anterior wall STEMI, patients presenting with signs or symptoms of HF, and those with a left ventricular ejection fraction (LVEF) of less than 40% unless contraindication present (class I).
      b. Continue indefinitely in all patients with LVEF of less than 40% and in those with HTN, diabetes, or CKD, unless contraindicated (class I).

    c. Reasonable for all patients with ASCVD to continue indefinitely if no contraindications present (class IIa)

    d. Largest benefit is for patients with a reduced LVEF of less than 40% (class I vs. class IIa recommendation in 2011 AHA Secondary Prevention guidelines).

  2. Efficacy and treatment goals: Meta-analysis (J Am Coll Cardiol 2006;47:1576-83)

    a. A total of 33,500 patients (in six trials) with CAD and preserved LVEF randomly assigned to receive ACE inhibitor or placebo and monitored for a median of 4.4 years

    b. Thirteen percent reduction in all-cause mortality (RR 0.87; 95% CI, 0.81–0.94; p=0.0003), 17% reduction in CV mortality (RR 0.83; 95% CI, 0.72–0.96; p=0.01), 16% reduction in nonfatal MI (RR 0.84; 95% CI, 0.75–0.94; p=0.003), 7% reduction in revascularization rates (RR 0.93; 95% CI, 0.87–1.00; p=0.04)

M. Angiotensin Receptor Blockers *(Domain 1)*

  1. Guideline recommendations

    a. ACCF/AHA guidelines: As an alternative for patients intolerant of ACE inhibitor; same recommendations apply (see above)

    b. No benefit and increased harm (increased adverse effects and study drug discontinuation) if added to ACE inhibitor after MI (Valsartan in Acute Myocardial Infarction Trial [VALIANT])

  2. Efficacy and treatment goals: Valsartan noninferior to captopril in patients with systolic dysfunction after MI in VALIANT

N. Aldosterone Antagonists (mineralocorticoid receptor antagonists [MRAs]) *(Domain 1)*

  1. Guideline recommendations

    a. Eplerenone or spironolactone

    b. For patients post MI without significant renal dysfunction (creatinine values above 2.5 mg/dL in men or above 2.0 mg/dL in women) or hyperkalemia (K greater than 5.0 mEq/L) already receiving therapeutic doses of ACE inhibitor and a β-blocker and with an LVEF of 40% or less, HF, or DM

  2. Efficacy and treatment goals

    a. Eplerenone Post–Acute Myocardial Infarction Heart Failure Efficacy and Survival Study (EPHESUS) of eplerenone (mean dose of about 40 mg/day starting 3–14 days post MI) versus placebo showed a 15% reduction in all-cause mortality with eplerenone at a mean follow-up of 16 months when added to standard care that included antiplatelets, β-blockers, and ACE inhibitors.

    b. No benefit observed in the subgroup of patients with DM, and FDA approval does not include DM without HF symptoms in labeling.

    c. Clinical pearl: Initiate in selected patients as soon as hemodynamically stable after initiation of ACE inhibitor and β-blockers and preferably before hospital discharge. Often, initiation occurs after hospital discharge at the first outpatient appointment.

O. Nitrates *(Domains 1, 2)*

  1. ACCF/AHA guideline recommendations: Not indicated for secondary prevention

  2. Efficacy and treatment goals

    a. Do not reduce mortality

    b. Are indicated for treatment of chronic stable angina as an addition to a β-blocker or calcium channel blocker (CCB)

  3. All patients who are post ACS should be given sublingual or spray nitroglycerin with verbal and written instructions for use.

P. Calcium Channel Blockers *(Domain 1)*
1. ACCF/AHA guideline recommendations
   a. Do not use immediate-release (IR) nifedipine (reflex tachycardia and hypotension).
   b. Are not indicated for secondary prevention of MI
2. Efficacy and treatment goals
   a. Do not reduce mortality
   b. Are indicated for chronic stable angina in a patient with a contraindication to a β-blocker or in combination with a β-blocker

Q. Immunizations *(Domains 1, 2, 5)*
1. Guideline recommendations: Annual influenza vaccination
2. Efficacy and treatment goals
   a. Suggestion that infections, especially influenza and pneumococcal pneumonia, are triggers of plaque rupture and MI
   b. Systematic review reported two small randomized trials of influenza vaccine for secondary prevention with divergent results, leading to a nonsignificant benefit in CV death (RR 0.51;95% CI, 0.15–1.76) (Lancet Infect Dis 2009;9:601-10).
   c. Dual immunization with 23-valent pneumococcal vaccine plus influenza vaccination reduces mortality, pneumonia, MI, and intensive care unit admissions (including for coronary events) compared with placebo in 36,000 Chinese subjects 65 years and older (Clin Infect Dis 2010;51:1007-15).
   d. Kaiser Permanente study of more than 84,000 enrollees found no benefit of pneumococcal vaccination on risk of MI and stroke in patients 45–69 years (JAMA 2010;303:1699-706).

R. Patients with Systolic HF *(Domain 1)*
1. Other than the agents listed above, hydralazine plus nitrate is recommended as an addition to ACE inhibitor, β-blockers (metoprolol succinate, carvedilol, bisoprolol), and diuretics.
2. No trials have addressed which is preferred—An MRA or hydralazine plus nitrate—To add first to ACE inhibitor and β-blocker therapy; however, no MI studies have documented mortality benefit with hydralazine plus nitrates, and less than 25% of patients who enrolled in the African-American Heart Failure Trial (AHeFT) had ischemic heart disease. Therefore, would suggest an MRA before hydralazine plus nitrate for patient post MI

V. HYPERTENSION

Guidelines:
Joint National Committee on Prevention, Detection, and Treatment of High Blood Pressure (JNC) 7 (2002)
AHA/ACCF update (2007)
AHA/ACCF secondary prevention and risk reduction in patients with atherosclerotic vascular disease (2011)
AHA/ACCF updated guideline for the diagnosis and management of patients with stable ischemic heart disease (2012)
ADA Clinical Practice Recommendations (2016)
Kidney Disease: Improving Global Outcomes Clinical Practice Guideline for the Management of Blood Pressure in Chronic Kidney Disease (2012)
JNC 8 (December 2013) - Guideline not sanctioned by National Heart, Lung, and Blood Institute (NHLBI)
American Society of Hypertension (ASH)/International Society of Hypertension (ISH) Clinical Practice Guidelines for the Management of Hypertension in the Community (December 2013)

A. Epidemiology of HTN in the United States
   1. Almost 1 in 3 U.S. adults has HTN.
   2. In adults 18 years and older, the overall prevalence of HTN was 30.4% (66.9 million) in 2003–2010.
      a. An estimated 35.8 million (53.5%) people did not have their HTN controlled (less than 140/90 mm Hg). This may be because of inadequate lifestyle modifications or inadequate antihypertensive drug doses or combinations.
         i. Of these, 39.4% (14.1 million) were unaware of their HTN.
         ii. Of these, 15.8% (5.7 million) were aware of their HTN but were not receiving pharmacologic treatment.
         iii. Of these, 44.8% (16.0 million) were aware of their HTN and were being treated with medication.
      b. Of the 35.8 million U.S. adults with uncontrolled HTN, 89.4% reported having a usual source of health care, and 85.2% reported having health insurance.
   3. Most common primary diagnosis during office visits

B. Classification and Management of BP for Adults – From JNC 7 and ASH/ISH Guidelines (not defined in JNC 8) *(Domain 1)*
   1. Pre-HTN: SBP 120–139 mm Hg; diastolic BP (DBP) 80–89 mm Hg
   2. Stage 1 HTN: SBP 140–159 mm Hg; DBP 90–99 mm Hg
   3. Stage 2 HTN: SBP 160 mm Hg or greater; DBP 100 mm Hg or greater
   4. If the SBP and DBP fall into different classifications, the patient's condition is staged according to the higher category.

C. Identifiable Causes of HTN *(Domain 1)*
   1. Sleep apnea
   2. Drug-induced or related causes (see section L.3.d for specific drugs)
   3. Chronic kidney disease
   4. Primary aldosteronism
   5. Renovascular disease
   6. Chronic steroid therapy or Cushing syndrome
   7. Pheochromocytoma
   8. Coarctation of the aorta
   9. Thyroid or parathyroid disease

D. Risks of HTN *(Domain 1)*
   1. The relationship between BP and CVD events is continuous, consistent, and independent of other risk factors.
   2. For people 40–70 years of age, each increment of 20 mm Hg in SBP or 10 mm Hg in DBP doubles the risk of CVD across the range of 115/75–185/115 mm Hg.
   3. Target organ damage
      a. Heart
         i. Left ventricular hypertrophy
         ii. Angina or MI
         iii. Coronary revascularization
         iv. Heart failure
            (a) Reduced LVEF
            (b) Preserved LVEF
      b. Brain: Stroke or TIA
      c. Chronic kidney disease
      d. Peripheral arterial disease
      e. Retinopathy

E. Benefits of Lowering BP *(Domain 1)*
   1. Associated with relative risk reductions in the incidence of the following conditions:
      a. Stroke: 35%–40%
      b. MI: 20%–25%
      c. HF: Greater than 50%
   2. In patients with stage 1 HTN and additional cardiac risk factors, achieving a sustained 12-mm-Hg reduction in SBP for 10 years will prevent one death for every 11 patients treated. In the presence of CVD or other target organ damage, only nine patients would require such a BP reduction to prevent a death.

Patient Case

6. M.P., a 52-year-old Asian woman, presents to the clinic to discuss her heartburn symptoms. Her primary care physician has been running late, and she was rushed back to her examination room a few minutes ago. Her BP is 151/84 mm Hg. She has no history of HTN, and the only drug she takes is OTC famotidine. Which is the next best action to take for M.P.?

   A. Recheck her BP after she has been seated quietly for 5 minutes.
   B. Initiate hydrochlorothiazide 12.5 mg/day.
   C. Initiate lisinopril 10 mg/day.
   D. There is no need for concern with her BP because she does not have HTN.

F. Accurate BP Measurement *(Domain 1)*
   1. Seated quietly for 5 minutes with feet on floor, back supported, and arm supported at heart level
   2. Appropriate-sized cuff: Cuff width should be ⅓ to ½ of limb circumference, and bladder length should be about 80% of the arm circumference.
   3. At least two measurements should be made.
   4. Clinicians should provide to patients, both verbally and in writing, their specific BP readings and goals.

G. Self-Measurement of BP *(Domains 1, 2)*
   1. Helpful in evaluating white-coat HTN and long-term BP monitoring
      a. White-coat HTN: Uncontrolled office BP with a controlled average BP by 24-hour ambulatory blood pressure monitoring (ABPM) (below 130/80 mm Hg) or home BP above 135/85 mm Hg
   2. Home measurement devices should be checked regularly for accuracy.
   3. Automatically inflating arm devices are preferred to wrist monitors or manual inflation devices for accuracy.

H. Ambulatory Blood Pressure Monitoring *(Domains 1, 2)*
   1. Devices should meet validation standards (www.dableducational.org).
   2. Systolic ABPM has been found to statistically significantly predict stroke and other CV outcomes independently of office BP monitoring (Ann Int Med 2015;162:192-204).
   3. For groups where office BP below 140/90 mm Hg is defined as controlled, the 24-hour mean BP should be below 130/80 mm Hg, with a corresponding mean daytime BP below 135/85 mm Hg and mean nighttime BP below 120/70 mm Hg (J Hypertens 2014;32:1359-66).

I. Patient Evaluation *(Domain 1)*
   1. Assess lifestyle and identify other CV risk factors or concomitant disorders that may affect prognosis and treatment.
   2. Evaluate for identifiable causes of elevated BP.
   3. Assess for the presence of CVD or other target organ damage.

J. BP Goals – Variation in National Guidelines *(Domains 1, 3)*
   1. 2014 Evidence-Based Guideline for the Management of High Blood Pressure in Adults (JNC 8 Committee) - Guideline not sanctioned by NHLBI
      a. Goal less than 150/90 mm Hg for patients 60 years and older who do not have DM or CKD
      b. Goal less than 140/90 mm Hg for patients younger than 60 years
      c. Goal less than 140/90 mm Hg for patients with CKD or diabetes
   2. 2013 ASH/ISH HTN guidelines
      a. Goal less than 150/90 mm Hg for patients 80 years and older
      b. Goal less than 140/90 mm Hg for patients younger than 80 years
      c. Goal less than 140/90 mm Hg for patients with CKD or DM
   3. 2013 ACC/AHA: "An effective approach to high blood pressure control": No specific BP goals mentioned beyond less than 140/90 mm Hg
   4. 2011 AHA/ACCF secondary prevention update and 2012 AHA/ACCF ischemic heart disease update – Goal less than 140/90 mm Hg for patients with coronary and other atherosclerotic vascular disease
   5. 2016 ADA clinical practice recommendations update
      a. Goal less than 140/90 mm Hg for patients with DM
      b. Lower systolic targets (e.g., less than 130 mm Hg) may be appropriate for certain individuals (e.g., younger patients) if they can be achieved without undue treatment burden.
   6. 2013 KDIGO
      a. Goal less than 140/90 mm Hg: For adults with and without diabetes who have CKD and urine albumin excretion less than 30 mg/24 hours (or equivalent)
      b. Goal less than 130/80 mm Hg: For adults with and without diabetes who have CKD and urine albumin excretion greater than 30 mg/24 hours (or equivalent)

Patient Case

7. A 50-year-old African American woman with no significant medical history presents to your clinic for her BP assessment. When she participated in a health fair in the past week, she was told her BP was "too high." Today, her BP is 150/85 mm Hg, with repeat of 147/83 mm Hg. Her HR is 72 beats/minute. She currently takes vitamin D supplementation daily and acetaminophen as needed. Laboratory test results reveal SCr 0.9 mg/dL, K 4.0 mEq/L, and Na 141 mEq/L. Her BMI is 26.0 kg/m². Which is the next best action that should be taken for her?

    A. Treat with education on diet and exercise only.
    B. Treat with education on diet and exercise, and initiate terazosin 1 mg/day.
    C. Treat with education on diet and exercise, and initiate hydrochlorothiazide 12.5 mg/day.
    D. No action is needed.

K. Treatment *(Domains 1, 3)*
    1. 2014 Evidence-Based Guideline for the Management of High Blood Pressure in Adults (by the JNC 8 Committee)
        a. In non–African American populations, initial antihypertensive therapy should include a thiazide-type diuretic, a CCB, an ACE inhibitor, or an ARB.
        b. In the African American population, initial antihypertensive therapy should include a thiazide-type diuretic or CCB.
        c. For adult patients with CKD, initial or add-on antihypertensive therapy should include an ACE inhibitor or an ARB.
        d. No specific therapy recommendations for patients with diabetes or CVD
    2. 2013 ASH/ISH HTN guidelines
        a. Stage I (140–159/90–99 mm Hg) – May delay therapy until after trial of lifestyle modification
            i. African American patients
                (a) Initial therapy: CCB or thiazide diuretic (combine if necessary)
                (b) Subsequent therapy: Add ACE inhibitor or ARB.
            ii. Non–African American patients
                (a) Age younger than 60 years
                    (1) Initial therapy: ACE inhibitor or ARB
                    (2) Subsequent therapy: Add CCB or thiazide diuretic (combine if necessary).
                (b) Age 60 years or older
                    (1) Initial therapy: CCB or thiazide diuretic (combine if necessary)
                    (2) Subsequent therapy: Add ACE inhibitor or ARB.
        b. Stage II (160/100 mm Hg or greater) – Therapy initiated for all patients
            i. Start with two drugs: CCB or thiazide diuretics plus ACE inhibitor or ARB.
            ii. If necessary, combine CCB, thiazide diuretic, and ACE inhibitor or ARB.
        c. Comorbid conditions
            i. Chronic kidney disease
                (a) Initial therapy: ACE inhibitor or ARB
                (b) Subsequent therapy: Add a CCB or thiazide diuretic (combine if necessary).
            ii. Diabetes
                (a) Initial therapy: ACE inhibitor or ARB
                (b) Subsequent therapy: Add CCB or thiazide diuretic (combine if necessary).

   iii. Coronary disease
       (a) Initial therapy: β-Blocker with ACE inhibitor or ARB
       (b) Subsequent therapy: Add CCB or thiazide diuretic (combine if necessary).
   iv. Stroke
       (a) Initial therapy: ACE inhibitor or ARB
       (b) Subsequent therapy: Add CCB or thiazide diuretic (combine if necessary).
   v. Symptomatic HF
       (a) Regardless of BP, should receive ACE inhibitor or ARB plus a β-blocker plus a diuretic plus spironolactone
       (b) If BP is elevated, add dihydropyridine CCB.
3. 2013 ACC/AHA: "An effective approach to high blood pressure control"
   a. For stage 1 HTN, thiazide diuretic recommended as initial therapy (other drug classes not mentioned)
   b. ACE inhibitors, ARBs, and CCB recommended as subsequent therapy
   c. For stage 2 HTN, two-drug therapy preferred
       i. Thiazide plus ACE inhibitor, ARB, or CCB
       ii. ACE inhibitor plus CCB
   d. Certain disease states with specific medication recommendations
       i. CAD: β-Blockers and ACE inhibitors
       ii. Systolic HF: ACE inhibitors or ARBs, β-blockers (metoprolol succinate, carvedilol, bisoprolol), aldosterone antagonists, thiazide diuretics
       iii. Diastolic HF: ACE inhibitors, ARBs, β-blockers, thiazide diuretics
       iv. Diabetes: ACE inhibitors, ARBs, thiazide diuretics, β-blockers, CCBs
       v. Renal disease: ACE inhibitors, ARBs
       vi. Stroke or TIA: Thiazide diuretics, ACE inhibitors
4. Landmark trial: Primary outcomes in high-risk hypertensive patients randomly assigned to receive ACE inhibitor or CCB versus diuretic: The Antihypertensive and Lipid-Lowering Treatment to Prevent Heart Attack Trial (ALLHAT) – 2002
   a. More than 33,000 individuals, 55 years and older, with HTN and one additional risk factor
   b. Participants were randomly assigned to receive chlorthalidone 12.5–25 mg/day (n=15,255), amlodipine 2.5–10 mg/day (n=9048), lisinopril 10–40 mg/day (n=9054).
   c. The primary outcome was combined fatal CHD or nonfatal MI, analyzed by intent-to-treat.
   d. No differences were found in the primary CHD outcome or in mortality between the thiazide-type diuretic chlorthalidone; the ACE inhibitor lisinopril; or the CCB amlodipine.
   e. Original authors' conclusion: Thiazide-type diuretics are superior in preventing one or more major forms of CVD and are less expensive.
   f. Limitations of the study include the following:
       i. Atenolol was added as a second drug (may not be the most appropriate).
       ii. Mean SBPs were higher in the amlodipine-treated arm (0.8 mm Hg; p=0.03) and the lisinopril arm (2 mm Hg; p<0.001) than in chlorthalidone-treated patients.
       iii. New-onset DM was higher in the chlorthalidone arm.
       iv. Chlorthalidone is not the most common thiazide used in the United States, and the clinical implications of comparing hydrochlorothiazide with other antihypertensives are unknown.
       v. Started with monotherapy, although much shifting has been toward combination therapy in recent years (supported by the benazepril plus amlodipine or hydrochlorothiazide for HTN in a high-risk patient trial [ACCOMPLISH]).
   g. Thiazide-type diuretics may no longer be less expensive than other generically available antihypertensive medications.

5. Lifestyle modification
    a. Weight reduction: Can reduce SBP by 5–20 mm Hg for every 10 kg of weight loss
    b. Diet
        i. Dietary Approaches to Stop Hypertension (DASH) diet – Can reduce SBP by 8–14 mm Hg
        ii. Sodium restriction – Can reduce SBP by 2–8 mm Hg
    c. Exercise: 30 minutes/day of aerobic activity on most days of the week can reduce SBP by 4–9 mm Hg.
    d. Moderation of alcohol consumption: Limiting consumption to no more than two drinks a day for men or one drink a day for women can reduce SBP by 2–4 mm Hg.
6. Pharmacotherapy
    a. ACE inhibitors (e.g., lisinopril, enalapril, captopril, ramipril, trandolapril)
        i. Mechanism of action – Prevent conversion of angiotensin I to angiotensin II (potent vasoconstrictor) by competitive inhibition of ACE. Results in lower BP secondary to lower levels of angiotensin II, increased levels of plasma renin activity, and a reduction in aldosterone secretion
        ii. Evidence
            (a) Effects of an ACE inhibitor, ramipril, on CV events in high-risk patients: the Heart Outcomes Prevention Evaluation Study (HOPE)
            (b) Efficacy of Perindopril in Reduction of Cardiovascular Events Among Patients with Stable Coronary Artery Disease: Randomized, double-blind, placebo-controlled, multicenter trial (EUROPA)
            (c) ACE inhibitor in stable CAD (PEACE)
            (d) Randomized trial of a perindopril-based blood pressure–lowering regimen among 6105 individuals with previous stroke or TIA (PROGRESS)
            (e) Effect of captopril on mortality and morbidity in patients with left ventricular dysfunction after MI: Results of the Survival And Ventricular Enlargement trial (SAVE)
            (f) A comparison of outcomes with ACE inhibitors and diuretics for HTN in the elderly (ANBP2)
        iii. Clinical use
            (a) Indications to use ACE inhibitors first line
                (1) Non–African American patients
                (2) DM – Reduce the progression of nephropathy and albuminuria
                (3) CKD – Reduce the progression of diabetic and nondiabetic renal disease
                (4) HF or left ventricular dysfunction with an LVEF of 40% or less
                (5) CAD
                (6) Recurrent stroke prevention – Reduce recurrence when used in combination with thiazide diuretics
            (b) Recommended add-on therapy for African American patients
        iv. Contraindications
            (a) Bilateral renal artery stenosis
            (b) Pregnancy
            (c) Angioedema
        v. Important adverse drug reactions (ADRs)
            (a) Increasing creatinine (Cr) – Limited rise as much as 30% above baseline is acceptable. This becomes the patient's new baseline Cr concentration.
            (b) Hyperkalemia
            (c) Angioedema – Occurs 2–4 times more often in African Americans
            (d) Cough, dry (11% with 2.5% discontinuation)

    vi. Dosing and monitoring

        (a) Consider avoiding in women during childbearing years.

        (b) Consider starting at lower-than-average dose if patient is elderly, is receiving concomitant diuretic therapy, or has renal impairment.

        (c) Reassess SCr and K 1 to 2 weeks after initiation or dose titration.

Patient Case

8. A 60-year-old white man with type 2 DM is new to your clinic. Today, his BP is 155/78 mm Hg, with repeat of 151/73 mm Hg. His HR is 80 beats/minute. He reports intolerance to two different ACE inhibitors because of cough. He is currently taking metformin 850 mg three times/day, glipizide 10 mg twice daily, hydrochlorothiazide 25 mg/day, and omeprazole as needed. Laboratory test results are as follows: Cr 1.5 mg/dL (CrCl [IBW] 54 mL/minute), A1C 6.8%, K 4.0 mEq/L, and microalbumin/Cr 98.2. His BMI is 31.6 kg/m². Which option is best for addressing his elevated BP?

    A. No further treatment is needed.

    B. Initiate amlodipine 2.5 mg/day.

    C. Initiate losartan 25 mg/day.

    D. Initiate atenolol 25 mg/day.

---

    b. Angiotensin receptor blockers (e.g., losartan, irbesartan, candesartan, olmesartan, telmisartan)

      i. Mechanism of action – Selective, competitive angiotensin II receptor type 1 receptor antagonist, reducing the end-organ responses to angiotensin II. Results in decreased total peripheral resistance (afterload) and cardiac venous return (preload). Reduction in BP occurs independently of the status of the renin-angiotensin system.

      ii. Evidence

        (a) CV morbidity and mortality in the Losartan Intervention For Endpoint reduction in hypertension study (LIFE): A randomized trial against atenolol

        (b) Valsartan, captopril, or both, in MI complicated by HF, left ventricular dysfunction, or both (VALIANT)

      iii. Clinical use

        (a) Indications to use ARBs first line

          (1) Non–African American patients

          (2) DM – Reduce the progression of nephropathy and albuminuria

          (3) CKD– Reduce the progression of diabetic and nondiabetic renal disease

          (4) HF or left ventricular dysfunction with LVEF of 40% or less

          (5) CAD

          (6) Recurrent stroke prevention – Reduce recurrence when used in combination with thiazide diuretics

        (b) Recommended add-on therapy for African American patients

      iv. Contraindications

        (a) Bilateral renal artery stenosis

        (b) Pregnancy

        (c) Angioedema (ARB-induced or idiopathic) – Although ARBs may be considered alternative therapy for patients who have developed angioedema while taking an ACE inhibitor, patients have also developed angioedema with ARBs, and extreme caution is advised when substituting an ARB for a patient who has had angioedema associated with ACE inhibitor use. Must weigh risk versus benefit of use.

      v.   Important ADRs – Similar to those with ACE inhibitors except for cough

         (a) Increasing SCr – Limited rise of as much as 30% above baseline is acceptable. This becomes the patient's new baseline SCr value.

         (b) Hyperkalemia

         (c) Angioedema – Less than with ACE inhibitors

      vi. Dosing and monitoring

         (a) Consider avoiding in women during childbearing years.

         (b) Monitor SCr and K values for 7–10 days after initiation or titration.

c. Renin inhibitor (aliskiren)

    i. Mechanism of action – Direct renin inhibition, decreasing plasma renin activity and inhibiting the conversion of angiotensinogen to angiotensin I

    ii. Evidence

         (a) No outcomes data available for aliskiren monotherapy

         (b) Aliskiren Trial in Type 2 Diabetes Using Cardiovascular and Renal Disease Endpoints (ALTITUDE) – Study terminated early

            (1) Aliskiren added to ACE inhibitor or ARB therapy in patients with type 2 DM and renal impairment compared with a placebo add-on

            (2) An increase in adverse events (nonfatal stroke, renal complications, hyperkalemia, and hypotension) and no apparent benefits among patients randomly assigned to aliskiren group

    iii. Contraindication

         (a) Pregnancy

         (b) Do not use with ARBs or ACE inhibitors in patients with diabetes.

    iv. Important ADRs

         (a) Angioedema

         (b) Hyperkalemia if used concomitantly with ACE inhibitor

    v. Dosing and monitoring

         (a) Consider avoiding in women during childbearing years.

         (b) High-fat meals decrease absorption substantially.

         (c) Patients with renal insufficiency were excluded from trials.

d. β-Blockers (e.g., metoprolol, atenolol, bisoprolol, carvedilol, labetalol, nebivolol)

    i. Mechanism of action – Selective (β_1 only) or nonselective (β_1 and β_2) receptor blocker results in negative inotropic and chronotropic actions. Some β-blockers (e.g., pindolol, acebutolol) exhibit intrinsic sympathomimetic activity, meaning they are capable of exerting low-level agonist activity at the β-adrenergic receptor while simultaneously acting as a receptor site antagonist. Cardioselective agents without intrinsic sympathomimetic activity are usually used for HTN. Carvedilol and labetalol also have α_1-blocking activity.

    ii. Evidence – ACCF/AHA guidelines since the 1980s

    iii. Clinical use

         (a) Indications

             (1) HF or left ventricular systolic dysfunction with LVEF of 40% or less – First line (metoprolol, carvediolol, bisoprolol) with ACE inhibitors

            (2) Post MI (within first 3 years) – First line

         (b) β-Blockers with α_1-blocking activity are likely more effective antihypertensive agents than β-blockers without this mechanism.

    iv. Contraindications

         (a) Sinoatrial or atrioventricular (AV) node dysfunction

         (b) Decompensated HF

         (c) Severe bronchospastic disease

v. Important ADRs
  (a) Bradycardia – Adjust doses for symptomatic bradycardia only.
  (b) Heart block – Adjust doses for greater than first-degree heart block.
  (c) Bronchospastic disease
  (d) Exercise intolerance, sexual dysfunction, fatigue

vi. Dosing and monitoring
  (a) Relative contraindications include significant sinus or AV node dysfunction, hypotension, decompensated HF, and severe bronchospastic lung disease.
  (b) Monitor HR regularly.

Patient Case

9. A 65-year-old African American woman with progressing renal insufficiency presents to the clinic. Today, her BP is 128/65 mm Hg, with repeat of 129/66 mm Hg. She is currently taking hydrochlorothiazide 25 mg/day, lisinopril 10 mg/day, amlodipine 5 mg/day, and a multivitamin daily. At her previous clinic visit 2 months ago, her Cr was 1.5 mg/dL (CrCl [IBW] 35 mL/minute). Today, laboratory test results reveal Cr 2.0 mg/dL (CrCl [IBW] 26.3 mL/minute), K 3.3 mEq/L, Na 133 mEq/L, and microalbumin/Cr 65. Her BMI is 21.9 kg/m². Which change, if any, would be best for her medication regimen?

A. Discontinue hydrochlorothiazide.

B. Discontinue amlodipine.

C. Increase amlodipine to 10 mg/day.

D. No change in her current regimen is warranted.

---

e. Diuretics
  i. Thiazides (e.g., hydrochlorothiazide, chlorthalidone, metolazone, indapamide)
    (a) Mechanism of action – Act on the kidneys to reduce Na reabsorption in the distal convoluted tubule. By impairing Na transport in the distal convoluted tubule, natriuresis and concomitant water loss are induced.
    (b) Evidence
      (1) ALLHAT
      (2) Prevention of stroke by antihypertensive drug treatment in older people with isolated systolic HTN: Final results of the Systolic Hypertension in the Elderly Program (SHEP)
      (3) Medical Research Council (MRC) trial of treatment of mild HTN: Principal results
    (c) Clinical use
      (1) Option as first-line therapy for most patients with HTN, either alone or in combination with one of the other drug classes (ACE inhibitors, ARBs, CCBs)
      (2) Enhances the efficacy of multidrug regimens
    (d) Contraindication – Anuria
    (e) Important ADRs
      (1) Electrolyte abnormalities (hypokalemia, hyponatremia)
      (2) Hyperuricemia
    (f) Dosing and monitoring
      (1) Ineffective for patients with a GFR less than 30 mL/minute
      (2) Monitor SCr, Na, and K for 7–10 days after initiation or titration.

ii. Loop (e.g., furosemide, bumetanide, torsemide, ethacrynic acid)
   (a) Mechanism of action – Act by reversibly binding to the Na, K, chloride cotransport mechanism on the luminal side of the ascending loop of Henle, thereby inhibiting the active reabsorption of these ions
   (b) Clinical use: HTN management for patients with HF and CKD, using scheduled twice-daily dosing
   (c) Contraindication – Anuria
   (d) Important ADRs
      (1) Electrolyte abnormalities (hypokalemia, hyponatremia, hypomagnesemia)
      (2) Dehydration
   (e) Dosing and monitoring
      (1) Monitor SCr, Na, and K for 7–10 days after initiation or titration.
      (2) Approximate dose equivalence
         (A) Furosemide 40 mg
         (B) Bumetanide 1 mg
         (C) Torsemide 10-20 mg
   (f) Ethacrynic acid 25–50 mg (may be useful for patients with allergic reactions to other loop diuretics caused by sulfa moiety)
iii. Potassium-sparing (e.g., triamterene, amiloride)
   (a) Mechanism of action – Block the epithelial Na channel on the lumen side of the kidney collecting tubule. Sodium channel blockers directly inhibit the entry of Na into the Na channels.
   (b) Clinical use: Typically used in combination with thiazide diuretic for K balance
   (c) Contraindication
      (1) Anuria
      (2) Hyperkalemia
      (3) Severe renal or hepatic disease
   (d) Important ADRs – Hyperkalemia
   (e) Dosing and monitoring
      (1) Avoid in patients with a CrCl less than 10 mL/minute.
      (2) Monitor SCr and K for 7–10 days after initiation or titration.
f. Calcium channel blockers
   i. Dihydropyridines (e.g., amlodipine, felodipine, nifedipine, nicardipine)
      (a) Mechanism of action – Act by relaxing the smooth muscle in the arterial wall, decreasing total peripheral resistance, and hence reducing BP. In angina, they increase blood flow to the heart muscle.
      (b) Evidence
         (1) ACCOMPLISH trial
         (2) Prevention of CV events with an antihypertensive regimen of amlodipine, adding perindopril as required versus atenolol, adding bendroflumethiazide as required, in the Anglo-Scandinavian Cardiac Outcomes Trial-Blood Pressure Lowering Arm (ASCOT-BPLA): a multicenter randomized controlled trial.
         (3) Outcomes in hypertensive patients at high CV risk treated with regimens based on valsartan or amlodipine (VALUE)
         (4) Effects of intensive BP lowering and low-dose aspirin in patients with HTN: Principal results of the Hypertension Optimal Treatment (HOT) randomized trial

   (c) Clinical use
    (1) Option as first-line therapy for most patients with HTN
    (2) Potent BP lowering
    (3) Improve anginal symptoms
   (d) Important ADRs – Peripheral edema, orthostasis, reflex tachycardia
   (e) Dosing and monitoring – Start at a low dose for elderly patients.
  ii. Non-dihydropyridines (verapamil, diltiazem)
   (a) Mechanism of action – Act as a potent vasodilator of coronary vessels, increasing blood flow and decreasing the HR by strong depression of AV node conduction. In addition, act as a potent vasodilator of peripheral vessels, reducing peripheral resistance and afterload. They have negative inotropic effects.
   (b) Evidence
    (1) Principal results of the Controlled Onset Verapamil Investigation of Cardiovascular End Points trial (CONVINCE)
    (2) A CCB versus a non-CCB treatment strategy for patients with CAD: The International Verapamil-Trandolapril Study (INVEST): A randomized controlled trial
    (3) Randomized trial of effects of CCBs compared with diuretics and β-blockers on CV morbidity and mortality in HTN: The Nordic Diltiazem study (NORDIL)
   (c) Clinical use: Used for HTN in patients with concomitant conditions (e.g., atrial fibrillation or stable angina) who would benefit from these medications
   (d) Contraindications
    (1) Heart block
    (2) Sick sinus syndrome
   (e) Important ADRs
    (1) Bradycardia
    (2) Heart block
    (3) Constipation
   (f) Dosing and monitoring
    (1) Potent cytochrome P450 (CYP) inhibitors; source of potentially serious drug-drug interactions
    (2) Do not use with concomitant systolic dysfunction HF (ejection fraction less than 40%).
    (3) Use with caution in patients receiving concomitant β-blocker therapy.
 g. α_1-Blockers (e.g., terazosin, doxazosin, prazosin)
  i. Mechanism of action – Selective α_1-antagonists that work by blocking the action of adrenaline on smooth muscle of the blood vessel walls
  ii. Evidence – ALLHAT showed a 25% higher rate of combined CVD and a 2-fold higher rate of HF compared with the diuretic arm.
  iii. Clinical use
   (a) In general, reserved for hypertensive male patients with concomitant benign prostatic hyperplasia
   (b) Usually viewed as fourth- or fifth-line agent for HTN
  iv. Important ADRs – Dizziness and orthostatic hypotension
  v. Dosing and monitoring: Start with a very low dose. Patient should consider taking the first dose at night while in bed. Titrate slowly over time as needed.

h. Aldosterone receptor blockers (spironolactone, eplerenone)

   i. Mechanism of action – Inhibit the effect of aldosterone by competing for intracellular aldosterone receptors in the cortical collecting duct. This decreases the reabsorption of Na and water while decreasing the secretion of K.

   ii. Evidence

      (a) Efficacy of low-dose spironolactone in subjects with resistant HTN

      (b) The role of spironolactone in the treatment of patients with refractory HTN

   iii. Clinical use

      (a) Resistant HTN

      (b) Patients with HTN and HF

   iv. Contraindications

      (a) Anuria

      (b) Acute renal insufficiency – Avoid if CrCl is 30 mL/minute or less.

      (c) Hyperkalemia – Avoid if K is 5.0 mEq/L or greater.

   v. Important ADRs

      (a) Hyperkalemia

      (b) Gynecomastia and mastodynia with spironolactone

   vi. Dosing and monitoring: Monitor Cr and K for 3 days, 7 days, and monthly for the first 3 months after initiation or titration, then periodically thereafter.

i. Central α_2-agonists (e.g., clonidine, methyldopa, guanfacine)

   i. Mechanism of action – Stimulate α_2-receptors in the brain, which decreases sympathetic outflow, cardiac output, and peripheral vascular resistance, lowering BP and HR

   ii. Clinical use

      (a) May be useful for resistant HTN

      (b) Beneficial for hypertensive urgency

   iii. Important ADRs

      (a) Dizziness and orthostatic hypotension

      (b) Drowsiness

      (c) Dry mouth

   iv. Dosing and monitoring

      (a) Rebound HTN possible if withdrawn too quickly, especially if taking concomitant β-blocker (except for carvedilol and labetalol, because of unopposed α-stimulation)

      (b) Avoid in patients with HF

j. Vasodilators (e.g., hydralazine, minoxidil)

   i. Mechanism of action – Direct-acting smooth muscle relaxants that act as a vasodilator primarily in arteries and arterioles

   ii. Clinical use

      (a) May be useful for resistant HTN

      (b) May be beneficial for patients with HTN and HF (hydralazine)

   iii. Important ADRs

      (a) Hydralazine

         (1) Tachycardia (use with β-blocker)

         (2) Drug-induced lupus-like syndrome

      (b) Minoxidil

         (1) Fluid retention (use with diuretic)

         (2) Pericardial effusion

         (3) Hirsutism

   iv. Dosing and monitoring – Can dose two to four times daily

Patient Case

10. A 58-year-old Hispanic woman with CAD and type 2 DM presents to the clinic with her home BP readings. She is frustrated because her BP is still not at goal. She is currently taking hydrochlorothiazide 25 mg/day, lisinopril 40 mg/day, amlodipine 10 mg/day, and metoprolol 25 mg twice daily. She tried terazosin but had to discontinue it because of dizziness. Today, her BP is 148/79 mm Hg, with repeat of 145/81 mm Hg. Her HR is 58 beats/minute. Laboratory test results today are as follows: Cr 1.2 mg/dL (CrCl [adjusted body weight {ABW}] 51.8 mL/minute), K 3.9 mEq/L, and Na 142 mEq/L. Her BMI is 27.5 kg/m², and her ejection fraction is 45%. Which regimen change, if any, would be the best intervention for this patient?

   A. Initiate spironolactone 25 mg/day.
   B. Discontinue hydrochlorothiazide and start spironolactone 25 mg/day.
   C. Increase metoprolol to 50 mg twice daily.
   D. No change in her current regimen is warranted.

7. Achieving BP control
   a. Most patients who are hypertensive will require two or more antihypertensive medications to achieve their BP goals.
   b. Addition of a second drug from a different class when use of a single drug in adequate doses fails to achieve the BP goal
   c. When BP is more than 20/10 mm Hg above goal, consider initiating therapy with two drugs. Use caution in patients at risk of orthostatic hypotension.
   d. Patients should return for follow-up and adjustment of medications at monthly intervals until goal is achieved. Appropriate laboratory tests (based on medications used) should be obtained and may be necessary at closer intervals after initiation of therapy.
   e. More frequent visits may be necessary for patients with stage 2 HTN or with complicating conditions.
   f. Once BP is at goal and stable, follow-up visits can occur at less frequent intervals.
   g. Referral to HTN specialist may be indicated for patients in whom goal BP cannot be attained with several medications at maximum effective and/or tolerated doses.

L. Specific Indications *(Domains 1–3)*
   1. Ischemic heart disease
      a. Most common form of target organ damage associated with HTN
      b. 2011 AHA/ACCF secondary prevention update
         i. Patients with coronary and other atherosclerotic vascular disease
         ii. For BP readings of 140/90 mm Hg or greater, patients should be treated with BP medication, as tolerated, treating initially with β-blockers and/or ACE inhibitors, with the addition of other drugs as needed to achieve goal BP.
      c. 2012 AHA/ACCF on stable ischemic heart disease
         i. For patients with stable ischemic heart disease having a BP of 140/90 mm Hg or higher, antihypertensive drug therapy should be instituted in addition to or after a trial of lifestyle modifications.
         ii. The specific medications used for treatment of high BP should be based on specific patient characteristics and may include ACE inhibitors and/or β-blockers, with the addition of other drugs (e.g., thiazide diuretics, CCBs) if needed to achieve a goal BP of less than 140/90 mm Hg.

2. Heart failure
   a. No specific BP goal
   b. Asymptomatic individuals with demonstrable ventricular dysfunction: ACE inhibitors and β-blockers
   c. Symptomatic ventricular dysfunction or end-stage heart disease: ACE inhibitor (or ARB), β-blocker (metoprolol succinate, carvedilol, bisoprolol), aldosterone antagonists (with loop diuretics)
3. HTN in patients with diabetes
   a. ADA Standards of Medical Care in Diabetes 2016: BP goal less than 140/90 mm Hg
   b. Cochrane review 2009: No significant reduction in total mortality, MI, stroke, HF, or CVD events with lower BP target.
   c. European Society of Cardiology 2012 guidelines on primary prevention recommend a BP goal of less than 140/80 mm Hg for patients with DM, according to results from the ACCORD (Action to Control Cardiovascular Risk in Diabetes) BP study, which showed a small reduction in stroke (secondary end point), no reduction in the primary end point, and increased adverse effects when antihypertensive therapy was targeted to a BP of less than 120 mm Hg (Eur Heart J 2012;33:1635-701).
   d. Combinations of two or more drugs are usually needed to achieve a goal of less than 140/90 mm Hg. Combinations should include an ACE inhibitor or an ARB (but not both), if no contraindications.
   e. ACE inhibitors, ARBs, thiazide diuretics, β-blockers, and dihydropyridine CCBs are beneficial in reducing CVD and stroke incidence in patients with DM.
   f. ACE inhibitor– and ARB-based treatments favorably affect the progression of diabetic nephropathy and reduce albuminuria.
   g. Administer one or more antihypertensive medications at bedtime.
4. Chronic kidney disease (GFR less than 60 mL/minute or the presence of albuminuria)
   a. According to the KDIGO guidelines, BP management depends on whether patients have proteinuria. This is based, in part, on the African American Study of Kidney Disease (AASK) study, which showed that the benefit of lower BP in preventing the progression of renal disease was limited to patients with a urinary protein/Cr ratio greater than 0.22. Treatment is as follows:
      i. ACE inhibitors/ARBs preferentially used
         (a) Suggest use in adults with and without diabetes who have CKD and urine albumin excretion greater than 30 mg/24 hours (or equivalent)
         (b) Recommend use in adults with and without diabetes who have CKD and urine albumin excretion greater than 300 mg/24 hours (or equivalent)
      ii. No preferred antihypertensive medication: Patients with CKD but no significant proteinuria (as described above)
   b. BP management often requires three or more antihypertensive drugs.
   c. A limited rise in SCr of as much as 30% above baseline is acceptable with ACE inhibitors and ARBs.
5. Cerebrovascular disease
   a. Recurrent stroke rates are lowered by the combination of an ACE inhibitor and a thiazide diuretic.
   b. 2011 AHA/ACCF secondary prevention update: Patients with atherosclerotic vascular disease with BP readings of 140/90 mm Hg or greater should be treated, as tolerated.

M. Causes of Resistant HTN (failure to reach goal BP in patients who are prescribed full doses of an appropriate three-drug regimen that includes a diuretic) *(Domains 1, 2)*
   1. Improper BP measurement
   2. Volume overload and pseudotolerance
      a. Excessive Na intake
      b. Volume retention from kidney disease
      c. Inadequate diuretic therapy

3. Drug-induced causes
    a. Nonadherence
        i. Educate patient on benefits of HTN control. Solicit patient buy-in for BP goals, develop patient-centered treatment strategies, and explain the importance of BP self-monitoring.
        ii. Ensure regimen is affordable and well tolerated.
        iii. Adjust treatments on the basis of cultural beliefs and attitudes.
        iv. Use all members of the health care team.
    b. Inadequate doses
    c. Inappropriate drug combinations
    d. Specific drugs
        i. NSAIDs
        ii. Cocaine, amphetamines
        iii. Sympathomimetics
        iv. Oral contraceptives
        v. Adrenal steroids
        vi. Cyclosporine or tacrolimus
        vii. Erythropoietin
        viii. Licorice
        ix. Dietary supplements
4. Associated conditions
    a. Obesity
    b. Alcoholism
5. Identifiable causes of HTN (described above, see section C B)
6. Clinical inertia by the provider may be caused by failure to titrate or combine medications, even though the patient is not at goal. Decision support systems, in addition to involvement of nurse clinicians and pharmacists, can be helpful.

N. Treatment of Resistant HTN *(Domain 1)*
1. Rule out and/or treat, if possible, causes of resistant HTN.
2. For patients with uncontrolled HTN who are taking ACE inhibitor (or ARB) plus thiazide-like diuretic plus CCB, consider adding one (or more) of the following:
    a. Aldosterone antagonist
    b. β-Blocker
    c. α-Blocker
    d. Vasodilator
    e. Centrally acting agent

O. Special Cases *(Domains 1, 2)*
1. Ethnic and socioeconomic considerations
    a. Lowest BP control rates are in Mexican American and Native American people.
    b. Socioeconomic factors and lifestyle may be barriers to BP control.
    c. African American people experience an increase in severity, prevalence, and impact of HTN and have a reduced response to some antihypertensive therapy (β-blockers, ACE inhibitors, and ARBs). Recommend starting with a thiazide diuretic or a dihydropyridine CCB.
2. Obesity (BMI of 30 kg/m² or more)
    a. Prevalent risk factor for HTN and CVD
    b. Intensive lifestyle modification recommended

3. Left ventricular hypertrophy
    a. Independent risk factor for CVD
    b. Regression may occur with aggressive BP management.
4. Older individuals (older than 65 years)
    a. HTN occurs in two-thirds of people older than 65 years.
    b. Lowest rate of BP control
    c. Lower initial drug doses may be indicated, but standard doses and several drugs are usually needed to reach BP goals.
    d. For patients older than 80 years, the HYVET trial (Hypertension in the Very Elderly Trial) showed that targeting a BP of less than 150/80 mm Hg significantly decreases the risk of stroke and all-cause mortality.
5. Postural hypotension
    a. Decrease in standing BP of more than 10 mm Hg, when associated with dizziness, occurs more often in older patients with systolic HTN and DM and in those taking diuretics, vasodilators, and psychotropic drugs.
        i. Orthostatic hypotension is a decrease in SBP of at least 20 mm Hg or a decrease in DBP of at least 10 mm Hg.
    b. Use caution to avoid volume depletion and rapid-dose titration of antihypertensive drugs.
6. Women
    a. Oral estrogen-containing contraceptives may increase BP, and the risk can increase with the duration of use.
    b. HTN increases the risk to mother and fetus in women who are pregnant. Preferred medications include methyldopa, β-blockers (especially labetalol), and vasodilators. ACE inhibitors and ARBs should not be used because of the potential for fetal defects. Avoid atenolol because it can cause intrauterine growth restriction.
7. Hypertensive urgencies – Patients with markedly elevated BP (greater than 180 mm Hg/greater than 120 mm Hg) without acute target organ damage usually do not require hospitalization, but they should receive immediate combination oral antihypertensive therapy. Oral agents typically used include captopril, clonidine, and labetalol. Markedly elevated BP with acute target organ damage is deemed a hypertensive emergency and is not traditionally treated in an ambulatory care setting.

P. Other Potential Effects of Antihypertensive Drug Choices *(Domain 1)*
    1. Favorable
        a. Thiazides – Slow demineralization in osteoporosis
        b. β-Blockers – Treat atrial fibrillation and tachyarrhythmias, angina, migraine prophylaxis, and essential tremor
        c. CCBs – Treat Raynaud syndrome and certain arrhythmias, migraine prophylaxis
        d. α-Blockers – Used in prostatism
        e. ACE inhibitors – May show favorable effects on blood glucose
    2. Unfavorable
        a. Thiazides – Use caution with gout or hyponatremia; may negatively affect blood glucose
        b. β-Blockers – Use caution with asthma or heart block; may negatively affect blood glucose (except carvedilol)
        c. ACE inhibitors or ARBs – Avoid in women who are, or are likely to become, pregnant.
        d. Aldosterone antagonists and K-sparing diuretics – Avoid in patients with K values greater than 5.0 mEq/L or CrCl less than 30 mL/minute.

Patient Case

11. A 72-year-old white man is new to your clinic. He has not seen a health care provider for the past 7 years because of financial issues. Today, his BP is 175/100 mm Hg, with repeat of 169/99 mm Hg. He takes no medications, although he reports taking a drug for his BP "years ago." He reports no symptoms of illness or of feeling bad. Today, laboratory test results are as follows: Cr 1.6 mg/dL (CrCl [ABW] 56.4 mL/minute), K 4.0 mEq/L, and Na 142 mEq/L. His BMI is 30.2 kg/m². Which option is the best intervention to treat this patient's HTN?

   A. Initiate lisinopril/hydrochlorothiazide 10/12.5 mg/day.
   B. Initiate lisinopril 10 mg/day.
   C. Initiate hydrochlorothiazide 12.5 mg/day.
   D. Send him to the emergency department for hypertensive emergency.

VI. DYSLIPIDEMIA

Guidelines:
2013 ACC/AHA Guideline on the Treatment of Blood Cholesterol to Reduce Atherosclerotic Cardiovascular Risk in Adults
2013 KDIGO Clinical Practice Guidelines for Lipid Management in Chronic Kidney Disease
2016 ADA Standards of Medical Care in Diabetes

Patient Case

12. A 62-year-old white man who smokes 1 pack/day presents to your clinic taking no medications. His medical history includes an MI 5 years ago, at which time a stent was placed. The primary care physician would like your help in addressing his cholesterol status. The patient would prefer to lower his cholesterol without medications, if possible. Fasting laboratory results are as follows: TC 187 mg/dL, TG 157 mg/dL, HDL-C 43 mg/dL, LDL-C 113 mg/dL, non–HDL-C 144 mg/dL, SCr 1.0 mg/dL, ALT 25 IU/L, Na 140 mEq/L, and K 4.7 mEq/L. His BMI is 32.5 kg/m², and his BP is 115/65 mm Hg. Which is the best recommendation to treat his cholesterol?

   A. Diet, exercise, and weight loss only.
   B. Diet, exercise, weight loss, and simvastatin 40 mg/day.
   C. Diet, exercise, weight loss, and atorvastatin 80 mg/day.
   D. Diet, exercise, weight loss, and pravastatin 20 mg/day.

   A. Components of a Fasting Lipid Panel *(Domain 1)*
      1. Total cholesterol: Cholesterol
         a. Fat-like substance (lipid) present in cell membranes and a precursor of bile acids and steroid hormones
         b. Travels in the blood in distinct particles containing both lipid and proteins (lipoproteins)
      2. Triglycerides
         a. Found in chylomicrons and very low-density lipoprotein (VLDL)
         b. Treatment
            i. Diet (limit alcohol and simple carbohydrates [e.g., sugar, rice, pasta, and bread])
            ii. Exercise
            iii. Weight loss if BMI greater than 25 kg/m²
            iv. Smoking cessation

      v.   Adequate glucose control for patient with diabetes

      vi. Fibrates (for values greater than 500 mg/dL)

      vii. Niacin

      viii. Omega-3 fatty acids (fish oil)

      ix. If possible, eliminate drug therapy that may contribute to hypertriglyceridemia (e.g., estrogens, corticosteroids)

3. High-density lipoprotein cholesterol
   a. "Good cholesterol"
   b. The major apolipoproteins are apo AI and apo AII
   c. Inversely correlated with risk of CHD
4. Low-density lipoprotein cholesterol
   a. "Bad cholesterol"
   b. Contains a single apolipoprotein (apo B100 [apo B]), which is the major atherogenic lipoprotein
5. Non–HDL-C
   a. Other "bad cholesterol" (TC minus HDL-C)
   b. Combination of LDL-C and VLDL. Because VLDL cholesterol is highly correlated with atherogenic remnant lipoproteins, it is combined with LDL-C to enhance risk prediction when serum TG values are high.

B. Practice Guidelines: 2013 ACC/AHA Guideline on the Treatment of Blood Cholesterol to Reduce ASCVD in Adults RCTs *(Domain 1)*
   1. Identified four groups that benefit from statin therapy to reduce ASCVD events for primary and secondary prevention
      a. Clinical ASCVD – Acute coronary syndromes, or a history of MI, stable or unstable angina, coronary or other arterial revascularization, stroke, TIA, or atherosclerotic PAD
         i. Age 75 or younger – High-intensity statin recommended
         ii. Older than 75 years – Moderate-intensity statin recommended
      b. Primary elevations of LDL-C greater than 190 mg/dL – High-intensity statin recommended
      c. Patients with diabetes, 40–75 years of age, with LDL-C of 70–189 mg/dL and without clinical ASCVD
         i. Estimated 10-year risk of ASCVD at least 7.5% – High-intensity statin recommended
         ii. Estimated 10-year risk of ASCVD less than 7.5% – Moderate-intensity statin recommended
      d. No clinical ASCVD or diabetes with LDL-C of 70–189 mg/dL and estimated 10-year ASCVD risk greater than 7.5%, age 40–75 years – Moderate- to high-intensity statin recommended
         i. Can consider moderate-intensity statin therapy if ASCVD risk ranges from 5% to less than 7.5%.
         ii. The potential for adverse effects may outweigh the potential for ASCVD risk reduction in the group with ASCVD risk of 5% to less than 7.5%.
   2. ASCVD prevention benefit of statin therapy may be less clear in other groups.
   3. May consider other risk factors for ASCVD risk
      a. Primary LDL-C of 160 mg/dL or greater or other evidence of genetic hyperlipidemias
      b. Family history of premature ASCVD with onset before 55 years of age in a first-degree male relative or before 65 years of age in a first-degree female relative
      c. hs-CRP greater than 2 mg/L
      d. Coronary artery calcium score of 300 Agatston units or greater or 75th percentile or greater for age, sex, and ethnicity
      e. ABI less than 0.9
      f. Elevated lifetime risk of ASCVD

4. Consider possible adverse effects, drug-drug interactions, and patient preferences for statin treatment.
5. There is no RCT evidence to support LDL-C or non–HDL-C treatment targets or goals. No recommendations for or against specific LDL-C or non–HDL-C targets were given for any patient population.
   a. Adherence to medication and lifestyle, therapeutic response to statin therapy, and safety should be regularly assessed.
   b. This should also include a fasting lipid panel performed within 4–12 weeks after initiation or dose adjustment and every 3–12 months thereafter.
6. Except for ezetimibe, the benefit of non-statin therapies for ASCVD risk reduction has not been shown to exceed the risk of potential adverse effects.
   a. In individuals with a higher ASCVD risk who are receiving the maximum-tolerated intensity of statin therapy and who continue to have a less-than-anticipated therapeutic response, adding a non-statin cholesterol-lowering drug(s) may be considered if the ASCVD risk-reduction benefits outweigh the potential for adverse effects.
   b. Higher-risk individuals include the following:
      Individuals with clinical ASCVD and younger than 75 years
      Individuals with baseline LDL-C of 190 mg/dL or higher
      Individuals 40–75 years of age with DM
7. The Pooled Cohort Equations are recommended to estimate the 10-year risk of ASCVD in both white and African American men and women.
8. Statin adverse effects should be effectively managed.
9. Additional guidance is needed.
   a. Treatment of hypertriglyceridemia
   b. Role of non–HDL-C
   c. Role of apo B, lipoprotein(a), or LDL-C particles
   d. Role of noninvasive imaging in contributing to risk estimates
   e. Role of lifetime ASCVD risk and optimal age for statin therapy in reducing lifetime risk of ASCVD
   f. Subgroups such as patients with HF or patients on hemodialysis that may benefit from statin therapy
   g. Long-term effects of statin-associated new-onset diabetes and management
   h. Efficacy and safety of statins in patient groups excluded from RCTs
   i. Role of pharmacogenetic testing

Patient Case

13. A 62-year-old woman who underwent three-vessel CABG 5 years earlier and with a history of diabetes completes her fasting laboratory testing. Medications have been stable since her CABG and include simvastatin 80 mg/day, glipizide 5 mg twice daily, metoprolol SR 25 mg/day, and aspirin 81 mg/day. During the past year, she has seen a steady decline in her renal function (6 months ago her SCr was 1.5 mg/dL). Laboratory results are as follows: TC 143 mg/dL, TG 160 mg/dL, HDL-C 42 mg/dL, LDL-C 63 mg/dL, non–HDL-C 101 mg/dL, SCr 2.3 mg/dL, CrCl (IBW) 21.9 mL/minute, ALT 45 IU/L, Na 144 mEq/L, K 4.9 mEq/L, and A1C 7.5%. She weighs 81 kg and is 64 inches tall. Which is the best recommendation for this patient?

A. Add omega-3 fatty acids, with eicosapentaenoic acid (EPA)/docosahexaenoic acid (DHA) at least 1 g/day.
B. Add fenofibrate 160 mg/day.
C. Continue therapy.
D. Change simvastatin to atorvastatin 20 mg/day.

C. Pharmacotherapy *(Domains 1, 3)*
 1. LDL-C–lowering drugs
  a. Statins (HMG-CoA reductase inhibitors) – Rosuvastatin, atorvastatin, simvastatin, pravastatin, lovastatin, fluvastatin, pitavastatin
   i. Mechanism of action – Reduce hepatic cholesterol synthesis and lower intracellular cholesterol, which stimulates the up-regulation of the LDL-C receptor and increases the uptake of non–HDL-C particles from systemic circulation
   ii. Evidence
    (a) Landmark – Primary prevention
     (1) Prevention of CHD with pravastatin in men with hypercholesterolemia (WOSCOPS trial)
      (A) Pravastatin 40 mg versus placebo for 5 years in 6595 male patients
      (B) Reduction in acute coronary event: 31%; reduction in death from CV causes: 32%; reduction in all-cause mortality not statistically significant
     (2) Primary prevention of acute coronary events with lovastatin in men and women with average cholesterol concentrations: Results of AFCAPS/TexCAPS
      (A) Lovastatin 20–40 mg versus placebo for 5.2 years in 6605 patients with average or below-average cholesterol concentrations
      (B) Reduction in acute coronary event: 37%; no change in all-cause mortality
     (3) Pravastatin in elderly individuals at risk of vascular disease (PROSPER trial)
      (A) Pravastatin 40 mg versus placebo for 3.2 years in 5804 older patients (about 45% had preexisting vascular disease)
      (B) Reduction in coronary events/stroke: 15%; reduction in CHD mortality: 24%
     (4) Major outcomes in moderately hypercholesterolemic, hypertensive patients randomly assigned to receive pravastatin versus usual care: The Antihypertensive and Lipid-Lowering Treatment to Prevent Heart Attack trial (ALLHAT-LLT trial)
      (A) Pravastatin 40 mg versus usual care for 4.8 years in 10,355 hypertensive patients
      (B) No difference in mortality or coronary events
     (5) Prevention of coronary and stroke events with atorvastatin in hypertensive patients who have average or lower-than-average cholesterol concentrations, in the Anglo-Scandinavian Cardiac Outcomes Trial–Lipid Lowering Arm (ASCOT-LLA trial)
      (A) Atorvastatin 10 mg versus placebo for 3.3 years in 19,342 hypertensive patients
      (B) Reduction in coronary events: 29%; no difference in all-cause mortality
     (6) Rosuvastatin to prevent vascular events in men and women with elevated CRP (JUPITER trial)
      (A) Rosuvastatin 20 mg versus placebo in healthy men and women with LDL-C less than 130 mg/dL and CRP greater than 1.9 mg/L
      (B) Primary end points: Composite of MI, stroke, revascularization, hospitalization for UA, or death from CV causes
      (C) Reduction in composite end point (MI, stroke, arterial revascularization, hospitalization for UA, or death from CV causes): 44%; number needed to treat: 25
      (D) Reduction in all-cause mortality: 20%
      (E) Study was terminated early because of the observed treatment benefit, as well as the effects on death rates and other secondary end points.
      (F) The FDA approved the expanded indication.

 (b) Meta-analyses – Primary prevention

  (1) Arch Intern Med 2006;166:2307-13

   (A) Seven studies with at least 80% of population free of CVD at baseline

   (B) Statins reduced risk of MI and stroke.

   (C) Statins did not reduce total mortality or CHD mortality.

  (2) Meta-analysis (Arch Intern Med 2010;170:1024-31)

   (A) Eleven studies restricted to enrollment of patients without prior CVD, including JUPITER

   (B) Statins did not reduce all-cause mortality.

   (C) No relationship between baseline LDL-C concentration and relative reduction in mortality

 (c) Landmark – Secondary prevention

  (1) Randomized trial of cholesterol lowering in 4444 patients with CHD: The Scandinavian Simvastatin Survival Study (4S trial)

   (A) Simvastatin 10–40 mg versus placebo for 5.4 years in 4444 patients

   (B) Reduction in coronary events: 34%; reduction in all-cause mortality: 30%

  (2) Prevention of CV events and death with pravastatin in patients with CHD and a broad range of initial cholesterol concentrations (Long-Term Intervention with Prevastatin in Ischaemic Disease [LIPID] trial)

   (A) Pravastatin 40 mg versus placebo for 6 years in 9014 patients

   (B) Reduction in coronary events (fatal CHD or nonfatal MI): 24%; reduction in all-cause mortality: 22%

  (3) The effect of pravastatin on coronary events after MI in patients with average cholesterol concentrations (Cholesterol and Recurrent Events [CARE] trial)

   (A) Pravastatin 40 mg versus placebo for 5 years in 4159 patients

   (B) Reduction in coronary events: 24%; no difference in all-cause mortality

  (4) MRC/BHF (British Heart Foundation) Heart Protection Study of cholesterol lowering with simvastatin in 20,536 high-risk individuals: A randomized placebo-controlled trial (HPS trial)

   (A) Simvastatin 40 mg versus placebo for 5 years in 20,536 patients

   (B) Reduction in major vascular events: 24%; reduction in all-cause mortality: 13%

   (C) Statin therapy is beneficial for high-risk patients with low-normal cholesterol concentrations as well as for patients older than 70 years.

   (D) Consider statin therapy for anyone who is at increased risk of vascular disease regardless of cholesterol concentrations.

  (5) Intensive versus moderate lipid lowering with statins after ACSs (PROVE-IT – TIMI 22 trial)

   (A) Within 10 days of MI, patients randomly assigned to receive 40 mg of pravastatin (median achieved LDL-C 95 mg/dL) versus 80 mg of atorvastatin (median achieved LDL-C 62 mg/dL)

   (B) Compared with the pravastatin group, 16% reduction in primary end point (all-cause mortality, MI, revascularization) in the atorvastatin group. Absolute risk reduction of 3.9% in the atorvastatin group.

   (C) Initiate statin therapy immediately after ACS event, regardless of lipid status.

   (D) Consider a lower LDL-C goal, especially in very high-risk patients.

(6) Intensive lipid lowering with atorvastatin in patients with stable coronary disease (Treating to New Targets [TNT] trial)

    (A) Atorvastatin 10 mg versus 80 mg for 4.0 years in 10,001 patients

    (B) Mean LDL-C concentrations were 77 mg/dL during treatment with 80 mg of atorvastatin and 101 mg/dL during treatment with 10 mg of atorvastatin.

    (C) Reduction in major vascular events: 22%; no difference in reduction of mortality

(d) Meta-analysis – Primary and secondary prevention

    (1) Cholesterol Treatment Trialists Collaboration (Lancet 2010;376:1670-81) included 26 randomized trials

        (A) More intensive versus less intensive cholesterol lowering comparing statin doses (five trials of 39,612 patients)

        (B) 19.7-mg/dL difference in LDL-C

        (C) Reductions in major coronary events (RR 0.87; 95% CI, 0.81–0.93), coronary revascularizations (RR 0.81; 95% CI, 0.76–0.85), and stroke (RR 0.86; 95% CI, 0.77–0.96)

        (D) Reduction in events proportional to LDL-C reduction and not dependent on baseline LDL-C. A 39-mg/dL reduction reduces the risk by 20%. A 77- to 116-mg/dL reduction would reduce the risk by 40%–50%.

        (E) Conclusion: Any statin that achieves significant LDL-C reduction remains the cornerstone of therapy for reducing CV risk.

iii. Clinical use – Recommended first line for dyslipidemia in primary and secondary prevention because of the cardioprotective benefits shown in clinical trials

(a) Lipid lowering

    (1) Lower LDL-C 21%–63%; for each doubling of a statin dose (e.g., simvastatin, from 10 mg to 20 mg), anticipate about 6% additional LDL-C reduction.

    (2) Lower TG 8%–37%; atorvastatin and rosuvastatin generally more effective at lowering TG than other statins

    (3) Raise HDL-C 3%–16%

Table 12. Relative LDL-C–Lowering Efficacy of Statin and Statin-Based Therapies

Atorva, mg	Fluva, mg	Pitava, mg	Lova, mg	Prava, mg	Rosuva, mg	Ezetimibe/ Simva, mg	Simva, mg	%↓ LDL-C
	40	1	20	20	—	—	10	30
10	80	2	40	40	—	—	20	38
20	—	4	80	80	5	10/10	40	41
40	—		—	—	10	10/20	—	47
80	—		—	—	20	10/40	—	55
	—		—	—	40	—	—	63

Denotes high-intensity statin; lowers LDL-C by ≥50%.

Denotes moderate-intensity statin; lowers LDL-C by 30% to <50%.

Denotes low-intensity statin.

Atorva = atorvastatin; Fluva = fluvastatin; LDL-C = low-density lipoprotein cholesterol; Lova = lovastatin; Pitava = pitavastatin;

Prava = pravastatin; Rosuva = rosuvastatin; Simva = simvastatin.

(b) Pleiotropic effects

    (1) Improve endothelial function

    (2) Inhibit platelet aggregation

    (3) Decrease LDL-C oxidation

    (4) Reduce vascular inflammation

    (5) Stabilize atherosclerotic plaques

iv. Contraindications

  (a) Pregnancy and lactation

  (b) Active liver disease

v. Important ADRs

  (a) In general, well tolerated

  (b) Elevated liver function test (LFT) results (0.1%–2.3%)

    (1) No link between statins and life-threatening liver damage

    (2) Elevations greater than 3 times the upper limit of normal (ULN) occur in less than 1% of patients across the range for marketed statins.

    (3) Mild, asymptomatic transaminase elevations in 1 patient per 100,000 person-years within clinical trials

    (4) Elevations usually transient and resolve without intervention

  (c) Myalgias (0.5%–5%)

    (1) Risk factors for statin myopathy

      (A) Advanced age (older than 65 years)

      (B) Increased statin (and metabolite) concentrations

      (C) Increased dose

      (D) Concomitant fibrate or niacin

      (E) Other drug-drug interactions (see Table 13)

      (F) Uncontrolled hypothyroidism

      (G) Alcohol abuse

      (H) Crack cocaine use

      (I) Genetic variants affecting statin pharmacokinetics: SLCO1B1 reduced-function alleles

    (2) FDA Drug Safety Communication: Simvastatin (June 2011)

      (A) The FDA's review of the Study of the Effectiveness of Additional Reductions in Cholesterol and Homocysteine (SEARCH) trial and other data prompted label changes for simvastatin.

      (B) SEARCH was a 7-year, randomized, double-blind clinical trial comparing the efficacy and safety of simvastatin 80 mg with simvastatin 20 mg in survivors of MI.

        • Safety

          ○ Myopathy: Fifty-two patients (0.9%) in the 80-mg group versus one patient (0.02%) in the 20-mg group

          ○ Rhabdomyolysis: Twenty-two patients (0.4%) in the 80-mg group versus no patient in the 20-mg group

          ○ The risks of myopathy and rhabdomyolysis with simvastatin 80 mg were highest in the first 12 months of treatment.

          ○ The findings from the SEARCH trial are supported by analyses of the FDA's Adverse Event Reporting System database.

- Efficacy
  - Nonsignificant 0.6% absolute risk reduction in the primary end point of CV death, MI, stroke, or arterial revascularization (24.5% vs. 25.7%; RR 0.94; 95% CI, 0.88–1.01) with 80 mg versus 20 mg of simvastatin treatment for a mean of 6.7 years
  - Nonfatal MI reduced from 7.7% to 6.6% with high-dose simvastatin (RR 0.85; 95% CI, 0.75–0.99)
  - (C) FDA recommendations
    - Maintain patients on a regimen of simvastatin 80 mg/day only if patients have been taking this dose more than 12 months without evidence of muscle toxicity. Do not initiate simvastatin 80 mg/day for new patients.
    - Limit simvastatin doses, or avoid completely if interacting medications (see Table 13) are used concomitantly, to decrease the risk of myopathy.
  - (3) Myalgias usually occur without CK elevation.
    - (A) Manage by holding drug for a few weeks to see whether symptoms improve.
    - (B) Consider a retrial (with a lower dose of original statin or a different statin). Hydrophilic statins (e.g., pravastatin and rosuvastatin) theoretically decrease statin entry into the skeletal muscle and may be tried in patients with a history of myalgias. However, hydrophilic statins have not been studied in a direct comparison with more lipophilic statins to determine whether this theory holds.
  - (4) Rhabdomyolysis (0.002%)
    - (A) CK greater than 10,000 IU/L OR
    - (B) CK greater than 10 times the ULN plus an elevation in SCr or medical intervention with intravenous hydration therapy
    - (C) Risk factors: Advanced age (older than 65 years), small body frame, renal insufficiency, diabetes, hypothyroidism, drug interactions
    - (D) Reversible with drug discontinuation
  - (d) Others adverse events added to the statin labels in February 2012
    - (1) In general nonserious and reversible cognitive adverse effects (e.g., memory loss, confusion)
    - (2) Increased blood glucose and A1C values
      - (A) For patients treated with statin for 1 year, the excess risk of diabetes is the main consideration in about 0.1 excess cases per 100 individuals with moderate-intensity statin and 0.3 excess cases per 100 individuals with high-intensity statin.
    - (3) The FDA continues to believe that the CV benefits of statins outweigh these small increased risks.
- vi. Monitoring
  - (a) Lipid panel
    - (1) Check 4–12 weeks after statin initiation or titration.
    - (2) Check every 3 to 12 months thereafter, mainly to assess for adherence.
    - (3) Decrease in statin dose may be considered when two consecutive LDL-C values are below 40 mg/dL.
  - (b) LFTs (usually ALT): The FDA revised labels in February 2012 to remove the need for routine periodic monitoring of liver enzymes in patients taking statins.
    - (1) LFTs performed before starting statin therapy and as clinically indicated thereafter
    - (2) Serious liver injury with statins is rare and unpredictable in individual patients, and routine periodic monitoring of liver enzymes does not appear to be effective in detecting or preventing serious liver injury.
    - (3) If liver enzymes are elevated, important to exclude other etiologies such as viral hepatitis, alcohol consumption, steatosis, or other drug-related causes

(c) Creatine kinase
  (1) Baseline levels not necessary unless patient is at risk of myopathy (renal or hepatic dysfunction; concomitant agent that affects statin metabolism; personal or family history of statin intolerance or muscle disease)
  (2) Routine monitoring not necessary in asymptomatic patients. Most CK elevations during statin therapy are benign and caused by other factors such as physical exertion, infection, long periods of immobility, seizures, drugs/toxins, trauma, electrolyte abnormalities, and low thyroid hormone level.
  (3) Monitor CK in symptomatic patients, in addition to evaluating thyroid function, renal and hepatic function, rheumatologic disorders, vitamin D deficiency, and exacerbating factors (drug-drug interactions, including OTC medications [red yeast rice] and foods [grapefruit juice]). If patient has intolerable muscle symptoms do the following:
    (A) Hold statin regardless of CK value until patient is asymptomatic. If symptoms do not resolve within a few weeks, then they are not likely caused by statin therapy.
    (B) Once the symptoms have resolved (or a few weeks have passed without change in symptoms), the same statin (at a lower dose) or another statin can be reinitiated to test the reproducibility of symptoms.
    (C) Recurrence of symptoms with many statins and statin doses requires the use of other lipid-lowering agents.
  (4) If patient has no muscle symptoms or if muscle symptoms are tolerable and CK elevation is mild (less than 10 times the ULN), statin therapy can be continued at the same or reduced dose.
  (5) If the CK elevation is moderate or severe or if rhabdomyolysis occurs, statin therapy should be discontinued, and the risk-benefit of statin therapy should be weighed.
(d) Other laboratory values to consider: Renal function (see Chronic Kidney Disease section), thyroid function, glucose
  vii. Drug interactions with statins

Table 13. Statin Dosing with Interacting Drugs

Interacting Drug	Atorvastatin	Fluvastatin	Lovastatin	Pitavastatin	Pravastatin	Rosuvastatin	Simvastatin
Amiodarone			40 mg[c]				20 mg[g]
Amlodipine							20 mg[g]
Atazanavir + ritonavir			CI[c,h]			10 mg[f,g]	CI[g,h]
Boceprevir			CI[c,h]				CI[g,h]
Clarithromycin	20 mg[a]		CI[c]		40 mg[e]		CI[g]
Colchicine		Use caution[b]					Use caution[g]
Cyclosporine	Avoid use[a]	20 mg BID[b]	Avoid use[c]	CI[d]	20 mg[e]	5 mg[f]	CI[g]
Erythromycin			CI[c]	1 mg[d]			CI[g]
Danazol			20 mg[c]				CI[g]
Darunavir + ritonavir	20 mg[a,h]		CI[c,h]				CI[g,h]
Diltiazem			20 mg[c]				10 mg[g]
Dronedarone							10 mg[i]

Table 13. Statin Dosing with Interacting Drugs *(continued)*

Interacting Drug	Atorvastatin	Fluvastatin	Lovastatin	Pitavastatin	Pravastatin	Rosuvastatin	Simvastatin
Gemfibrozil	Avoid use[a]	Avoid use[b]	Avoid use[c]	Avoid use[d]	Avoid use[e]	10 mg[f]	CI[g]
Grapefruit juice	Avoid >1.2 L/day[a]		Avoid >1 qt/day[c]				Avoid >1 qt/day[g]
Fenofibrate	Use caution[a]	Use caution[b]	Use caution[c]	Use caution[d]	Use caution[e]	Use caution[f]	Use caution[g]
Fluconazole		20 mg BID[b]					
Fosamprenavir	20 mg[a,h]		CI[c,h]				CI[g,h]
Fosamprenavir + ritonavir	20 mg[a,h]		CI[c,h]			Use caution[f,h]	CI[g,h]
Itraconazole	20 mg[a]		CI[c]				CI[g]
Ketoconazole			CI[c]				CI[g]
Nefazodone			CI[c]				CI[g]
Nelfinavir	40 mg[a]		CI[c,h]				CI[g,h]
Niacin (>1 g/day)	Use caution[a]	Use caution[b]	Use caution[c]	Use caution[d]	Use caution[e]	Use caution[f]	Use caution[g]
Lopinavir + ritonavir	Use lowest dose[a,h]		CI[c,h]			10 mg[f,h]	CI[g,h]
Posaconazole			CI[c]				CI[g]
Ranolazine			Consider dose adjustment[c]				20 mg[g]
Rifampin	Simultaneous coadmin-istration[a]			2 mg[d]			
Saquinavir + ritonavir	20 mg[a,h]		CI[c,h]				CI[g,h]
Telaprevir	Avoid use[a,h]		CI[c,h]				CI[g,h]
Telithromycin			CI[c]				CI[g]
Ticagrelor			40 mg[j]				40 mg[j]
Tipranavir + ritonavir	Avoid use[a,h]		CI[c,h]			Use caution[f,h]	CI[g,h]
Verapamil			20 mg[c]				10 mg[g]

[a]Lipitor (atorvastatin calcium) tablets [prescribing information]. New York: Pfizer, February 2012.

[b]Lescol (fluvastatin sodium) capsules/Lescol XL (fluvastatin sodium) extended-release tablets [prescribing information]. East Hanover, NJ: Novartis Pharmaceuticals, February 2012.

[c]Mevacor (lovastatin) tablets [prescribing information]. Whitehouse Station, NJ: Merck & Co., February 2012.

[d]Livalo (pitavastatin) tablets [prescribing information]. Montgomery, AL: Kowa Pharmaceuticals America, February 2012.

[e]Pravachol (pravastatin sodium) tablets [prescribing information]. Princeton, NJ: Bristol-Myers Squibb, February 2012.

[f]Crestor (rosuvastatin calcium) tablets [prescribing information]. Wilmington, DE: AstraZeneca Pharmaceuticals LP, February 2012.

[g]Zocor (simvastatin) tablets [prescribing information]. Cramlington, Northumberland, UK: Merck Sharp & Dohme, February 2012.

[h]FDA Drug Safety Communication (3-1-12): Interactions Between Certain HIV or Hepatitis C Drugs and Cholesterol-Lowering Statin Drugs Can Increase the Risk of Muscle Injury. Available at www.fda.gov/Drugs/DrugSafety/ucm293877.htm. Accessed May 1, 2012.

[i]Multaq (dronedarone) tablets [prescribing information]. Bridgewater, NJ: sanofi-aventis U.S., January 2012.

[j]Brilinta (ticagrelor) tablets [prescribing information]. Wilmington, DE: AstraZeneca Pharmaceuticals, July 2011.

BID = twice daily; CI = contraindicated.

b. Niacin (vitamin B$_3$) (examples include IR niacin, Slo-Niacin, and Niaspan)

    i. Mechanism of action – Inhibits the hepatic production of VLDL and consequently its metabolite, LDL-C

    ii. Evidence

        (a) Clofibrate and niacin in the Coronary Drug Project

            (1) IR niacin versus placebo in 8341 patients with a history of MI

            (2) The niacin treatment arm had an 11% decrease in coronary mortality.

        (b) Extended-release (ER) niacin or ezetimibe and carotid intima-media thickness (ARBITER-6 trial)

            (1) Niaspan 2 g/day versus ezetimibe in 363 patients with CHD or a CHD risk equivalent

            (2) Baseline LDL-C less than 100 mg/dL; HDL-C less than 50 mg/dL when taking statins

            (3) Niaspan significantly reduced carotid artery intima-media thickness progression compared with ezetimibe when used in combination with statins. (Unknown whether improvement in carotid artery intima-media thickness or as revealed by intravascular ultrasound translates to improved clinical outcomes)

        (c) Niacin for patients with low HDL-C concentrations receiving intensive statin therapy (AIM HIGH trial)

            (1) A total of 3414 patients with established heart disease, low HDL-C concentrations, and raised TG values were randomly assigned to receive ER niacin (1500–2000 mg/day) or placebo. All patients received simvastatin 40–80 mg/day, plus ezetimibe 10 mg/day, if needed, to maintain an LDL-C concentration of 40–80 mg/dL.

            (2) Trial terminated early after a mean follow-up of 3 years because niacin showed no additional benefits over placebo, and there was also a small, insignificant increase in ischemic stroke in the niacin group.

            (3) At 2 years, niacin therapy had increased HDL-C values from a median of 35–42 mg/dL, lowered TG values from 164 mg/dL to 122 mg/dL, and lowered LDL-C values from 74 mg/dL to 62 mg/dL.

            (4) The primary end point, the first event of a composite of CHD death, nonfatal MI, ischemic stroke, hospitalization for ACS, or symptom-driven coronary or cerebral revascularization, was similar in the two groups, occurring in 282 patients (16.4%) in the niacin group versus 274 patients (16.2%) receiving placebo.

        (d) Heart Protection Study 2–Treatment of HDL to Reduce the Incidence of Vascular Events [HPS2-THRIVE] trial

            (1) More than 38,000 patients were assessed for adherence to a regimen of ER niacin 2 g plus laropiprant 40 mg daily; about one-third were excluded largely because of niacin adverse effects.

            (2) A total of 25,673 patients were randomly assigned to receive ER niacin plus laropiprant daily or placebo and followed up for a median of 3.9 years.

            (3) There was no significant benefit of ER niacin/laropiprant on the primary outcome of major vascular events when added to effective statin-based LDL-C–lowering therapy.

            (4) Significant excesses of serious niacin-related adverse events occurred (about 30 patients per 1000).

    iii. Clinical use – Consider after statins (unable to tolerate) for LDL-C lowering

        (a) Lowers LDL-C by 5%–25%

        (b) Lowers TG by 20%–50%

        (c) Raises HDL-C by 15%–35%

    iv. Contraindications

        (a) Active hepatic disease

        (b) Active peptic ulcer

    v. Important ADRs
      (a) Flushing/itching
        (1) Less common in controlled-release preparations
        (2) Food, aspirin 30 minutes before administration, nighttime administration, and slow-dose titration can improve symptoms.
      (b) Elevated LFT results: Less common in IR preparations
      (c) Increases glucose values – Importance is controversial
      (d) Induces hyperuricemia – In general, avoided in patients with a history of gout
      (e) Myopathy (especially if combined with statin therapy)
      (f) GI distress – Caution in patients with history of peptic ulcer disease

    vi. Dosing and monitoring
      (a) OTC and prescription (Niaspan) products available
        (1) ER products may be better tolerated, but they may cause more liver dysfunction than IR products.
        (2) IR products likely to cause flushing/itching.
        (3) Flush-free niacin (inositol hexaniacinate) has no impact on lipids.
      (b) Fasting lipid panel, ALT and A1C assessment 6–8 weeks after initiation or titration. Consider CK test if used concomitantly with statins.

c. Ezetimibe
    i. Mechanism of action – Selective inhibitor of dietary and biliary cholesterol absorption
    ii. Evidence
      (a) Simvastatin with or without ezetimibe in familial hypercholesterolemia (ENHANCE trial)
        (1) Simvastatin 80 with or without ezetimibe for 2 years in 720 patients with familial dyslipidemia
        (2) Primary end point was the change in carotid artery intima-media thickness.
        (3) Baseline LDL-C 319 mg/dL
        (4) LDL-C reduced by 39% with simvastatin monotherapy and 56% with ezetimibe/simvastatin
        (5) No statistically significant difference found for primary end point
      (b) Intensive lipid lowering with simvastatin and ezetimibe in aortic stenosis (SEAS trial)
        (1) Ezetimibe/simvastatin 10/40 mg versus placebo
        (2) A total of 1873 older patients with aortic valve stenosis
        (3) Primary end point: Aortic stenosis and CV events
        (4) LDL C reduced by 4% in the placebo group and 54% with ezetimibe/simvastatin
        (5) No statistically significant difference found in primary end point. Cancer occurred statistically more often in the ezetimibe/simvastatin group (likely incidental finding).
      (c) The effects of lowering LDL-C with simvastatin plus ezetimibe in patients with CKD (Study of Heart and Renal Protection [SHARP] trial): A randomized placebo-controlled trial
        (1) Simvastatin 20 mg plus ezetimibe 10 mg/day versus matching placebo
        (2) A total of 9270 patients with CKD (3023 on dialysis and 6247 not) with no known history of MI or coronary revascularization
        (3) Outcome was the first major atherosclerotic event (nonfatal MI or coronary death, nonhemorrhagic stroke, or any arterial revascularization procedure).
        (4) Seventeen percent proportional reduction in major atherosclerotic events (526 [11.3%] simvastatin plus ezetimibe versus 619 [13.4%] placebo; RR 0.83; 95% CI, 0.74–0.94; log-rank p=0.0021)
        (5) In November 2011, FDA advisers recommended Vytorin for CVD prevention at predialysis for patients with CKD.

    (d) The IMProved Reduction of Outcomes: Vytorin Efficacy International Trial (IMPROVE-IT): A multicenter randomized controlled trial

        (1) Simvastatin 40 mg plus ezetimibe 10 mg/day versus simvastatin 40 mg/day

        (2) A total of 18,144 high-risk patients who were enrolled within 10 days after hospitalization for ACS. Patients were followed up an average of 7 years.

        (3) The primary outcome (composite CV death, MI, UA, and coronary revascularization) was reduced in the ezetimibe/simvastatin group as compared to the simvastatin-alone group (32.7% vs. 34.7%; hazard ratio 0.94; 95% CI, 0.89–0.99; p=0.016).

        (4) Compared to simvastatin alone, the simvastatin/ezetimibe group had a 6.4% lower risk of all CV events, 14% lower risk of heart attack or stroke, and a 21% lower risk of ischemic stroke. There was no significant difference in CV death between the two groups.

        (5) This is the first trial to show a decrease in CV outcomes when adding a non-statin lipid-lowering agent to statin therapy.

  iii. Clinical use

    (a) Lowers LDL-C about 17% as monotherapy, or an additional 14%–20% when added to statin therapy.

    (b) Agent for LDL-C lowering used after statins maximized or not tolerated. May consider ezetimibe/simvastatin in patients with CKD.

    (c) More research is needed to further define the role of ezetimibe.

  iv. Contraindication: Active hepatic disease

  v. Important ADRs: In general well tolerated

  vi. Dosing and monitoring

    (a) Consider trial of 5 mg/day; efficacy in LDL-C lowering similar to 10 mg (26.1% vs. 25.8%)

    (b) Fasting lipid panel and LFTs at 6–8 weeks after initiation or titration

d. Bile acid sequestrants (examples include cholestyramine, colestipol, and colesevelam)

  i. Mechanism of action – Bind bile acids in the intestine, decreasing biliary cholesterol absorption

  ii. Evidence: The Lipid Research Clinics Coronary Primary Prevention Trial results (LRC-CPPT trial)

    (a) Cholestyramine 24 g (six packets daily) versus placebo for 7 years in 3806 patients

    (b) Reduction in coronary events: 19%

  iii. Clinical use

    (a) Agent for LDL-C lowering used after statins and niacin maximized or not tolerated. Tolerability issues and drug-drug interactions may limit use.

    (b) Lowers LDL-C by 15%–30%

    (c) Raises HDL-C by 3%–5%

    (d) May raise TG

    (e) Colesevelam lowers glucose levels.

  iv. Cotraindication: Complete biliary obstruction

  v. Important ADRs: GI effects (e.g., constipation, obstruction)

  vi. Dosing and monitoring

    (a) Requires 3–20 g/day to be effective

    (b) Can bind many drugs, resulting in decreased absorption. Recommend dosing other drug 2 hours before or 4–6 hours after administering bile acid sequestrant

    (c) Fasting lipid panel 6–8 weeks after initiation or titration

e. Proprotein convertase subtilisin kexin type 9 (PCSK9) inhibitors (alirocumab and evolocumab)

  i. Mechanism of action – Bind to PCSK9. PCSK9 binds to LDL receptors (LDLRs) on the surface of hepatocytes to promote LDLR degradation within the liver. LDLR is the primary receptor that clears circulating LDL-C; the decrease in LDLR by PCSK9 results in higher serum LDL-C values. By binding PCSK9, more LDLRs are available to clear LDL-C.

  ii. Evidence: No current evidence to demonstrate reduction in CV events

  iii. Clinical use

   (a) Adjunct to maximally tolerated statin therapy in adults with heterozygous or homozygous familial hypercholesterolemia or clinical atherosclerotic vascular disease who require additional LDL-C lowering

   (b) Lowers LDL-C by an additional 50%–70% when added to statin therapy

   (c) Lowers triglycerides 12%–17% and increases HDL-C 4%–7%

   (d) Reduces non–HDL-C by about 50% and apolipoprotein B by 47%–54%

   (e) Potential role in statin-intolerant patients

  iv. Contraindication: History of hypersensitivity reaction to either medication

  v. Important ADRs: Allergic reactions, injection site reactions, nasopharyngitis, upper respiratory infection, myalgia, skeletal muscle pain, diarrhea, cough, elevated LFT results

  vi. Dosing and monitoring

   (a) Alirocumab: 75 mg subcutaneously every 2 weeks; increase to 150 mg if LDL-C elevated after 8 weeks.

   (b) Evolocumab: 140 mg subcutaneously every 2 weeks or 420 mg subcutaneously every month

   (c) If a dose is missed, instruct the patient to administer the injection within 7 days from the missed dose and then resume original schedule.

   (d) Fasting lipid panel 4–8 weeks after initiation or titration

 f. Other OTC options

  i. Plant stanols/sterols

   (a) The National Cholesterol Education Program (NCEP) recommends as adjuncts to diet

   (b) Fifteen percent to 20% LDL-C reduction possible if taken as directed (usually in large quantities)

  ii. Red yeast rice

   (a) May contain lovastatin

   (b) Caution warranted: Lack of regulatory oversight and quality control (cases of hepatic failure)

Patient Case

14. A 50-year-old African American woman with no significant medical history presents for her annual well woman examination. Fasting laboratory test results are as follows: TC 157 mg/dL, TG 277 mg/dL, HDL-C 39 mg/dL, LDL-C 63 mg/dL, non–HDL-C 118 mg/dL, SCr 0.9 mg/dL, ALT 20 IU/L, Na 144 mEq/L, K 4.5 mEq/L, and FBG 99 mg/dL. Her BMI is 30.3 kg/m², and her BP is 110/60 mm Hg. Which is the best recommendation to manage her elevated TG?

 A. Diet, exercise, and weight loss.

 B. Fenofibrate 160 mg/day.

 C. Gemfibrozil 600 mg twice daily.

 D. Pravastatin 80 mg every evening.

2. TG-lowering drugs
   a. Fibrates – Examples include fenofibrate, gemfibrozil
      i. Mechanism of action
         (a) Peroxisome proliferator-activated receptor α activation
         (b) Reduced hepatic secretion of VLDL
         (c) Induction of lipoprotein lipase–mediated lipolysis and clearance of TG
      ii. Evidence
         (a) Helsinki Heart Study: Primary prevention trial with gemfibrozil in middle-aged men with dyslipidemia
             (1) Gemfibrozil versus placebo in 4081 primary prevention patients with non–HDL-C of 200 mg/dL or greater
             (2) Showed a reduction of 34% in the cumulative rate of cardiac end points at 5 years
         (b) Gemfibrozil for the secondary prevention of CHD in men with low levels of HDL-C (Veterans Affairs High-Density Lipoprotein Cholesterol Intervention Trial [VA-HIT])
             (1) Gemfibrozil versus placebo in 2531 secondary prevention patients with low HDL-C and high TG for 5 years
             (2) The combined primary end point of cardiac death and nonfatal MI occurred less often in the gemfibrozil-treated group (17% vs. 22%).
         (c) Effect of fenofibrate on the need for laser treatment for diabetic retinopathy (Fenofibrate Intervention and Event Lowering in Diabetes [FIELD] study)
             (1) Fenofibrate versus placebo in 9795 patients with type 2 DM
             (2) The treatment arm had nonsignificantly lower rates of coronary events, but it had nonsignificantly higher rates of coronary death and all-cause mortality.
      iii. Clinical use – In general, fibrates are reserved for patients with high TG values (above 500 mg/dL), despite implementation of lifestyle modifications. Gemfibrozil should not be used in combination with statin therapy owing to risk of myopathy (2013 AHA/ACC guidelines).
         (a) Lower LDL-C by 5%–20% (with normal TG concentration)
         (b) May raise LDL-C (with high TG concentration)
         (c) Lower TG by 20%–50%
         (d) Raise HDL-C by 10%–20%
      iv. FDA Drug Safety Communication: Fenofibric acid (November 2011)
         (a) According to data from the Action to Control Cardiovascular Risk in Diabetes (ACCORD) lipid trial, which evaluated the efficacy and safety of fenofibrate and simvastatin combination therapy compared with simvastatin alone in patients with type 2 DM, fenofibric acid may not lower a patient's risk of having an MI or stroke.
         (b) The benefits and risks of fenofibric acid should be considered when deciding to prescribe the drug.
      v. Contraindications
         (a) Significant renal or hepatic dysfunction
         (b) Gallbladder disease
         (c) Biliary cirrhosis
      vi. Important ADRs
         (a) In general, well tolerated; most common ADR is GI upset
         (b) More severe (but rarer) ADRs: Elevated LFT results, myopathy, increases in SCr
      vii. Dosing and monitoring
         (a) Fasting lipid panel and ALT assessment 6–8 weeks after initiation or titration; patients should report unusual muscle pain or weakness immediately, and CK concentration should be assessed.

(b) Adjust dose for renal insufficiency.

(1) Fenofibrate should not be used when eGFR is below 30 mL/minute/1.73 m^2

(2) Fenofibrate dose should not exceed 54 mg if GFR is between 30–59 mL/minute/1.73 m^2.

b. Omega-3 fatty acids – DHA and EPA

i. Mechanism of action – Inhibit hepatic secretion of TG and promote metabolism of TG

ii. Evidence

(a) Dietary supplementation with n-3 polyunsaturated fatty acids and vitamin E after MI: Results of the GISSI-Prevenzione trial – Showed a significant reduction in the risk of sudden death associated with the use of 850 mg/day of DHA/EPA combined

(b) Other trials examining omega-3 fatty acid supplementation have failed to confirm this finding.

iii. Clinical use

(a) TG lowering (20%–30%): Literature reports doses of 3–15 g/day. Can initiate at DHA/EPA 1 g/day to see TG lowering

(b) Cardioprotection

iv. Important ADRs

(a) Fishy taste/burping

(b) Antiplatelet effects

v. Dosing and monitoring

(a) OTC (choose concentrated products) and prescription products available

(b) Base the dose on the amount of DHA/EPA per capsule.

c. Niacin – See previous section (C.1.b).

3. Novel lipid-lowering medications

a. Mipomersen

i. Mechanism of action – Inhibits apo B (major component of LDL-C) production by binding to apo B messenger RNA

ii. Evidence - Studied in small trials, mainly in patients with familial hypercholesterolemia. LDL-C significantly lowered

iii. Clinical use - Indicated for patients with homozygous familial hypercholesterolemia

iv. Important ADRs

(a) Injection site reactions

(b) Elevated LFT results; greater than 3 times the upper limit of normal

(c) High discontinuation rate in some trials

v. Dosing and monitoring

(a) Given once weekly by subcutaneous injection

(b) Very expensive

b. Lomitapide

i. Mechanism of action – Inhibits microsomal triglyceride transfer protein, which participates in the forming of VLDL particles

ii. Evidence – Studied in small trials, mainly in patients with familial hypercholesterolemia. LDL-C significantly lowered

iii. Clinical use – Indicated for patients with homozygous familial hypercholesterolemia

iv. Important ADRs

(a) Black box warning for serious risk of liver toxicity

(b) Teratogenic

(c) GI symptoms, including elevated LFT results

v. Dosing and monitoring
   (a) Dose by mouth once daily and titrate as tolerated.
   (b) Very expensive
   (c) LFTs and pregnancy tests (as indicated) must be routinely performed.
   (d) Fat-soluble nutrients must be supplemented to avoid deficiency.

D. Comorbid Conditions *(Domains 1, 3)*
   1. Diabetes
      a. 2016 ADA Standards of Medical Care in Diabetes
      b. Statins added to lifestyle changes, regardless of LDL-C concentrations, in those 40 years and older who have at least one additional major risk factor for ASCVD
         i. Family history of premature ASCVD
         ii. Hypertension
         iii. Smoking
         iv. LDL of 100 mg/dL or above
         v. Overweight and obesity
      c. Statin recommendations
         i. High-intensity statin recommended for:
            (a) Clinical ASCVD
            (b) Patients 40 to 75 years of age with ASCVD risk factors
         ii. Moderate- to high-intensity statin recommended for:
            (a) Patients younger than 40 years or older than 75 years with ASCVD risk factors
         iii. Moderate-intensity statins recommended for:
            (a) Patients 40 years of age and older without any ASCVD risk factors
         iv. Moderate-intensity plus ezetimibe recommended for:
            (a) Patients 40 years of age and older with acute coronary syndrome (ACS) and LDL above 50 mg/dL who cannot tolerate high-intensity statin therapy
            (b) Meet IMPROVE-IT eligibility
      d. 2008 Cholesterol Treatment Trialists' Collaborators meta-analysis
         i. Diabetic subgroup analysis of 18,686 patients from 14 clinical trials
         ii. Sixty-three percent of patients without prior atherosclerotic vascular disease
         iii. Statistically significant reduction in 5-year risk of major vascular events in subgroup of patients with DM and no prior vascular disease as compared with control (15.6% vs. 19.2%; RR 0.73; 95% CI, 0.66–0.82).
         iv. Benefit similar irrespective of baseline LDL-C
   2. Chronic kidney disease
      a. KDIGO dyslipidemia guidelines 2013
         i. No specific LDL-C target is recommended, and titrating statin doses according to LDL-C concentration is not recommended.
         ii. Patients older than 50 years with an eGFR of less than 60 mL/minute but not treated with dialysis or kidney transplant: Treatment with a recommended dosed statin or statin/ezetimibe combination is advised.
         iii. Patients older than 50 years with CKD and eGFR greater than 60 mL/minute: Treatment with a recommended dosed statin is advised.
         iv. Adults younger than 50 years with CKD but not treated with dialysis or kidney transplant: Statin treatment is recommended if patient has at least one of the following concomitant conditions:
            (a) Known coronary disease (MI or coronary revascularization)
            (b) Diabetes mellitus
            (c) Prior ischemic stroke
            (d) Estimated 10-year incidence of coronary death or nonfatal MI greater than 10%

    v. Statins should not be initiated for patients undergoing dialysis. However, if patients undergoing dialysis are already receiving statins or a statin/ezetimibe combination when dialysis is initiated, statins should be continued.

    vii. Statins should be used post kidney transplantation in adults.

    viii. Recommended doses of statins in adults with CKD are as follows:

        (a) Atorvastatin 20 mg/day

        (b) Fluvastatin 80 mg/day

        (c) Lovastatin – Not studied

        (d) Pitavastatin 2 mg/day

        (e) Pravastatin 40 mg/day

        (f) Rosuvastatin 10 mg/day

        (g) Simvastatin 40 mg/day

        (h) Simvastatin/ezetimibe 20/10 mg/day

b. 2008/2009 Cochrane systematic reviews

    i. Insufficient data to assess mortality in patients receiving dialysis

    ii. Statins reduce all-cause and CVD deaths in patients with CKD not receiving dialysis.

    iii. Many patients had established CVD.

    iv. Insufficient evidence for primary prevention

c. 2009 Study to Evaluate the Use of Rosuvastatin in Subjects on Regular Hemodialysis: An Assessment of Survival and Cardiovascular Events (AURORA trial)

    i. n=2776 patients receiving dialysis; mean LDL-C concentration at baseline was 100 mg/dL

    ii. More than a 3.8-year follow-up; no benefit in CV death, MI, or stroke versus placebo with rosuvastatin 10 mg/day versus placebo

d. 2011 Study of Heart and Renal Protection (SHARP)

    i. n=9270 patients with CKD (3023 receiving dialysis); mean LDL-C concentration at baseline was 112 mg/dL and 100 mg/dL (receiving dialysis)

    ii. 4.9-year follow-up; 17% reduction in major atherosclerotic events (RR 0.83; 95% CI, 0.74–0.94; p=0.0021) with simvastatin 20 mg plus ezetimibe 10 mg/day versus placebo

    iii. Fourteen percent of placebo-treated patients were taking a non-study statin by the end of study.

e. Dose modifications based on package labeling

    i. Estimated CrCl less than 30 mL/minute

        (a) Lovastatin 10–40 mg/day

        (b) Simvastatin 10–40 mg/day

        (c) Atorvastatin 10–80 mg/day

        (d) Rosuvastatin 5–10 mg/day

        (e) Pravastatin 10–80 mg/day

        (f) Pitavastatin 1–2 mg/day

        (g) Fluvastatin – No dosage adjustment necessary

    ii. Estimated CrCl 30–60 mL/minute: Pitavastatin 1–2 mg/day

    iii. Estimated CrCl less than 50 mL/minute – Initiate lower-dose fenofibrate (54 mg/day) and gemfibrozil (300 mg twice daily), and titrate as needed.

    iv. No dose adjustment needed for people receiving dialysis, except for pitavastatin (1–2 mg/day) and fenofibrate (avoid).

Patient Case

15. A 52-year-old man with a history of symptomatic atrial fibrillation and hypothyroidism presents to the clinic. For the past month he has been out of normal sinus rhythm, with unsuccessful cardioversion. His cardiologist initiated chronic amiodarone therapy today. Medications include simvastatin 40 mg/day, levothyroxine 137 mcg/day, warfarin as directed, and metoprolol SR 50 mg/day. Laboratory test results are as follows: TC 131 mg/dL, TG 100 mg/dL, HDL-C 32 mg/dL, LDL-C 79 mg/dL, non–HDL-C 99 mg/dL, SCr 1.8 mg/dL, CrCl 37 mL/minute, ALT 52 IU/L, Na 142 mEq/L, K 4.8 mEq/L, INR 2.3, and TSH 4.32 μIU/mL. Which is the best treatment recommendation for this patient?

A. Discontinue simvastatin because it cannot be used concomitantly with amiodarone.

B. Increase simvastatin to 80 mg every evening because the patient's LDL-C will increase once amiodarone therapy is started.

C. Lower simvastatin to 20 mg every evening to reduce the risk of a drug-drug interaction.

D. Add niacin 500 mg twice daily to increase his HDL-C.

---

3. Mixed dyslipidemia
    a. Treatment not discussed in updated AHA/ACC guidelines
        i. Niacin or fibrate added to statin for markedly elevated TG (greater than 500 mg/dL)
        ii. Product labeling for omega-3 acid ethyl esters suggests about a 25% reduction in TG when added to a statin.
    b. Monitoring for toxicity with combinations of statins and fibrates or niacin
        i. Niacin, fenofibrate, fenofibric acid, and gemfibrozil increase the risk of myopathy.
        ii. Gemfibrozil
            (a) Limit doses of rosuvastatin to 10 mg orally daily.
            (b) Simvastatin, lovastatin, atorvastatin: Avoid/contraindicated because of the risk of rhabdomyolysis.
        iii. Fenofibrate – Patients should report unusual muscle pain or weakness immediately, and CK level should be assessed.
        iv. Niacin – Consider checking CK after initiating or titrating combination therapy. For Chinese patients:
            (a) Limit niacin dose to less than 1 g orally daily if receiving simvastatin 80 mg orally daily.
            (b) If using niacin 1 g/day or more orally, limit simvastatin dose to 40 mg orally daily.

Patient Case

16. A 76-year-old man with a history of CAD and diabetes completes his fasting laboratory testing. For the past 2 months, he has been treated for a diabetic foot ulcer. After interviewing the patient, you discover he just had helped his wife tear down her jewelry display at a convention and has been feeling achy during the past week. Medications include atorvastatin 80 mg/day, niacin 500 mg twice daily, fish oil supplement 1000 mg/day, metoprolol SR 25 mg/day, lisinopril 20 mg/day, and aspirin 81 mg/day. Laboratory test results are as follows: TC 148 mg/dL, TG 146 mg/dL, HDL-C 37 mg/dL, LDL-C 82 mg/dL, non–HDL-C 111 mg/dL, CK 1064 U/L, SCr 1.7 mg/dL, CrCl 37 mL/minute, ALT 36 IU/L, Na 144 mEq/L, and K 5.0 mEq/L. Which strategy is best to address his laboratory test results?

A. Discontinue atorvastatin because of his elevated CK. The patient will be unable to take statin therapy in the future.

B. Hold atorvastatin because of his elevated CK, and monitor his CK.

C. Continue therapy because the elevated CK is likely caused by his diabetic foot ulcer and recent strenuous activity.

D. Change his therapy to ezetimibe/simvastatin 10/80 mg/day because his LDL-C is not at goal.

E. Other Disease States That Can Affect Lipids
1. Diabetes – Elevated TG
2. Hypothyroidism – Elevated TG and LDL-C
3. Alcoholism – Elevated TG
4. Recent cardiac event – Falsely lowers lipids up to 12 weeks after event

VII. PERIPHERAL ARTERIAL DISEASE

Guideline:
2013 ACCF/AHA Management of Patients With Peripheral Artery Disease (compilation of 2005 and 2011 guideline recommendations)

A. Resting ABI *(Domain 1)*
1. Diagnosis – ABI is used to establish the lower-extremity PAD diagnosis in patients with suspected lower-extremity PAD, defined as individuals with one or more of the following:
   a. Exertional leg symptoms
   b. Non-healing wounds
   c. Age 65 years or older
   d. Age 50 years or older with a history of smoking or diabetes
2. Classification *(Domain 1)*
   a. Greater than 1.40 – Arteries noncompressible
   b. 1.0–1.40 – Normal
   c. 0.91–0.99 – Borderline
   d. 0.90 or less – Abnormal
   e. Fontaine classification
      i. Stage I: Asymptomatic
      ii. Stage II: Intermittent claudication
         (a) Stage IIa: Intermittent claudication after more than 200 m of pain-free walking
         (b) Stage IIb: Intermittent claudication after less than 200 m of walking.
      iii. Stage III: Rest pain
      iv. Stage IV: Ischemic ulcers or gangrene

B. Smoking Cessation *(Domains 1, 2, 5)*
1. Patients who are smokers or former smokers should be asked about their smoking status at each visit.
2. Patients who use tobacco should be advised to quit at each visit and should be offered help in developing a smoking cessation plan, which may include the following:
   a. Pharmacotherapy (varenicline, bupropion, and/or nicotine replacement)
   b. Behavioral treatment
   c. Referral to a smoking cessation program

C. Antiplatelet Therapy *(Domain 1)*
1. Indicated to reduce the risk of MI, stroke, or vascular death in patients with symptomatic, atherosclerotic lower-extremity PAD
   a. Intermittent claudication
   b. Critical limb ischemia
   c. Prior lower-extremity revascularization
   d. Prior amputation of a lower extremity
2. Aspirin, dosed 75–325 mg/day, is recommended as a safe and effective therapy.
3. Clopidogrel, dosed 75 mg/day, is the recommended alternative antiplatelet therapy when aspirin is contraindicated.
4. Aspirin and clopidogrel combination therapy may be considered for patients without increased risk of bleeding who are perceived to be high CV risk (class IIb recommendation).

D. Claudication Therapy *(Domain 1)*
1. Cilostazol 100 mg twice daily is indicated to improve symptoms and increase walking distance in patients with lower-extremity PAD (class I recommendation).
2. Pentoxifylline 400 mg three times daily may be considered as a second-line therapy to improve walking distance (class IIb recommendation).

E. Statins for CV Risk Reduction in Patients with Atherosclerotic PAD *(Domain 1)*
1. Age 75 years or younger – High-intensity statin recommended
2. Older than 75 years – Moderate-intensity statin recommended

F. HTN Therapy *(Domain 1)*
1. Goal: Less than 140/90 mm Hg
2. Drugs of choice: β-Blockers and ACE inhibitors

VIII. ATHEROSCLEROTIC (NON-CARDIOEMBOLIC ISCHEMIC) STROKE OR TIA

Guideline:
2014 ACCF/AHA Guideline for the Prevention of Stroke in Patients with Stroke and Transient Ischemic Attack

A. Antiplatelet Therapy
   1. Antiplatelet therapy is recommended over oral anticoagulation therapy to reduce the risk of recurrent atherosclerotic stroke and other CV events.
   2. After a TIA or atherosclerotic stroke, aspirin (50–325 mg/day) monotherapy or the combination of aspirin 25 mg and ER dipyridamole 200 mg twice daily is recommended as initial therapy.
   3. Another reasonable option for initial therapy is clopidogrel 75 mg/day monotherapy for secondary prevention of stroke. Clopidogrel is the drug of choice for patients who are allergic to aspirin.
   4. The combination of aspirin and clopidogrel might be considered for initiation within 24 hours of a minor ischemic stroke or TIA and for continuation for 21 days.
   5. The combination of aspirin and clopidogrel is not recommended for long-term use for secondary prevention of a stroke because of potential to increase the risk of hemorrhage.
   6. For patients who have had a stroke or TIA while receiving aspirin, there is no evidence that increasing the aspirin dose is an effective strategy to decrease the risk of subsequent strokes or TIAs. Although alternative antiplatelet agents may be considered, these agents have not been adequately studied in patients who have had a TIA or stroke while receiving aspirin.

B. Statins for CV Risk Reduction in Patients with a History of Atherosclerotic Stroke
   1. Age 75 years or younger – High-intensity statin recommended
   2. Older than 75 years – Moderate-intensity statin recommended

C. HTN Therapy
   1. Goal: Less than 140/90 mm Hg; for a recent lacunar stroke, consider SBP goal below 130 mm Hg
   2. Drugs of choice: ACE inhibitors and thiazide diuretics

REFERENCES

Primary Prevention

1. American Diabetes Association (ADA). Standards of medical care in diabetes – 2016. Diabetes Care 2016;39(suppl 1):S1-112.

2. Appel LJ, Wright JT Jr, Greene T, et al. Intensive blood-pressure control in hypertensive chronic kidney disease. N Engl J Med 2010;363:918-29.

3. Arguedas JA, Perez MI, Wright JM. Treatment blood pressure targets for hypertension. Cochrane Database Syst Rev 2009;3:CD004349.

4. Campbell CL, Smyth S, Montelescot G, et al. Aspirin dose for the prevention of cardiovascular disease: a systematic review. JAMA 2007;297:2018-24.

5. Cholesterol Treatment Trialists' Collaborators. Efficacy of cholesterol-lowering therapy in 18686 people with diabetes in 14 randomized trials of statins: a meta-analysis. Lancet 2008;371:117-25.

6. De Berardis G, Sacco M, Strippoli GF, et al. Aspirin for primary prevention of cardiovascular events in people with diabetes: meta-analysis of randomised controlled trials. BMJ 2009;339:b4531.

7. Fellström BC, Jardine AG, Schmieder RE, et al. Rosuvastatin and cardiovascular events in patients undergoing hemodialysis. N Engl J Med 2009;360:1395-407.

8. Framingham Heart Study. Coronary Heart Disease 10-Year Risk. Available at www.framinghamheartstudy.org/risk/coronary.html. Accessed February 11, 2013.

9. Go AS, Mozaffarian D, Roger VL. 2013 update: a report from the American Heart Association. Circulation 2013;127:e6-245.

10. Jardine MJ, Ninomiya T, Perkovic V, et al. Aspirin is beneficial in hypertensive patients with chronic kidney disease: a post-hoc subgroup analysis of a randomized controlled trial. J Am Coll Cardiol 2010;56:956-65.

11. Lloyd-Jones DM, Hong Y, Labarthe D, et al. Defining and setting national goals for cardiovascular health promotion and disease reduction: the American Heart Association's strategic impact goal through 2020 and beyond. Circulation 2010;121:586-613.

12. Marrs JC, Saseen JJ. Effects of lipid-lowering therapy on reduction of cardiovascular events in patients with end-stage disease requiring hemodialysis. Pharmacotherapy 2010;30:823-9.

13. National Cholesterol Education Program. Third Report of the Expert Panel on Detection, Evaluation, and Treatment of High Blood Cholesterol in Adults (Adult Treatment Panel III). Risk Assessment Tool for Estimating 10-Year Risk of Developing Hard CHD (Myocardial Infarction and Cardiac Death). Available at http://hp2010.nhlbihin.net/atpiii/calculator.asp?usertype=prof. Accessed February 11, 2013.

14. Navaneethan SD, Nigwekar SU, Perkovic V, et al. HMG CoA reductase inhibitors (statins) for dialysis patients. Cochrane Database Syst Rev 2009;2:CD004289.

15. Navaneethan SD, Pansini F, Perkovic V, et al. HMG CoA reductase inhibitors (statins) for people with chronic kidney disease not requiring dialysis. Cochrane Database Syst Rev 2009;2:CD007784.

16. Pignone M, Alberts MJ, Colwell JA, et al. Aspirin for primary prevention of cardiovascular events in people with diabetes. J Am Coll Cardiol 2010;55:2878-86.

17. Ray KK, Seshasai SR, Erqou S, et al. Statins and all-cause mortality in high-risk primary prevention: a meta-analysis of 11 randomized controlled trials involving 65,229 participants. Arch Intern Med 2010;170:1024-31.

18. Redberg RF, Benjamin EJ, Bittner V, et al. ACCF/AHA 2009 performance measures for primary prevention of cardiovascular disease in adults: a report of the American College of Cardiology Foundation/American Heart Association Task Force on Performance Measures (Writing Committee to Develop Performance Measures for Primary Prevention of Cardiovascular Disease) developed in collaboration with the American Academy of Family Physicians; American Association of Cardiovascular and Pulmonary Rehabilitation; and Preventive Cardiovascular Nurses Association: endorsed by the American College of Preventive Medicine, American College of Sports Medicine, and Society for Women's Health Research. J Am Coll Cardiol 2009;54:1364-405.

19. Siu AL. Behavioral and Pharmacotherapy Interventions for Tobacco Smoking Cessation In Adults, Including Pregnant Women: U.S. Preventative Services Task Force Recommendation Statement. Ann Int Med 2015;163:622-34. doi: 10.7326/M15-2023.

20. Thavendiranathan P, Bagai A, Brookhart MA, et al. Primary prevention of cardiovascular diseases with statin therapy: a meta-analysis of randomized controlled trials. Arch Intern Med 2006;166:2307-13.

21. United States Preventive Services Task Force (USPSTF). Aspirin for the Prevention of Cardiovascular Disease. March 2009. Available at www.uspreventiveservicestaskforce.org/uspstf/uspsasmi.htm. Accessed February 11, 2013.

22. United States Preventative Services Taks Force (USPSTF). Topic Update in Progress: Aspirin to Prevent Cardiovascular Disease and Cancer. September 2015. Available at http://www.uspreventiveservicestaskforce.org/Page/Document/Update-SummaryDraft/aspirin-to-prevent-cardiovascular-disease-and-cancer. Accessed September 21, 2015.

23. US Preventive Services Task Force (USPSTF). Screening for Lipid Disorders in Adults. June 2008. Available at www.uspreventiveservicestaskforce.org/uspstf/uspschol.htm. Accessed February 11, 2013.

24. Western States Stroke Consortium. Framingham Stroke Risk Calculator. Available at http://hp2010.nhlbihin.net/atpiii/calculator.asp?usertype=prof. Accessed February 11, 2013.

25. Younis N, Williams S, Ammori B, et al. Role of aspirin in the primary prevention of cardiovascular disease in diabetes mellitus. Expert Opin Pharmacother 2010;11:1459-66.

Secondary Prevention

1. Amsterdam EA, Wenger NK, Brindis RG, et al. 2014 ACC/AHA guideline for the management of patients with non–ST-elevation acute coronary syndromes: a report of the American College of Cardiology/American Heart Association TaskForce on Practice Guidelines. Circulation. 2014;64:e139-228.

2. Antman EM, Anbe DT, Armstrong PW, et al. ACC/AHA guidelines for the management of patients with ST-elevation myocardial infarction – executive summary: a report of the American College of Cardiology/American Heart Association Task Force on Practice Guidelines (Writing Committee to Revise the 1999 Guidelines for the Management of Patients with Acute Myocardial Infarction). Circulation 2004;110:588-636.

3. Antman EM, Hand M, Armstrong PW, et al. 2007 focused update of the ACC/AHA 2004 guidelines for the management of patients with ST-elevation myocardial infarction: a report of the American College of Cardiology/American Heart Association Task Force on Practice Guidelines: developed in collaboration with the Canadian Cardiovascular Society endorsed by the American Academy of Family Physicians: 2007 Writing Group to Review New Evidence and Update the ACC/AHA 2004 guidelines for the management of patients with ST-elevation myocardial infarction, Writing on Behalf of the 2004 Writing Committee. Circulation 2008;117:296-329.

4. Balady GJ, Williams MA, Ades PA, et al. Core components of cardiac rehabilitation/secondary prevention programs: 2007 update: a scientific statement from the American Heart Association Exercise, Cardiac Rehabilitation, and Prevention Committee, the Council on Clinical Cardiology; the Councils on Cardiovascular Nursing, Epidemiology and Prevention, and Nutrition, Physical Activity, and Metabolism; and the American Association of Cardiovascular and Pulmonary Rehabilitation. Circulation 2007;115:2675-82.

5. Bell AD, Roussin A, Cartier R, et al. The use of antiplatelet therapy in the outpatient setting: Canadian Cardiovascular Society guidelines. Can J Cardiol 2011;27(suppl A):S1-59.

6. Bonaca MP, Deepak L, Bhatt MD, et al. Long-term use of ticagrelor in patients with prior myocardial infarction. N Engl J Med 2015;372:1791-800.

7. Cholesterol Treatment Trialists' (CTT) Collaboration; Baigent C, Blackwell L, Emberson J, et al. Efficacy and safety of more intensive lowering of LDL cholesterol: a meta-analysis of data from 170,000 participants in 26 randomised trials. Lancet 2010;376:1670-81.

8. Cohen DE, Anania FA, Chalasani N; National Lipid Association Statin Safety Task Force Liver Expert Panel. An assessment of statin safety by hepatologists. Am J Cardiol 2006;97:77C-81C.

9. Ducrocq G, Wallace JS, Baron G, et al. Risk score to predict serious bleeding in stable outpatients with or at risk of atherothrombosis. Eur Heart J 2010;31:1257-65.

10. Fihn SD, Gardin JM, Abrams JA, et al. 2012 ACCF/AHA/ACP/AATS/PCNA/SCAI/STS Guideline for the Diagnosis and Management of Patients with Stable Ischemic Heart Disease. J Am Coll Cardiol 2012;60:e44-e164.

11. Hung IF, Leung AY, Chew EW, et al. Prevention of acute myocardial infarction and stroke among elderly persons by dual pneumococcal and influenza vaccination: a prospective cohort study. Clin Infect Dis 2010;51:1007-16.

12. Levine GN, Bates ER, Blankenship JC, et al. 2011 ACCF/AHA/SCAI guideline for percutaneous coronary intervention: a report of the American College of Cardiology Foundation/American Heart Association Task Force on Practice Guidelines and the Society for Cardiovascular Angiography and Interventions. Circulation 2011;124:2574-609.

13. Mauri L, Kereiakes DJ, Yeh RW, et al. Twelve or 30 months of dual antiplatelet therapy after drug-eluting stents. N Engl J Med 2014;371:2155-66. doi:10.1056/NEJMoa1409312.

14. Morrow DA, Braunwald MD, Bonaca MP, et al. Vorapaxar in the secondary prevention of atherothrombotic events. N Engl J Med 2012;366:1404-13.

15. National Institute for Health and Clinical Excellence (NICE) CG108 Full Guideline and Appendices. Available at http://guidance.nice.org.uk/CG108/Guidance. Accessed March 12, 2012.

16. O'Gara PT, Kushner FG, Ascheim DD, et al. 2013 ACCF/AHA guideline for the management of ST-elevation myocardial infarction: a report of the American College of Cardiology Foundation/American Heart Association Task Force on Practice Guidelines. J Am Coll Cardiol 2013;61:e78-140.

17. Smith SC Jr, Benjamin EJ, Bonow RO, et al. AHA/ACCF secondary prevention and risk reduction therapy for patients with coronary and other atherosclerotic vascular disease: 2011 update: a guideline from the American Heart Association and American College of Cardiology Foundation. Circulation 2011;124:2458-73.

18. Study of the Effectiveness of Additional Reductions in Cholesterol and Homocysteine (SEARCH) Collaborative Group. Intensive lowering of LDL cholesterol with 80 mg versus 20 mg simvastatin daily in 12,064 survivors of myocardial infarction: a double-blind randomised trial. Lancet 2010;376:1658-69.

19. Task Force for Diagnosis and Treatment of Acute and Chronic Heart Failure 2008 of European Society of Cardiology; Dickstein K, Cohen-Solal A, Filippatos G, et al. ESC guidelines for the diagnosis and treatment of acute and chronic heart failure 2008: the Task Force for the Diagnosis and Treatment of Acute and Chronic Heart Failure 2008 of the European Society of Cardiology: developed in collaboration with the Heart Failure Association of the ESC (HFA) and endorsed by the European Society of Intensive Care Medicine (ESICM). Eur Heart J 2008;29:2388-442.

20. Thompson PD, Clarkson PM, Rosenson RS; National Lipid Association Statin Safety Task Force Muscle Safety Expert Panel. An assessment of statin safety by muscle experts. Am J Cardiol 2006;97:69C-76C.

21. Tricoci P, Huang Z Held C, et al. Thrombin-receptor antagonist vorapaxar in acute coronary syndromes. N Engl J Med 2012;366:20-33.

22. Tseng HF, Slezak JM, Quinn VP, et al. Pneumococcal vaccination and risk of acute myocardial infarction and stroke in men. JAMA 2010;303:1699-706.

23. Winchester DE, Xen X, Xie L, et al. Evidence of pre-procedural statin therapy a meta-analysis of randomized trials. J Am Coll Cardiol 2011;14:1099-109.

24. Wright RS, Anderson JL, Adams CD, et al. 2011 ACCF/AHA focused update of the guidelines for the management of patients with unstable angina/non-ST-elevation myocardial infarction (updating the 2007 guideline): a report of the American College of Cardiology Foundation/American Heart Association Task Force on Practice Guidelines. Circulation 2011;123:2022-60.

Hypertension

1. The ACCOMPLISH Trial Investigators. Benazepril plus amlodipine or hydrochlorothiazide for hypertension in high-risk patients. N Engl J Med 2008;359:2417-28.

2. The ACCORD Study Group. Effects of intensive blood pressure control in type 2 diabetes mellitus. N Engl J Med 2010;362:1575-85.

3. ALLHAT Officers and Coordinators for the ALLHAT Collaborative Research Group. Major outcomes in high-risk hypertensive patients randomized to angiotensin-converting enzyme inhibitor or calcium channel blocker vs diuretic: the antihypertensive and lipid-lowering treatment to prevent heart attack trial (ALLHAT). JAMA 2002;288:2981-97.

4. American Diabetes Association (ADA). Standards of medical care in diabetes – 2015. Diabetes Care 2015;38(suppl 1):S49–57.

5. Bakris GL, Fonseca V, Katholi RE, et al. Metabolic effects of carvedilol vs metoprolol in patients with type 2 diabetes mellitus and hypertension: a randomized controlled trial. JAMA 2004;292:2227-36.

6. Beckett NS, Peters R, Fletcher AE, et al. Treatment of hypertension in patients 80 years of age or older. N Engl J Med 2008;358:1887-98.

7. Black HR, Elliott WJ, Grandits G, et al.; CONVINCE Research Group. Principal results of the Controlled Onset Verapamil Investigation of Cardiovascular End Points (CONVINCE) trial. JAMA 2003;289:2073-82.

8. Braunwald E, Domanski MJ, Fowler SE, et al.; PEACE Trial Investigators. Angiotensin-converting-enzyme inhibition in stable coronary artery disease. N Engl J Med 2004;351:2058-68.

9. Chobanian AV, Bakris GL, Black HR, et al. Seventh report of the Joint National Committee on Prevention, Detection, Evaluation, and Treatment of High Blood Pressure. Hypertension 2003;42:1206-52.

10. Dahlof B, Devereux RB, Kjeldsen SE, et al.; LIFE Study Group. Cardiovascular morbidity and mortality in the Losartan Intervention For Endpoint reduction in hypertension study (LIFE): a randomised trial against atenolol. Lancet 2002;359:995-1003.

11. Dahlof B, Sever PS, Poulter NR, et al.; ASCOT Investigators. Prevention of cardiovascular events with an antihypertensive regimen of amlodipine adding perindopril as required versus atenolol adding bendroflumethiazide as required, in the Anglo-Scandinavian Cardiac Outcomes Trial-Blood Pressure Lowering Arm (ASCOT-BPLA): a multicentre randomised controlled trial. Lancet 2005;366:895-906.

12. Fihn SD, Gardin JM, Abrams J, et al. 2012 ACCF/AHA/ACP/AATS/PCNA/SCAI/STS guideline for the diagnosis and management of patients with stable ischemic heart disease. Circulation 2012;126:3097-137.

13. Fox KM; EURopean trial On reduction of cardiac events with Perindopril in stable coronary Artery disease Investigators. Efficacy of perindopril in reduction of cardiovascular events among patients with stable coronary artery disease: randomised, double-blind, placebo-controlled, multicentre trial (the EUROPA study). Lancet 2003;362:782-8.

14. Go AS, Bauman MA, Coleman King SM, et al. An effective approach to high blood pressure control: a science advisory from the American Heart Association, the American College of Cardiology, and the Centers for Disease Control and Prevention. J Am Coll Cardiol. 2014;63:1230-8.

15. Hansson L, Hedner T, Lund-Johansen P, et al. Randomised trial of effects of calcium antagonists compared with diuretics and beta-blockers on cardiovascular morbidity and mortality in hypertension: the Nordic Diltiazem (NORDIL) study. Lancet 2000;356:359-65.

16. Hansson L, Zanchetti A, Carruthers SG, et al. Effects of intensive blood-pressure lowering and low-dose aspirin in patients with hypertension: principal results of the Hypertension Optimal Treatment (HOT) randomised trial: HOT Study Group. Lancet 1998;351:1755-62.

17. James PA, Oparil S, Carter BL, et al. 2014 evidence-based guideline for the management of high blood pressure in adults: report from the panel members appointed to the Eighth Joint National Committee (JNC 8). JAMA 2014;311:507-20.

18. Julius S, Kjeldsen SE, Weber M, et al.; VALUE Trial Group. Outcomes in hypertensive patients at high cardiovascular risk treated with regimens based on valsartan or amlodipine: the VALUE randomised trial. Lancet 2004;363:2022-31.

19. KDIGO clinical practice guideline for the management of blood pressure in chronic kidney disease. Kidney Int 2013;5:337-414.

20. Medical Research Council Working Party. MRC trial of treatment of mild hypertension: principal results. Br Med J (Clin Res Educ) 1985;291:97-104.

21. Nishizaka MK, Zaman MA, Calhoun DA. Efficacy of low-dose spironolactone in subjects with resistant hypertension. Am J Hypertens 2003;16:925-30.

22. Ouzan J, Pérault C, Lincoff AM, et al. The role of spironolactone in the treatment of patients with refractory hypertension. Am J Hypertens 2002;15:333-9.

23. Packer M, Fowler MB, Roecker EB, et al.; Carvedilol Prospective Randomized Cumulative Survival (COPERNICUS) Study Group. Effect of carvedilol on the morbidity of patients with severe chronic

heart failure: results of the Carvedilol Prospective Randomized Cumulative Survival (COPERNICUS) Study. Circulation 2002;106:2194-9.

24. Pepine CJ, Handberg EM, Cooper-DeHoff RM, et al.; INVEST Investigators. A calcium antagonist vs a non-calcium antagonist treatment strategy for patients with coronary artery disease: the International Verapamil-Trandolapril Study (INVEST): a randomized controlled trial. JAMA 2003;290:2805-16.

25. Pfeffer MA, Braunwald E, Moye LA, et al.; for the SAVE Investigators. Effect of captopril on mortality and morbidity in patients with left ventricular dysfunction after myocardial infarction: results of the Survival And Ventricular Enlargement trial. N Engl J Med 1992;327:669-77.

26. Pfeffer MA, McMurray JJ, Velazquez EJ, et al.; Valsartan in Acute Myocardial Infarction Trial Investigators. Valsartan, captopril, or both in myocardial infarction complicated by heart failure, left ventricular dysfunction, or both. N Engl J Med 2003;349:1893-906.

27. PROGRESS Collaborative Group. Randomised trial of a perindopril-based blood-pressure-lowering regimen among 6,105 individuals with previous stroke or transient ischaemic attack. Lancet 2001;358:1033-41.

28. Rosendorff C, Black HR, Cannon CP, et al. Treatment of hypertension in the prevention and management of ischemic heart disease: a scientific statement from the American Heart Association Council for High Blood Pressure Research and the Councils on Clinical Cardiology and Epidemiology and Prevention. Circulation 2007;115:2761-88.

29. SHEP Cooperative Research Group. Prevention of stroke by antihypertensive drug treatment in older persons with isolated systolic hypertension: final results of the Systolic Hypertension in the Elderly Program. JAMA 1991;265:3255-64.

30. Smith SC, Benjamin EJ, Bonow RW, et al. AHA/ACCF secondary prevention and risk reduction therapy for patients with coronary and other atherosclerotic vascular disease: 2011 update. Circulation 2011;124:2458-73.

31. Smith SC Jr, Allen J, Blair SN, et al.; AHA/ACC; National Heart, Lung, and Blood Institute. AHA/ACC guidelines for secondary prevention for patients with coronary and other atherosclerotic vas

cular disease: 2006 update [published correction appears in Circulation 2006;113:e847]. Circulation 2006;113:2363-74.

32. Wang JG, Staessen JA. Benefits of antihypertensive pharmacologic therapy and blood pressure reduction in outcome trials. J Clin Hypertens (Greenwich) 2003;5:66-75.

33. Weber MA, Schiffrin EL, White WB, et al. Clinical practice guidelines for the management of hypertension in the community: a statement by the American Society of Hypertension and the International Society of Hypertension. J Hypertens. 2014;32:3-15.

34. Wing LM, Reid CM, Ryan P, et al.; Second Australian National Blood Pressure Study Group. A comparison of outcomes with angiotensin-converting-enzyme inhibitors and diuretics for hypertension in the elderly. N Engl J Med 2003;348:583-92.

35. Yusuf S, Sleight P, Pogue J, et al. Effects of an angiotensin-converting-enzyme inhibitor, ramipril, on cardiovascular events in high-risk patients: the Heart Outcomes Prevention Evaluation Study. N Engl J Med 2000;342:145-53.

Dyslipidemia

1. The AIM-HIGH Investigators. Niacin in patients with low HDL cholesterol levels receiving intensive statin therapy. N Engl J Med 2011;365:2255-67.

2. The ALLHAT Officers and Coordinators for the ALLHAT Collaborative Research Group. Major outcomes in moderately hypercholesterolemic, hypertensive patients randomized to pravastatin vs usual care: the antihypertensive and lipid-lowering treatment to prevent heart attack trial (ALLHAT-LLT). JAMA 2002;288:2998-3007.

3. American Diabetes Association (ADA). Standards of medical care in diabetes – 2015. Diabetes Care 2015;38(suppl 1):S49–57.

4. Baigent C, Landray MJ, Reith C, et al. The effects of lowering LDL cholesterol with simvastatin plus ezetimibe in patients with chronic kidney disease (Study of Heart and Renal Protection): a randomized placebo-controlled trial. Lancet 2011;377:2181-92.

5. Baruch L, Gupta B, Lieberman-Blum SS, et al. Ezetimibe 5 and 10 mg for lowering LDL-C: potential billion-dollar savings with improved tolerability. Am J Manag Care 2008;14:637-41.

6. Bowman L, Armitage J, Bulbulia R, et al. Study of the effectiveness of additional reductions in cholesterol and homocysteine (SEARCH): characteristics of a randomized trial among 12064 myocardial infarction survivors. Am Heart J 2007;154:815-23.

7. Cannon CP, Braunwald E, McCabe CH, et al.; Pravastatin or Atorvastatin Evaluation and Infection Therapy-Thrombolysis in Myocardial Infarction 22 Investigators. Intensive versus moderate lipid lowering with statins after acute coronary syndromes. N Engl J Med 2004;350:1495-504.

8. Cohen DE, Anania FA, Chalasani N. An assessment of statin safety by hepatologists. Am J Cardiol 2006;97(suppl):77C-81C.

9. The Coronary Drug Project Research Group. Clofibrate and niacin in coronary heart disease. JAMA 1975;231:360-81.

10. Downs JR, Clearfield M, Weis S, et al. Primary prevention of acute coronary events with lovastatin in men and women with average cholesterol levels: results of AFCAPS/TexCAPS. JAMA 1998;279:1615-22.

11. The ENHANCE Investigators. Simvastatin with or without ezetimibe in familial hypercholesterolemia. N Engl J Med 2008;358:1431-43.

12. Expert Panel on Detection, Evaluation, and Treatment of High Blood Cholesterol in Adults. Executive Summary of the Third Report of the National Cholesterol Education Program (NCEP) Expert Panel on Detection, Evaluation, and Treatment of High Blood Cholesterol in Adults (Adult Treatment Panel III). JAMA 2001;285:2486-97.

13. Frick MH, Elo O, Haapa K, et al. Helsinki heart study: primary-prevention trial with gemfibrozil in middle-aged men with dyslipidemia. N Engl J Med 1987;317:1237-45.

14. GISSI-Prevenzione Investigators. Dietary supplementation with n-3 polyunsaturated fatty acids and vitamin E after myocardial infarction: results of the GISSI-Prevenzione trial. Lancet 1999;354:447-55.

15. Grundy SM, Cleeman JI, Bairey Merz CN, et al. Implications of recent clinical trials for the National Cholesterol Education Program Adult Treatment Panel III guidelines. Circulation 2004;110:227-39.

16. Heart Protection Study Collaborative Group. MRC/BHF Heart Protection Study of cholesterol lowering with simvastatin in 20,536 high-risk individuals: a randomised placebo-controlled trial. Lancet 2002;360:7-22.

17. IMPROVE-IT (IMProved Reduction of Outcomes: Vytorin Efficacy International Trial). Available at http://newsroom.heart.org/news/cholesterol-lowering-drug-with-different-action-adds-to-statins-reduction-of-cardiovascular-risk. Accessed November 24, 2014.

18. Keech AC, Mitchell P, Summanen PA, et al. Effect of fenofibrate on the need for laser treatment for diabetic retinopathy (FIELD study): a randomised controlled trial. Lancet 2007;370:1687-97.

19. Kidney Disease: Improving Global Outcomes. KDIGO clinical practice guidelines for lipid management in chronic kidney disease. Kidney Int 2013;3:1-56.

20. LaRosa JC, Grundy SM, Waters DD, et al. Intensive lipid lowering with atorvastatin in patients with stable coronary disease. N Engl J Med 2005;352:1425-35.

21. Lipid Research Clinics Program. The lipid research clinics coronary primary prevention trial results. JAMA 1984;251:365-74.

22. The Lipid Study Group. Prevention of cardiovascular events and death with pravastatin in patients with coronary heart disease and a broad range of initial cholesterol levels. N Engl J Med 1998;339:1349-57.

23. Pedersen TR, Kjekshus J, Berg K, et al. Randomised trial of cholesterol lowering in 4444 patients with coronary heart disease: the Scandinavian Simvastatin Survival Study (4S). Lancet 1994;344:1383-9.

24. Ridker PM, Danielson E, Fonseca FAH, et al. Rosuvastatin to prevent vascular events in men and women with elevated C-reactive protein. N Engl J Med 2008;359:2195-207.

25. Rossebo AB, Pedersen TR, Boman K, et al. Intensive lipid lowering with simvastatin and ezetimibe in aortic stenosis. N Engl J Med 2008;359:1343-56.

26. Rubins HB, Robins SJ, Collins D, et al. Gemfibrozil for the secondary prevention of coronary heart disease in men with low levels of high-density lipoprotein cholesterol: Veterans Affairs High-Density Lipoprotein Cholesterol Intervention Trial Study Group. N Engl J Med 1999;341:410-8.

27. Sacks FM, Pfeffer MA, Moye LA, et al. The effect of pravastatin on coronary events after myocardial infarction in patients with average cholesterol levels. N Engl J Med 1996;335:1001-9.

28. Sever PS, Dahlof B, Poulter NR, et al.; ASCOT investigators. Prevention of coronary and stroke events with atorvastatin in hypertensive patients who have average or lower-than-average cholesterol concentrations, in the Anglo-Scandinavian Cardiac Outcomes Trial – Lipid Lowering Arm (ASCOT-LLA): a multicentre randomised controlled trial. Lancet 2003;361:1149-58.

29. Shepherd J, Blauw GJ, Murphy MB, et al. Pravastatin in elderly individuals at risk of vascular disease (PROSPER): a randomised controlled trial. Lancet 2002;360:1623-30.

30. Shepherd J, Cobbe SM, Ford I, et al. Prevention of coronary heart disease with pravastatin in men with hypercholesterolemia. N Engl J Med 1995;333:1301-7.

31. Stone NJ, Robinson J, Lichtenstein AH, et al.; American College of Cardiology/American Heart Association Task Force on Practice Guidelines. 2013 ACC/AHA guideline on the treatment of blood cholesterol to reduce atherosclerotic cardiovascular risk in adults: a report of the American College of Cardiology/American Heart Association Task Force on Practice Guidelines. Circulation. 2014;129(25 suppl 2):S1-45.

32. Taylor AJ, Villines TC, Stanek EJ, et al. Extended-release niacin or ezetimibe and carotid intima-media thickness. N Engl J Med 2009;361:2113-22.

33. Thompson PD, Clarkson PM, Rosenson RS. An assessment of statin safety by muscle experts. Am J Cardiol 2006;97(suppl):69C-76C.

34. Tonkin AM, Chen L. Effects of combination lipid therapy in the management of patients with type 2 diabetes mellitus in the Action to Control Cardiovascular Risk in Diabetes (ACCORD) trial. Circulation 2010;122:850-2.

Peripheral Arterial Disease

1. Anderson JL, Halperin JL, Albert NM, et al. Management of patients with peripheral artery disease (compilation of 2005 and 2011 ACCF/AHA guideline recommendations): a report of the American College of Cardiology Foundation/American Heart Association Task Force on Practice Guidelines. Circulation 2013;127:1425-43.

Atherosclerotic (Non-Cardioembolic Ischemic) Stroke or TIA

1. Kernan WN, Ovbiagele B, Black HR, et al; on behalf of the American Heart Association Stroke Council, Council on Cardiovascular and Stroke Nursing, Council on Clinical Cardiology, and Council on Peripheral Vascular Disease. Guidelines for the prevention of stroke in patients with stroke and transient ischemic attack: a guideline for healthcare professionals from the American Heart Association/American Stroke Association. Stroke. 2014;45:2160–236.

ANSWERS AND EXPLANATIONS TO PATIENT CASES

1. Answer: D

Using the Pooled Cohort Equation, his 10-year risk of ASCVD is 51.4%. Because Hispanic is not an option under the race category, it is most appropriate to use the white category.

2. Answer: B

For a 58-year-old man, the USPSTF recommends aspirin for primary prevention if the risk of MI is 4% or greater (see Table 3). The 2012 ACCP guidelines recommend aspirin for primary prevention in patients older than 50 years. Using the 2008 modified Framingham risk score (www.framinghamheartstudy.org/risk/index.html), his 10-year risk of a CHD event is as follows: Age 58 years = 4 points; LDL-C 110 mg/dL = 0 point; HDL-C 50 mg/dL = 0 point; BP: SBP 135 mm Hg = 1 point and DBP 85 mm Hg = 1 point, so for BP, use 1 point; DM no = 0 points; smoking yes = 2 points; step 7 total score = 7 points corresponding in step 8 to a 10-year risk of CHD = 14%. Therefore, aspirin is indicated for preventing an MI, and Answer B is correct (Option C and Option D are incorrect). Neither data from clinical trials nor the guidelines support a role for aspirin in stroke prevention in men; thus, Option A is incorrect.

3. Answer: A

The 2016 ADA Standards of Medical Care recommend low-dose aspirin 75–162 mg/day orally for patients with DM if the 10-year risk of CHD is greater than 10%. You may use either the modified risk score for CHD events or the Reynolds risk score for stroke (for women). Using the 2008 modified Framingham risk score (www.framinghamheartstudy.org/risk/index.html), calculate the number of LDL-C points as follows: Age 56 years = 7 points; LDL-C 110 mg/dL = 0 points; HDL-C 51 mg/dL = 0 points; BP: SBP 145 mm Hg = 2 points and DBP 89 mm Hg = 2 points, so for BP, use 2 points; DM yes = 4 points; smoking no = 0 points; step 7 total score = 13 points corresponding in step 8 to a 10-year risk of CHD = 17%. Because the patient's risk is greater than 10%, aspirin 75–162 mg/day is indicated for this patient currently, making Answer A correct and Option D incorrect. The aspirin doses in Option C and Option D are too high.

4. Answer: A

According to the ADA, the goal BP for a patient with DM is less than 140/80 mm Hg, and this patient's BP is 145/89 mm Hg (similar to an office BP reading taken 6 months ago). Therefore, initial treatment of HTN is indicated currently. The ADA guidelines recommend initial therapy with an ACE inhibitor or an ARB over other agents, making Option B and Option D incorrect. According to the ADA, a statin is indicated for all patients with DM older than 40 years who have at least one additional risk factor for CVD. This patient has three additional risk factors: HTN, dyslipidemia, and a family history of premature CVD. According to the AHA, a statin is recommended for patients with diabetes, 40–75 years of age, with an LDL-C of 70–189 mg/dL; and a high-intensity statin is recommended for patients with a 10-year ASCVD risk greater than 7.5%. Therefore, a high-intensity statin is indicated. Because Option C includes a moderate-intensity statin plus an ACE inhibitor, whereas Answer A includes an ACE inhibitor plus a high-intensity statin, Answer A is a better choice than Option B.

5. Answer: D

After placement of a BMS or a DES for ACS, a $P2Y_{12}$ inhibitor is indicated for at least 1 year; therefore, Option A and Option B are incorrect. No current data support DAPT for more than 1 year compared with longer therapy durations; therefore, Option C is incorrect.

6. Answer: A

At least two BP measurements should be made to accurately assess BP. A BP measurement is likely inaccurate if the patient has not been seated quietly for at least 5 minutes. Determinations for therapy can be made after accurate BP readings have been obtained. This patient may have undiagnosed HTN.

7. Answer: C

Because the patient's BMI is near goal, diet and exercise only will not likely get her BP to goal. Thiazide diuretics are a recommended first-line therapy, whereas verapamil is not. Because her BP is above goal (goal is less than 140/90 mm Hg), treatment is necessary.

8. Answer: C

Angiotensin receptor blockers are the best replacement medications for ACE inhibitors in this patient because DM is a compelling indication for their use, especially in patients with microalbuminuria. Treatment is needed because the patient's BP is above goal (goal is less than 140/80 mm Hg per ADA).

9. Answer: A

The patient's hydrochlorothiazide dose should be discontinued because her CrCl is now less than 30 mL/minute; hydrochlorothiazide is probably not providing any benefit, but it may contribute to electrolyte abnormalities. Amlodipine should be continued for BP control, but the amlodipine dose does not have to be increased currently because her BP is at goal (i.e., less than 130/80 mm Hg per KDIGO).

10. Answer: A

This patient has resistant HTN, which is the inability to reach goal BP with full doses of an appropriate three-drug regimen that includes a diuretic. Spironolactone is beneficial for resistant HTN. Therapy change is needed because her BP remains above goal (goal is less than 140/80 mm Hg per ADA). Metoprolol cannot be increased because of her HR. Discontinuing hydrochlorothiazide may further increase her BP.

11. Answer: A

Initiation of a two-drug regimen is required for this patient to control his BP in a reasonable time. This patient's BP is not high enough to qualify as a hypertensive emergency (or urgency).

12. Answer: C

Because this patient has CAD and is younger than 75 years, a high-intensity statin (e.g., atorvastatin 80 mg/day) is indicated. Simvastatin 40 mg/day is a moderate-intensity statin, and pravastatin 20 mg/day is a low-intensity statin.

13. Answer: D

Because this patient has ASCVD, a high-intensity statin would normally be recommended. However, she also has renal insufficiency. Per the simvastatin package label, patients with CrCl less than 30 mL/minute should not take simvastatin 80 mg/day, so Option C would be incorrect. However, atorvastatin 20 mg/day would be a safe

dose for her, so Answer D is correct. Fenofibrate would not be of benefit because her TG concentrations are not elevated above 500 mg/dL, so Option B is incorrect. Adding omega-3 fatty acids would have less of a benefit than changing the patient's regimen to an appropriately dosed statin, so Option A is not the best answer.

14. Answer: A

Because this patient's TG values are less than 500 mg/dL, she does not require fibrate therapy currently, so Options B and C are incorrect, nor does she require statin therapy because her 10-year ASCVD risk is less than 7.5% (currently 1.4%); therefore, Option D would be incorrect. Answer A is correct because this patient's TG would likely lower as a result of weight loss and lifestyle modification.

15. Answer: C

This patient's simvastatin dose should be reduced to decrease the likelihood of a drug interaction with amiodarone. He requires statin therapy for lipid control. Increasing the simvastatin dose would increase the likelihood of an interaction. Although niacin can improve his HDL-C, this is not his primary concern currently.

16. Answer: B

Because the patient is symptomatic, it is recommended to hold statin therapy to ascertain whether symptoms resolve or CK improves. Future CK readings will dictate whether statin therapy should be discontinued. His LDL-C can be addressed once the CK issue has been resolved. Although infection and strenuous activity can contribute to elevated CK, it is important to rule in/out the statin as the cause.

ANSWERS AND EXPLANATIONS TO SELF-ASSESSMENT QUESTIONS

1. Answer: D

The patient's BP is above his goal of less than 140/90 mm Hg (per ADA), so antihypertensive therapy should be initiated. The preferred first-line agent for patients with diabetes is ACE inhibitor therapy. Using the 2013 AHA/ACC guideline risk calculator, this patient has an estimated 10-year ASCVD risk of 15.8%. Because this patient is 40–75 years of age with diabetes and an LDL-C concentration between 70 and 189 mg/dL, a high-intensity statin is indicated. For patients with DM, the ADA recommends aspirin 75–162 mg for patients with a CHD risk greater than 10%. If no risk assessment is available, aspirin may be considered for men older than 50 years who have at least one other risk factor for CHD. If indicated, aspirin 81 mg may be used for primary prevention. Option B is incorrect because it does not contain a statin or treatment for HTN. Option A is incorrect because it does not contain aspirin or a statin. Option C is incorrect because the initial statin dose of simvastatin 80 mg is too high (risk of rhabdomyolysis), and there is no aspirin. Answer D is correct because the regimen contains low-dose aspirin, an ACE inhibitor, and a statin.

2. Answer: D

Aspirin reduces stroke risk as primary prevention in women; therefore, Option B and Option C are incorrect (no benefit in reducing risk of MI or CHD). This is a female patient, and the USPSTF recommends using the Western States Stroke Consortium calculator (Framingham stroke risk score) to estimate the patient's risk of stroke. Using the online calculator, her estimated 10-year risk is 1.8%. According to the USPSTF recommendations in Table 6, aspirin is not indicated for a 56-year-old woman unless the estimated 10-year stroke risk is 3% or greater because the benefit for the strokes prevented exceeds the risk of bleeding, making Answer D correct.

3. Answer: A

The patient's HR is at goal of less than 60 beats/minute. Therefore, the metoprolol dose should not be increased because of the risk of worsening bradycardia and heart block, making Option B and Option C incorrect. Because the patient is taking a high-intensity statin, with an adequate response in his LDL-C (currently less than 70 mg/dL), an increase in his statin dose is not needed, making Option B and Option D incorrect. The patient's BP is not at goal (goal is less than 140/90 mm Hg). An

ACE inhibitor guideline is a class I recommendation for secondary prevention in patients with HTN. The aspirin dose after PCI that is associated with the lowest bleeding risk is 81 mg. Therefore, Answer A is correct. Clopidogrel is indicated for at least 1 year after PCI in the setting of ACS; therefore, Option D is incorrect.

4. Answer: D

Patients with a DES should take aspirin 81 mg indefinitely. This change, giving a preference to low-dose aspirin over full-dose aspirin, differs from the 2007 PCI guidelines, which recommended 325 mg for 1 month and low-dose aspirin thereafter; thus, Option A and Option B are incorrect. Option A is also incorrect because ticagrelor should not be administered with aspirin doses higher than 100 mg orally daily. Because the patient had a recent MI, $P2Y_{12}$ inhibitor therapy is indicated for at least 12 months, making Option B and Option C incorrect.

5. Answer: C

Vorapaxar is indicated for the reduction of thrombotic CV events in patients with a history of MI or PAD and should be used with aspirin and/or clopidogrel on the basis of the TRACER and TRA 2P-TIMI 50 studies, making Answer C correct. It has not been studied with ticagrelor or prasugrel, making Option D incorrect. Studies with vorapaxar included patients taking both aspirin and clopidogrel, so neither need to be discontinued in patients at low risk of bleeding, making Options A and B incorrect.

6. Answer: D

Patients who have recently (less than 1 year) undergone DES placement are at higher risk of stent thrombosis after the cessation of $P2Y_{12}$ inhibitor therapy. Both the Society of Thoracic Surgeons and the 2012 ACCP guidelines recommend continuing DAPT in this setting; thus, Answer D is correct. The 2011 ACCF/AHA PCI guidelines give the option of discontinuing the $P2Y_{12}$ inhibitor. However, Option A and Option C are incorrect because the proper timing of clopidogrel discontinuation would have been 5 days, not 7 days. Option B is incorrect because aspirin should be continued in the setting of recent ACS.

7. Answer: A

Angiotensin-converting enzyme inhibitors have both renal- and cardiac-protective properties in patients with DM. α-Blockers were shown to be associated with a higher rate of CVD in the ALLHAT trial. Atenolol is not a first-line antihypertensive drug for this patient because of his low HR. This patient requires medications because his BP is above his goal of less than 140/80 mm Hg (according to the ADA).

8. Answer: D

A thiazide diuretic is the next best step for this patient because this agent will help prevent CVD complications and increase the efficacy of her other BP medications. Her metoprolol dose cannot be increased because of her low HR. Terazosin has been associated with more CVD events than thiazide diuretics. Her BP has to be treated because it is above her BP goal (goal is less than 140/90 mm Hg).

9. Answer: D

Oral contraceptives, specifically estrogen, may increase BP, and risk can increase with duration of use. An alternative contraceptive without estrogen would be less likely to contribute to her HTN. Option A and Option B are incorrect because her BP requires better control, but weight loss is unlikely to help because her BMI is normal. Option C is incorrect because hydrochlorothiazide is no more potent than chlorthalidone.

10. Answer: B ·

Angiotensin-converting enzyme inhibitor therapy is contraindicated in pregnancy, and discontinuing ramipril is the most important next step, making Option A and Option C incorrect. Option D is incorrect because this patient will require very good BP control during her pregnancy.

11. Answer: C

Nonsteroidal anti-inflammatory drugs and CKD are identifiable causes of HTN. Option A is incorrect; the patient likely adheres to her therapy because she has been on the same regimen without problems for 5 years. Option D is incorrect; her TSH is normal, so she is unlikely to have thyroid disease. Option B is incorrect; her BMI is within normal limits, so her HTN is unlikely to be caused by poor lifestyle.

12. Answer: B

Because the patient has proteinuria, her BP goal is less than 130/80 mm Hg according to the KDIGO guidelines, and additional treatment is needed. Loop diuretics (Answer B) work well for patients with renal insufficiency. Option A is incorrect because this patient would benefit most from add-on diuretic therapy, but her CrCl is too low to realize benefit from thiazide diuretics. Option C is incorrect because changing from lisinopril to losartan would probably not result in lower BP. Option D is incorrect because her HR is too low to increase her atenolol dose.

13. Answer: D

According to the pooled cohort equations, this patient's 10-year ASCVD risk is 21.6%. According to the 2013 ACC/AHA lipid guideline, patients with diabetes whose 10-year ASCVD risk is greater than 7.5% should receive a high-intensity statin. Because simvastatin 40 mg/day is a moderate-dose statin, it should be changed to a high-dose statin (e.g., atorvastatin 40 mg/day). Option A and Option C are incorrect because a mild, chronic ALT elevation will not be adversely affected by statin therapy, and lowering the dose will not likely improve this. Option B is incorrect because ezetimibe has not shown reduced morbidity or mortality in clinical trials to date.

14. Answer: B

Option A is incorrect; a therapy change must be made because simvastatin is metabolized primarily by the CYP3A4 isoenzyme system, and verapamil competes for this same metabolic pathway. Option C is incorrect; the maximal dose of lovastatin has similar risks. Option D is incorrect; although the coadministration of simvastatin and verapamil is not contraindicated, the simvastatin dose should be decreased to 10 mg/day to reduce the risk of rhabdomyolysis (the 40-mg/day dose is still too high). Rosuvastatin is metabolized through an alternative pathway and does not interact with verapamil.

15. Answer: A

This patient is asymptomatic; thus, she can continue her current statin therapy because it is controlling her LDL-C. Option B is incorrect because a mildly elevated CK concentration alone does not justify discontinuing therapy. She should be receiving high-intensity statin therapy because of her history of CAD. Option C and Option D are incorrect because there would be no benefit to switching to lovastatin or lowering her atorvastatin dose.

16. Answer: A

The patient is currently taking a recommended dosed statin (simvastatin 40 mg/day), so no change in therapy is needed. Option B is incorrect because her renal function is insufficient to safely use maximal-dose simvastatin. According to the 2013 KDIGO lipid guidelines, statin therapy should not be based on LDL-C (only dosed appropriately). Per KDIGO, atorvastatin 40 mg/day exceeds the recommended dosing for patients with CKD, so Option C is incorrect. Option D is incorrect because simvastatin 20 mg/day is below the recommended dosing for simvastatin.

17. Answer: B

Because the patient's LDL-C remains greater than 190 mg/dL, the 2013 ACC/AHA lipid guidelines recommend starting a high-intensity statin such as atorvastatin 80 mg/day. Option C and Option D are incorrect because they recommend initiating moderate- and low-intensity statins, respectively.

18. Answer: A

The patient is currently receiving maximum doses of both atorvastatin and ezetimibe. PCSK9 inhibitors lower LDL-C values an additional 50% to 70% when added to statin therapy. Answer A is correct because alirocumab is a PCSK9 inhibitor that is dosed every 2 weeks. Option B is incorrect because the 140-mg dose of evolocumab should be given every 2 weeks, not monthly. Fenofibrate is primarily used for TG lowering and can increase LDL-C values, making Option C incorrect. Although bile acid sequestrants do provide additional LDL-C lowering, they can also increase TG values and have a relative contraindication with TG concentrations above 200 mg/dL, making Option D incorrect.

Obstetrics and Gynecology

Alicia B. Forinash, Pharm.D., BCPS,BCACP

St. Louis College of Pharmacy
Saint Louis, Missouri

Obstetrics and Gynecology

Alicia B. Forinash, Pharm.D., BCPS,BCACP

St. Louis College of Pharmacy
Saint Louis, Missouri

Learning Objectives

1. Recommend therapy for contraception, infertility, menstrual disorders, endometriosis, and symptoms of menopause on the basis of patient-specific information.
2. Recommend appropriate treatment for common acute and chronic conditions in pregnancy and lactation.
3. Develop patient education regarding medication use during pregnancy and lactation, contraception, infertility, menstrual disorders, endometriosis, and postmenopausal therapy.
4. Identify additional resources for health care providers and patients on contraception, infertility, pregnancy and lactation, menstrual disorders, endometriosis, and postmenopausal therapy.

Self-Assessment Questions

Answers and explanations to these questions may be found at the end of the chapter.

The following case pertains to questions 1 and 2.

A 36-year-old woman is in the clinic for her 2-week postpartum checkup, wanting to know which contraceptive method she should use. She had to stop breastfeeding when she was 5 days postpartum, after she suffered a stroke. Her medical history is significant for morbid obesity, a tilted and bicornate uterus, allergic rhinitis, and a cerebrovascular accident (5 days postpartum). She is allergic to latex. Current medications are lisinopril 5 mg/day, hydrochlorothiazide 12.5 mg/day, simvastatin 20 mg every night, and aspirin 81 mg/day (all medications initiated 1.5 weeks ago).

1. Which is the best contraceptive recommendation for this woman?

   A. Depot medroxyprogesterone acetate.
   B. Levonorgestrel intrauterine device (IUD).
   C. Contraceptive sponge.
   D. Male polyurethane condom.

2. The patient calls to ask for another contraceptive choice because she cannot afford the item you recommended. She states that the free clinic does not carry the item either. Of the alternative contraceptives that can be provided free from either your clinic or the free clinic, which is the best recommendation?

   A. Female condom.
   B. Male latex condom.
   C. Yaz (ethinyl estradiol and drospirenone).
   D. Ella (ulipristal).

3. A double-blind randomized trial is under way to evaluate the effects of depot medroxyprogesterone, leuprolide, and placebo on the bone mineral density of 600 patients with endometriosis. Which statistical test is most appropriate?

   A. Student t-test.
   B. Fisher exact test.
   C. Kruskal-Wallis test.
   D. Analysis of variance.

4. A 40-year-old woman asks to see the pharmacist after her physician's appointment. She states that she was prescribed a new drug during her pregnancy. She is uncomfortable taking medications during her pregnancy because her family said that they all carry risk. Which is the best information to include when educating the patient on the risks and benefits of the drug?

   A. Rate of birth defects in studies of animals.
   B. Gestational timing of risks and pregnancy.
   C. Molecular weight of the drug.
   D. Half-life of the medication.

5. A 32-year-old woman who is 4 weeks postpartum calls your office asking whether it is okay for her to start terbinafine therapy for 6 months for toe onychomycosis that began during the pregnancy. She states that she consulted a podiatrist yesterday and that the podiatrist gave her this prescription. She reports no pain, redness, or difficulty walking but states she does not like how her toes look when wearing sandals. She is currently breastfeeding every 2 hours. You will find the following information regarding use in breastfeeding in the reference *Medications and Mothers' Milk* (Hale 2008): milk/plasma ratio, unknown; relative infant dose, unknown; half-life, 26 hours; 99% protein bound; molecular weight, 291 daltons. Which is the best recommendation?

A. Delay treatment until finished with breastfeeding.
B. Change to itraconazole.
C. Use topical terbinafine.
D. Schedule doses right after feedings.

6. A 21-year-old woman is in the office for a follow-up of her dysmenorrhea. She states that because ibuprofen has only slightly improved her pain, she would like something else. She is currently in a monogamous relationship and would like contraceptive protection as well. Her vital signs today include the following: height 63 inches, weight 99 kg (220 lb), blood pressure 118/68 mm Hg, and heart rate 72 beats/minute. Which is the best recommendation?

A. Ethinyl estradiol and norelgestromin (Ortho-Evra): Apply one patch every week for 3 weeks; then repeat after a 1-week hormone-free interval.
B. Ethinyl estradiol and norelgestromin (Ortho-Evra): Apply one patch every week for 11 weeks; then repeat after a 1-week hormone-free interval.
C. Ethinyl estradiol 35 mcg and ethynodiol diacetate 1 mg (Demulen 1/35): Take one tablet every days for 3 weeks; then repeat after a 7-day hormone-free interval.
D. Ethinyl estradiol 35 mcg and ethynodiol diacetate 1 mg (Demulen 1/35): Take one tablet every day for 11 weeks; then repeat after a 7-day hormone-free interval.

7. A 49-year-old woman is initiating therapy with estradiol valerate and dienogest (Natazia) for perimenopausal symptoms and contraceptive needs. You are asked to educate her about this product. Which option provides the best information for the patient regarding the minimal time a backup method of contraception should be used after initiation?

A. 48 hours.
B. 7 days.
C. 9 days.
D. 28 days.

8. A 38-year-old woman is calling because of the intolerable vasomotor symptoms she is experiencing, which interfere with her daily activities. She states her hot flashes occur at least 12 times a day and cause her to change clothes often. She would like additional therapy. Her medical history includes breast cancer (diagnosed 1 month ago). She takes trastuzumab. Blood pressure is 104/64 mm Hg, and heart rate is 66 beats/minute. Which is the best recommendation?

A. Conjugated equine estrogens.
B. Venlafaxine.
C. Clonidine.
D. Black cohosh.

9. A 25-year-old woman was recently given a diagnosis of endometriosis. She is having trouble coping with the diagnosis and wants to find a support group. Which is the best resource for finding local support groups?

A. Association of Reproductive Healthcare Professionals.
B. American Congress of Obstetricians and Gynecologists (ACOG).
C. Endometriosis Association.
D. National Women's Health Network.

I. CONTRACEPTION

Patient Case

A 39-year-old woman is requesting hormonal contraception. She plans to start attempting conception in about 12 months. The woman is currently 6 weeks postpartum, and she is feeding formula to the infant. Her medical history is significant for gestational diabetes, hypertension, and hyperthyroidism. She states she is concerned about losing her pregnancy weight. Current medications are propylthiouracil 100 mg three times daily, lisinopril 10 mg/day, hydrochlorothiazide 25 mg/day, and a prenatal vitamin one tablet daily. With respect to social history, the patient reports no tobacco use, uses ethanol socially, and reports not using illegal drugs. Her height is 65 inches; her weight today is 131 kg (290 lb) (pre-pregnancy weight of 104 kg [230 lb]). Blood pressure is 178/96 mm Hg today (188/102 mm Hg 2 weeks ago).

1. Which is the most appropriate hormonal contraceptive recommendation?
   A. Depo-Provera (medroxyprogesterone acetate).
   B. Ortho-Evra (ethinyl estradiol and norelgestromin).
   C. Yaz (ethinyl estradiol and drospirenone).
   D. Micronor (norethindrone).

   A. Product Overview

Table 1. Hormonal Contraceptive Comparison

Product	Hormones	Route	Administration (standard)	Return of Ovulation	Notes
Monophasic oral contraceptives	Estrogen-progestin	Oral	Daily for 21 days or see below	3 months	Some products have added iron (e.g., Loestrin Fe) or levomefolate (Beyaz, Safyral)
	Mircette: 21 active tablets, 2 placebo tablets, and 5 tablets of 10 mcg of estrogen: Decrease estrogen withdrawal symptoms during menses Yaz and Loestrin 24, Beyaz: 24 active tablets; lighter, shorter menses Seasonale: 84 active tablets to have menses every 3 months Seasonique: 84 active tablets; then 10 mcg of estrogen for 7 days for menses every 3 months and fewer estrogen withdrawal symptoms during menses Lybrel: 30 active tablets for no menses; high rates of breakthrough bleeding					
Multiphasic oral contraceptives	Estrogen-progestin	Oral	Daily for 21 days	3 months	Biphasic, triphasic, and quadriphasic
Ethinyl estradiol and etonogestrel vaginal ring (NuvaRing)	Estrogen-progestin	Vaginal	3 weeks	3 months	Only one strength available Can safely be removed for up to 3 hours during intercourse; rinse product then reinsert Squeeze ring and insert into vagina while sitting, squatting, or standing with one leg up; if discomfort arises, push further back into the vagina

Table 1. Statistical Content of Original Articles in The New England Journal of Medicine, 2004–2005 *(continued)*

Product	Hormones	Route	Administration (standard)	Return of Ovulation	Notes
Ethinyl estradiol and norelgest-romin patch (Ortho-Evra)	Estrogen-progestin	Topical	Weekly for 3 weeks	3 months	Only one strength available Higher cumulative estrogen exposure than most oral contraceptives Reduced efficacy for body weight > 90 kg Apply to clean and dry area on body that will not be rubbed by tight fitting clothing (i.e., avoid waistband); rotate patch site; avoid cream/lotion/powder at the patch site
Progestin-only pills	Progestin	Oral	Daily for 28 days	1 month	Must be taken within 3 hours of usual time or backup method of contraception needed for 48 hours
Medroxy-progesterone acetate (Depo-Provera, Depo SubQ Provera)	Progestin	IM, SC	Every 12 ± 2 weeks	9 months	Risk of bone loss after 2 years of continued use, although reversible on discontinuation Weight gain
Etonogestrel (Implanon/ Nexplanon)	Progestin	Intradermal	Every 3 years	1 month	
Levonorgestrel IUD (Mirena)	Progestin	Intrauterine	Every 5 years	1 month	FDA-approved labeling recommends use in parous women only
Levonorgestrel IUD (Skyla)	Progestin	Intrauterine	Every 3 years	1 month	Smaller than Mirena and intended for use in nulliparous women although FDA does not comment on use in parous or nulliparous women
Levenorgestrel IUD (Liletta)	Progestin	Intrauterine	Every 3 years	1 month	Studied in both parous and nulliparous women

FDA = U.S. Food and Drug Administration; IM = intramuscular; IUD = intrauterine device; SC = subcutaneous.

B. Extended-Interval Dosing (i.e., stacking packs)
   1. Monophasic oral contraceptives
      a. Take 3 weeks of active pills from pack 1.
      b. Throw out placebo tablets from pack 1. Start active pills from pack 2 immediately.
      c. Extends cycle by 3 weeks
      d. Can use several packs in a row to extend cycle

2. Multiphasic oral contraceptives
   a. Option 1 (to extend cycle by 5–11 days, depending on brand of contraceptive)
      i. Take 3 weeks of active pills from pack 1.
      ii. Throw out the placebo tablets from pack 1. Start highest-progestin-concentration active pills in pack (usually 7 [range 5–11] tablets, depending on brand).
      iii. Use of each additional pack extends the cycle by 1 week.
   b. Option 2 (to extend cycle by several weeks)

Table 2. Using Several Packs of Multiphasic Contraceptives (example of two packs)

Steps	Directions
1	Take level 1 tablets (e.g., week 1—Low-estrogen, low-progestin tablets) of pack 1
2	Take level 1 tablets of pack 2; repeat with number of packs using to extend cycle
3	Take level 2 tablets (e.g., week 2—High-estrogen, low-progestin tablets) of pack 2
4	Take level 2 tablets of pack 2; repeat with number of packs using to extend cycle
5	Take level 3 tablets (e.g., week 3—High-estrogen, high-progestin tablets) of pack 1
6	Take level 3 tablets of pack 2; repeat with number of packs using to extend cycle

3. Ethinyl estradiol and etonogestrel vaginal ring (NuvaRing)
   a. Insert vaginal ring for 3 weeks then remove.
   b. Immediately insert a new ring for 3 weeks.
   c. May use several rings in a row to extend cycle
4. Ethinyl estradiol and norelgestromin patch (Ortho-Evra)
   a. Place on one patch for 1 week and remove.
   b. Immediately place on a new patch for 1 week.
   c. May use several patches in a row to extend cycle

C. Advantages/Disadvantages of Products *(Domain 1; Tasks 1, 3)*
   1. Estrogen-progestin products
      a. Advantages
         i. High efficacy if taken as instructed
         ii. Improved menstrual symptoms; decreased amount of blood loss and length of menses
         iii. Decreased risk of ectopic pregnancies
         iv. Safe throughout reproductive years
         v. Readily reversible on discontinuation (average 3 months)
         vi. Cycle manipulation
         vii. Decreased incidence and severity of pelvic inflammatory disease (PID); decreased menstrual blood loss, which may act as a medium for bacterial growth
         viii. Decreased risk of ovarian and endometrial cancer
         ix. Decreased risk of functional ovarian cysts
         x. Decreased risk of fibrocystic breast disease
         xi. Helpful for patients with polycystic ovary syndrome (PCOS)
            (a) Decreased stimulation of androgen production in the ovaries
            (b) Decreases free testosterone by increasing sex hormone–binding globulin
         xii. Decreased acne

      b. Disadvantages
          i. No protection against sexually transmitted infections
          ii. Pills require timely daily administration.
          iii. Increased blood pressure
             (a) Increased angiotensinogen
             (b) Sodium and water retention
          iv. Increased risk of stroke and myocardial infarction
             (a) Mainly with 50-mcg ethinyl estradiol products and concomitant risk factors
             (b) Smokers older than 35 years
          v. Increased risk of thromboembolic disorders
          vi. Increased risk of glucose intolerance
          vii. Increased risk of chlamydial infections
             (a) Associated with cervical ectopy (cervical surface becomes covered with mucus-secreting cells that normally line the cervical canal), increasing the risk of chlamydial infections
             (b) PID infection rate is not increased.
          viii. Increased risk of gallbladder disease

2. Progestin-only products
      a. Advantages of progestin-only pills
          i. Used for patients with contraindications to estrogen products (e.g., older than 35 years and who smoke 15 or more cigarettes per day, history of thromboembolism)
          ii. Good for patients with intolerable adverse events to estrogen products
          iii. Less risk of myocardial infarction and stroke in patients older than 35 years
          iv. Safe for breastfeeding patients; progestin has no effect on milk production, whereas estrogen decreases milk production
      b. Disadvantages of progestin-only pills
          i. Timely daily administration
          ii. Irregular menses and increased risk of breakthrough bleeding and spotting
          iii. Increased risk of ectopic pregnancy
          iv. Increased need for adherence and consistent administration time (use backup method of contraception for 48 hours if dose is taken 3 or more hours late)
          v. Increased risk of ovulation because of lower progestin dose
      c. Advantages of depot medroxyprogesterone acetate
          i. Progestin-only pill advantages
          ii. Less user variance/error with less frequent administration
          iii. Scant to light menstrual bleeding with continued use; this characteristic makes it advantageous in the treatment of endometriosis
          iv. Decreased risk of anemia secondary to decreased menstrual bleeding
          v. Decreased menstrual cramps and mittelschmerz pain
          vi. Decreased risk of endometrial and ovarian cancer
          vii. Decreased risk of PID
          viii. No drug interactions
      d. Disadvantages of depot medroxyprogesterone acetate
          i. Delayed onset of returned fertility
          ii. Menstrual irregularities with first several injections
          iii. Increased risk of bone loss
              (a) Package insert: After 2 years of use, bone density monitoring recommended
             (b) Reversible on discontinuation
             (c) World Health Organization does not recommend product discontinuation.

       iv. Decreases high-density lipoproteins

       v. Weight gain (year 1: 2.45 kg [5.4 lb]; year 2: 3.68 kg [8.1 lb]; year 4: 6.27 kg [13.8 lb]; year 6: 7.5 kg [16.5 lb])

  e. Advantages of progestin-only IUD

       i. Progestin-only pill advantages

       ii. Levonorgestrel IUD (Mirena) can be left in place for up to 5 years; levonorgestrel IUD (Skyla and Liletta) can be left in place for up to 3 years.

       iii. Provides two mechanisms of action

          (a) Progestin-only product mechanisms

          (b) IUD mechanisms

       iv. Amenorrhea

          (a) Mirena—20% at 1 year

          (b) Skyla—6% at 1 year

  f. Disadvantages of progestin-only IUD

       i. Must check daily for strings

       ii. Cautions: Increased risk of PID; do not initiate if active chlamydia, gonorrhea, or purulent cervicitis infection

       iii. Heavy menstrual bleeding and cramping after placement (improves with continued use)

D. Adverse Events: Adjusting Products *(Domain 1, Task 3)*

Patient Case

A 21-year-old woman has been taking contraceptive X for the past 8 months. She calls today because she has been experiencing breakthrough bleeding for 2 days, and then her menses begin 4–5 days later. She states it is bothersome to have so much bleeding in the past two cycles. Her medical history includes dysmenorrhea.

Product	Estrogen Activity	Progestin Activity	Androgenic Activity
X	++	++	++
A	++	+++	++
B	+++	++	++
C	+	++	++
D	++	+	++

2. Which contraceptive product is the best recommendation?

  A. A.

  B. B.

  C. C.

  D. X

Table 3. Signs/Symptoms of Hormone Excesses and Deficiencies

Estrogen Excess	Progestin Excess	Androgen Excess	Estrogen Deficiency	Progestin Deficiency
Nausea	Moodiness	Increased appetite	Irritability	Weight loss
Dizziness	Noncyclic weight gain	Noncyclic weight gain	Nervousness	Heavy menstrual
Edema	Fatigue	Increased libido	Vasomotor	bleeding
Bloating	Depression	Oily skin	symptoms	Late-cycle
Cyclic weight gain	Increased libido	Hirsutism	Early- to mid-cycle	breakthrough
Chloasma	Alopecia	Acne	breakthrough	bleeding/
Uterine cramps	Decreased menstrual	Pruritus	bleeding/spotting	spotting
Irritability	bleeding length		Decreased libido	Delayed onset
Depression	Insulin resistance		Headaches	of menstrual
Poor contact lens fit	Headaches between		Depression	bleeding
Headaches during	pill packs		Dry vaginal mucosa	
active pill regimen	Vaginal candidiasis		Atrophic vaginitis	
Hypertension	Hypertension		Dyspareunia	
Breast tenderness	Breast tenderness		Uterine prolapse	
Increased breast size	Leg vein dilation			
Thrombophlebitis	Decreased breast size			
Stroke				
Myocardial				
infarction				
Decreased lactation				

1. Identify whether an adverse event is related to hormone deficiency/excess; need to rule out that the adverse event is related to incorrect use or timing of administration (i.e., nausea with morning dose)
2. Select a product with more or less activity than the hormone abnormality thought to be causing the adverse event.
3. If you choose a replacement product with higher endometrial activity, you can switch products at any time in the pack. If the new product has less endometrial activity, wait until the next cycle before changing.
4. Use Dickey's Managing Contraceptive Pill Patients reference tables.

E.   Contraindications *(Domain 1; Tasks 3, 5)*

Table 4. Contraindications to Hormonal Contraceptives (U.S. Medical Eligibility Criteria and World Health Organization)

Contraindications to the Various Hormonal Contraceptives and Copper IUD				
Definitions 3 = A condition for which the theoretical or proven risks usually outweigh the advantages of using the method 4 = A condition that represents an unacceptable health risk if the contraceptive method is used				
	Estrogen-Progestin	Progestin Only	LNG-IUD	Copper IUD
Breast cancer -Disease free for greater than 5 years -Current breast cancer	3 4	3 4	3 4	
Cerebrovascular -Stroke	4	3		
Diabetes mellitus -Diagnosed >20 years ago -Diabetes with end-organ damage	3/4 3/4	3 3		
Gallbladder -Symptomatic gallstones without cholecystectomy -Hormone-related gallstones	3 3			
Heart disease -Ischemic heart disease -Complicated valvular heart disease -Several risk factors	4 4 3/4	3	3	
Hypertension -Well-controlled blood pressure -SBP 140–160 mm Hg or DBP 90–100 mm Hg -SBP > 160 mm Hg or DBP > 100 mm Hg -Hypertension + vascular disease	3 3 4 4	3 (DMPA) 3 (DMPA)		
Inflammatory bowel disease[a] -Moderate disease or increased risk of VTE	3			
Liver -Severe cirrhosis -Tumors (hepatocellular adenoma or malignant) -Acute or flare viral hepatitis	4 4 4	3 3	3 3 3	
Migraines -Without aura and >35 years of age -With aura (all ages)	3 4			
Rheumatoid arthritis -Receiving immunosuppressive therapy		DMPA 3[c,d]		

Table 4. Contraindications to Hormonal Contraceptives (U.S. Medical Eligibility Criteria and World Health Organization) *(continued)*

Contraindications to the Various Hormonal Contraceptives and Copper IUD				
Definitions 3 = A condition for which the theoretical or proven risks usually outweigh the advantages of using the method 4 = A condition that represents an unacceptable health risk if the contraceptive method is used				
	Estrogen-Progestin	Progestin Only	LNG-IUD	Copper IUD
Systemic lupus erythematosus -Positive antiphospholipid antibodies -Severe thrombocytopenia	4	3 3[c]	3[c]	
Thromboembolism -History of DVT/PE with ≥1 risk factor -History of DVT/PE without risk factor -DVT/PE during anticoagulation therapy -Known thrombogenic mutations	4 3 4 4			
Tobacco use <15 cigarettes/day and ≥35 years of age ≥15 cigarettes/day and ≥35 years of age	3 4			
Transplant -Complicated[e]	4		3[c]	3[c]
Genitourinary -Unexplained vaginal bleeding -Gestational trophoblastic disease +No hCG or decreasing hCG +hCG persistently elevated -Endometrial/cervical cancer awaiting treatment -Ovarian cancer -Uterine fibroids with torsion -Distorted uterine cavity		3 (DMPA)	4[c] 3 4 4[c] 3[c] 4 4	4[c] 3 4 4[c] 3[c] 4 4

[a]Increased risk of inflammatory bowel disease: Active or extensive disease, surgery, immobilization, corticosteroid use, vitamin deficiencies, fluid depletion.

[b]Risk factors include age 5 years or older, previous thromboembolism, thrombophilia, immobility, transfusion at delivery, BMI 30 kg/m² or greater, postpartum hemorrhage, post cesarean delivery, preeclampsia, or smoking.

[c]Initiation of product.

[d]Only if taking steroids long term or patient has other risk factors for bone fracture.

[e]Complicated transplant: Graft failure, rejection, cardiac allograft vasculopathy.

AIDS = acquired immunodeficiency syndrome; BMI = body mass index; DBP = diastolic blood pressure; DMPA = depot medroxyprogesterone acetate; DVT = deep venous thrombosis; hCG = human chorionic gonadotropin; IUD = intrauterine device; LNG-IUD = levonorgestrel IUD; PE = pulmonary embolism; SBP = systolic blood pressure; VTE = venous thromboembolism.

F. Drug Interactions *(Domain 1, Task 3)*

Table 5. Drug Interactions with Hormonal Contraceptives

Interacting Agent	Estrogen-Progestin Oral	Estrogen-Progestin Vaginal Ring	Estrogen-Progestin Patch	POP	SPRM	DMPA	Implantable Progestin	LNG-IUD
Anticonvulsants Barbiturates Phenytoin Carbamazepine Felbamate Lamotrigine[a] Oxcarbazepine Primidone Topiramate Vigabatrin	✓	✓	✓	✓	✓		✓	✓[a]
Anti-infectives (see note below) Rifampin[b]	✓	✓	✓	✓	✓		✓	✓
Nonnucleoside reverse transcriptase inhibitors Delavirdine Efavirenz Nevirapine	✓	✓	✓	Probable ✓[c]	Probable		✓	Probable
Protease inhibitors Amprenavir Atazanavir Indinavir Lopinavir Ritonavir	✓	✓	✓	Probable	Probable		✓	Probable
Herbal products St. John's wort	✓	✓	✓	✓	✓		✓	Probable
P-glycoprotein substrates					✓[d]			

[a]Lamotrigine concentrations are significantly reduced when used as monotherapy with estrogen-progestin contraceptives.

[b]Note: Antibiotics: The American Congress of Obstetricians and Gynecologists states that penicillin, ampicillin, doxycycline, fluconazole, miconazole, metronidazole, fluoroquinolones, and tetracycline do not interact with hormone concentrations. The American Medical Association and the Centers for Disease Control and Prevention Medical Eligibility Criteria for hormonal contraceptives state that rifampin is the only major interacting anti-infective but that patients should be notified of low potential interactions with other anti-infectives.

[c]Carten ML, Kiser JJ, Kwara A, et al. Pharmacokinetic interactions between the hormonal emergency contraception, levonorgestrel (Plan B), and efavirenz. Infect Dis Obstet Gynecol 2012;2012:137192. Study found that levonorgestrel EC AUC was decreased 56% after coadministration with efavirenz.

[d]SPRM is an inhibitor of P-glycoprotein, so object drugs may have increased concentrations.

AUC = area under the curve; DMPA = depot medroxyprogesterone acetate; EC = emergency contraception; LNG-IUD = levonorgestrel-releasing intrauterine device; POP = progestin-only pill; SPRM = selective progesterone receptor modulator.

G. Product Initiation *(Domain 1, Tasks 1, 2, 4; Domain 2, Tasks 2, 3)*
   1. Interview the patient.
      a. Preferences (e.g., personal, religious), plans for future pregnancy (if/when)
      b. History with previous products
      c. Purpose of product (e.g., contraceptive, sexually transmitted infection protection, cycle control, treatment of menstrual-related disorder)
      d. Importance of product reversibility
      e. Adherence, partner's (or partners') support for various methods
      f. Cost
      g. No need to perform any laboratory tests or examinations before initiation of products, except baseline blood pressure for estrogen-progestin products. Consider baseline weight and body mass index (BMI) to monitor changes.
   2. Review patient-specific factors to aid with initiation.
      a. Can use adverse event table to help with initiation. For example, if patient has heavy menses, choose a product with moderate to high progestin activity.
      b. Contraindications
      c. Drug interactions

H. Education *(Domain 2, Task 5)*
   1. Purpose
   2. Proper use
      a. Initiation if reasonably certain the patient is not pregnant (patient has to meet one criterion below [i–v]): Products can be initiated on the first day of menses, first Sunday after menses, or day prescribed (quick jump-start) (from Centers for Disease Control and Prevention [CDC] U.S. Practice Recommendations, 2013)
         i. 7 days or less from onset of menses, spontaneous abortion, or elective abortion
         ii. No intercourse since onset of latest menses
         iii. Has been correctly and consistently using current form of contraception
         iv. Is within 4 weeks postpartum
         v. Is currently breastfeeding at least 85% of time, is still experiencing amenorrhea, and is less than 6 months postpartum
      b. Can initiate if uncertain about pregnancy status: Benefits of initiating a contraceptive likely outweigh any potential risk, except with IUD. If a product is started (except IUD), consider checking a pregnancy test result in 2–4 weeks to confirm pregnancy status.
      c. Take at any time of the day, but bedtime administration may help with nausea. Patient to select administration time for ease/convenience to improve adherence
      d. Backup method of contraception with initiation (see below)
   3. Potential adverse drug reactions
      a. Common
         i. Breakthrough bleeding, spotting, nausea, breast tenderness, weight gain (cyclic vs. noncyclic), fluid retention, dizziness, sexual adverse drug events, mood changes
         ii. Symptoms may improve after three cycles, so generally wait until after three cycles before changing.
      b. Serious: Warrant emergency department visit
         i. A   Abdominal pain
         ii. C   Chest pain (severe), cough, shortness of breath
         iii. H Headache (severe), dizziness, weakness, or numbness
         iv. E   Eye problems (vision loss or blurring), speech problems
         v. S   Severe leg pain (calf or thigh)

4. Missed doses *(Domain 1, Task 3)*

Table 6. Instructions for Missed Estrogen-Progestin Contraceptive Tablets

Consecutive OCs Omitted	Time in Cycle	Instructions for the Patient
Most Monophasic and Multiphasic Products		
1 pill	Anytime	Take missed OC immediately and next OC at regular time
2 pills	First 2 weeks	Take 2 OCs daily for next 2 days; then resume taking OCs on regular schedule; use backup method for 7 days
2 pills ≥3 pills	Third week Anytime	-Sunday start—Take 1 OC daily until Sunday, dispose of current pack; then begin next OC pack without placebo pills; backup method required for 7 days -Other—Dispose of current OCs and begin new OC (no missed days); backup method required for 7 days
Natazia		
1 pill (<12 hours late)	Days 1–17	Take missed OC immediately and next OC at regular time
1 pill (>12 hours late)	Days 1–17	Take missed OC immediately and next OC at regular time; use backup method for 9 days
1 pill (>12 hours late)	Days 18–24	Throw out current pack; start day 1 of a new pack; use backup method for 9 days
1 pill (>12 hours late)	Days 25–28	Take missed OC immediately and next OC at regular time
2 pills	Days 1–17	Throw out missed pills; take next OC at regular time and use backup method for 9 days
2 pills	Days 17–25	Throw out current pack; start day 3 of a new pack; use backup method for 9 days
2 pills	Days 25–28	Throw out current pack; start day 1 of a new pack
Seasonale/Seasonique		
1 pill	Anytime	Take missed pill as soon as remembered; take next OC at regular time
2 pills	Anytime	Take 2 OCs daily for next 2 days; then resume taking OCs on regular schedule; use backup method for 7 days
≥3 pills	Anytime	Throw out missed pills; take next OC at the regular time and use backup method for 7 days

OC = oral contraceptive.

5. Use of backup methods
   a. Product initiation if initiating after cycle day 5 or unknown cycle day
      i. All products except for progestin-only pills: 7 days (for Natazia: 9 days)
      ii. Progestin-only pill initiation: 48 hours
   b. With drug interactions that decrease efficacy: During interacting drug and for 7 days afterward (Natazia is for a minimum of 9 days afterward)
   c. If severe diarrhea and/or vomiting
      i. Oral estrogen-progestin: 7 days
      ii. Progestin-only pills: 48 hours
   d. If progestin-only pill dose is more than 3 hours late, use backup method for 48 hours.
   e. With missed doses (as above)
6. Follow-up appointments
   a. Any time patient wants to discuss adverse events or alternative choices
   b. At routine visits: Review satisfaction, adverse events, concerns, and changes in health status. Review drug interactions and contraindications for changes in health status. Change as appropriate.

I. Suggestions for Improving Contraceptive Adherence *(Domain 1, Task 3; Domain 2, Tasks 3, 4)*
   1. Recommend long-acting reversible methods whenever appropriate. Individually adjust contraceptive choice; help each woman think through the choice according to her background and individual needs and concerns.
   2. Stress the importance of daily routine for pill-taking; importance of timeliness (decreased effectiveness if not timely).
   3. Discuss the transient nature of most adverse effects in new users, especially spotting and bleeding.
   4. Dispel myths and misinformation: Discuss the non-contraceptive health benefits of contraception.
   5. Demonstrate correct use of the specific contraceptive. Obtain and use demonstration devices when available. Manufacturers can provide demonstration devices (e.g., NuvaRing, IUDs, Ortho-Evra, Implanon).
   6. Provide easy-to-understand instructions in both oral and written forms on proper use and dealing with missed doses.
   7. Suggest backup contraceptive method (provide condoms).
   8. Provide a means for patient to get additional information about the chosen method and its use.
   9. Use follow-up contact to look for signs of nonadherence (e.g., calls about spotting should be a flag for inconsistent use and an opportunity to review instructions) (Am J Obstet Gynecol 1999;180:S276-9).

J. Permanent Contraception
   1. Essure: Microinsert is inserted bilaterally into the fallopian tubes, stimulating tissue growth to occlude the fallopian tube and permanently block oocyte transport.
   2. Surgery (tubal ligation, total abdominal hysterectomy with or without bilateral salpingo-oophorectomy)

K. Emergency Contraception *(Domain 1, Tasks 4, 6; Domain 2, Task 5)*
   1. Product dosing

Table 7. EC Options

Class	Drug	Dose	Initiate Within...	MOA	Notes
Progestin only	Levonorgestrel (Plan B) (Plan B One-Step)	0.75 mg q12h × 2 doses, 1.5 mg × 1 dose (regimens equally effective, single-dose regimen preferred)	72 h per FDA; studies support 120 h	<u>Before ovulation</u> + Prevent/delay ovulation <u>After ovulation</u> + Limited to no effects + May prevent implantation	-Plan B One-Step is OTC and has no age or storage restrictions -Plan B is OTC only if 17 years or older -May be less effective with increasing body weight/BMI
Selective progestin receptor modulator	Ulipristal (Ella)	30 mg × 1 dose	120 h	<u>If embryo implanted</u>, EC will not interrupt; this is not an abortifacient	Prescription only
Yuzpe	Estrogen-progestin (ethinyl estradiol plus levonorgestrel or norgestrel)	One dose q12h × 2 doses (number of tablets per dose varies depending on product used; see note)	72 h		Uses current OC if patient receives at least 100 mcg of ethinyl estradiol and 500 mcg of levonorgestrel
IUD	Copper IUD	IUD	120 h	Prevent implantation	Serves as regular contraceptive afterward

BMI = body mass index; EC = emergency contraception; FDA = U.S. Food and Drug Administration; h = hours; IUD = intrauterine device; MOA = mechanism of action; OC = oral contraceptive; OTC = over the counter; q = every.

Patient Case

A 17-year-old patient is crying in the waiting room, saying she needs help. The front desk asks you to talk to her. She states that a condom broke during intercourse 4 days ago and that she wants to use emergency contraception. She states that the pharmacy down the road refused to provide Plan B One-Step (levonorgestrel 1.5 mg) and told her she should not have sex until she is older. She has been unable to tolerate the vomiting with the Yuzpe method for emergency contraception in the past. Her medical history includes PID (treated and resolved 2 months ago) and several sexual partners.

3. Which is the best action to take?
   A. Refer her to another pharmacy to get over-the-counter (OTC) levonorgestrel 1.5 mg every 12 hours for two doses.
   B. Recommend that her physician insert an IUD.
   C. Have her physician prescribe ulipristal 30 mg for one dose.
   D. Refuse emergency contraception because it has been too long since she took it.

2. Contraindication: Pregnancy, but no harm to pregnancy or fetus if used while currently pregnant
3. Education
   a. Purpose
   b. Proper use
4. Potential adverse events (Yuzpe method > progestin only > selective progestin receptor modulator)
   a. Nausea (50% > 23% > 12%) for up to 2 days, bloating, menstrual cramps, headache
   b. Give an antiemetic (e.g., metoclopramide 10 mg, meclizine 50 mg, or other antiemetic) 1 hour before Yuzpe method or other methods if there is concern about nausea. Meclizine available OTC in 25-mg tablets
   c. IUD: Abdominal cramping, heavy bleeding, spotting, and breakthrough bleeding
5. Menstrual changes
   a. Start date and amount of blood loss during menses vary after progestin-only pill emergency contraception.
   b. If taken before ovulation, early onset of menses (3–7 days) is common.
   c. If taken post ovulation, normal to late onset of menses is common.
   d. Ulipristal extends cycle by a mean of 2.5 days.
   e. The ACOG recommends taking a pregnancy test if menses does not start within 21 days or if menses is more than 1 week late.
6. Restarting regular contraceptives
   a. Barrier method immediately
   b. Hormonal contraception the day after Yuzpe or levonorgestrel. Wait until the next cycle for ulipristal.

L. Nonhormonal Contraception Options (independent study) *(Domain 1; Tasks 3, 4, 6)*

Table 8. Comparison of Nonhormonal Contraceptives

Product	Failure Rate in Typical Use/ Perfect Use	Sexually Transmitted Infection Protection	Minimum Time Before Efficacy	Use for Single or Several Acts of Intercourse	Notes
Male latex condoms	14%/3%	Yes	Immediate	Single	Avoid oil-based lubricants
Male polyurethane condoms	14%/3%	Probable	Immediate	Single	Can use water- or oil-based lubricants
Male lamb cecum condoms	14%/3%	No	Immediate	Single	Can use water- or oil-based lubricants
Female polyurethane or nitrile (FC2 formulation) condoms	25%/5%	Yes	Immediate	Single	Can insert for maximum of 8 hours Do not use in combination with male condoms Use lubricant if squeaking occurs
Spermicidal foam/gel	26%/6%	No	Immediate	Single	Can use if condom breaks Check dosing for individual products Re-dose after 60 minutes
Spermicidal film	26%/6%	No	15 minutes	Single	Re-dose after 60 minutes
Spermicidal suppository	26%/6%	No	10–15 minutes	Single	Re-dose after 60 minutes

Table 8. Comparison of Nonhormonal Contraceptives *(continued)*

Product	Failure Rate in Typical Use/ Perfect Use	Sexually Transmitted Infection Protection	Minimum Time Before Efficacy	Use for Single or Several Acts of Intercourse	Notes
Contraceptive sponge	36%/26%	No	Immediate	Several	Do not use if structural abnormalities, history of toxic shock syndrome Leave in place for 6–8 hours after intercourse (max 24 hours)
IUD (copper)	0.8%/0.6%	No	Immediate	Several	Check for strings daily
Diaphragm	16%/6%	No	Immediate	Several	Use with spermicidal gel Reapply gel with each act Leave in place for 6 hours
Lactational amenorrhea	N/A	No	See notes	–	Need to have exclusive breastfeeding (no pumping) Can provide effects for 6 months but generally need backup method after 6 weeks postpartum
Calendar method	N/A	No	See notes	–	To calculate time that is unsafe for intercourse (fertile time): First fertile day: Average cycle length (days) – 18 Last fertile day: Average cycle length (days) – 11 Intercourse should be avoided during these days of the cycle
Basal body temperature	N/A	No	See notes	–	Check temperature daily before any movement An increase of 0.4°X–1°X notes ovulation; safe time is 3 days after this day to menses
Cervical mucus method	N/A	No	See notes	–	Check cervical mucus daily for amount and characteristics Unsafe from detection of cervical mucus until 3 days after peak mucus Peak mucus is clear, increased production and elasticity Postovulation mucus thickens and turns white

IUD = intrauterine device; max = maximum; N/A = not applicable.

II. MENSTRUAL DISORDERS (INDEPENDENT STUDY)

A. Amenorrhea *(Domain 1; Tasks 2–5)*
   1. Definitions
      a. Primary: Absence of menarche by 16 years of age with the presence of secondary development or absence of menarche by 14 years of age in the absence of secondary development
      b. Secondary: Absence of menses for 6 months or three cycles
   2. Treatment
      a. Always rule out pregnancy.
      b. Ensure intake of at least 1000 mg of elemental calcium and 400 IU of vitamin D.
      c. Correct underlying etiology.
         i. Primary: Estrogen-progestin contraceptives
         ii. Decrease exercise and encourage weight gain.
            (a) Estrogen-progestin contraceptives
            (b) Conjugated equine estrogens 0.625–1.25 mg/day on cycle days 1–25
            (c) Ethinyl estradiol patch 50 mcg/day
         iii. Hyperprolactinemia
            (a) Cabergoline 0.25 mg twice weekly; then titrated as needed: Has higher efficacy and improved tolerability compared with bromocriptine (N Engl J Med 1994;331:904-9)
            (b) Bromocriptine 2.5 mg three times daily
         iv. Polycystic ovary syndrome (see lecture for more details)
            (a) Clomiphene if attempting pregnancy (see infertility)
            (b) Metformin
            (c) Thiazolidinediones
            (d) Estrogen-progestin contraceptives
         v. Unknown secondary
            (a) Medroxyprogesterone acetate 5–10 mg every day on cycle days 14–25 (95% efficacy to induce menses)
            (b) Micronized progesterone 400 mg/day (90% efficacy to induce menses)
            (c) Estrogen-progestin contraceptives

B. Anovulatory Bleeding/Dysfunctional Uterine Bleeding *(Domain 1; Tasks 2, 4, 5)*
   1. Definition: Menstrual bleeding that occurs because of disorganized menstrual system from absences of ovulation
      a. Without ovulation, progesterone is not produced, and the endometrium continues to thicken without regulation. Eventually, the thickened endometrium irregularly sloughs off, causing irregular and sometimes heavy bleeding.
      b. Adolescent anovulatory bleeding is normal for up to 5 years because of an immature hypothalamus-pituitary-ovarian axis.
   2. Treatment
      a. Ensure intake of at least 1000 mg of elemental calcium and 400 IU of vitamin D.
      b. Estrogen-progestin contraceptives
      c. Progestin-only contraceptives, including the levonorgestrel IUDs
      d. Treat any underlying etiologies (PCOS, hyperprolactinemia).
      e. Dilation and curettage
      f. Intrauterine trichloroacetic acid

C. Dysmenorrhea *(Domain 1; Tasks 2, 4, 5)*
   1. Definition: Cramping and pain just before and/or during menses
      a. Primary: Normal pelvic anatomy
      b. Secondary: Pelvic abnormalities
   2. Treatment
      a. Nonpharmacologic
         i. Exercise
         ii. Topical heat
         iii. Low-fat vegetarian diet
      b. Nonsteroidal anti-inflammatory drugs (NSAIDs) started 1–2 days before menses
         i. Naproxen 550 mg twice daily for 1–2 days before menses; then 275 mg every 6–12 hours
         ii. Ibuprofen 800 mg three times daily
         iii. Diclofenac 50 mg three times daily
      c. Estrogen-progestin contraceptives
         i. Prefer levonorgestrel or norgestrel products
         ii. Prefer extended-interval dosing
      d. Medroxyprogesterone acetate (Depo-Provera)
      e. Levonorgestrel IUD

D. Menorrhagia *(Domain 1; Tasks 2, 4, 5)*
   1. Definition: Menstrual blood loss of at least 80 mL per cycle
   2. Treatment
      a. Contraception desired
         i. Levonorgestrel IUD
         ii. Estrogen-progestin contraceptive
         iii. Surgery
      b. Contraception not desired
         i. NSAIDs during menses. Effective compared with placebo but less effective than tranexamic acid and levonorgestrel IUD (Cochrane Database Syst Rev 2013;1:CD000400)
         ii. Progesterone for 21 days starting on cycle day 5
         iii. Tranexamic acid 1.3 g three times daily during menses (maximum 5 days). May increase risk of thrombosis
         iv. Ulipristal 10 mg daily for 3 months (for uterine fibroids)
         v. Surgery (endometrial ablation, hysterectomy)

E. Premenstrual Syndrome and Premenstrual Dysphoric Disorder *(Domain 1; Tasks 2, 4, 5)*
   1. Definition
      a. Premenstrual syndrome: Physical symptoms with mild mood disorder that resolves with the onset of menses. Please refer to ACOG Practice Bulletin No. 15: Premenstrual Syndrome, 2000 (www.acog.org/publications/pdfs/pb015.pdf).
      b. Premenstrual dysphoric disorder: Severe mood disorder that occurs during the luteal phase of the menstrual cycle and that interferes with work or social life. Please refer to the Diagnostic and Statistical Manual of Mental Disorders, 5th edition (DSM-V) for full criteria (American Psychiatric Association 2013).
   2. Treatments
      a. Nonpharmacologic
         i. Well-balanced diet that includes complex carbohydrates and that is low in fat and low in caffeine
         ii. Smoking cessation
         iii. Alcohol restriction

        iv. Exercise

        v. Adequate sleep

        vi. Stress reduction

        vii. Anger management

        viii. Support groups and counseling

    b. Nutritional supplements

        i. Vitamin B_6 up to 100 mg/day

        ii. Calcium elemental 600–1000 mg/day

    c. Antidepressants daily during at least the luteal phase

        i. Citalopram 10–30 mg

        ii. Escitalopram 10–20 mg

        iii. Fluoxetine 10–20 mg

        iv. Fluvoxamine 50 mg

        v. Paroxetine 10–30 mg

        vi. Sertraline 25–150 mg

        vii. Venlafaxine 50–200 mg/day

        viii. Clomipramine 25–75 mg/day

        ix. Buspirone 10 mg

    d. Estrogen-progestin contraceptives containing drospirenone: Consider continuous use or stacking packs for longer cycles.

    e. Leuprolide 3.75 mg intramuscularly every 3 months

  F. Resources *(Domain 5; Task 2)*

    1. American Congress of Obstetricians and Gynecologists

      a. Patient education

      b. Practice bulletins

    2. Association of Reproductive Healthcare Professionals

      a. Patient education

      b. Continuing education

Patient Case

A 42-year-old woman and her husband have tried to conceive but have been unsuccessful after 6 months. Her medical history includes amenorrhea. Current medications are a prenatal vitamin daily and clomiphene 25 mg/day on cycle days 5–9. She states she was instructed to check for ovulation.

4. Which is the best method for detecting ovulation?

    A. Cervical mucus monitoring.

    B. Basal body temperature.

    C. Urine luteinizing hormone (LH) kits.

    D. Ultrasonography.

5. The patient's condition does not respond to clomiphene, so treatment with follicle-stimulating hormone (FSH) and LH is initiated. With respect to monitoring for ovarian hyperstimulation, it would be best to educate the patient about which of the following symptoms?

    A. Constipation.

    B. Polyuria.

    C. Double vision.

    D. More than a 2.25-kg weight gain.

III. INFERTILITY

A. Evaluation *(Domain 1, Task 2)*
   1. Infertility is a challenge for the couple, not just the woman; abnormalities occur in 40%–50% of male partners.
   2. Evaluation begins after 12 months unless the woman
      a. Is 35 years or older
      b. Has a history of oligomenorrhea/amenorrhea
      c. Has known/suspected uterine/tubal disease
      d. Has endometriosis or PCOS
      e. Has a subfertile partner

B. Types of Infertility *(Domain 1, Task 1)*
   1. Tubal/peritoneal
      a. Endometriosis: Endometrial tissue outside uterus that increases risk of blockage and scar tissue
      b. Pelvic inflammatory disease
      c. Treatment: Surgical
   2. Ovulatory
      a. Hypothalamus-pituitary-ovary axis abnormalities
      b. Hyperprolactinemia (suppresses ovulation)
      c. Polycystic ovarian syndrome
      d. Treatment: Medications
   3. Pelvic/uterine
      a. Polyps
      b. Fibroids
      c. Congenital/structural abnormalities
      d. Diethylstilbestrol exposure
      e. Treatment: Surgical
   4. Immune: Immune system attacks sperm.
   5. Infectious: Chlamydia, ureaplasma, mycoplasma, gonorrhea
   6. Unknown: Treatment: Medications
   7. Male infertility
      a. Spermatogenesis: Medications and lifestyle modifications
      b. Transport
      c. Ejaculation abnormalities
      d. Structural abnormalities
      e. Hormonal abnormalities of hypothalamus-pituitary-testicular axis
      f. Immunologic
      g. Infection

C. Nonpharmacologic Treatment *(Domain 1, Task 5)*
   1. Avoid medications, products, and activities known to interfere with fertility (e.g., nicotine, alcohol, illicit drugs).
   2. Achieve a BMI of less than 27 kg/m^2, but avoid excessive dieting or overstrenuous exercise.
   3. Eat a well-balanced diet.
   4. Take a multivitamin with at least 0.4 mg of folic acid (preferably 1 mg).
   5. Avoid water-based lubricants. If a lubricant is needed, use hydroxyethylcellulose-based products.
   6. Have intercourse every 1–2 days in the 6 days before expected ovulation, as desired.

D. Medications Known to Decrease Fertility *(Domain 1; Tasks 2, 3)*

Table 9. Medications Known to Increase Prolactin Values

Chlorpromazine	Cimetidine	Estrogen	Haloperidol
Medroxyprogesterone acetate	Methyldopa	Phenothiazines	Pimozide
Reserpine	Tricyclic antidepressants	Verapamil	

Table 10. Medications and Substances Known to Decrease Sperm Activity

Allopurinol	Anabolic/ androgenic steroids	Caffeine	Calcium channel blockers	Chemotherapeutic agents
Colchicine	Nitrofurantoin	Spironolactone	Sulfasalazine	Tetracycline

E. Pharmacologic Treatment *(Domain 1; Tasks 4, 6, 7)*
  1. Risks associated with treatment
    a. Multiple gestation
    b. Ovarian hyperstimulation syndrome
      i. Risk with high-dose gonadotropins or gonadotropin-releasing hormone (GnRH) agents
      ii. Exact mechanism unknown
      iii. Symptoms begin 3–10 days after ovulation or human chorionic gonadotropin (hCG) injection.
        (a) Weight gain greater than 2.25 kg and increased abdominal girth
        (b) Abdominal or pelvic pain
        (c) Nausea, vomiting, diarrhea
        (d) Dyspnea, dizziness
        (e) Oliguria
      iv. Discontinue current cycle. Restart next cycle with lower doses and/or slower titration.
  2. Role of hormones
    a. FSH: Matures egg
    b. LH: Stimulates ovulation
    c. Human chorionic gonadotropin
      i. Structurally similar to LH
      ii. Mimics LH
    d. Progesterone: Induces menses
  3. Ovulation induction
    a. Clomiphene
    b. Metformin
    c. Aromatase inhibitors
    d. FSH/LH
    e. FSH plus hCG
    f. Pulsatile GnRH
  4. Suppress endogenous hormones; then use ovulation induction.
    a. Continuous GnRH
    b. GnRH antagonist, followed by ovulation induction (usually FSH plus hCG)
  5. Luteal support
    a. Progesterone
    b. Required with FSH/LH, FSH plus hCG, pulsatile gonadotropin

6. Hyperprolactinemia
   a. Bromocriptine
   b. Cabergoline
7. Assistive technologies
   a. Intrauterine insemination
   b. In vitro fertilization and embryo transfer
   c. Gamete intrafallopian transfer
   d. Zygote intrafallopian transfer

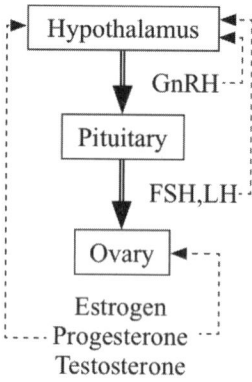

Figure 1. Hypothalamus-pituitary-ovary axis.

Table 11. Comparison of Medications for Infertility (independent study)

Step	Drug	Adverse Events	Miscellaneous
Ovulation induction level 1 (ovulatory dysfunction and unexplained infertility)	Clomiphene 80%–85% of patients will ovulate 40%–50% of patients will become pregnant in 6 months	Multiple gestation (5%–12.3%) Vaginal dryness, moodiness (10%) Thickened cervical mucus Visual disturbances (2%) + D/C if patient experiences: Weight gain Increased mittelschmerz Abdominal symptoms (discomfort, distention, bloating, abnormal uterine bleeding) (6%)	25–50 mg/day on cycle days 5–9; increase by 25 mg/day per cycle to maximum 250 mg/day until ovulation occurs Basal body temperature monitoring not recommended If no pregnancy within 6–12 months, consider alternative therapy Need normal LFT results and estrogen values before therapy initiation Use for >12 months increases risk of ovarian cancer
Ovulation induction level 1 (ovulatory dysfunction and unexplained infertility)	Letrozole, anastrazole 44%–90% of patients with PCOS will ovulate 9.7%–40% of patients with PCOS will become pregnant	Vasomotor symptoms, headache, breast tenderness (>10%)	Letrozole 5 mg/day on cycle days 3–7 Anastrazole 1 mg/day on cycle days 3–7 Higher efficacy than clomiphene in treatment-naive patients[a] Effective in clomiphene-resistant patients Limited data for safety in pregnancy after exposure, but potential for increased spontaneous abortions Generics available, so may have financial advantage over clomiphene

Table 11. Comparison of Medications for Infertility (independent study) *(continued)*

Step	Drug	Adverse Events	Miscellaneous
Ovulation induction level 1 (ovulatory dysfunction and unexplained infertility)	Metformin 90% ovulation in combination with clomiphene	Abdominal symptoms (nausea, diarrhea) Often continued through first trimester of pregnancy because it can decrease risk of spontaneous abortion	500 mg PO daily with meals titrated to 850–1000 mg PO bid with meals 2012 Cochrane database review found no increase in live births and limited role May have benefit in combination with clomiphene
Ovulation induction level 2 (ovulatory dysfunction, clomiphene failure, unexplained infertility, assistive technologies)	Gonadotropins (FSH + LH, FSH only) Success rate: 50% pregnancy after 12 cycles	Hyperstimulation Multiple gestation (11%–44%) Febrile reaction (10%–15%) Abdominal pain, nausea, vomiting, diarrhea (10%–12%) Injection site reaction Dry skin, rash, alopecia, hives	Dosage customized to patient Trials investigating low-dose FSH as first-line therapy: Higher ovulation, pregnancy, and live birth rates compared with clomiphene; cost may limit use Avoid if first degree of ovarian failure (FSH > 30 mIU/mL) Requires ultrasound monitoring for follicular development Requires luteal support Men: Decreased spermatogenesis from primary or secondary pituitary dysfunction
Ovulation induction level 2 (used in combination with FSH products)	hCG	Hyperstimulation (3%) Enlargement or rupture of preexisting ovarian cysts Headache Irritability Aggressive behavior Restlessness, fatigue Depression Edema (especially with long periods in patients with epilepsy, migraines, asthma, or cardiac or renal disease) Injection site reactions (10%–13%)	5000–10,000 international units OR 250 mcg (recombinant) 3–4 days after clomiphene or if follicle is 16–18 mm on ultrasonography Requires ultrasound monitoring Luteal support needed
Ovulation (failure of gonadotropin)	GnRH	Hyperstimulation Multiple gestation (8%–12%) Pump-related issues Injection site reactions	Pulsatile release by pump customized
Suppress female hypo-thalamus-pituitary-ovarian axis	GnRH agonist Nafarelin Leuprolide	Ovarian cysts (15%) Multiple gestation (8%) Bone loss Vaginal bleeding Pelvic pain Breast tenderness Estrogen deficiency	Given in long or short protocol Expense limits use Requires patient to use FSH/LH or FSH + hCG products; then progesterone support

Table 11. Comparison of Medications for Infertility (independent study) *(continued)*

Step	Drug	Adverse Events	Miscellaneous
Suppress female hypo-thalamus-pituitary-ovarian axis	GnRH antagonist Ganirelix Cetrorelix	Ovarian hyperstimulation (2.4%–3.5%) Nausea, abdominal pain (4.8%) Fetal death (3.7%) Headache (3%) Vaginal bleeding (1.8%) Injection site reactions	Patient-specific dosage Discontinue when hCG is given Axis returns to baseline 1–2 months after discontinuation Requires patient to use FSH/LH or FSH + hCG products; then progesterone support
Luteal support and/or induce menses	Progesterone	Visual disturbances D/C product Insomnia or somnolence Depression Dermatologic (rash, acne, melasma) Injection site reactions Changes in weight Breakthrough bleeding Galactorrhea Cervical mucus Fluid retention	Luteal support for 10–12 weeks Induce menses for 10–14 days Products: Progesterone 50–100 mg IM daily Vaginal suppositories bid–tid Crinone gel qday-bid Micronized progesterone 200-mg capsules inserted vaginally bid–tid
Hyperpro-lactinemia	Bromocriptine Cabergoline	Nausea, vomiting, constipation (49%) Headache (19%) Dizziness (17%) Orthostatic hypotension (6%)	Bromocriptine 1.25 mg qHS × 1 week and titrate Cabergoline 0.25 mg twice weekly and titrate Slow titration to decrease adverse events Administer qHS with food Barrier contraception often used until normal ovulation pattern established

[a]Franik S, Kremer JAM, Nelen WLDM, et al. Aromatase inhibitors for subfertile women with polycystic ovary syndrome. Cochrane Database Syst Rev 2014;2:CD010287.

bid = twice daily; D/C = discontinue; FSH = follicle-stimulating hormone; GnRH = gonadotropin-releasing hormone; hCG = human chorionic gonadotropin; HS = bedtime; IM = intramuscularly; LFT = liver function test; LH = luteinizing hormone; PCOS = polycystic ovary syndrome; PO = by mouth; q = every; tid = three times daily.

    F.   Role of the Pharmacist in Infertility Treatments: Education *(Domain 1, Task 5; Domain 2, Tasks 1, 5; Domain 5, Task 2)*

        1.   Proper use of ovulation detection

            a.   Cervical mucus monitoring

            b.   Basal body temperature monitoring

                i.   Oral monitoring

                ii.   Vaginal monitoring (OvuSense device approved 2013)

            c.   Urine LH kits

            d.   Ultrasound monitoring

                * Considerations when selecting methods: Accuracy, cost, ease of use, interactions with conditions and medications

        2.   Medications: Purpose, proper use, and potential adverse events and risks

3. When to notify physician
   a. Abnormal increase in circumference
   b. Nausea
   c. Pelvic pain
   d. Decreased urine output
   e. Weight gain greater than 2.25 kg
   f. Dizziness
   g. Shortness of breath
4. Support groups (RESOLVE: The National Infertility Association) and counseling

IV. ENDOMETRIOSIS (INDEPENDENT STUDY)

A. Definition: Endometrial Tissue Found Outside the Uterus; associated with pain, scarring, and infertility

B. Treatment *(Domain 1; Tasks 5, 6)*
   1. Asymptomatic patients: No treatment and monitor for pain
   2. Symptomatic
      a. Nonsteroidal anti-inflammatory drugs
         i. Role: Decrease pain
         ii. Agents
            (a) Ibuprofen 400 mg every 4–6 hours
            (b) Naproxen 250 mg every 4–6 hours
         iii. Cost: Low
      b. Estrogen-progestin contraceptives
         i. Role: Decrease pain, menstrual flow, decrease endometrial implants. Can use contraceptives continuously to suppress menses
         ii. Cost: Low
      c. Progestins
         i. Role: Decrease pain, menstrual flow, and atrophy of endometrial implants
         ii. Agents
            (a) Depot medroxyprogesterone acetate 150 mg intramuscularly or 104 mg subcutaneously every 12 weeks
            (b) Levonorgestrel 20 mcg/day IUD
         iii. Cost: Low
      d. Gonadotropin-releasing hormone agonist
         i. Role: Decrease pain, suppress menses, and induce atrophy of endometrial implants
         ii. Agents
            (a) Leuprolide 11.25 mg intramuscularly every 3 months
            (b) Goserelin 3.6 mg subcutaneously every month
            (c) Nafarelin 200 mcg one spray intranasally twice daily
         iii. Adverse events: Estrogen deficiency effects such as vasomotor symptoms, vaginal dryness, bone loss
         iv. Cost: High

    e. Danazol 600–800 mg/day in divided doses

        i. Role: Decrease pain and induce endometrial atrophy

        ii. Adverse events

            (a) Androgenic effects such as acne, weight gain, increase in low-density lipoprotein cholesterol

            (b) Estrogen deficiency effects such as vasomotor symptoms, breast reduction, vaginal dryness, bone loss

        iii. Cost: Moderate

    f. Surgery

3. Efficacy

    a. Similar efficacy between 28-day cycles and extended-interval dosing with estrogen-progestin contraceptives

    b. Similar efficacy between estrogen-progestin contraceptives, progestin contraceptives, GnRH agonists, and danazol for pain

4. Other: Ensure adequate calcium and vitamin D intake to help maintain bone health.

C. Resources *(Domain 5, Task 2)*

1. Endometriosis.org (www.endometriosis.org/)

    a. Patient information

    b. Listing for support groups

    c. Clinical trial information

2. Endometriosis Association (www.endometriosisassn.org/)

    a. Patient information

    b. Listing for support groups

    c. Clinical trial information

V. PREGNANCY AND LACTATION *(Domain 1, Task 4)*

A. Diagnosis of Pregnancy (independent study) *(Domain 1, Task 5)*

1. Confirmed by the presence of hCG in the serum or urine

2. Human chorionic gonadotropin

    a. Concentration doubles every 2–3 days and peaks at 8–12 weeks.

    b. Composed of α and β subunits

    c. The α subunit has cross-reactivity with LH, thyroid-stimulating hormone, and FSH and may produce false-positive results.

    d. The β subunit is specific to hCG; used in newer pregnancy tests

3. Home pregnancy tests

    a. Ninety-seven percent accurate but 25% false negative

    b. Ectopic pregnancies

    c. According to U.S. Food and Drug Administration (FDA) minimum sensitivity requirements, devices may take up to 11 days after conception to detect pregnancy.

B. Patient Interactions *(Domain 2; Tasks 2–5)*

1. Establish trust.

    a. Do not impose your values on the patient with drug and disease treatment during pregnancy.

    b. Actively listen to the patient.

    c. Teratogenicity (72% idiopathic, 25% genetic, and 3% medications)

    d. May seek treatment with other medications, herbal products, or illicit drugs

    e. May never take prescribed therapy because patient believes all medications are harmful

2. Evaluating medication risk
   a. Medications
      i. When deciding about medications, evaluate risks with specific percentage, prevalence, etc.
      ii. Risk of the same abnormality in the general population with specific percentage, prevalence, etc.
      iii. Stage of development compared with patient's current gestational age
      iv. Dosage-related risks
   b. Untreated disease
      i. Risks of abnormal pregnancy outcomes
      ii. Risks of malformations
   c. Decide on risks versus benefit.

3. Educate.
   a. Purpose
   b. Proper use
   c. Potential adverse events
      i. Maternal
      ii. Fetal
   d. Potential risks of untreated conditions
   e. Incorporate specific information when possible.
      i. Timing (risk time for adverse event and current gestational week)
      ii. Present risk in understandable terms (percentage, prevalence).

C. Principles of Medication Use in Pregnancy *(Domain 1, Tasks 3, 4; Domain 3, Task 3)*
  1. Factors influencing teratogenicity
   a. Stage at the time of exposure
   b. Maternal and fetal genotypes
   c. Dose and duration of exposure
   d. Specificity of the agent
   e. Other simultaneous exposures (other drugs or environmental agents)
  2. Possible complications of medication exposure
   a. No effect
   b. Premature or delayed labor
   c. Spontaneous abortion
   d. Malformations—Major or minor
   e. Altered fetal growth
   f. Functional deficit
   g. Carcinogenesis
   h. Mutagenesis
  3. Mechanisms of substance transfer
   a. Simple diffusion (most drugs)
      i. Molecular weight (low [defined as less than 600 Da] > high)
      ii. Lipid solubility (lipophilic > hydrophilic)
      iii. Ionization (nonionized > ionized)
      iv. Protein binding (free > low > high)
      v. Maternal and fetal blood flow (high > low)
      vi. Placental diffusion distance (thin > thick)
      vii. Placental villi exchange area (large > small)
      viii. Efflux proteins (no activity > high activity)
   b. Facilitated diffusion (glucose)

c. Active transport (some vitamins, amino acids)

d. Pinocytosis (immune antibodies)

e. Breaks between cells (erythrocytes)

4. Physiologic changes affecting medication use in pregnancy

Table 12. Effects of Physiologic Changes During Pregnancy on Medications

	Physiologic Change	Pharmacokinetic Effects	Potential Therapeutic Effects
Metabolic	↑ Hepatic metabolism ↓ Hepatic metabolism	↑ Drug metabolism ↓ Metabolism	↓ Drug concentrations ↑ Drug concentrations
Placental	Thinning of fetal-maternal barrier	↑ Distribution	↑ Fetal concentrations ↓ Maternal concentrations
Renal	↑ Renal blood flow	↑↑ GFR and drug elimination	↓ Maternal concentrations
Volume	↑ Blood volume ↓ Albumin and α1-glycoprotein ↑ Body fat	↑ Distribution ↓ Protein binding ↑ Distribution of lipophilic medications	↓ Concentration ↑ Free drug ↓ Concentration of lipophilic medications
Gastro-intestinal	↓ Motility and intestinal blood flow	↑ Drug absorption	↑ Concentration

GFR = glomerular filtration rate.

5. FDA pregnancy categories for medication use in pregnancy

a. Old system has many faults and should not be the only piece of information used to determine safety.

b. New system approved by FDA and effective for all products approved after June 30, 2015

Table 13. New and Old FDA Pregnancy Categories

OLD System (before June 30, 2015)		NEW System (after June 30, 2015)	
Category	Description	Category	Description

A	- Adequate, well-controlled studies of pregnant women have not shown an increased risk of fetal abnormalities	Pregnancy	- Required to provide registry and contact information if available
			- Risk summary
			- Clinical considerations
			  + Disease-associated maternal and/or embryo/fetal risk
			  + Dose adjustments during pregnancy and the postpartum period
			  + Maternal adverse reactions
			  + Fetal/neonatal adverse reactions
			  + Labor or delivery
			- Human and animal data

B	- Animal = no risk; human = no controlled studies - Animal = risk; human = controlled studies have no risk		

C	- Animal = risk; human = no controlled studies
	- Studies of women or animals are unavailable
		Lactation	- Risk summary
			- Clinical considerations
			  + Minimizing exposure
			  + Monitoring adverse effects

D	- Known risk; benefit of medicine greater than risk	Female and male individuals with fertility potential	- Pregnancy testing - Contraception Infertility
X	- Known risk; risk greater than benefit		

FDA = U.S. Food and Drug Administration.

D. Acute Conditions *(Domain 1, Tasks 3–7; Domain 2, Task 5)*
   1. Nausea and vomiting
      a. Nonpharmacologic
         i. Light snack 15–20 minutes before getting out of bed
         ii. Small, dry, more frequent meals
         iii. Prevent stomach from completely emptying.
         iv. Avoid spicy or fatty foods and strong odors.
         v. High protein and/or high carbohydrate
         vi. Ginger
      b. Vitamin B_6 (category A) with or without doxylamine (category A). Now available in a combination tablet
      c. Metoclopramide (category B)
      d. Promethazine or prochlorperazine (category C)
      e. Ondansetron (category B)
   2. Gastroesophageal reflux disease
      a. Nonpharmacologic
         i. Smaller, more frequent meals
         ii. Avoid caffeine.
         iii. Avoid foods and liquids (other than water) for at least 3 hours before bedtime.
         iv. Elevate head of bed.
         v. Avoid foods and beverages that can trigger symptoms (e.g., tomato products, chocolate, spicy foods, peppermint, acidic items such as orange juice).
      b. Antacids (category B)
      c. Histamine-2 antagonists (category B)
      d. Metoclopramide (category B)
      e. Proton pump inhibitors (category B; except for omeprazole, category C)
      f. Avoid: Sodium bicarbonate
   3. Constipation
      a. Nonpharmacologic
         i. Add bulky, high-fiber foods to diet.
         ii. Increase fluid intake.
         iii. Moderate exercise
         iv. Sitz baths for hemorrhoids
      b. Fiber bulk-forming laxatives (category C)
      c. Polyethylene glycol (category C)
      d. Docusate sodium (category C)
      e. Senna (category C)
      f. Bisacodyl (category C)
      g. Lactulose (category C)
      h. Avoid: Castor oil and mineral oil
   4. Diarrhea
      a. Nonpharmacologic
         i. Maintain hydration.
         ii Correct electrolyte abnormalities.
      b. Fiber bulk-forming agents
      c. Loperamide (category B)
      d. Avoid: Diphenoxylate plus atropine, paregoric

5. Pain
   a. Acetaminophen (category B)
   b. Acetaminophen plus narcotics (category C/D)
   c. Avoid: NSAIDs, aspirin, NSAIDs plus narcotics
6. Headaches
   a. Acetaminophen (category B)
   b. Acetaminophen plus caffeine plus butalbital (category C)
   c. Acetaminophen plus narcotics (category C/D)
   d. Avoid: NSAIDs (especially in third trimester), aspirin, NSAIDs plus narcotics, aspirin plus caffeine plus butalbital, ergotamine
7. Smoking cessation
   a. Nonpharmacologic (see smoking cessation lecture)
   b. Nicotine replacement therapy (category D)
   c. Bupropion (category C)
8. Preterm labor/delivery (before 37 weeks' gestation)
   a. Prophylaxis if patient has a history of preterm labor/delivery
      i. Progesterone from 16 weeks' to 36 weeks' gestation
         (a) 17-Hydroxyprogesterone acetate 250 mcg intramuscularly every week
         (b) Vaginal progesterone suppository 100 mg every day
         (c) Micronized oral capsule 200 mg intravaginally every day
      ii. Surgical procedure (cerclage)
      iii. Inflatable pessary
      iv. Modified bed rest
      v. Hydration
   b. Abortive treatment
      i. Calcium channel blockers (nifedipine immediate release 10–20 mg every 4–6 hours)
      ii. NSAIDs (indomethacin 50 mg × 1; then 25 mg every 6 hours). Not recommended after 31–32 weeks
      iii. β-Adrenergic receptor agonists (terbutaline 0.25 mg subcutaneously). Not recommended for use longer than 48 hours (boxed warning)
      iv. Magnesium sulfate (inpatient before 32 weeks for neuroprotection)
   c. Preterm premature rupture of membranes
      i. Ampicillin 2 g × 1; then 1 g every 6 hours
      ii. Azithromycin 500 mg × 1; then 250 mg every day
   d. Prevention of hyaline membrane disease
      i. Betamethasone 12 mg intramuscularly every 24 hours × 2 doses
      ii. Dexamethasone 6 mg intramuscularly every 12 hours × 4 doses
      iii. No other steroids cross the placenta for effects.

E. Chronic Conditions *(Domain 1, Tasks 2–7; Domain 2, Task 5)*
   1. Balance risks of uncontrolled disease versus medication risk.
   2. Hypertension

Table 14. Hypertension in Pregnancy

Type	Definition (2 BP readings at least 6 hours apart)	Complications	Severe Complications
Gestational or pregnancy induced	>140/90 mm Hg After 20 weeks	-Low risk (if not severe BP) -↑ Cesarean delivery rate	-Maternal and fetal death -Target organ damage -Pulmonary edema, cyanosis -Placental abruption -Hemorrhage
Chronic	>140/90 mm Hg Preexisting or onset <20 weeks' gestation	IUGR, low birth weight, premature birth, target organ damage	
Preeclampsia	>140/90 mm Hg plus one of the following: At least 300 mg of proteinuria in 24 hours -Platelets < 100,000/mm3 -LFTs 2 x ULN -New development of renal dysfunction (SCr > 1.1 mg/dL or doubling of previous SCr value) -Pulmonary edema -Cerebral or visual disturbances After 20 weeks	Headache, visual disturbance, oliguria, upper quadrant pain, LFT, HELLP syndrome	
Eclampsia	Preeclampsia + seizures		

BP = blood pressure; HELLP syndrome = hemolysis, elevated liver enzymes, low platelets; IUGR = intrauterine growth restriction; LFT = liver function test; ULN = upper limit of normal; SCr = serum creatinine.

a. Prevention of preeclampsia
    i. Aspirin 81 mg every day starting at week 12 (U.S. Preventive Services Task Force [USPSTF] 2014 and ACOG 2013)
    ii. Calcium 500 mg twice daily for patients with low calcium intake
b. Initiate therapy.
    i. Goal blood pressure of less than 140/90 mm Hg
    ii. In general, initiate treatment when greater than 150/100 mm Hg unless there is preexisting vascular disease or diabetes.
c. Treatment
    i. Methyldopa: Most studied but limited use because not potent and high potential for adverse events (somnolence, depression)
    ii. Dihydropyridine calcium channel blockers (nifedipine preferred)
    iii. Some β-blockers (avoid atenolol because of risk of intrauterine growth restriction)
    iv. Hydralazine
    v. Nondihydropyridine calcium channel blockers
    vi. Avoid: Angiotensin-converting enzyme inhibitor, angiotensin receptor blocker, minoxidil, aliskiren

3. Diabetes

Table 15. Risks of Uncontrolled Diabetes During Pregnancy

	Any MCM	**Cardiac**	**Neural Tube Defects**	**Macrosomia**	**Other**
Pregnancy rate	1%–3%	0.8%	0.2%	10%	-Central nervous system abnormalities -Stillbirth -Respiratory distress -Intrauterine growth restriction -Polyhydramnios -Progression of retinopathy
Risk time	—	0–12 weeks	0–5 weeks	Second/third trimester	
Uncontrolled DM	18.4%	8.5%	1%	12%–35%	

DM = diabetes mellitus; MCM = major congenital malformation.

a. Definitions: Gestational diabetes
    i.   Routine screening at 24–28 weeks using the two-step method (ACOG) or the one-step method (American Diabetes Association [ADA])
    ii. Screening during first trimester if a history of gestational diabetes or obesity
    iii. One-step method (ADA 2012)
        (a) 75-g glucose tolerance test after 8-hour fast
        (b) Diagnosed if one reading is as follows: Fasting blood glucose (BG) 92 mg/dL or greater; BG 180 mg/dL or greater at 1 hour, 153 mg/dL or greater at 2 hours
    iv. Two-step method (ACOG recommends not following ADA one-step method)
        (a) Glucose challenge (50 g) abnormal if BG 130 mg/dL or greater at 1 hour
        (b) Then, glucose tolerance test (100 g). Diagnosed if any two readings are as follows: Fasting BG 95 mg/dL or greater; BG 180 mg/dL or greater at 1 hour, 155 mg/dL or greater at 2 hours, 140 mg/dL or greater at 3 hours
b. Treatment
    i.   Neutral protamine Hagedorn or detemir plus aspart/lispro/regular insulin (increased requirement with increased gestational age)
    ii. Limited data in pregnancy for glargine
    iii. Glyburide can be considered an alternative to insulin. Not associated with malformations and not detected in cord blood samples likely because of high placental efflux protein activity
    iv. Metformin can be considered an alternative to insulin. Not associated with malformations and when continued in the first trimester can decrease the risk for spontaneous abortions. Not very potent during pregnancy

Patient Case

6. A patient is 18 weeks pregnant and here for her prenatal visit. You discover that she has not been taking lamotrigine because of a fear of birth defects. Her last seizure was 6 months ago. Which represents the best way to educate the patient on the risk of birth defects?

    A. Risk is low because she is past the stage when cleft palate/lip develops.
    B. Risk is low because intrauterine growth restriction is similar to uncontrolled epilepsy.
    C. Risk is high because lamotrigine is associated with the development of cardiac abnormalities during second trimester.
    D. Risk is high because neurodevelopmental delays are associated with exposure to lamotrigine during the second and third trimesters.

4. Epilepsy
    a. Risks of uncontrolled epilepsy
        i. Maternal: Preterm labor, anemia, hypertension, urinary tract infections, nausea/vomiting, vaginal bleeding
        ii. Fetal: Placental abruption or detachment, premature membrane rupture, significant fetal heart rate decelerations, decreased IQ with five seizures during gestation
    b. If recurrent epilepsy while taking medications
        i. Ninety percent chance of having a normal child
        ii. Monotherapy is preferred.

Table 16. Preventive Recommendations for Patients Taking Seizure Medications During Pregnancy

Preconception care	If >2 years since last seizure, consider trial off for 6 months If <2 years, continue therapy
Decrease risk of complications	Folic acid 4 mg/day recommended (0.4 mg required) Vitamin K after delivery Adequate calcium and vitamin D intake
Therapy	Continue therapy; monotherapy preferred Avoid phenobarbital, phenytoin, and valproic acid in women of childbearing age, if possible

Table 17. Risks Associated with Epilepsy Medications During Pregnancy[a]

	Major Malformations	Neural Tube Defects	Cleft Palate/ Lip	Cardiac	Neuro-developmental Delays	Anti-convulsant Syndrome[b]	Other
General pregnancy risk	1%–3%	0.2%	0.14%	0.5%–0.8%		0%	
Risk time	—	0–5 weeks	0–9 weeks	0–12 weeks	Second to third trimester	Any	
Phenytoin (D)	3.67%–4.7%	0	1.2%	1.2%	No	11%	
Phenobarbital, primidone (D)	6.5%			1.1%	No	6.5%	
Carbamazepine, oxcarbazepine (D)	2.2%–4.5%	0.2%–1%	0.4%	0.7%–0.9%	No	4%	
Valproic acid (D)	6.2%–17.1%	1%–2%	1.5%	0.7%–0.9%	Yes	>4%	IUGR, hernia, hypospadia
Gabapentin, pregabalin (C)	3.2%					Possible	↓ Birth weight, preterm delivery
Topiramate (D)	7.1%		0.23%				Hirsutism, third fontanelle, hypospadia
Lamotrigine (C)	2.8%–3.2%		0.2%		No		↓ Concentrations
Levetiracetam (C)	2%						↓ Birth weight, ↓ Concentrations
Felbamate (C)	Unknown	Only 10 reported exposures in literature					
Zonisamide (C)	Unknown	Only 28 reported exposures in literature	↓ Concen-trations				
Tiagabine (C)	Unknown	Only 23 reported exposures in literature					
Ethosuccimide (C)	Unknown	Only 18 reported exposures in literature					
Lacosamide (C)	Unknown	No reports					

[a]Pregnancy category in italics.

[b]Fetal anticonvulsant syndrome: Craniofacial abnormalities (drug-specific), growth restriction, limb defects, cardiac lesions, hernias, and distal digital and nail hypoplasia.

IUGR = intrauterine growth restriction.

5. Thyroid disorders
    a. Hyperthyroidism

Table 18. Hyperthyroidism in Pregnancy

	Medication Risk	**Maternal Risk**	**Fetal Risk**
Untreated hyperthyroidism (0.2%)	–	Heart failure, preeclampsia, preterm delivery	Stillbirth, imperforate anus, anencephaly, cleft lip, ↑ thyroidism, craniosynostosis, hydrops, advanced bone age
Propylthiouracil Preferred first trimester	D	Usual ADRs (see thyroid lecture)	Fetal hypothyroidism, goiter
Methimazole Preferred second and third trimesters	D		Aplasia cutis, fetal hypothyroidism, goiter Rare: Esophageal atresia, transesophageal fistula

ADRs = adverse drug reactions.

b. Hypothyroidism

Table 19. Hypothyroidism in Pregnancy

	Medication Risk	**Maternal Risk**	**Fetal Risk**
Untreated hypothyroidism	–	Hypertension, preeclampsia, preterm delivery, placental abruption	-Spontaneous abortion -Heart failure -Low birth weight -Cretinism -Low IQ
Levothyroxine	A	Safe and effective Usually requires 30% higher dosage	

6. Asthma

Table 20. Risks of Asthma in Pregnancy

	Maternal Risks	**Fetal Risks**
Uncontrolled asthma	-Antepartum/postpartum hemorrhage -Cesarean delivery -Hypertension -Premature labor -Premature rupture of membranes	-Intrauterine growth restriction -Low birth weight -Fetal hypoxia -Perinatal death

Table 21. Safety of Asthma Medications in Pregnancy

Medication	Category	Risks	Notes
Albuterol	B	Minimal	2% of dose absorbed systemically

Beclomethasone
Budesonide
Flunisolide
Fluticasone
Mometasone
Triamcinolone
	C
	B
	C
	C
	C
	C
		Minimal	2%–20% of dose absorbed systemically
			Budesonide preferred for new starts;
			  do not need to change products if
			  previously well controlled with an
			  alternative ICS

Salmeterol Formoterol	C C	Minimal	No to low dose absorbed systemically Do not use as monotherapy
Montelukast Zafirlukast Zileuton	B B C	Minimal data Minimal data Low birth weight, skeletal	Montelukast has more data than others
Cromolyn	C	Minimal	1%–4% of dose absorbed systemically
Theophylline	C	Tachycardia, hypertension	Therapeutic serum concentration: 5–12 µg/mL
Prednisone	C	Oral clefts (0–9 weeks) Diabetes mellitus	Preferred steroid

ICS = inhaled corticosteroid.

7. Coagulation disorders

Table 22. Treatment of Coagulation Disorders in Pregnancy

Place in Therapy	Medication	Category	Risks	Notes
First line -Preferred ≥36 weeks	Heparin	C	None to PG/fetus	-Readily reversed with protamine

First line
-Preferred <36 weeks
	LMWH	B		-Less risk of heparin-induced
				  thrombocytopenia, bone loss
				-Daily bid dosing
				-Antifactor-Xa monitoring
				  4 hours post dose for at least
				  therapeutic dosing
				Expensive

Avoid
Alternative for second/
third trimester
	Warfarin	X	Warfarin syndrome
			Ophthalmic
			  abnormalities,
			  mental retardation	

Alternatives	Lepirudin Bivalirudin Others	C	Limited data	Use if patient unable to use heparin/LMWH

bid = twice daily; daily = every day; LMWH = low-molecular-weight heparin; PG = pregnancy.

F. Pregnancy Termination *(Domain 1; Tasks 5, 6)*
    1. Ectopic pregnancy: Methotrexate
    2. Intrauterine
        a. Misoprostol
        b. Mifepristone

G. Lactation *(Domain 1, Task 4; Domain 2, Task 3; Domain 3, Task 3; Domain 5, Task 2)*
    1. Rule of thumb: Hale TW. Lactational pharmacology. In: Walker M, ed. Core Curriculum for Lactation Consultant Practice. Sudbury, MA: Jones & Bartlett, 2002:356-91.
        a. In general, less than 1% of the maternal dose will reach the infant.
        b. The American Academy of Pediatrics considers most medications safe for use in lactation, except for radioactive compounds; however, still check LactMed or other reference for safety (Pediatrics 2013;132:e796-809).
        c. Watch for exceptions to the rule.
    2. Things to consider when determining medication use in lactation
        a. Evaluate mother's need to use the medication.
            i. Can treatment be delayed?
            ii. Is the treatment effective for the condition?
        b. Safety to the infant
            i. Relative infant dose is calculated by dividing the infant dose in the milk (mg/kg/day) by the maternal dose (mg/kg/day).
            ii. If the relevant infant dose is less than 10%, it is generally safe.
            iii. Infant age
                (a) Medications cross easiest in the first 0–14 days postpartum.
                (b) Ability to metabolize medications: Adverse events tend to be higher when the infant is younger than 2 months or if the infant has certain medical conditions.
                (c) Oral absorption rate
        c. Effects on milk production
    3. Medication management during breastfeeding
        a. Acute, short-term drug therapy: If drug is contraindicated during lactation, keep pumping breast milk and discard until drug therapy is complete.
        b. Chronic medical condition treated with drug therapy
            i. Has the infant been exposed throughout pregnancy? If so, less likely to have problems during lactation
            ii. Is breastfeeding safe with this chronic condition?
            iii. Evaluate risks versus benefits.
    4. Minimizing effects of drug therapy on breastfeeding
        a. Minimize sustained-release preparations or drugs with long half-life values.
        b. Schedule doses immediately after feeding or before a long sleep period. Difficult to do with newborns because they eat about every 2 hours
        c. If there are several similar, equally effective medications from which to choose, choose the agent with the lowest concentration in breast milk and the least effect on the infant.
        d. Always consider—Can the medication be given to neonates?

Table 23. Potential Effects of Drugs on Lactation

Drugs That ↑ Milk Production	Drugs That ↓ Milk Production	Medications to Avoid During Lactation
Amoxapine	Androgens	Bromocriptine
Antipsychotics	Bromocriptine	Cyclosporine
Cimetidine	Estrogens	Cyclophosphamide
Methyldopa	Ergot alkaloids	Doxorubicin
Metoclopramide	Levodopa	Ergotamine
Reserpine	Monoamine oxidase inhibitors	Lithium
	Nicotine	Methotrexate
	Pyridoxine	Nicotine
	Sympathomimetics	Retinoids
	Dopaminergics	Iodine
	Diuretics	Illicit drugs
	Alcohol	
	Anticholinergics	
	Pseudoephedrine	

5. Relactation
   a. Nonpharmacologic therapy
      i. Education with lactation specialist to review technique for proper latching, positioning, length of feeding
      ii. Adequate nutrition/fluid intake and rest overall. Try eating or drinking enjoyable foods during lactation.
      iii. Increased nipple stimulation by nursing or pumping (pump after nursing)
      iv. Relaxation techniques, including deep breathing, gentle massage, listening to favorite music, and decreased stress
      v. Massage and warm the breast during feeding.
      vi. Increase feeding/pumping time, decrease intervals between feeding/pumping. Look at a photograph of the baby or the baby's items while pumping.
   b. Medications
      i. Minimal efficacy and safety data
      ii. If nonpharmacologic methods fail, consider metoclopramide 10 mg three times daily before eating for 7–14 days.
      iii. Anecdotal evidence: Fenugreek 580–610 mg two or three capsules three or four times daily
6. Mastitis
   a. Infection of the milk ducts
   b. Symptoms: Pain, tenderness, redness, warmness of the breast, fever, and flulike symptoms
   c. Etiology: Clogged milk ducts, cracked nipples or other breaks in the skin, breast engorgement
   d. Nonpharmacologic
      i. Keep breastfeeding, and start each feeding on the infected breast.
      ii. Use a warm compress.
      iii. Wear a bra.
   e. Treatment: Cephalosporins (cephalexin) or penicillinase-resistant penicillins (dicloxacillin, cloxacillin, oxacillin) for 10–14 days

H. Resources *(Domain 5, Task 2)*
1. Drugs in Pregnancy and Lactation (Briggs 2014)
2. Medications and Mothers' Milk (Hale 2008)
3. Committee on Drugs of the American Academy of Pediatrics. Transfer of drugs and other chemicals into human milk. Pediatrics 2001;108:776-89.
4. LactMed (http://toxnet.nlm.nih.gov/cgi-bin/sis/htmlgen?LACT)
5. Organization of Teratology Information Specialists (www.otispregnancy.org)
   a. Patient information handouts
   b. Local teratology information services
   c. Toll-free patient counselors available
   d. Members have access to e-mail list.
   e. Provider information
6. Motherisk (www.motherisk.org/women/index.jsp)
   a. Patient information
   b. Toll-free patient access lines (general and disease state–specific)
   c. Clinical trials
   d. Patient discussion forums
7. Textbooks
   a. Creasy and Resnik's Maternal-Fetal Medicine
   b. Women's Health Across the Lifespan
   c. Diseases, Complications, and Drug Therapy in Obstetrics
   d. Core Curriculum for Lactation Consultant Practice

Patient Cases

7. A 44-year-old woman is experiencing vasomotor symptoms that disrupt her ability to complete work activities and get a good night's sleep. Her medical history is significant for hyperlipidemia and total abdominal hysterectomy with bilateral salpingo-oophorectomy (2 months ago). Laboratory values include total cholesterol 198 mg/dL, triglycerides 225 mg/dL, and high-density lipoprotein cholesterol 44 mg/dL. Which product is most appropriate for this patient?

   A. Estinyl tablet (ethinyl estradiol) 0.02 mg/day.
   B. Vivelle patch (17□-estradiol) 0.025 mg/day twice weekly.
   C. Prempro tablet (conjugated equine estrogens plus medroxyprogesterone) 0.45 mg/1.5 mg/day.
   D. Estratest tablet (esterified estrogens plus testosterone) 0.625 mg/1.25 mg/day.

8. A 66-year-old woman is experiencing vaginal dryness and painful intercourse. She states her symptoms are bothersome but not horrible. She would like therapy to help relieve the symptoms. Her medical history includes hyperlipidemia, hypertension, low bone mass, and coronary artery disease (myocardial infarction 3 years ago). Her allergies include adhesives (reaction is rash). Which is the best recommendation?
   A. Estrogel (17β-estradiol gel) 0.75 mg daily.
   B. Venlafaxine XR (extended release) 37.5 mg daily.
   C. Ospemifene 60 mg daily.
   D. Lubricating gel three times daily.

VI. MENOPAUSAL SYMPTOMS

A. Estrogen and Estrogen plus Progestin *(Domain 1; Tasks 4, 6)*
   1. Indications
      a. Moderate to severe symptoms associated with menopause
      b. Moderate to severe vulvar and vaginal atrophy associated with menopause
      c. Prevention of postmenopausal osteoporosis
   2. Benefits
      a. Vasomotor symptoms: Systemic estrogens are the most effective treatment to decrease frequency and severity, but they can require 2–6 weeks to achieve effects.
      b. Genitourinary symptoms: Estrogens administered by any route is the most effective treatment.
         i. Genitourinary atrophy
         ii. Vaginal dryness
         iii. Dyspareunia
         iv. Increased risk of urinary tract infections. Only local estrogen has shown decreased risk in a randomized controlled trial.
      c. Osteoporosis prevention
      d. Quality of life
      e. Mood stability
      f. Fatigue
      g. Insomnia
   3. Risks
      a. Cardiovascular risk
         i. Estrogen-progestin primary prevention: No overall increase in cardiovascular events or death, but hazard ratio (HR) 1.29 (95% confidence interval [CI], 1.02–1.63) with absolute risk of 7 per 10,000 person-years (Women's Health Initiative [WHI] trial; JAMA 2002;288:321-33)
         ii. Estrogen-progestin secondary prevention: Increased risk of myocardial infarction during first year of use (HR 1.52 [95% CI, 1.01–2.29]), but no overall difference for 6.8 years. HR 0.99 (95% CI, 0.80–1.22) (Heart and Estrogen/Progestin Replacement Study [HERS], JAMA 1998;280:605-13; HERS II, JAMA 2002;288:49-57)
         iii. Estrogen primary prevention: No overall increase in cardiovascular events or death (HR 0.91 [95% CI, 0.75–1.12]) (WHI-ET; JAMA 2004;291:1701-12)
         iv. Factors to consider when evaluating cardiovascular risk: Timing (age and years since onset of menopause)
      b. Cerebrovascular risk
         i. Estrogen-progestin: Increased risk with HR 1.41 (95% CI, 1.07–1.85) with absolute risk of 8 per 10,000 person-years (WHI; JAMA 2002;288:321-33)
         ii. Estrogen: Significant increased risk with HR 1.39 (95% CI, 1.10–1.77). Absolute risk of 12 per 10,000 person-years (WHI-ET; JAMA 2004;291:1701-12)
      c. Thromboembolism
         i. Estrogen increases vitamin K–dependent clotting factors.
         ii. Increased risk adjusted HR 2.11 (95% CI, 1.26–3.55) absolute risk of pulmonary embolism of 8 per 10,000 person-years (WHI; JAMA 2002;288:321-33)
         iii. Overall, increases risk of deep venous thrombosis by 2–3.5, but the absolute risk is relatively small (20 per 100,000 cases)
      d. Breast cancer
         i. Estrogen-progestin: 15% higher rate for the first 5 years (nonsignificant) and 54% higher rate for greater than 5 years of use (WHI; JAMA 2002;288:321-33, Lancet 1997;350:1046-59)
         ii. Estrogen: Risk of breast cancer increases after 10–15 years of use.

e. Endometrial cancer
    i. Estrogen stimulates endometrial cell mitosis and hyperproliferation.
    ii. Increased risk after 1 year of unopposed estrogen in patients who still have a uterus
    iii. Using progestins (medroxyprogesterone acetate 5–10 mg/day or equivalent) 10–14 days/month prevents hyperproliferation.
f. Gallbladder dysfunction
g. Cognitive decline: Increased risk in patients receiving estrogen-progestin for dementia in women older than 65 years. HR 2.05 (95% CI, 1.21–3.48). Absolute risk of 12 per 10,000 person-years (Women's Health Initiative Memory Study [WHIMS]; JAMA 2003;289:2651-62)
h. Ovarian cancer: Meta-analysis, case-control, and cohort trials show both estrogen and estrogen-progestin therapy increase the risk of ovarian cancer. However, only one randomized controlled trial evaluated the risk and did not show increased risk.

4. Routes of administration
a. Oral
    i. Advantages: Greater increase in effect on hepatic lipoproteins, ease of administration
    ii. Disadvantages: Liver effects greater (thromboembolism, lipoprotein changes)
b. Transdermal/topical
    i. Advantages: Decreased or no liver effects, useful in patients with gastrointestinal absorption problems, stable concentrations of estrogen
    ii. Disadvantages: Skin irritation, less significant effects on lipids, still need to give progestins for women with an intact uterus, sunscreen applied near administration time can affect estrogen absorption
c. Vaginal
    i. Advantages: Useful for symptoms of vaginal atrophy
    ii. Disadvantages: Erratic absorption, long-term use may increase risk of endometrial hyperplasia (especially with ring with systemic effects), no bone density benefit

5. Regimens
a. Choice 1: Continuous estrogen and cyclic progestin
    i. Estrogen is given every day at a set dose.
    ii. Progestin is added for 10–14 days/month.
    iii. Advantages: No return of menopausal symptoms because estrogen is given each day
    iv. Disadvantages: Bleeding each month (usually begins 1–2 days after last progestin dose)
b. Choice 2: Continuous estrogen and progestin
    i. Thought to create an atrophic endometrium and induce amenorrhea
    ii. Advantages: 75% of women have amenorrhea at 1 year.
    iii. Disadvantages: Unpredictable spotting or breakthrough bleeding when beginning therapy
c. Choice 3: Continuous long-cycle estrogen-progestin (rare)
    i. Estrogen is given every day at a set dose.
    ii. Progestin is added six times per year (every other month) for at least 12 days.
    iii. Advantages: Known times for menstrual bleeding and less often than continuous estrogen-cyclic progestin regimens
    iv. Disadvantages: Still causes withdrawal bleeding that is heavier than continuous estrogen-cyclic progestin. Effects on long-term endometrial protection unknown
d. Choice 4: Intermittent combined estrogen-progestin
    i. Estrogen only for 3 days; then estrogen plus progestin for 3 days in rotating pattern
    ii. Advantages: Less progestin exposure and decreased risk of menstrual bleeding
    iii. Disadvantages: Effects on long-term endometrial protection unknown

e. Choice 5: Continuous estrogen and bazedoxifene
  i. Bazedoxifene is an estrogen agonist/antagonist that provides endometrial protection.
  ii. Advantages: Relieves moderate to severe vasomotor symptoms and prevents osteoporosis
  iii. Disadvantages: Limited data
f. Unopposed estrogen: ONLY for women WITHOUT a uterus

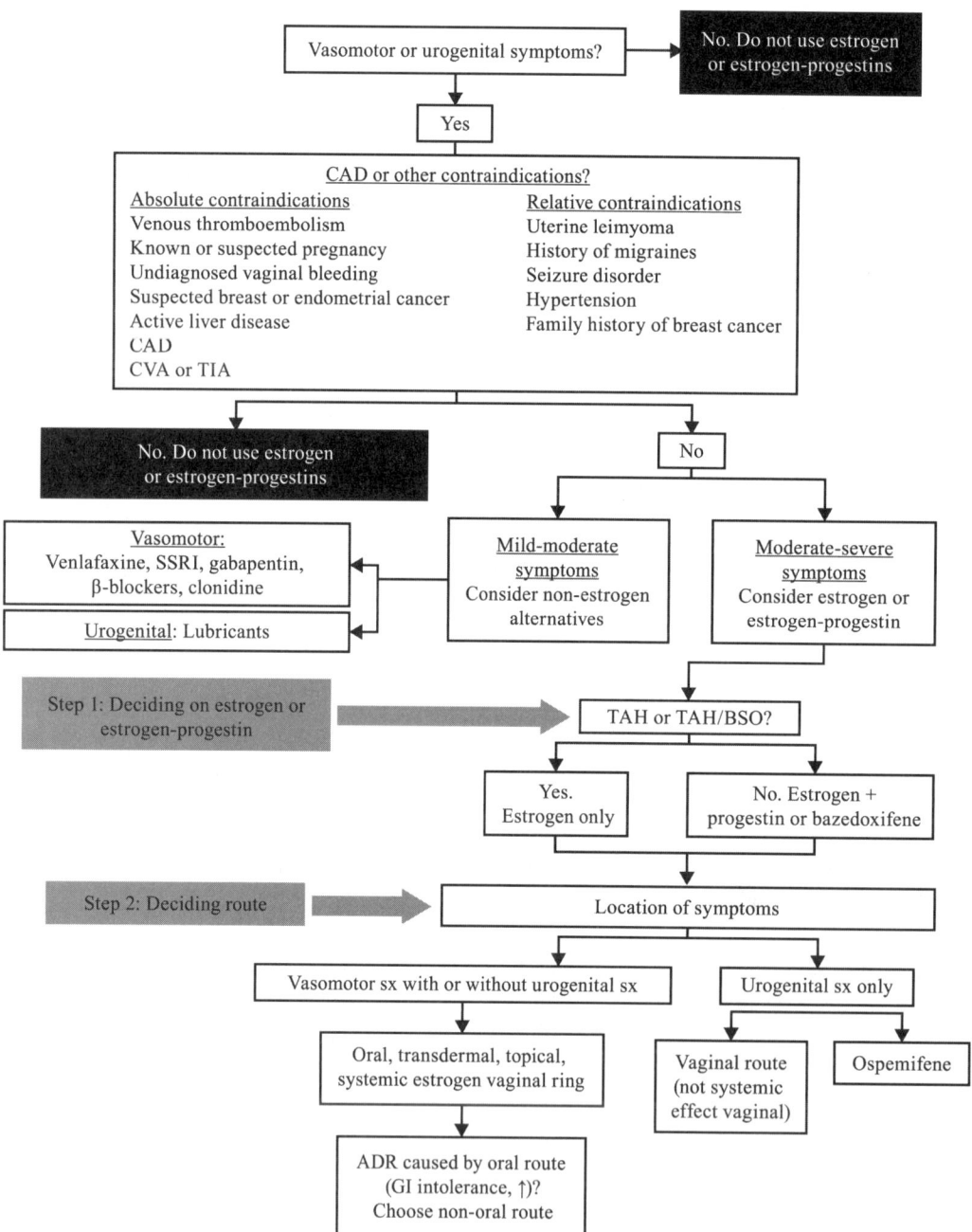

Figure 2. Determining who should be prescribed HT/ET.

ADR = adverse drug reaction; CAD = coronary artery disease; CVA = cerebrovascular accident; ET = estrogen therapy; GI = gastrointestinal; HT = hormone therapy; SSRI = selective serotonin receptor antagonist; sx = symptoms; TAH = total abdominal hysterectomy; TAH/BSO = total abdominal hysterectomy and bilateral salpingo-oophorectomy; TG = triglycerides; TIA = transient ischemic attack.

Table 24. Estrogen and Estrogen-Progestin Combination Products Available

Composition	Product	Doses
Oral Estrogen		
Conjugated equine estrogens	Premarin	0.3, 0.45, 0.625, 0.9, 1.25 mg
Synthetic conjugated estrogens A (contains nine estrogens)	Cenestin	0.3, 0.45, 0.625, 0.9, 1.25 mg
Synthetic conjugated estrogens B (contains 10 estrogens)	Enjuvia	0.3, 0.45, 0.625, 0.9, 1.25 mg
Esterified	Menest	0.3, 0.625, 1.25, 2.5 mg
17β-Estradiol	Estrace Various generics	0.5, 1, 2 mg 0.5, 1, 2 mg
Estropipate	Ortho-Est Ogen Various generics	0.75, 1.5 mg 0.75, 1.5, 3, 6 mg 0.625, 1.25 mg
Ethinyl estradiol	Estinyl	0.02, 0.05 mg
Estradiol acetate	Femtrace	0.45, 0.9, 1.8 mg
Oral Combination Products		
Conjugated equine estrogens and medroxyprogesterone	Prempro	0.3/1.5, 0.45/1.5, 0.625/2.5, 0.625/5 mg
Conjugated equine estrogens and medroxyprogesterone	Premphase	0.625/0 mg for 14 d; then 0.625/5 mg for 14 d
Estradiol and drospirenone	Angeliq	1/0.5 mg
Ethinyl estradiol and norethindrone acetate	Femhrt	2.5 mcg/0.5 mg, 5 mcg/1 mg
Estradiol and norethindrone acetate	Activella	0.5/0.1 mg, 1/0.5 mg
Estradiol and norgestimate	Prefest	1/0 mg for 15 d; then 1/0.09 mg for 15 d
Oral Estrogen + Estrogen Agonist/Antagonist		
Conjugated equine estrogens + bazedoxifene	Duavee	0.45/20 mg
Oral Estrogen and Testosterone Combination Products		
Esterified estrogens and methyltestosterone	Estratest, Covaryx, EEMT Estratest HS, Covaryx HS < EEMT HS	1.25/2.5 mg 0.625/1.25 mg
Testosterone Products in Varying Routes of Administration		
Mixed testosterone esters (IM)		50, 100 mg IM q4–6 weeks
Testosterone pellets (SC)		50 mg SC q6 months
Nandrolone decanoate (IM)		50 mg IM q8–12 weeks
Transdermal testosterone system		150, 300 mcg/d topically q3–4d
Transdermal Estrogen		

Table 24. Estrogen and Estrogen-Progestin Combination Products Available *(continued)*

Composition	Product	Doses
Testosterone Products in Varying Routes of Administration		
17β Matrix patch	Alora (two times/week)	0.025, 0.05, 0.075, 0.1 mg
	Climara (once weekly)	0.025, 0.05, 0.075, 0.1 mg
	Esclim (two times/week)	0.025, 0.0375, 0.05, 0.075, 0.1 mg
	Vivelle (two times/week)	0.05 mg
	Vivelle Dot (two times/week)	0.025, 0.0375, 0.05, 0.075, 0.1 mg
	Various generics (two times/ week)	0.05, 0.1 mg
	Menostar (once weekly)	0.014 mg
17β Reservoir	Estraderm (two times/week)	0.025, 0.05, 0.1 mg
17β Gel	Estrogel (daily)	0.75 mg
	Elestrin (daily)	0.52 mg
	Divigel (daily)	0.25, 0.5, 1 mg
17β Topical emulsion	Estrasorb (two packets daily)	0.05 mg
17β Transdermal spray	Evamist (initial 1 spray daily, may increase to 2 or 3 sprays/d)	0.021 mg/spray
Transdermal Combination		
Estradiol and levonorgestrel	Climara Pro	0.045/0.015 mg/d
Estradiol and norethindrone acetate	CombiPatch	0.05/0.14 mg and 0.05/0.25 mg/d
Vaginal		
17β Cream	Estrace cream	2–4 g/d for 2–4 weeks, 1 g/d for 1–3 weeks
Conjugated equine estrogens cream	Premarin cream	0.5–2 g/d for 3 weeks; then off 1 week
Estrone cream	Neo-Estrone cream	1 mg/g
17β Ring	Estring	7.5 mcg/d for 90 d
Estradiol ring	Femring	5, 10 mcg/d for 90 d
Estradiol tablet	Vagifem	10 mcg, one tablet vaginally daily for 2 weeks then one tablet vaginally twice weekly

d = day(s); IM = intramuscularly; q = every; SC = subcutaneously.

Table 25. Progestin Availability and Minimal Doses for Endometrial Protection

Generic	Brand Name	Minimal Dose for Continuous Estrogen and Progestin, mg	Minimal Dose for Continuous Estrogen and Cyclic Progestin, mg	Available, mg
Oral				
Medroxyprogesterone	Provera	2.5	5	2.5, 5, 10
Norethindrone	Micronor, Nor-QD	0.35	0.35	0.35
Norethindrone acetate	Aygestin	5	5	5
Micronized progestin	Prometrium	100	200	100, 200
Vaginal/Intrauterine				
Levonorgestrel	Mirena IUD	0.20 mcg	N/A	20 mcg/day
Progesterone gel	Crinone	45 mg	45 mg	(4%) 45 mg

IUD = intrauterine device; N/A = not applicable.

B. Nonhormonal Options for Vasomotor Symptoms *(Domain 1; Tasks 5, 6)*
  1. Antidepressants
     a. Venlafaxine 75 mg/day: Efficacy in patients with breast cancer
     b. Paroxetine 7.5–30 mg/day
     c. Sertraline 25–50 mg/day
     d. Fluoxetine 20 mg/day
  2. Antihypertensives
     a. Clonidine 0.1 mg every day or twice daily
     b. β-Blockers
  3. Other
     a. Gabapentin 300 mg three times daily
     b. Megestrol
  4. Herbal products
     a. Soy (isoflavones)
     b. Black cohosh: Studies have not shown efficacy in patients with breast cancer.

C. Nonhormonal Options for Vulvovaginal Symptoms *(Domain 1; Tasks 5, 6)*
  1. Lubricating gels
  2. Ospemifene 60 mg daily

D. Resources: North American Menopause Society (www.menopause.org/) *(Domain 5, Task 2)*
  1. Patient information
  2. Position statements
  3. Certified menopause provider

VII. GENERAL RESOURCES FOR WOMEN'S HEALTH

    A. Patient Resources *(Domain 5, Task 2)*
1. American Congress of Obstetricians and Gynecologists (www.acog.org): Patient information
2. FDA Office of Women's Health: Patient information
3. Medline Plus: Patient information
4. National Women's Health Network: Patient information
5. Massachusetts General Hospital Center for Women's Health
   a. Patient information
   b. Clinical trial information
6. Association of Reproductive Healthcare Professionals: Patient education

    B. Provider Resources *(Domain 5, Task 2)*
1. American Congress of Obstetricians and Gynecologists (www.acog.org): Practice bulletins
2. FDA Office of Women's Health
   a. Approval information
   b. MedWatch updates
3. Association of Reproductive Healthcare Professionals

REFERENCES

Contraception

1. ACOG Committee on Practice Bulletins—Gynecology. ACOG practice bulletin No. 73: use of hormonal contraception in women with coexisting medical conditions. Obstet Gynecol 2006;107:1453-72.

2. American Congress of Obstetricians and Gynecologists. ACOG practice bulletin No. 112: emergency contraception. Obstet Gynecol 2010;115:1100-9.

3. Archer JSM, Archer DF. Oral contraceptive efficacy and antibiotic interaction: a myth debunked. J Am Acad Dermatol 2002;46:917-23.

4. Blumenthal PD, Edelman A. Hormonal contraception. Obstet Gynecol 2008;112:670-84.

5. Centers for Disease Control and Prevention (CDC). Update to CDC's U.S. medical eligibility criteria for contraceptive use, 2010: revised recommendations for the use of contraceptive methods during the postpartum period. MMWR 2011;60:878-83.

6. Centers for Disease Control and Prevention (CDC). U.S. medical eligibility criteria for contraceptive use, 2010. MMWR 2010;59(RR-4):1-4.

7. Centers for Disease Control and Prevention (CDC). U.S. selected practice recommendations for contraceptive use, 2013. MMWR 2013;62:1-64.

8. Dickey RA. Managing Contraceptive Pill Patients, 14th ed. New Orleans: Emis Medical Publishers, 2010.

9. Dickinson BD, Altman RD, Nielson NH. Drug interactions between oral contraceptives and antibiotics. Obstet Gynecol 2001;98:853-60.

10. Hatcher RA, Trussell J, Stewart F, et al. Contraceptive Technology, 19th ed. New York: Ardent Media, 2007.

11. Leung VWY, Levine M, Soon JA. Mechanisms of action of hormonal emergency contraceptives. Pharmacotherapy 2010;30:158-68.

12. Rosenberg M, Waugh MS. Causes and consequences of oral contraceptive noncompliance. Am J Obstet Gynecol 1999;180:S276-9.

13. Selbert C, Barbouche E, Fagan J, et al. Prescribing oral contraceptives for women older than 35 years of age. Ann Intern Med 2003;138:54-64.

14. World Health Organization. Reproductive Health and Research. Medical Eligibility Criteria for Contraceptive Use, 4th ed. Geneva: Reproductive Health and Research, World Health Organization, 2009.

Postmenopausal Therapy

1. Grady D, Herrington D, Bittner V, et al. Cardiovascular disease outcomes during 6.8 years of hormone therapy: Heart and Estrogen/Progestin Replacement Study follow-up (HERS II). JAMA 2002;288:49-57.

2. Hulley S, Grady D, Bush T, et al. Randomized trial of estrogen plus progestin for secondary prevention of coronary heart disease in postmenopausal women: Heart and Estrogen/Progestin Replacement Study (HERS) research group. JAMA 1998;280:605-13.

3. North American Menopause Society. Estrogen and progestogen use in postmenopausal women: 2010 position statement from the North American Menopause Society. Menopause 2010;17:242-55.

4. Rapp SR, Espeland MA, Shumaker SA. Effect of estrogen plus progestin on global cognitive function in postmenopausal women: the Women's Health Initiative Memory Study: a randomized controlled trial. JAMA 2003;289:2663-72.

5. Schierbeck LL, Rejnmark L, Tofteng CL, et al. Effect of hormone replacement therapy on cardiovascular events in recently postmenopausal women: randomized trial. BMJ 2012;345:e6409.

6. Shumaker SA, Legault C, Rapp SR. Estrogen plus progestin and the incidence of dementia and mild cognitive impairment in postmenopausal women: the Women's Health Initiative Memory Study: a randomized controlled trial. JAMA 2003;289:2651-62.

7. Vickers MR, MacLennan AH, Lawton B, et al. Main morbidities recorded in the Women's International Study of Long Duration Oestrogen After Menopause (WISDOM): a randomised controlled trial of hormone replacement therapy in postmenopausal women. BMJ 2007;335:239.

8. Women's Health Initiative Steering Committee. Effects of conjugated equine estrogen in postmenopausal women with hysterectomy: the Women's Health Initiative randomized controlled trial. JAMA 2004;291:1701-12.

9. Writing Group for the PEPI Trial. Effects of estrogen or estrogen/progestin regimens on heart disease risk factors in postmenopausal women: the Postmenopausal Estrogen/Progestin Interventions (PEPI) Trial. JAMA 1995;273:199-208.

10. Writing Group for the Women's Health Initiative Investigators. Risks and benefits of estrogen plus progestin in healthy postmenopausal women: principal results from the Women's Health Initiative randomized controlled trial. JAMA 2002;288:321-33.

Menstrual Disorders

1. Abdellah MS, Elsaman AM. Trichloroacetic acid for the treatment of dysfunctional uterine bleeding: a pilot prospective clinical trial. Eur J Obstet Gynecol Reprod Biol 2012;165:280-3.

2. ACOG Committee on Practice Bulletins—Gynecology. ACOG practice bulletin: management of anovulatory bleeding. Int J Gynecol Obstet 2001;72:263-71.

3. ACOG Practice Bulletin No. 15: Premenstrual Syndrome. 2000. Available at www.acog.org/publications/pdfs/pb015.pdf. Accessed November 27, 2011.

4. Battino S, Ben-Ami M, Geslevich Y, et al. Factors associated with withdrawal bleeding after administration of oral dydrogesterone or medroxyprogesterone acetate in women with secondary amenorrhea. Gynecol Obstet Invest 1996;42:113-6.

5. Bhatia SC, Bhatia SK. Diagnosis and treatment of premenstrual dysphoric disorder. Am Fam Physician 2002;66:1239-48, 1253-4.

6. Cohen LS, Soares CN, Lyster A, et al. Efficacy and tolerability of premenstrual use of venlafaxine (flexible dose) in the treatment of premenstrual dysphoric disorder. J Clin Psychopharmacol 2004;24:540-3.

7. European Multicentre Study Group for Cabergoline in Lactation Inhibition. Single dose cabergoline versus bromocriptine for inhibition of puerperal lactation: randomized, double-blind, multicenter study. BMJ 1991;302:1367-71.

8. Freeman EW, Kroll R, Rapkin A, et al. Evaluation of a unique oral contraceptive in the treatment of premenstrual dysphoric disorder. J Womens Health Gend Based Med 2001;10:561-9.

9. Freeman EW, Rickels K, Sondheimer SJ, et al. Differential response to antidepressants in women with premenstrual syndrome/premenstrual dysphoric disorder: a randomized controlled trial. Arch Gen Psychiatry 1999;56:932-9.

10. Freeman EW, Rickels K, Yonkers KA, et al. Venlafaxine in the treatment of premenstrual dysphoric disorder. Obstet Gynecol 2001;98:737-44.

11. Freeman EW, Sondheimer SJ, Sammel MD, et al. A preliminary study of luteal phase versus symptom-onset dosing with escitalopram for premenstrual dysphoric disorder. J Clin Psychiatry 2005;66:769-73.

12. French L. Dysmenorrhea. Am Fam Physician 2005;71:285-91.

13. Grady-Weliky TA. Premenstrual dysphoric disorder. N Engl J Med 2003;348:433-8.

14. Halbreich U, Bergeron R, Yonkers KA, et al. Efficacy of intermittent, luteal phase sertraline treatment of premenstrual dysphoric disorder. Obstet Gynecol 2002;100:1219-29.

15. Kletzky OA, Davajan V, Nakamura RM, et al. Clinical categorization of patients with secondary amenorrhea using progesterone-induced uterine bleeding and measurement of serum gonadotropin levels. Am J Obstet Gynecol 1975;121:695-703.

16. Kornstein SG, Pearlstein TB, Fayyad R, et al. Low-dose sertraline in the treatment of moderate-to-severe premenstrual syndrome: efficacy of 3 dosing strategies. J Clin Psychiatry 2006;67:124-32.

17. Matteson KA, Rahn DD, Wheeler TL II, et al. Nonsurgical management of heavy menstrual bleeding: a systematic review. Obstet Gynecol 2013;121:632-43.

18. Roy SN, Bhattacharya S. Benefits and risks of pharmacological agents used for the treatment of menorrhagia. Drug Saf 2004;27:75-90.

19. Shangold MM, Tomai TP, Cook JD, et al. Factors associated with withdrawal bleeding after administration of oral micronized progesterone in women with secondary amenorrhea. Fertil Steril 1991;56:1040-7.

20. Simon JA. Progestogens in the treatment of secondary amenorrhea. J Reprod Med 1999;44(2 suppl):185-90.

21. Steiner M, Hirschberg AL, Begeron R, et al. Luteal phase dosing with paroxetine controlled release (CR) in the treatment of premenstrual dysphoric disorder. Am J Obstet Gynecol 2005;193:352-60.

22. Stevinson C, Ernst E. Complementary/alternative therapies for premenstrual syndrome: a systematic review of randomized clinical trials. Am J Obstet Gynecol 2001;185:227-35.

23. Umland EM, Klootwyk J. Umland E.M., Klootwyk J Umland, Elena M., and Jacqueline Klootwyk.Chapter 63. Menstruation-related disorders. In: DiPiro JT, Talbert RL, Yee GC, et al., DiPiro J.T., Talbert R.L., Yee G.C., Matzke G.R., Wells B.G., Posey L Eds. Joseph T. DiPiro, et al.eds. Pharmacotherapy: A Pathophysiologic Approach, 9th ed. New York: McGraw-Hill, 2014:XXX-XXX. Available at http://accesspharmacy.mhmedical.com/content.aspx?bookid=689&Sectionid=45310516. Accessed January 18, 2016.

24. Warren MP, Biller BM, Shangold MM. A new clinical option for hormone replacement therapy in women with secondary amenorrhea: effects of cyclic administration of progesterone from the sustained-release vaginal gel Crinone (4% and 8%) on endometrial morphologic features and withdrawal bleeding. Am J Obstet Gynecol 1999;180(1 pt 1):42-8.

25. Webster J, Piscitelli G, Polli A, et al. A comparison of cabergoline and bromocriptine in the treatment of hyperprolactinemic amenorrhea. N Engl J Med 1994;331:904-9.

26. Yonkers KA, Holthausen GA, Poschman K, et al. Symptom-onset treatment for women with premenstrual dysphoric disorder. J Clin Psychopharmacol 2006;26:198-202.

Endometriosis

1. Alison E, Gallo MF, Jensen JT, et al. Continuous or extended cycle vs. cyclic use of combined hormonal contraceptives for contraception. Cochrane Database Syst Rev 2010;3:CD004695.

2. Prentice A, Deary AJ, Bland E. Progestogens and anti-progestogens for pain associated with endometriosis. Cochrane Database Syst Rev 2000;2:CD002122.

3. Prentice A, Deary AJ, Goldbeck-Wood S, et al. Gonadotrophin-releasing hormone analogues for pain associated with endometriosis. Cochrane Database Syst Rev 2000;2:CD000346.

4. Selak V, Farquhar C, Prentice A, et al. Danazol for pelvic pain associated with endometriosis. Cochrane Database Syst Rev 2000;2:CD000068.

5. Selak V, Farquhar C, Prentice A, et al. Danazol for pelvic pain associated with endometriosis. Cochrane Database Syst Rev 2009;1:CD000068.

6. Sturpe DA, Pincus KJ. Sturpe D.A., Pincus K.J. Sturpe, Deborah A., and Kathleen J. Pincus.Chapter 64. Endometriosis. In: DiPiro JT, Talbert RL, Yee GC, et al., DiPiro J.T., Talbert R.L., Yee G.C., Matzke G.R., Wells B.G., Posey L Eds. Joseph T. DiPiro, et al.eds. Pharmacotherapy: A Pathophysiologic Approach, 9th ed. New York: McGraw-Hill, 2014:XXX-XXX. Available at http://accesspharmacy.mhmedical.com/content.aspx?bookid=689&Sectionid=45310517. Accessed January 13, 2015.

7. Vercellini P, Trespidi L, Colombo A, et al. A gonadotropin-releasing hormone agonist versus a low-dose oral contraceptive for pelvic pain associated with endometriosis. Fertil Steril 1993;60:75-9.

Pregnancy and Lactation

1. American Academy of Neurology (AAN). Practice parameter: management issues for women with epilepsy (summary statement): report of the Quality Standards Subcommittee of the American Academy of Neurology. Neurology 1998;51:944-8.

2. American Academy of Pediatrics (AAP). Committee on Genetics: folic acid for the prevention of neural tube defects. Pediatrics 1999;104(2 pt 1):325-7.

3. American Congress of Obstetrics and Gynecology (ACOG). ACOG Practice Bulletin No. 44: Neural Tube Defects. Washington, DC: ACOG, 2003.

4. American Congress of Obstetrics and Gynecology (ACOG). ACOG practice bulletin No. 123: thromboembolism in pregnancy. Obstet Gynecol 2011;118:718-29.

5. Bates SM, Greer IA, Pabinger I, et al. Venous thromboembolism, thrombophilia, antithrombotic therapy, and pregnancy: American College of Chest Physicians Evidence-Based Clinical Practice Guidelines (8th edition). Chest 2008;133(6 suppl):S844-86.

6. Briggs GG, Freeman RK, Yaffe SJ. Drugs in Pregnancy and Lactation, 8th ed. Philadelphia: Lippincott Williams & Wilkins, 2008.

7. Briggs GG, Nageotte M. Diseases, Complications, and Drug Therapy in Obstetrics. Bethesda, MD: ASIIP, 2009.

8. Forinash AB, Pitlick JM, Clark K, et al. V. Nicotine replacement therapy effect on pregnancy outcomes. Ann Pharmacother 2010;44:1817-21.

9. Hale TW. Lactational pharmacology. In: Walker M, ed. Core Curriculum for Lactation Consultant Practice. Sudbury, MA: Jones & Bartlett, 2002:356-91.

10. Loebstein R, Lalkin A, Koren G. Pharmacokinetic changes during pregnancy and their clinical relevance. Clin Pharmacokinet 1997;33:328-43.

11. Longo B, Forinash AB, Murphy JA. Levetiracetam use in pregnancy. Ann Pharmacother 2009;43:1692-5.

12. Morrow J, Russell A, Guthrie E, et al. Malformation risks of antiepileptic drugs in pregnancy: a prospective study from the UK Epilepsy and Pregnancy Register. J Neurol Neurosurg Psychiatry 2006;77:193-8.

13. Pennell PB. 2005 AES annual course: evidence used to treat women with epilepsy. Epilepsia 2006;47(suppl 1):46-53.

14. Sachs CH, Committee on Drugs. The transfer of drugs and therapeutics into human breast milk: an update on selected topics. Pediatrics 2013;132:e796-809.

15. Tatum WO. Use of antiepileptic drugs in pregnancy. Expert Rev Neurother 2006;6:1077-86.

Infertility

1. Badawy A, Shokeir T, Allam AF, et al. Pregnancy outcome after ovulation induction with aromatase inhibitors or clomiphene citrate in unexplained infertility. Acta Obstet Gynecol Scand 2009;88:187-91.

2. Burney RO, Schust DJ, Yao MWM. Infertility. In: Berek JS, ed. Novak's Obstetrics and Gynecology, 14th ed. Philadelphia: Lippincott Williams & Wilkins, 2009:1185-275.

3. Eckmann KR, Kockler DR. Aromatase inhibitors for ovulation and pregnancy in polycystic ovary syndrome. Ann Pharmacother 2009;43:1338-46.

4. Hughes E, Collins J, Brown J, et al. Clomiphene citrate for unexplained subfertility in women. Cochrane Database Syst Rev 2010;1:CD000057.

5. Hughes E, Collins J, Vandekerckhove P. Clomiphene citrate for ovulation induction in women with oligo-amenorrhoea. Cochrane Database Syst Rev 2008;4:CD000056.

6. Kocak M, Caliskan E, Simsir C, et al. Metformin therapy improves ovulatory rates, cervical scores, and pregnancy rates in clomiphene citrate-resistant women with polycystic ovary syndrome. Fertil Steril 2001;77:101-6.

7. Lieu CL, Yoshida T. Infertility. In: DiPiro JT, Talbert RL, Yee GC, et al., eds. Pharmacotherapy: A Pathophysiologic Approach, 5th ed. New York: McGraw-Hill, 2002:1431-43.

8. Nestler JE, Jakubowicz DJ, Evans WS, et al. Effects of metformin on spontaneous and clomiphene-induced ovulation in the polycystic ovary syndrome. N Engl J Med 1998;338:1876-80.

9. Nugent D, Vanderkerchove P, Hughes E, et al. Gonadotrophin therapy for ovulation induction in subfertility associated with polycystic ovary syndrome. Cochrane Database Syst Rev 2009;1:CD000410.

10. Pritts EA. Letrozole for ovulation induction and controlled ovarian hyperstimulation. Curr Opin Obstet Gynecol 2010;22:289-94.

11. Smith S, Pfeifer SM, Collins JA. Diagnosis and management of female infertility. JAMA 2003;290:1767-70.

12. Stachnik JM, Krueger CD. Infertility in women. In: Murphy JE, Lee MW, eds. Pharmacotherapy Self-assessment Program, 2013, Book 2, Special Populations. Lenexa, KS: American College of Clinical Pharmacy, 2013:61-79.

13. Vandermolen DT, Ratts VS, Evans WS, et al. Metformin increases the ovulatory rate and pregnancy rate from clomiphene citrate in patients with polycystic ovary syndrome who are resistant to clomiphene citrate alone. Fertil Steril 2001;75:310-5.

ANSWERS AND EXPLANATIONS TO PATIENT CASES

1. Answer: D

This patient currently has contraindications to using an estrogen-containing contraceptive because her systolic blood pressure is greater than 160 mm Hg (Answer B and Answer C are incorrect). Medroxyprogesterone acetate (Answer A) would not be the best choice because the patient is already overweight, and this product causes significant weight gain. In addition, medroxyprogesterone has an average return of fertility of 9 months after the last injection. Because the patient wants to attempt conception in 12 months, she would receive only a few injections and would then need to consider alternative agents. Norethindrone (Answer D) does not contain estrogen and is not associated with significant weight gain.

2. Answer: A

Late-cycle breakthrough bleeding is a result of progestin deficiency. The patient must start using a different product that has higher progestin activity (+++) than her current product (++) (Answer A). Answers B, C, and D do not increase progestin activity, so these are incorrect.

3. Answer: C

Answer A is incorrect because this patient is past the optimal dosing window of 72 hours for Plan B One-Step. Studies have shown continued efficacy for up to 120 hours after unprotected intercourse. However, the patient would have to find another pharmacy and begin taking the product soon. She is not a candidate for IUD therapy (new guidelines say if PID is resolved, it can potentially be used, but it is not the best choice) because of her history of PID (Answer B). Ulipristal (Answer C) can be given up to 120 hours after unprotected intercourse and could be initiated immediately if samples are available. In addition, it has the lowest risk for nausea and vomiting of the emergency contraceptive products. Answer D is incorrect because she can still receive emergency contraception because it has been less than 120 hours since unprotected intercourse.

4. Answer: C

Clomiphene can elevate the body temperature, making basal body temperature monitoring inaccurate (Answer B). Cervical mucus monitoring is an option for detecting ovulation; however, it requires practice by the patient for several cycles to increase correct interpretation

(Answer A). Urine LH kits are readily available and are not affected by clomiphene (Answer C). Ultrasonography will detect follicular development and ovulation, but it requires several visits and is costly (Answer D).

5. Answer: D

Ovarian hyperstimulation symptoms include weight gain greater than 2.25 kg and increased abdominal girth, abdominal or pelvic pain, nausea, vomiting, diarrhea, dyspnea, dizziness, and oliguria (Answer D). This is an important education point for patients receiving gonadotropin therapy because they have increased risk with this class of medications. Answers A, B, and C do not match ovarian hyperstimulation symptoms.

6. Answer: A

Lamotrigine is associated with an increased risk of cleft palate/lip; however, the palate and lip are developed by 9 weeks' gestation. The patient is currently at 18 weeks' gestation, so lamotrigine could not cause cleft palate/lip (Answer A). Lamotrigine has not been associated with intrauterine growth restriction, cardiac abnormalities, or neurodevelopment delays (Answers B, C, and D).

7. Answer: B

The patient does not require progestin therapy because she has had her uterus removed (Answer C). Testosterone therapy is not required because she is not experiencing decreased libido (Answer D). A non-oral route would be preferred because of her elevated triglyceride values (Answer B). Oral therapy has the highest effects on the cholesterol panel, including increasing the concentration of triglycerides (Answer A).

8. Answer: D

The options in Answer A and Answer C are contraindicated for this patient because of her history of myocardial infarction. In addition, Answer A is incorrect because this patient still has her uterus and would need a progestogen with the estrogen for protection against endometrial hyperplasia. Although ospemifene is indicated for moderate to severe dyspareunia, it would be inappropriate for this patient. Answer B is incorrect because this is a nonhormonal product used for vasomotor, not genitourinary, symptoms. Patients with mild to moderate genitourinary symptoms should start with a vaginal lubricating gel.

ANSWERS AND EXPLANATIONS TO SELF-ASSESSMENT QUESTIONS

1. Answer: D

Depot medroxyprogesterone acetate (Answer A) causes considerable weight gain, making it a less-than-optimal choice for this patient. Cerebrovascular accident is also a relative contraindication for progestin-only contraceptives. The levonorgestrel IUD (Answer B) should not be used because the patient has structural abnormalities of the uterus. The contraceptive sponge (Answer C) should be avoided because of the patient's uterine structural abnormalities and because she is recently postpartum. The polyurethane condom (Answer D) is the best option because the patient has no contraindications or allergies that would prohibit its use.

2. Answer: A

The patient has no contraindications or allergies to the female condom (Answer A). However, she has a latex allergy, so the male latex condom (Answer B) would not be a good choice. Estrogen-containing contraceptives (Answer C) are contraindicated for patients with stroke, according to the CDC and the World Health Organization. Ulipristal (Answer D) is a form of emergency contraception; it should not be used as a regular form of contraception.

3. Answer: D

Analysis of variance (Answer D) would be most appropriate because the trial consists of more than two groups and involves continuous data that are most likely normally distributed (n=600). Although the Student t-test (Answer A) is for continuous data, it should be used only if two groups are being compared. Both the Fisher exact test (Answer B) and the Kruskal-Wallis test (Answer C) are for nonparametric data.

4. Answer: B

Although molecular weight is an important factor in determining whether a drug will cross the placenta, the risk of malformations is not directly addressed (Answer C is incorrect). The information obtained in studies of animals is helpful as a guide to determine the potential risks of drugs in humans, but it does not confer exact risks in humans (Answer A is incorrect). Educating the patient on the gestational timing of risks and on the current stage of pregnancy is imperative to an understanding of whether the patient has any chance of experiencing that birth defect (Answer B is correct). The half-life of a medication does not affect the risk of medication exposure during pregnancy (Answer D is incorrect).

5. Answer: A

The best recommendation is to delay the treatment until after she stops breastfeeding (Answer A is correct).

The drug is likely to cross into breast milk, but exact concentrations are unknown. Because of its long half-life and therapy duration, the infant would be exposed to the drug. The patient, who is currently asymptomatic, is seeking treatment only for cosmetic reasons. Itraconazole is an option for treating onychomycosis; however, it has decreased efficacy compared with terbinafine (Answer B is incorrect). Topical terbinafine is not effective for treating onychomycosis (Answer C is incorrect). Scheduling the doses right after feedings is recommended to minimize infant exposure; however, because the half-life is long and the baby is feeding every 2 hours, this recommendation is unlikely to decrease infant exposure (Answer D is incorrect).

6. Answer: D

Because the patient weighs more than 90 kg, Ortho-Evra is not recommended because of decreased efficacy, making Answer A and Answer B incorrect. Estrogen-progestin contraceptives (Answer C and Answer D) are second-line agents after NSAIDs for treating dysmenorrhea because they can decrease menstrual length and volume. Extended-interval dosing is preferred because it decreases the frequency of menses, making Answer D correct.

7. Answer: C

Natazia is a quadriphasic hormonal contraceptive that requires 9 days of backup contraception. The first two pills contain only estrogen, and ovulation protection does not occur until after the seventh dose. Sperm can remain active for 48 hours in the body, so 9 days (Answer C) are required to provide pregnancy protection.

8. Answer: B

Estrogens should be avoided because of the patient's active breast cancer (Answer A is incorrect). Venlafaxine has shown efficacy in decreasing vasomotor symptoms in patients with and without breast cancer (Answer B is correct). Clonidine improves vasomotor symptoms but may not be the best choice because this patient's blood pressure is low (Answer C is incorrect). Black cohosh has not been effective in reducing vasomotor symptoms in patients with breast cancer (Answer D is incorrect).

9. Answer: C

The Endometriosis Association (Answer C) provides contact information for local support groups and patient information. The Association of Reproductive Healthcare Professionals (Answer A), ACOG (Answer B), and the National Women's Health Network (Answer D) provide patient information and health care–related information.

Infectious Diseases I

Shellee A. Grim, Pharm.D., MSCTS, BCPS

Loyola University Medical Center
Maywood, Illinois

Infectious Diseases I

Shellee A. Grim, Pharm.D., MSCTS, BCPS

Loyola University Medical Center

Maywood, Illinois

Learning Objectives

1. Design appropriate treatment regimens for patients with sexually transmitted diseases.
2. Explain common routes of transmission of HIV and current screening guidelines.
3. Explain the mechanisms of action of antiretroviral agents and commonly encountered adverse effects.
4. Formulate treatment strategies for the management of HIV and commonly encountered opportunistic infections.
5. Select appropriate ancillary medications and immunizations as needed for the management of HIV infection and its associated morbidities.
6. Explain the epidemiology of influenza and herpesviruses and formulate appropriate strategies for treatment of infection.
7. Explain the risk factors for superficial and invasive fungal infections and design corresponding treatment regimens.
8. Identify and manage the drug interactions associated with anti-infective medications.

Self-Assessment Questions

Answers and explanations to these questions can be found at the end of the chapter.

1. A.A. is a 21-year-old college student who presents in the clinic with penile discharge and burning on urination. He reports drinking too much the past weekend (about 6 days ago) and to having unprotected intercourse with a girl he met at a party. A.A. is otherwise healthy with no comorbidities, chronic medications, or known drug allergies. A physical examination is performed, and a urethral discharge smear is taken. The smear reveals moderate gram-negative diplococci and many polymorphonuclear cells. Which is the most appropriate treatment recommendation for this patient?
   A. Ceftriaxone 250 mg intramuscularly once.
   B. Doxycycline 100 mg orally twice daily for 7 days.
   C. Ceftriaxone 250 mg intramuscularly once plus azithromycin 1 g orally once.
   D. Ceftriaxone 250 mg intramuscularly once plus doxycycline 1 g orally once.

2. B.B. is a 20-year-old woman who presents to her primary care provider with painful, ulcerative lesions on her labia bilaterally. Her physician makes the presumptive diagnosis of herpes labialis and requests your opinion on treatment. Which is the most appropriate therapy for this patient's first episode?
   A. Valacyclovir 1 g orally three times daily for 7 days.
   B. Valganciclovir 900 mg orally once daily for 7 days.
   C. Acyclovir 800 mg orally twice daily for 7 days.
   D. Acyclovir 400 mg orally three times daily for 7 days.

3. C.C. is a 30-year-old health care worker who is stuck by a needle that was being used to perform a venipuncture in a known HIV-seropositive patient. Which is the most important determinant with respect to the efficacy of postexposure prophylaxis (PEP)?
   A. The time elapsed since the needlestick injury occurred.
   B. The sex of the source patient.
   C. The nonprescription drug history of the source patient.
   D. The source patient's CD4+ cell count.

4. D.D. is a 30-year-old African American man with newly diagnosed HIV infection; his viral load is 250,000 copies/mL, and his CD4+ count is 220 cells/mm³. Which is the most appropriate next step in managing his disease?
   A. Obtain a genotype.
   B. Obtain a phenotype.
   C. Administer hepatitis B virus (HBV) vaccine.
   D. Administer influenza vaccine.

5. E.E. is referred to the pharmacotherapy clinic for the management of ongoing hyperlipidemia that has not responded to 6 months of diet and exercise. He is HIV seropositive and takes the following antiretroviral (ARV) regimen: zidovudine, lamivudine, and lopinavir/ritonavir. The only other medications the patient currently takes are citalopram for depression and zolpidem as needed for sleep. E.E.'s primary care

physician is concerned about his elevated low-density lipoprotein cholesterol (LDL-C) concentrations. Which intervention is most appropriate currently?

A. Initiate therapy with pravastatin.
B. Initiate therapy with simvastatin.
C. Discontinue zidovudine.
D. Discontinue lamivudine.

6. F.F. is a 26-year-old white man with HIV who presents today to begin a new ARV regimen. The patient has not previously been treated for HIV, and a genotypic resistance assay shows no resistance to any available ARV medication; his viral load is 76,300 copies/mL and CD4+ count is 355 cells/mm³. The patient is a graduate student who reports a very hectic work and school life. F.F. also reports that he has severe insomnia, which he attributes to "racing thoughts." He will consider only a once-daily regimen. Which is the best once-daily option for this patient?

A. Emtricitabine/tenofovir DF/rilpivirine.
B. Emtricitabine/tenofovir DF/efavirenz.
C. Emtricitabine/tenofovir DF/raltegravir.
D. Emtricitabine/tenofovir DF/cobistat/elvitegravir.

7. G.G. is a 49-year-old female renal transplant recipient who presents to the clinic for a routine follow-up. She has no food or drug allergies. G.G.'s allograft is functioning well, and she has not been treated for rejection. Because the influenza season has just begun, which is the most appropriate means of prevention for this patient?

A. Oseltamivir 75 mg orally once daily for the duration of the influenza season.
B. Inactivated influenza vaccine (IIV) and oseltamivir 75 mg orally once daily for 2 weeks.
C. IIV.
D. Live attenuated influenza vaccine (LAIV).

8. H.H. is 62-year-old woman who presents to her primary care provider for an annual follow-up. She states that she cannot recall ever having chickenpox or shingles. Which is the best option to prevent herpes zoster in this patient?

A. Obtain assay for varicella zoster virus (VZV) immunoglobulin G (IgG), and if negative result, give Varivax; if positive result, give Zostavax.
B. Give Varivax.
C. Give Zostavax.
D. Give varicella zoster immune globulin (VariZIG).

9. I.I. is a 56-year-old woman with diabetes mellitus and hypertension who is scheduled to receive a living related renal transplant from her niece. The donor's herpesvirus serologic profile is as follows: herpes simplex virus (HSV) positive, VZV positive, Epstein-Barr virus (EBV) positive, and cytomegalovirus (CMV) positive. The recipient's herpesvirus serologic profile is as follows: HSV positive, VZV positive, EBV positive, and CMV negative. Which is the best antiviral prophylaxis for this patient?

A. Ganciclovir 1 g orally twice daily.
B. Valganciclovir 900 mg orally once daily.
C. Acyclovir 400 mg orally twice daily.
D. Famciclovir 250 mg orally twice daily.

10. J.J. is a 22-year-old man with a 4-month history of pain and itching on the toes of both feet with noticeable peeling and scaling. In the past month, he has lost both toenails from his great toes. J.J. is otherwise in excellent health because he regularly competes in amateur triathlons. His primary care provider diagnoses tinea pedis. Which is the most likely cause of this patient's infection?

A. *Malassezia* spp.
B. Dermatophytes.
C. *Sporothrix schenckii.*
D. *Candida albicans.*

11. K.K. is a 67-year-old woman with diabetes mellitus who recently received two courses of high-dose steroids for chronic obstructive pulmonary disease (COPD) exacerbations. She presents to the pulmonary clinic with facial pain and increased nasal output for 1 week as well as a low-grade fever for the past 2 days. Sinus computed tomography (CT) reveals bony erosion, and a sinus biopsy reveals nonseptate hyphae. The pulmonologist calls his infectious diseases colleague, who recommends amphotericin B lipid complex 5 mg/kg intravenously once daily and surgical evaluation. With which

fungal pathogen is the infectious diseases specialist most likely concerned?

A. *Aspergillus fumigatus.*
B. *Blastomyces dermatitidis.*
C. *Cryptococcus neoformans.*
D. *Rhizopus.*

12. L.L. is a 42-year-old woman who underwent an allogeneic stem cell transplant for acute leukemia. Her initial posttransplant course was uncomplicated; however, 1 month after engraftment (7 weeks posttransplantation), the patient developed a fever and rash. A skin biopsy revealed graft-versus-host disease, for which the patient's tacrolimus dose was increased. L.L. also received high-dose steroids, which caused her fever to resolve and rash to improve. She received maintenance therapy with prednisone 30 mg orally once daily. One month later, L.L. presents to the hematology clinic with a worsening dry cough, shortness of breath, fever, and one episode of hemoptysis. Chest CT reveals a left-sided cavitary lesion. The hematologist would like to initiate anti-*Aspergillus* therapy. Which agent would be best to recommend?

A. Itraconazole.
B. Voriconazole.
C. Liposomal amphotericin B.
D. Caspofungin.

13. Which organism best fits the following description: endemic in the Ohio and Mississippi river valleys and may manifest as an acute pulmonary, chronic pulmonary, or disseminated infection?

A. *B. dermatitidis.*
B. *Histoplasma capsulatum.*
C. *Coccidioides immitis.*
D. *Coccidioides posadasii.*

I. SEXUALLY TRANSMITTED DISEASES

A. Introduction
   1. The Centers for Disease Control and Prevention (CDC) estimates that 20 million new sexually transmitted diseases (STDs) are diagnosed per year in the United States, half of which are among 15- to 24-year-olds. STDs may increase the risk of HIV infection and may cause infertility.
   2. All 50 states and the District of Columbia allow minors to consent for their own care of STDs.
   3. Syphilis, gonorrhea, chlamydia, chancroid, and HIV infection are reportable diseases in every state. The requirements for reporting other STDs vary by state.
   4. Many cases of chlamydia, gonorrhea, and syphilis go underdiagnosed and underreported, and because data on other STDs are not routinely reported to the CDC, surveillance data fail to capture the true burden of STDs.

B. Screening *(Domain 5, Task 2)*
   1. Routine annual screening for *Chlamydia trachomatis* in sexually active female individuals up to 25 years of age and women older than 25 years with new or several sexual partners is recommended.
   2. Routine screening of male individuals is not recommended, though screening should be considered in settings associated with a high prevalence of *Chlamydia* (e.g., adolescent clinics, correctional facilities, STD clinics, young men who have sex with men [MSM]).
   3. Routine annual screening for *Neisseria gonorrhoeae* in sexually active female individuals up to 25 years of age, in women older than 25 years at risk of gonorrhea (e.g., previous gonorrheal infection, other STDs, new or several sex partners, inconsistent condom use, commercial sex work, drug use), and in young MSM
   4. HIV screening should be offered to all adolescents (see HIV chapter).
   5. The routine screening of asymptomatic adolescents for syphilis, trichomoniasis, bacterial vaginosis, HSV, human papillomavirus (HPV), and hepatitis A and B viruses is not recommended, although a more thorough evaluation of young MSM and pregnant adolescent females may be considered.
   6. The American Cancer Society recommends cervical cancer screening at 21 years of age. Women older than 65 years with previous normal cervical cancer screening results do not require further screening.
   7. HIV, syphilis, and HBV for all pregnant women and gonorrhea, chlamydia, and hepatitis C virus (HCV) screening for at-risk pregnant women, at the first prenatal visit
   8. At least once-yearly screening for HIV, syphilis, chlamydia, and gonorrhea for MSM. MSM who have several or anonymous partners or MSM who have sex in conjunction with illicit drug use should be screened more often, at 3- to 6-month intervals.

C. Prevention *(Domain 5, Task 1, 2)*
   1. HBV may be transmitted by percutaneous or mucous membrane exposure to infected blood or body fluids that contain blood.
      a. Risk factors for HBV transmission include unprotected sexual intercourse with infected partner, several partners, MSM, history of other STDs, and injection drug use.
      b. HBV vaccination is recommended as part of routine infant vaccination, to previously unvaccinated adolescents, and to previously unvaccinated adults at increased risk of infection.
      c. HBV vaccination series consists of a total of three doses given at 1, 2, and 6 months.
   2. HPV is common among sexually active adolescents and adults.
      a. Most HPV infections are asymptomatic or unrecognized. Oncogenic HPV types (e.g., HPV types 16 and 18) cause most cervical cancers as well as penile, vulvar, vaginal, anal, and oropharyngeal cancers. Nononcogenic HPV types (e.g., HPV types 6 and 11) cause genital warts.
      b. HPV vaccination is recommended routinely for boys and girls 11 or 12 years of age, although it may be given beginning at age 9 years.

    c.   Female patients may receive bivalent (Cervarix; HPV types 16 and 18), quadrivalent (Gardasil; HPV types 6, 11, 16, and 18), or 9-valent (Gardasil 9; HPV types 6, 11, 16, 18, 31, 33, 45, 52, 58) HPV vaccine, whereas only the quadrivalent or 9-valent vaccine is recommended for male patients.

    d.   HPV vaccination is recommended through age 26 years for female individuals and through age 21 years for male individuals who have not completed the vaccine series.

    e.   HPV vaccine series consists of a total of three doses given at 1, 2, and 6 months.

3.   Universal precautions

    a.   Practicing abstinence or maintaining a mutually monogamous sexual relationship with an uninfected partner is the best way to prevent STDs.

    b.   Barrier contraceptive methods – Condoms, dental dams

    c.   Latex condoms, with or without spermicide, are more effective than natural skin condoms.

    d.   Lubrication – Use water-based products because oil-based products can weaken latex.

    e.   Safe oral sex

D.   Gonorrhea and Chlamydia *(Domain 1, Task 1, 2, 3, 6, 7)*

   1.   Overview

      a.   Gonorrhea is caused by *N. gonorrhoeae*, a gram-negative diplococci, and humans are the only known host.

      b.   *C. trachomatis* is an obligate intracellular parasite that shares the properties of both viruses and bacteria.

      c.   Coinfection with *N. gonorrhoeae* and *C. trachomatis* occurs often; this coinfection should be assumed in patients who receive a diagnosis of gonorrhea.

      d.   Asymptomatic infection is common, highlighting the importance of screening (as above).

   2.   Clinical presentation and diagnosis

      a.   Gonorrhea: Incubation 1–14 days; symptom onset is 2–8 days for men and within 10 days for women

      b.   Chlamydia: Incubation 7–35 days; symptom onset is 7–21 days for men and women

      c.   Symptoms are more common with gonorrhea, especially among men.

         i.   Male individuals: Purulent urethral discharge or scant or profuse rectal discharge

        ii.   Female individuals: Abnormal vaginal discharge or uterine bleeding

        iii.   Both: Dysuria and urinary frequency

      d.   Diagnosis

         i.   Test for both pathogens.

        ii.   A Gram stain of a urethral specimen with polymorphonuclear leukocytes and gram-negative diplococci is diagnostic in symptomatic men (a negative Gram stain result does not rule out infection).

        iii.   Nucleic acid amplification tests (NAATs) are routinely done, having replaced culture for *C. trachomatis* because culture is less sensitive. Although NAATs are usually bundled together for *C. trachomatis* and *N. gonorrhoeae*, they are no better than culture for *N. gonorrhoeae*.

        iv.   In treatment failure or suspected drug resistance with gonococcal infection, a culture must be done to obtain antimicrobial susceptibility testing.

      e.   Treatment

         i.   Gonorrhea treatment, uncomplicated infection of the cervix, urethra, and rectum

            (a)   Ceftriaxone 250 mg intramuscularly in a single dose plus azithromycin 1 g orally in a single dose

(1) Because of the common coinfection with *N. gonorrhoeae* and *C. trachomatis*, it is recommended that patients being treated for gonococcal infection also be treated for chlamydial infection, even if the NAAT result for *C. trachomatis* is negative at the time of treatment.

(2) In addition, combination therapy may hinder the development of resistant *N. gonorrhoeae*.

(3) Due to increased tetracycline resistance among gonococcal isolates, doxycycline is no longer recommended.

(b) If ceftriaxone is unavailable, cefixime 400 mg orally in a single dose with a follow-up test of cure in 10 days (less effective than ceftriaxone; also given in combination with oral azithromycin)

(c) If the patient has a severe cephalosporin allergy, the following recently studied combinations may be considered: gemifloxacin 320 mg orally in a single dose plus azithromycin 2 g orally in a single dose OR gentamicin 240 mg intramuscularly in a single dose plus azithromycin 2 g orally in a single dose.

(d) Fluoroquinolones are not routinely recommended because of resistance to these antibiotics (especially in California and Hawaii). Resistance rates are available at the CDC website (www.cdc.gov).

(e) Rescreen 3 months after treatment.

(f) Expedited partner therapy (EPT) or patient-delivered partner therapy (PDPT)

(1) Unless prohibited by law, providers should routinely offer EPT to heterosexual patients with gonorrhea or chlamydia infection when the provider cannot ensure that all of the infected patient's sex partners within the past 60 days will be treated.

(2) If the infected patient has not had sex within 60 days of diagnosis, providers should try to treat the most recent sex partner.

(3) EPT is legal in most states (www.cdc.gov/std/ept).

(4) It is preferred to provide infected patients with appropriately labeled medication because the efficacy of PDPT using prescriptions is limited, and many individuals do not fill prescriptions given to them by a sex partner.

(5) Medications or prescriptions provided for PDPT should be accompanied by treatment instructions, appropriate warnings, general health counseling, and a statement advising partners to seek medical evaluation for STDs.

(6) No data support the routine use of PDPT for syphilis, and data for the use of PDPT for gonorrhea or chlamydia infection among MSM are limited (concern for new HIV infection); MSM partners should seek evaluation for STDs, including HIV.

ii. Chlamydia treatment

(a) Azithromycin 1 g orally in a single dose

(1) Azithromycin is preferred for patients with poor treatment adherence and/or an unpredictable follow-up because of its single dose and option for directly observed therapy.

(2) Azithromycin is also preferred for *Mycoplasma genitalium*, another cause of nongonococcal urethritis.

(b) OR, doxycycline 100 mg orally twice daily for 7 days

(c) Alternatives: Erythromycin base 500 mg orally four times daily for 7 days, erythromycin ethylsuccinate 800 mg orally four times daily for 7 days, levofloxacin 500 mg orally once daily for 7 days, or ofloxacin 300 mg orally twice daily for 7 days

(d) To minimize transmission to sex partners, abstain from sexual intercourse for 7 days after single-dose regimen or after completion of 7-day therapy.

Patient Case

1. J.C. is a 28-year-old woman who presents to her primary care physician because she had unprotected sex with a male acquaintance. Although she has no symptoms, she is concerned that she may have developed a sexually transmitted disease (STD) because this man is notorious for having several partners. J.C. takes oral birth control, although she reports often missing doses. An examination reveals a positive pregnancy test result, and a NAAT test result is positive for both *N. gonorrhoeae* and *C. trachomatis*. Which is the best treatment option for this patient?

   A. Levofloxacin 250 mg orally once plus azithromycin 1 g orally once.
   B. Cefixime 400 mg orally once plus azithromycin 1 g orally once.
   C. Ceftriaxone 250 mg intramuscularly once plus azithromycin 1 g orally once.
   D. Ceftriaxone 250 mg intramuscularly once plus doxycycline 100 mg orally twice daily for 7 days.

E. Syphilis *(Domain 1, Task 1, 2, 3, 6, 7)*
   1. Overview
      a. Local and systemic disease caused by the spirochete *Treponema pallidum*
      b. Infection divided into overlapping stages that affect treatment (see below)
      c. Rates of primary and secondary syphilis decreased in the 1990s, and in 2000, rates were lowest since reporting began in 1941. However, each year from 2001 to 2009, rates increased, plateauing in 2010–2011, but rates increased again in 2012 and 2013. Most cases in the United States are among MSM.
      d. Primarily acquired by sexual contact with infected mucous membranes or cutaneous lesions, but may be acquired by nonsexual contact (e.g., congenital, nonsexual contact in communities with poor hygiene conditions)
   2. Clinical presentation
      a. Primary syphilis
         i. Incubation period: Median 21 days (range 3–90 days)
         ii. Papule (usually painless) appears at the inoculation site. This soon ulcerates to form the classic chancre of primary syphilis, a 1- to 2-cm ulcer with a raised, indurated margin. However, the presentation of primary syphilis may be varied.
         iii. Usually associated with regional lymphadenopathy
      b. Secondary syphilis
         i. Develops 2–8 weeks after primary infection in about 25% of individuals with untreated or inadequately treated primary infection
         ii. Patients with secondary syphilis may not have a history of a chancre because the primary lesion may go unnoticed.
         iii. Secondary syphilis may occasionally develop when the primary chancre is still present; more common in patients with HIV infection
         iv. Infection may have multisystem involvement from hematogenous and lymphatic dissemination.
         v. Rash is the most characteristic finding of secondary syphilis; classically, a diffuse, symmetric macular or papular eruption involving the entire trunk and extremities, including palms and soles
         vi. Other manifestations include mucocutaneous lesions, lymphadenopathy, flu-like symptoms, and neurologic symptoms.

---

    c.   Tertiary syphilis: Involves the cardiovascular system, developing for a period of months to years and involving slow inflammatory tissue damage
- i. Gummatous syphilis (also called late benign)
  - (a) Characterized by granulomatous lesions called gummas, which have a center of necrotic tissue with a rubbery texture
  - (b) Gummas are primarily formed in the liver, bones, and testes, but they may affect any organ.
- ii. Cardiovascular syphilis
  - (a) Occurs many years after initial infection
  - (b) The most common manifestation is an ascending aortic aneurysm, which may result in aortic insufficiency.
- iii. Neurosyphilis
  - (a) Historically, neurosyphilis occurred late as a form of tertiary syphilis, but it can present at any stage of infection (especially in immunocompromised individuals).
  - (b) May manifest as meningitis, general paresis, dementia, and blindness
  - (c) Lumbar puncture should be performed in patients with neurologic, ophthalmic, or otologic symptoms.

    d.   Latent syphilis: Without clinical manifestations, detected by serologic testing
- i. Early latent infection: Infection acquired within the preceding year
- ii. Late latent infection: Infection acquired beyond the preceding year. Latent syphilis of unknown duration is treated as a late latent infection.

3. Diagnosis
    a.   *T. pallidum* is difficult to culture; therefore, serologic tests are used for diagnosis. The use of only one type of serologic test is insufficient for diagnosis.
    b.   Non-treponemal tests historically used for screening; antibody titers may correlate with disease activity and are used to follow treatment
- i. Venereal Disease Research Laboratory (VDRL) slide test
- ii. Rapid plasma reagin (RPR) card test

    c.   Treponemal tests historically used to confirm infection
- i. Fluorescent treponemal antibody absorption (FTA-ABS)
- ii. *T. pallidum* particle agglutination assay

    d.   Reverse screening algorithm may be replacing traditionally screening.
- i. Screening with treponemal tests with enzyme, chemiluminescence, or microbead immunoassay (automated tests that are easier to perform) followed by RPR or VDRL
- ii. Reverse screening algorithm can identify individuals previously treated for syphilis, those with untreated or incompletely treated syphilis, and those with false-positive tests that can occur with a low likelihood of infection.

4. Treatment
    a.   Penicillin is the drug of choice.
- i. Extended low-level penicillin concentrations are required to eradicate the slow-growing *T. pallidum*.
- ii. Penicillin is the only therapy with confirmed efficacy in pregnancy.
- iii. Penicillin-allergic patients
  - (a) Confirm penicillin allergy.
  - (b) Consider desensitizing penicillin-allergic patients, especially in pregnancy or cases of neurologic involvement.
- iv. Be aware of the Jarisch-Herxheimer reaction, which can occur within the first 24 hours of treatment. Occurs most often in early syphilis, presumably because of higher bacterial burden
  - (a) Transient immunologic reaction marked by fever, chills, headache, exacerbation of cutaneous lesions

(b) Caused by the release of antigenic toxic components of *T. pallidum*

b. Primary, secondary, and early latent syphilis

   i. Benzathine penicillin G 2.4 million units intramuscularly in a single dose

   ii. Penicillin-allergic patients

      (a) Doxycycline 100 mg orally twice daily for 14 days

      (b) Tetracycline 500 mg orally four times daily for 14 days

      (c) Ceftriaxone 1 g intramuscularly or intravenously daily for 8–10 days

c. Late latent syphilis

   i. Benzathine penicillin G 2.4 million units intramuscularly once weekly for 3 weeks

   ii. Penicillin-allergic patients

      (a) Doxycycline 100 mg orally twice daily for 28 days

      (b) Tetracycline 500 mg orally four times daily for 28 days

d. Tertiary syphilis

   i. Benzathine penicillin G 2.4 million units intramuscularly once weekly for 3 weeks

   ii. Penicillin-allergic patients should be treated in consultation with an infectious diseases specialist.

e. Neurosyphilis

   i. Aqueous crystalline penicillin G 18–24 million units per day, given as 3–4 million units intravenously every 4 hours or as a continuous infusion, for 10–14 days

   ii. Penicillin-allergic patients

      (a) Ceftriaxone 2 g once daily intramuscularly or intravenously for 10–14 days

      (b) Consider skin testing and penicillin desensitization in consultation with a specialist.

f. Follow-up quantitative non-treponemal tests are recommended 6 and 12 months after treatment for primary and secondary syphilis and again at 24 months for latent syphilis to ensure response to treatment. An adequate response is a 4-fold reduction in antibody titer, as measured by a VDRL or RPR test.

Patient Case

[handwritten: latent syphilis]

2. J.F. is a 39-year-old man with HIV (CD4+ count 225 cells/mm³, HIV viral load less than 48 copies/mL) who was treated for secondary syphilis because of the presence of a diffuse rash, generalized lymphadenopathy, and a previous primary genital chancre. His RPR titer was 1:64, and his FTA-ABS test result was positive. He reports no neurologic or ophthalmic concerns and receives benzathine penicillin G by intramuscular injection once. One and one-half years later, the patient has an RPR titer of 1:32 and a positive FTA-ABS test result. A lumbar puncture reveals the absence of white blood cells (WBCs), normal values of glucose and protein, and a negative VDRL test finding. Which is the most appropriate treatment currently?

A. Benzathine penicillin G 2.4 million units intramuscularly once.

B. Benzathine penicillin G 2.4 million units intramuscularly once weekly for 3 weeks.

C. Aqueous penicillin G 24 million units daily intravenously for 10 days.

D. Doxycycline 100 mg orally twice daily for 28 days.

F. Genital Herpes *(Domain 1, Task 1, 2, 6)*

   1. Overview

      a. Most common cause of genital ulceration in the United States

      b. More than 50 million Americans have genital herpes, which is a chronic, lifelong infection.

      c. Genital herpes is associated with a 2- to 4-fold increased risk of acquiring HIV infection if the individual is exposed when genital herpes is present.

2. Pathophysiology
   a. Caused by the herpes simplex viruses (HSVs)
      i. HSV-1: Most commonly causes oropharyngeal disease
      ii. HSV-2: Most commonly causes genital disease
      iii. Both HSV-1 and HSV-2 can cause disease in both anatomic areas.
      iv. Most cases of recurrent genital herpes are caused by HSV-2.
   b. HSV is transmitted by the inoculation of infected secretions on mucosal surfaces.
   c. Infection cycle
      i. Primary mucocutaneous infection
      ii. Infection of the ganglia
      iii. Establishment of lifelong latency
      iv. Reactivation
      v. Recurrent infection
3. Clinical presentation
   a. Incubation period: 2–14 days
   b. First-episode infection signs and symptoms
      i. Several painful pustular or ulcerative lesions on external genitalia; develop over 7–10 days and heal within 2–4 weeks
      ii. Flu-like symptoms during first few days of symptoms
      iii. Local itching and pain
      iv. Vaginal or urethral discharge
      v. Viral shedding lasts about 12 days.
   c. Recurrent infection signs and symptoms
      i. Prodrome symptoms before the appearance of lesions; mild burning, itching, or tingling
      ii. Fewer lesions than in primary infection and shorter duration (about 7 days for lesions to heal)
      iii. Viral shedding lasts about 4 days; shedding is more common the first year after primary infection.
      iv. Viral shedding may occur in the absence of signs and symptoms of infection.
      v. Recurrences and subclinical shedding is more common with HSV-2 than with HSV-1
4. Diagnosis
   a. Viral tissue culture is the current standard, but it has lower sensitivity than a polymerase chain reaction (PCR), which is often used.
   b. A PCR can be performed on the fluid collected from a lesion vesicle (or cerebrospinal fluid [CSF]), and this is the test of choice for HSV involving the central nervous system (CNS) and systemic infections.
   c. Direct fluorescent antibody test (can distinguish between HSV-1 and HSV-2)
      i. Tests for specific HSV antibodies
      ii. May be useful for patients with recurrent genital symptoms with negative culture results, for patients with a clinical diagnosis of genital herpes without laboratory confirmation, or for patients having a partner with a diagnosis of genital herpes
   d. Diagnosis is often made by obtaining a clinical history and noting characteristic physical findings.
5. Treatment
   a. Goal is to relieve symptoms and shorten clinical course.
   b. First episode
      i. Acyclovir 400 mg orally three times daily for 7–10 days
      ii. Acyclovir 200 mg orally five times daily for 7–10 days
      iii. Valacyclovir 1 g orally twice daily for 7–10 days
      iv. Famciclovir 250 mg orally three times daily for 7–10 days
      v. Antiviral therapy may be extended beyond 10 days if healing is incomplete.

    c. Recurrent infection

       i. Effective episodic treatment requires initiation within 1 day of lesion outbreak or during prodrome. The patient should be provided with a prescription in advance so that antiviral therapy can begin in a timely manner.

       ii. Acyclovir 400 mg orally three times daily for 5 days

       iii. Acyclovir 800 mg orally twice daily for 5 days

       iv. Acyclovir 800 mg orally three times daily for 2 days

       v. Valacyclovir 500 mg orally twice daily for 3 days

       vi. Valacyclovir 1 g orally once daily for 5 days

       vii. Famciclovir 125 mg orally twice daily for 5 days

       viii. Famciclovir 1 g orally twice daily for 1 day

       ix. Famciclovir 500 mg orally x 1 dose, followed by 250 mg orally twice daily for 2 days

    d. Suppressive therapy

       i. Reduces the frequency of recurrences by 70%–80% in patients who have frequent recurrences (although it is also effective in individuals with less frequent recurrences)

       ii. Decreases the rate of HSV-2 transmission in discordant couples and by individuals with multiple sexual partners

       iii. Periodically reassess need to continue suppressive therapy.

       iv. Consider cost and frequency of dosing.

       v. Acyclovir 400 mg orally twice daily

       vi. Valacyclovir 1 g orally once daily

       vii. Valacyclovir 500 mg orally once daily (might be somewhat less effective than valacyclovir 1 g or acyclovir in individuals who have 10 or more recurrences annually)

       viii. Famciclovir 250 mg orally twice daily (might be somewhat less effective for suppression of viral shedding)

Patient Case

3. K.D. is a 26-year-old woman with established HSV-2 infection, though she has had no visible lesions for more than 1 year. She is in a new relationship with a man who has never had genital or oral ulcers. Which is the best recommendation for K.D. to minimize the transmission of HSV-2 to her seronegative partner?

    A. Acyclovir 400 mg orally twice daily.

    B. Valacyclovir 500 mg orally once daily and consistent condom use.

    C. Acyclovir 800 mg orally twice daily during recurrences and avoidance of sexual activity during recurrences.

    D. Valacyclovir 500 mg orally once daily, consistent condom use, and avoidance of sexual activity during recurrences.

II. HUMAN IMMUNODEFICIENCY VIRUS

    A. Definitions

       1. HIV-1 infection: HIV-1 antibody and/or antigen positive

       2. AIDS: CD4+ cell count that is, or has ever been, less than 200 cells/mm^3 or development of an AIDS-defining illness (e.g., *Pneumocystis jiroveci* pneumonia [PJP], toxoplasmosis, Kaposi sarcoma, tuberculosis [TB], non-Hodgkin lymphoma, cryptococcal meningitis, *Mycobacterium avium* infection, CMV infection)

Patient Case

4. A.A. is a 29-year-old white man who has had a positive fourth-generation combination ELISA and an antibody differentiation assay positive for HIV-1. Today, his viral load is 58,525 copies/mL, and his CD4$^+$ cell count is 310 cells/mm^3. A WBC count is 9.8 x 10^3 cells/mm^3. The patient has fatigue and oral thrush. Which diagnosis is most appropriate for this patient?

    A. HIV.
    B. AIDS.
    C. Kaposi sarcoma.
    D. Immune reconstitution syndrome.

B. Historical Aspects of HIV
1. First U.S. cases reported in the early 1980s (June 1981 MMWR report)
2. Opportunistic infections in otherwise healthy white homosexual men
3. Early cases concentrated on the East and West coasts
4. Viral isolation in the mid-1980s
5. Disease has reached pandemic proportions, with an attached social stigma.

C. The Virus
1. HIV-1: Most common strain in the United States
2. HIV-2: Is predominant in Africa, less virulent
3. Retrovirus with RNA as baseline genetic material
4. Receptors
    a. CD4$^+$
    b. CCR5
    c. CXCR4
5. Enzymes (that serve as sites of action for current ARV agents)
    a. Reverse transcriptase
    b. Integrase
    c. Protease
6. Replication and mutation capabilities

D. Summary: Epidemiology *(Domain 5, Task 1)*
1. Global
    a. Significant impact on Africa (sub-Saharan regions)
    b. 50% of all infections in women
    c. 75% of infections are the result of heterosexual contact.
    d. Vertical transmission responsible for more than 95% of childhood infections
2. United States
    a. 2013: Estimated 50,000 new infections, 1.2 million infected
        i. 65% MSM
        ii. 17% heterosexual female individuals
        iii. 8% heterosexual male individuals
        iv. 6% intravenous drug users
        v. 3% MSM and intravenous drug users
        vi. Almost half of new infections in the United States are among African Americans.
    b. Rate of new infections has remained relatively stable since 2006.

    c.   An estimated 13% of infections are undiagnosed.

    d.   Since 1996, declines in AIDS diagnoses and deaths

    e.   Shifts in HIV infection toward women, minorities, and those residing in rural areas

E. Transmission *(Domain 1, Task 4; Domain 5, Task 1, 2)*
1. Classification
    a.   MSM
    b.   Heterosexual contact
2. Sexual practices
    a.   Anal intercourse (receptive: 0.3%; insertive: 0.06%)
    b.   Vaginal intercourse (receptive: 0.1%–0.2%; insertive: 0.03%–0.14%)
    c.   Oral sex (male receptive: 0.06%)
3. Injection drug use (transmission risk: 0.67%)
4. Perinatal/vertical
    a.   About a 25% risk of perinatal transmission without any ARV agents
    b.   AIDS Clinical Trials Group 076 was a pivotal study showing that the use of oral zidovudine beginning at 13–14 weeks' gestation (mother), zidovudine intravenous load and infusion during labor and delivery (mother), and oral zidovudine for first 6–8 weeks of life (neonate) reduced the risk to about 8% compared with placebo.
    c.   The current guidelines recommend that all women with HIV infection contemplating pregnancy receive a maximally suppressive ARV regimen and intravenous zidovudine added near delivery if the HIV RNA greater than 1000 copies/mL.
    d.   Breastfeeding is not recommended for women with HIV infection, regardless of antiretroviral therapy (ART).
    e.   Elective cesarean section: Viral load greater than 1000 copies/mL

Patient Cases

5.   B.T. is a 19-year-old white man who presents to your clinic for a baseline assessment. B.T. states that he regularly has sex with both men and women. You counsel him regarding safer sex practices. He asks, "What is my risk of contracting HIV from oral sex?" Which statement is most accurate?

    A.   The risk of acquiring HIV from oral sex is minimal, especially for the insertive partner.
    B.   Oral sex carries the same level of risk as other sexual practices.
    C.   Oral sex is associated with a high risk of acquiring HIV but a low risk with respect to other STDs.
    D.   The risk of oral sex is comparable with the risk of vaginal intercourse.

Patient Cases *(continued)*

6. C.C. is a 28-year-old white woman who acquired HIV from sharing needles with other injection drug users. Her viral load is 1000 copies/mL, and her CD4⁺ cell count is 400 cells/mm³. C.C. is in the 12th week of her first pregnancy. She is not taking ARV agents, and she refuses a complete HIV regimen because she "does not want to harm the baby." Which is the best advice for C.C.?

    A. Consider cesarean section instead of vaginal delivery to reduce HIV transmission risk.
    B. Consider initiating oral zidovudine monotherapy.
    C. Most ARV agents have been associated with fetal harm, and the risk of HIV transmission perinatally is very low; therefore, continue with the current course.
    D. Spontaneous abortion is common in women with HIV infection who are not taking ARV agents; consider starting therapy immediately.

    F. Prevention *(Domain 5, Task 2)*
        1. Standard precautions
        2. Latex condoms/polyurethane condoms
        3. Water-based lubricants
        4. Needle exchange programs (HIV, HBV, HCV)

Patient Cases

7. T.P. is a 45-year-old man who is HIV seronegative and has sex regularly with other men. He wishes to reduce his risk of acquiring HIV and other STDs. Which suggestion is the best counseling advice?

    A. Use oil-based lubricants accompanied by dental dams.
    B. No additional measures are necessary as long as serosorting is used with partners.
    C. Use water-based lubricants for oral sex and oil-based lubricants for all other exposures.
    D. Latex or polyurethane condoms should be used in all cases of exposure to sexual fluids.

8. Your municipality is considering the implementation of a needle exchange program. You are consulted on the merits of such a program. Which statement will best inform your opinion?

    A. An exchange program may reduce the community-wide incidence of HIV and hepatitis A.
    B. Exchange programs may reduce the transmission of HIV, HBV, and HCV.
    C. These programs may reduce the local incidence of syphilis and gonorrhea.
    D. Such programs have shown no significant reductions in the transmission of any disease.

    G. HIV Life Cycle/Pathophysiology *(Domain 1, Task 1)*
        1. CD4⁺ cells
        2. Coreceptors
        3. Conversion of viral RNA to viral DNA (reverse transcriptase)
        4. Integration of viral DNA into host cell DNA
        5. Translation of DNA and synthesis of proviral proteins
        6. Proteolytic conversion and activation of proteins
        7. Viral packaging and cellular departure

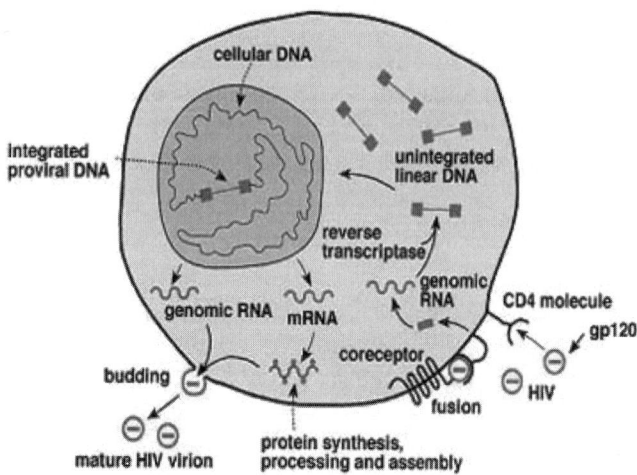

Figure 1. HIV replication cycle.

gp = glycoprotein; mRNA = messenger RNA.

Source: National Institute of Allergy and Infectious Diseases (NIAID)

[homepage on the Internet]. Bethesda, MD: National Institutes of Health. Available at www.niaid.nih.gov/topics/HIVAIDS/Understanding/howHIVCausesAIDS/pages/howhiv.aspx. Accessed September 15, 2015

Patient Cases

9. R.J. is a 23-year-old white man who regularly has sex with other men and recently moved to a large urban area for a new job. During the past 2–3 days, he has developed extreme malaise that has made it difficult for him to complete day-to-day tasks. He has missed 1 day of work. The malaise has been accompanied by intermittent fevers and a nonspecific rash. He presents to a local urgent care center, where an OraQuick assay is reactive. Which statement is most accurate?

    A. The symptoms described are most likely signs of an opportunistic infection.
    B. No confirmation of the OraQuick will be necessary because the patient is symptomatic.
    C. The patient is likely HIV seropositive with a high viral load.
    D. Confirmatory HIV testing should be performed with an HIV-1 NAAT. *ELISA*

10. M.C. is a 52-year-old white woman who lives in a large urban area in the United States where the HIV seroprevalence is estimated to be 1.3%. She is being seen by her primary care provider today. Which screening recommendation is best to make for this patient currently?

    A. Be screened at this time.
    B. Be screened only if she has had an episode of unprotected sex since the past visit.
    C. Be screened only as a component of perinatal care.
    D. Be screened at this visit unless she has previously been screened in the past 2 years.

11. A.D. is a 21-year-old college student who comes to your pharmacy and purchases an OraQuick test kit. Which is the most accurate counseling point?

    A. Whether negative or positive, the test results will require confirmation.
    B. The test kit is designed only to assay a fingerstick blood sample.
    C. Test results may not reflect any risk activities that occurred in the previous 3 months.
    D. After specimen acquisition, test results are available after a minimum of 1 hour.

H. Diagnosis and Screening *(Domain 1, Task 2; Domain 2, Task 5; Domain 5, Task 2)*
  1. High risk
      a. Men having sex with men
      b. Several sexual partners (male or female)
      c. Injection drug users
  2. Conversion syndrome (acute HIV infection)
      a. Occurs within days to weeks after initial infection
      b. High viral load
      c. Fever, rash, fatigue, malaise, lymphadenopathy
  3. Viral set point – Immune response to initial infection decreases viral load to set point.
  4. U.S. Preventive Services Task Force 2013: Routine screening for all Americans 15–64 years of age (annually for those at risk). Younger adolescents and older adults at increased risk should also be screened.
      a. Fourth-generation combination ELISA
          i. High sensitivity
          ii. Initial screening test; requires confirmation
          iii. Detects antibodies to HIV-1 and HIV-2 as well as p24 antigen (present in early infection)
          iv. If negative finding, no further testing
          v. If reactive, continue with antibody differentiation assay
      b. HIV-1/HIV-2 antibody differentiation assay
          i. Differentiates between HIV-1 and HIV-2; confirms infection
          ii. Detects HIV-1 antibodies earlier than the HIV-1 Western blot
          iii. Reduces indeterminate results
          iv. If negative or indeterminate findings, continue with HIV-1 NAAT test
      c. HIV-1 NAAT
          i. Distinguishes acute HIV-1 infection from false-positive initial immunoassay results in specimens with a reactive initial screening test result and nonreactive antibody differentiation assay result
          ii. Does not detect HIV-2
      d. Rapid HIV tests
          i. May make testing more accessible to at-risk populations
          ii. May test blood, plasma (or oral fluid for OraQuick)
          iii. Individuals with reactive test results should begin testing algorithm with fourth-generation combination assay.
          iv. Negative test results do not require confirmation, although it is recommended to repeat test in 6 months.
          v. Longer window period than newer tests (i.e., OraQuick detects antibodies 3 months after exposure)
  5. Window period – Time from infection to when testing will produce a positive result
      a. Combination assay with antigen detection reduces window from about 25 days to about 16 days.
      b. A NAAT reduces the window to 12 days.

I. Treatment Principles *(Domain 1, Task 2, 3, 4, 6)*
  1. Monotherapy is never appropriate (except in certain extenuating cases involving pregnancy).
  2. Standard of care consists of three active, concurrent ARV agents from at least two drug classes.
  3. HIV drug-resistance testing is indicated in treatment-naive patients initiating therapy and in treatment failure. Treatment failure: Inability to achieve undetectable viral load (less than 48 copies/mL) at 24 weeks or presence of a viremia in a patient who had previously achieved an undetectable viral load
  4. The primary goal of therapy is an undetectable viral load (lower limit of detection varies according to the assay); the secondary goal is an increase in the CD4$^+$ cell count.

5. Test for *HLA-B*5701* negativity before initiating any therapy that contains abacavir.
6. Therapy is lifelong and requires strict adherence.
7. For drug toxicity, it is acceptable to exchange a substitute drug from the same class as the offending agent without altering the entire ARV regimen.
8. Salvage therapy: Use of unconventional ARV combinations in an effort to achieve an undetectable viral load (usually in treatment-experienced patients)
9. Current treatment may reduce infectivity, but it is never curative.

J. HIV Drug-Resistance Testing *(Domain 1, Task 2, 6)*
    1. General principles
        a. Recommended for all individuals with HIV when they enter into care, regardless of ARV initiation
        b. If ART is deferred, repeated testing should be considered at the time of ARV initiation.
        c. Resistance testing should be done in patients whose therapy fails (ideally, while patients are taking current regimen or within 4 weeks of ARV discontinuation) and/or in cases of suboptimal viral load reduction.
        d. Requires a viral load of at least 1000 copies/mL to be performed (consider when viral load is 500–1000 copies/mL, though testing may be unsuccessful)
        e. Patients should continue receiving failing ARV regimens until test results are available.
    2. Genotype
        a. Analysis of viral genetic mutations known to be associated with resistance to particular ARV agents (standardly includes mutations in reverse transcriptase and protease genes; may add integrase strand transfer inhibitor [INSTI] genotype test)
        b. Less costly and quicker turnaround than phenotypic assays
        c. Provides resistant or susceptible data and the associated mutation present (e.g., M184V)
        d. May become particularly difficult to interpret when several mutations are present
        e. Preferred testing modality in treatment-naive and treatment-experienced patients
        f. Recommended for all pregnant women before initiation of ART and for those with detectable amounts of viral HIV RNA while on active therapy
    3. Phenotype
        a. Measure of direct susceptibility, which requires viral culture
        b. More costly and time-consuming than genotyping
        c. May account for "mixtures" of mutations that are synergistic or antagonistic
        d. Adding phenotypic testing to genotypic testing is generally preferred for patients with known or suspected complex drug resistance mutations, especially to protease inhibitors (PIs).

Table 1. Resistance Testing

	Relative Advantages	**Relative Limitations**
Genotypic	Ease of availability Shorter time to results (days) Less technically demanding Less costly	Indirect measure of susceptibility May not directly correlate with phenotype Expert interpretation required Insensitive to minor viral strains Reliance on mapped segments of HIV genome Lack of laboratory standardization
Phenotypic	Direct measure of susceptibility More familiar reporting results (IC_{50}, IC_{90})	Longer time to results Technically demanding Insensitive to minor viral strains Some clinically significant breakpoints undefined Costly

IC_{50}, IC_{90} = the concentration at which growth or activity is inhibited by 50% and 90%, respectively.

- K. ARV Agents
    1. Nucleoside reverse transcriptase inhibitors (NRTIs)
        a. Zidovudine
        b. Didanosine
        c. Stavudine
        d. Lamivudine
        e. Abacavir
        f. Emtricitabine
    2. Nucleotide reverse transcriptase inhibitor
        a. Tenofovir disoproxil fumarate (tenofovir DF)
        b. Tenofovir alafenamide fumarate (tenofovir AF)
    3. Nonnucleoside reverse transcriptase inhibitors (NNRTIs)
        a. Nevirapine
        b. Efavirenz
        c. Etravirine
        d. Rilpivirine
    4. PIs
        a. Saquinavir
        b. Ritonavir (primarily used as pharmacokinetic booster)
        c. Indinavir
        d. Nelfinavir
        e. Lopinavir
        f. Atazanavir
        g. Fosamprenavir
        h. Tipranavir
        i. Darunavir
    5. Fusion inhibitor: Enfuvirtide
    6. Coreceptor antagonist: Maraviroc
    7. INSTIs
        a. Raltegravir
        b. Dolutegravir
        c. Elvitegravir
    8. Pharmacokinetic booster (no ARV activity): Cobicistat

L. Initiating Therapy *(Domain 1, Task 3, 4, 6; Domain 2, Task 4)*

1. As of February 2013, ART is recommended for all HIV-seropositive patients.
   a. To reduce the risk of disease progression and HIV transmission
   b. Previous guidelines recommended treatment on the basis of specific CD4+ cell counts; the recommendation has changed because of the growing pool of data showing the consequences of uncontrolled HIV replication and the improved efficacy and tolerability of current therapies.
   c. Patients starting therapy should understand the risks and benefits of treatment and be willing and able to commit to therapy.
   d. Patients and/or providers may choose to defer or to initiate therapy on a case-by-case basis.

2. Recommended ARV combinations for patients who are ARV naive are as follows:
   a. PI-based regimen: Darunavir/ritonavir plus tenofovir DF/emtricitabine
   b. INSTI-based regimens
      i. Dolutegravir plus abacavir/lamivudine (only for patients who are *HLA-B*5701* negative)
      ii. Dolutegravir plus tenofovir DF/emtricitabine
      iii. Elvitegravir/cobicistat plus tenofovir DF/emtricitabine (only for patients with a creatinine clearance [CrCl] above 70 mL/minute/1.73 m^2 before ART)
      iv. Elvitegravir/cobicistat plus tenofovir AF/emtricitabine (only for patients with a CrCl above 30 mL/minute/1.73 m^2 before ART)
      v. Raltegravir plus tenofovir DF/emtricitabine
   c. Many alternative regimens may be considered the optimal regimen for some patients.
      i. Efavirenz plus tenofovir DF/emtricitabine
      ii. Rilpivirine plus tenofovir DF/emtricitabine (only for patients with a pretreatment HIV RNA less than 100,000 copies/mL and CD4 cell count greater than 200 cells/mm^3)
      iii. Atazanavir/cobicistat plus tenofovir DF/emtricitabine (only for patients whose CrCl is above 70 mL/minute/1.73 m^2 before ART)
      iv. Atazanavir/ritonavir plus tenofovir DF/emtricitabine
      v. Darunavir/cobicistat or darunavir/ritonavir plus abacavir/lamivudine (only for patients who are *HLA-B*5701* negative)
      vi. Darunavir/cobicistat plus tenofovir DF/emtricitabine (only for patients whose CrCl is above 70 mL/minute/1.73 m^2 before ART)
   d. ARV-naive pregnant women
      i. Preferred two-NRTI backbones (plus PI or NNRTI)
         (a) Abacavir plus lamivudine (only in patients who test negative for *HLA-B*5701* and not recommended with boosted atazanavir or efavirenz in patients with pretreatment HIV RNA more than 100,000 copies/mL)
         (b) Tenofovir DF plus emtricitabine
         (c) Tenofovir DF plus lamivudine
         (d) Zidovudine plus lamivudine
      ii. PI regimens
         (a) Ritonavir-boosted atazanavir plus a preferred two-NRTI backbone
         (b) Ritonavir-boosted darunavir plus a preferred two-NRTI backbone
      iii. NNRTI regimen: Efavirenz plus a preferred two-NRTI backbone; may be initiated after the first 8 weeks of pregnancy and requires postpartum contraception
      iv. INSTI regimen: Raltegravir plus a preferred two-NRTI backbone
   e. Factors to consider when selecting initial ARV regimen:
      i. Pretreatment HIV RNA level; do not use the following if greater than 100,000 copies/mL
         (a) Rilpivirine-based regimens
         (b) Abacavir/lamivudine plus efavirenz

       (c) Abacavir/lamivudine plus atazanavir/ritonavir

       (d) Darunavir/ritonavir plus raltegravir

   ii. Pretreatment CD4$^+$ cell count; do not use the following if less than 200 cells/mm^3

       (a) Rilpivirine-based regimens

       (b) Darunavir/ritonavir plus raltegravir

  iii. HIV genotypic drug resistance testing results

       (a) Use resistance testing to guide therapy.

       (b) Avoid NNRTI-based regimen if drug resistance tests not available

   iv. *HLA-B*5701* status; if positive, avoid abacavir

    v. Comorbidities

       (a) Chronic kidney disease: Consider avoiding tenofovir DF.

       (b) Osteoporosis: Consider avoiding tenofovir DF.

       (c) Psychiatric illness: Consider avoiding efavirenz.

       (d) Methadone: Consider avoiding efavirenz.

       (e) High cardiac risk: Consider avoiding abacavir or lopinavir/ritonavir.

       (f) Hyperlipidemia: The following drugs/drug classes have been associated with deleterious effects on lipids: ritonavir-boosted PIs, abacavir, efavirenz, elvitegravir/cobicistat

   vi. Pregnancy potential: See pregnancy section above.

  vii. Coinfections

       (a) HBV infection: Use tenofovir DF/emtricitabine or tenofovir DF/lamivudine, if possible.

       (b) HCV infection:

           (1) ART should be initiated in most HIV/HCV coinfected patients because the benefits of ARVs outweigh the risks (e.g., drug-induced liver toxicity).

           (2) ARV may slow the progression of liver disease by preserving immune function (HIV infection accelerates HCV infection).

           (3) Recommendations for initial ARVs are the same as for non–HCV-infected, but need to consider drug interactions and overlapping toxicities if HCV is being treated

           (4) It may be reasonable to delay ART in patients with CD4$^+$ counts greater than 500 cells/mm^3 until HCV treatment completed

           (5) In patients with CD4$^+$ counts less than 200 cells/mm^3, ART should be initiated promptly, and HCV treatment may be deferred until HIV treatment is stable.

           (6) Ledipasvir/sofosbuvir: No cytochrome P450 (CYP) interaction but increased tenofovir exposure

           (7) Ombitasvir/paritaprevir/dasabuvir/ritonavir: Substantial drug interactions

           (8) Simeprevir: Substantial drug interactions

       (c) TB: Consider drug interactions if using rifampin or rifabutin.

 viii. Regimen's genetic barrier to resistance

   ix. Potential adverse effects

    x. Drug interactions

   xi. Convenience (e.g., pill burden, dosing frequency, availability of fixed-dose combination product, food requirements)

       (a) One pill once-daily options include dolutegravir/abacavir/lamivudine, efavirenz/tenofovir DF/emtricitabine, elvitegravir/cobicistat/tenofovir DF/emtricitabine, rilpivirine/tenofovir DF/emtricitabine, and elvitegravir/cobicistat/tenofovir AF/emtricitabine.

       (b) To be taken with food: Boosted atazanavir, boosted darunavir, elvitegravir/cobicistat/tenofovir DF/emtricitabine, rilpivirine/tenofovir DF/emtricitabine, and elvitegravir/cobicistat/tenofovir AF/emtricitabine

       (c) To be taken on an empty stomach: Efavirenz

      xii.   Cost

      xiii. Patient preference

      xiv. Anticipated adherence

3. Several alternative and acceptable ARV regimens: Selected on a case-by-case basis; may be less satisfactory or offer disadvantages compared with recommended regimens

4. Other considerations

    a. Monotherapy should be avoided (although in unusual circumstances, zidovudine may be used alone in pregnancy to prevent perinatal transmission).

    b. NRTI-only regimens should be avoided.

    c. Efavirenz should not be used in the first 8 weeks of pregnancy or in women of childbearing potential who are not taking adequate contraception measures.

    d. Nevirapine should not be initiated in treatment-naive women with CD4$^+$ cell counts greater than 250 cells/mm^3 or in men with CD4$^+$ cell counts greater than 400 cells/mm^3.

    e. Zidovudine and stavudine should not be combined secondary to the risk of drug-drug antagonism.

    f. For other nuances, consult guidelines or HIV specialist.

Patient Cases

The following case pertains to questions 12–15:

P.R. is 32 years old with a history of methamphetamine abuse. He is given a diagnosis of HIV by his primary care provider and referred to your clinic for the potential initiation of ARV drug therapy. P.R. reports using no recreational drugs except for marijuana in the past 6 months. Laboratory values today include a viral load of 99,856 copies/mL and a CD4$^+$ cell count of 409 cells/mm^3.

12. Regarding the initiation of ARV drugs for this patient, which statement is most consistent with treatment consensus guidelines?

    A. ARV drugs are indicated to reduce the risk of disease progression and HIV transmission.

    B. ARV drugs are indicated on the basis of this patient's HIV viral load.

    C. ARV drugs are indicated because this patient's CD4$^+$ cell count is below a consensus treatment threshold.

    D. On the basis of the patient's laboratory values, ARV drugs are not indicated.

13. The decision is made to initiate ART for P.R. Which test is best to obtain in advance?

    A. Coreceptor tropism assay.

    B. Genotypic resistance testing.

    C. *HLA-B*5701* screening.

    D. Phenotypic resistance testing.

14. Which is the best ARV regimen for P.R.?

    A. Tenofovir DF/emtricitabine/efavirenz.

    B. Tenofovir DF/emtricitabine/nevirapine.

    C. Tenofovir DF/emtricitabine/dolutegravir.

    D. Tenofovir DF/emtricitabine/lopinavir/ritonavir.

Patient Cases (*continued*)

15. You sit down with P.R. to discuss his new medications, the possible adverse effects, and the importance of medication adherence. Which key point is best to include in P.R.'s counseling session?
    A. Therapy may be discontinued if the viral load remains undetectable for at least 1 year.
    B. If the patient experiences adverse events, he should seek medical attention before discontinuing the drug.
    C. The primary treatment goal will be to increase the CD4+ cell count.
    D. The primary treatment goal will be to reduce the viral load to fewer than 1000 copies/mL.

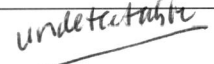

undetectable

Table 2. ARV Agents

Generic (Brand)	Adverse Effects	Dosing	Other
Nucleoside Reverse Transcriptase Inhibitors (NRTIs)			
Zidovudine (Retrovir)	Marrow suppression (especially anemia), N/V, headache	300 mg BID	Adjust for CrCl < 15 mL/min/1.73 m²; do not combine with stavudine
Didanosine EC (Videx EC)	Pancreatitis, peripheral neuropathy	400 mg/day	Take on an empty stomach, and do not crush or chew; adjust for CrCl < 60 mL/min/1.73 m²
Stavudine (Zerit)	Peripheral neuropathy	40 mg BID	Adjust for CrCl < 50 mL/min/1.73 m²
Lamivudine (Epivir)	Headache, nausea	150 mg BID or 300 mg/day	Adjust for CrCl < 50 mL/min/1.73 m²; active against HBV
Abacavir (Ziagen)	Hypersensitivity reaction (rash, shortness of breath)	300 mg BID or 600 mg/day	Hepatic dose adjustment, *HLA-B*5701* screening (positive test result precludes use)
Emtricitabine (Emtriva)	Headache, nausea	200 mg/day	Adjust for CrCl < 50 mL/min/1.73 m²; active against HBV
Nucleotide Reverse Transcriptase Inhibitor (NtRTI)			
Tenofovir DF (Viread)	Nephrotoxicity	300 mg/day	Adjust for CrCl < 50 mL/min/1.73 m²; active against HBV
NRTI/NtRTI Fixed-Dose Combinations			
Zidovudine/ lamivudine (Combivir)	Marrow suppression	1 capsule BID	Use individual agents if CrCl < 50 mL/min/1.73 m²
Zidovudine/ lamivudine/ abacavir (Trizivir)	Marrow suppression, hypersensitivity reaction, rash	1 capsule BID	Use individual agents if CrCl < 50 mL/min/1.73 m²; seldom used because of limited efficacy
Lamivudine/ abacavir (Epzicom)	Hypersensitivity reaction, rash	1 tablet daily	Use individual agents if CrCl < 50 mL/min/1.73 m²

Table 2. ARV Agents *(continued)*

Generic (Brand)	Adverse Effects	Dosing	Other
NRTI/NtRTI Fixed-Dose Combinations *(continued)*			
Emtricitabine/ tenofovir DF (Truvada)	Nephrotoxicity	1 tablet daily	Adjust for CrCl < 50 mL/min/1.73 m^2
Nonnucleoside Reverse Transcriptase Inhibitors (NNRTIs)			
Nevirapine (Viramune)	Rash (lower with dose titration), hepatotoxicity (risk based on sex and CD4$^+$ cell count)	200 mg/day x 2 wk; then 200 mg BID XR: 400 mg/day (only after 14-day 200-mg IR lead-in)	Contraindicated in moderate to severe liver impairment; low resistance ceiling
Efavirenz (Sustiva)	Rash, CNS disengagement (i.e., nightmares and vivid dreams)	600 mg at bedtime (to minimize CNS effects)	Take on an empty stomach; use with caution in liver dysfunction; avoid in patients with substance abuse or psychiatric issues
Etravirine (Intelence)	Rash, diarrhea	200 mg BID	Take after meals
Rilpivirine (Edurant)	Rash, headache	25 mg/day	Take with food; separate dose from antacids and H2-blockers, do not give with PPIs
NRTI/NtRTI/NNRTI Fixed-Dose Combinations			
Emtricitabine/ tenofovir DF/ efavirenz (Atripla)	Nephrotoxicity, CNS disengagement	1 tablet at bedtime	Take on an empty stomach; use individual agents if CrCl < 50 mL/min/1.73 m^2
Emtricitabine/ tenofovir DF/ rilpivirine (Complera)	Nephrotoxicity, rash	1 tablet daily	Take with food; separate dose from antacids and H2-blockers; do not give with PPIs
Protease Inhibitors			
Saquinavir (Invirase)	N/V, diarrhea	500 mg BID (boosted)	Take with food; use caution in hepatic impairment
Ritonavir (Norvir)	GI distress, perioral tingling	PK booster: 100–200 mg/day	Take with food; many drug interactions; used only as PK booster, no longer given in therapeutic doses
Indinavir (Crixivan)	Nephrolithiasis, increased bilirubin	800 mg BID (boosted)	Use caution in hepatic impairment; less commonly used because of toxicities; maintain hydration status

Table 2. ARV Agents *(continued)*

Generic (Brand)	Adverse Effects	Dosing	Other
Protease Inhibitors *(continued)*			
Nelfinavir (Viracept)	Diarrhea (amenable to OTC products), nausea	1250 mg BID	Take with food; do not use in moderate to severe hepatic dysfunction
Lopinavir/ ritonavir (Kaletra)	GI upset	2 tablets BID or 4 tablets daily	Use caution in hepatic impairment
Atazanavir (Reyataz)	Increased bilirubin	400 mg/day (boosting depends on concomitant acid suppression and ARV experience)	Take with food; separate dose from antacids and H2-blockers; do not give with PPIs; use caution in hepatic dysfunction; PI least likely to alter serum lipids
Atazanavir/ cobicistat (Evotaz)	Increased bilirubin, increased creatinine	1 tablet daily (ATV 300 mg plus COBI 150 mg)	Take with food
Fosamprenavir (Lexiva)	N/V, diarrhea	700 mg BID (boosting depends on drug interactions and ARV experience)	Hepatic dose adjustment
Tipranavir (Aptivus)	GI upset	500 mg BID (boosted)	Take with food; do not use in moderate to severe hepatic dysfunction; specific resistance profile
Darunavir (Prezista)	GI upset, rash	600 mg BID (boosted) or 800 mg/day (boosted)	Take with food; do not use in severe hepatic dysfunction; unique resistance profile
Darunavir/ cobicistat (Prezcobix)	GI upset, rash, increased creatinine	1 tablet once daily	Take with food
Fusion Inhibitor			
T-20, enfuvirtide (Fuzeon)	Injection-site reactions	90 mg subcutaneously BID	Reserved for salvage therapy; costly
CCR5 Inhibitor			
Maraviroc (Selzentry)	Cardiovascular, hepatotoxicity	150 mg BID	Adjust if CrCl < 30 mL/min/1.73 m^2; requires coreceptor tropism assay before use (need to confirm R5 virus); costly

Table 2. ARV Agents *(continued)*

Generic (Brand)	Adverse Effects	Dosing	Other
Integrase Inhibitors			
Raltegravir (Isentress)	Diarrhea, N/V, increased creatinine phosphokinase	400 mg BID	Minimal drug interactions
Dolutegravir (Tivicay)	Insomnia, headache, hypersensitivity reaction, hepatotoxicity	Integrase inhibitor naive (without concomitant rifampin, efavirenz, fosamprenavir/ritonavir, tipranavir/ritonavir): 50 mg/day All others: 50 mg BID	May retain activity against raltegravir- and elvitegravir-resistant strains
Elvitegravir (Vitekta)	Nausea, diarrhea	With once-daily atazanavir/ritonavir or BID lopinavir/ritonavir: 85 mg once daily; with BID darunavir/ritonavir, fosamprenavir/ritonavir, or tipranavir/ritonavir: 150 mg once daily	Take with food; unboosted elvitegravir is not recommended
Integrase Inhibitor Fixed-Dose Combination			
Elvitegravir/ cobicistat/ emtricitabine/ tenofovir DF (Stribild)	Diarrhea, nephrotoxicity	1 tablet daily	Take with food; separate from antacids, do not initiate if CrCl < 70 mL/min/1.73 m^2 and discontinue if CrCl < 50 mL/min/1.73 m^2; do not use in severe hepatic dysfunction
Abacavir/ lamivudine/ dolutegravir (Triumeq)	Insomnia, headache, fatigue, hypersensitivity reaction	1 tablet daily (if concomitant efavirenz, fosamprenavir/ritonavir, tipranavir/ritonavir, or rifampin; then an additional dose of dolutegravir 50 mg, separated 12 hr from Triumeq, should be taken)	*HLA-B*5701* screening (positive test result precludes use); take with or without food; use individual agents if CrCl < 50 mL/min/1.73 m^2; do not use in moderate or severe hepatic impairment
Elvitegravir/ cobicistat/ tenofovir AF/ emtricitabine (Genvoya)	Nausea, diarrhea, headache, fatigue, hyperlipidemia	1 tablet daily	Take with food; separate from antacids, do not initiate if CrCl < 30 mL/min/1.73 m^2; do not use in severe hepatic dysfunction

ARV = antiretroviral; CNS = central nervous system; CrCl = creatinine clearance; DF = disoproxil fumarate; EC = enteric coated; GI = gastrointestinal; HBV = hepatitis B virus; H$_2$ = histamine-2; IR = immediate release; N/V = nausea/vomiting; OTC = over-the-counter; PI = protease inhibitor; PK = pharmacokinetic; PPI = proton pump inhibitor; XR = extended release.

M. Common Drug-Drug Interactions *(Domain 1, Task 3)*
1. Interaction resources (www.hiv-druginteractions.org and HIV treatment guidelines)
2. NRTI/nucleotide reverse transcriptase inhibitor drug interactions
   a. Zidovudine should not be dosed with stavudine because of the competition for intracellular activation.
   b. Didanosine should not be dosed with tenofovir because of increased didanosine concentrations and risk of toxicity.
   c. Didanosine should be separated from atazanavir (give atazanavir with food 2 hours before or 1 hour after didanosine).
   d. When dosed with tenofovir, atazanavir will require dose adjustment; avoid unboosted atazanavir with tenofovir.
   e. Tenofovir exposure is increased when given with ledipasvir/sofosbuvir and rilpivirine, efavirenz, or boosted elvitegravir. The safety of tenofovir and ledipasvir/sofosbuvir with concomitant boosted PIs has not been established. Consider alternative HCV PIs or ARV drugs to avoid increased tenofovir exposure.
   f. Ribavirin increases concentrations of didanosine and zidovudine, and the combinations should not be coadministered.
3. NNRTI drug interactions
   a. The following ARV agents must be dose adjusted when dosed with efavirenz: all PIs, dolutegravir, maraviroc, and raltegravir. Elvitegravir/cobicistat is not recommended with efavirenz.
   b. The following ARV agents are not recommended with etravirine: efavirenz, nevirapine, atazanavir, fosamprenavir, indinavir, nelfinavir, tipranavir, saquinavir, indinavir, lopinavir/ritonavir, atazanavir, tipranavir, and elvitegravir/cobicistat. The following ARV agents must be dose adjusted with etravirine: ritonavir, rilpivirine, dolutegravir, and maraviroc.
   c. The following ARV agents must be dose adjusted when dosed with rilpivirine: atazanavir, fosamprenavir, indinavir, nelfinavir, ritonavir, saquinavir, tipranavir, all NNRTIs, and didanosine. Elvitegravir/cobicistat is not recommended with rilpivirine.
   d. Rilpivirine should not be dosed with proton pump inhibitors (PPIs); they should be spaced when dosing with antacids and/or histamine-2 receptor blockers.
   e. Interactions vary by individual agent, but in general, interactions occur with the following medications or classes: azole antifungal agents, benzodiazepines, HCV PIs, methadone, dexamethasone, clarithromycin, oral contraceptives, immunosuppressants, rifamycins, statins, anticonvulsants, antidepressants, and phosphodiesterase inhibitors.
4. PI drug interactions
   a. Unboosted atazanavir should not be given with PPIs, and regardless of boosting, concomitant PPIs should not be given to PI-experienced patients receiving atazanavir. In addition, atazanavir should be spaced when dosing with antacids and/or histamine-2 receptor blockers.
   b. Ritonavir has many drug-drug interactions, and references should always be consulted with respect to the drug's effects. In most cases, ritonavir acts as a potent CYP inhibitor and can be used in low doses to intentionally boost the concentrations of other PIs.
   c. Many interactions with PIs and other ARVs (especially NNRTIs, INSTIs, and maraviroc) require dosing adjustments.
   d. Boosted tipranavir significantly decreases concentrations of saquinavir, amprenavir, and lopinavir.
   e. Fluticasone inhalers should be avoided in combination with PIs. Concurrent dosing may result in a Cushing-like syndrome.
   f. Coadministration of salmeterol and PIs is not recommended for risk of supratherapeutic concentrations of the β_2-agonist.
   g. Concentrations of oral contraceptives are substantially reduced when given with ritonavir-boosted PIs. May need to recommend alternative or additional contraceptive method

    h.   Potential interactions with several classes of medications including statins, benzodiazepines, calcium channel blockers, calcineurin inhibitors, anticonvulsants, rifamycins, agents for erectile dysfunction, ergot derivatives, azole antifungal agents, macrolides, oral contraceptives, methadone, HCV PIs, and herbal products (e.g., St. John's wort)

5.   CCR5 antagonist interactions: Maraviroc is a CYP3A4 substrate and has several dosing schemes, depending on the coadministered ARV drugs.

6.   INSTIs

    a.   Dolutegravir and elvitegravir are CYP3A4 substrates and have several dosing schemes, depending on coadministered ARV drugs.

    b.   Raltegravir is not a CYP3A4 substrate and has minimal drug interactions.

    c.   Potential interactions with the following medications or classes: Azole antifungal agents, benzodiazepines, calcineurin inhibitors, erectile dysfunction agents, HCV PIs, rifamycins, salmeterol, and statins

7.   Fusion inhibitor interactions: None

8.   Pharmacokinetic boosters

    a.   Potential for increased nephrotoxicity with cobicistat (not recommended in combination with tenofovir DF in patients whose CrCl is less than 70 mL/minute/17.3 m^2)

    b.   Drug interactions with ritonavir discussed in PIs above

N.   Treatment Failure *(Domain 1, Task 6, 7)*

1.   When the viral load fails to become undetectable within 24 weeks of therapy or when a previously undetectable viral load becomes detectable (greater than 48 copies/mL)

2.   Assessment of virologic failure

    a.   Change in viral load/CD4$^+$ cell counts over time

    b.   History of ARV exposure

    c.   Resistance testing

    d.   Medication adherence/tolerability

    e.   Concomitant medications

    f.   Comorbidities

3.   Management

    a.   In general, ARV regimens should be changed as soon as possible.

    b.   New ARV regimen should contain at least two (ideally three) fully active ARV agents. A fully active ARV is one that is likely to have activity given the patient's history (drug-resistance testing results or the drug's novel mechanism of action).

    c.   Discontinuing or even briefly stopping therapy may result in a swift increase in HIV RNA, a decline in CD4$^+$ count, and an increase in the risk of disease progression. Therapy interruption is not recommended.

Patient Cases

16. T.T. is a patient with established HIV infection whose regimen is being changed from emtricitabine/tenofovir DF (Truvada) plus ritonavir-boosted darunavir to lamivudine/abacavir (Epzicom) plus ritonavir-boosted darunavir. The change is being made because the patient has developed some mild renal insufficiency. Which laboratory value is best to obtain currently?

    A. Renal ultrasonography.
    B. *HLA-B*5701* screen.
    C. Hepatitis B surface antibody.
    D. Bone density scan.

17. B.W. is a 42-year-old white woman with HIV whose condition is currently managed with the following ARV regimen: zidovudine, lamivudine, and atazanavir boosted with ritonavir. Which statement is most accurate regarding ritonavir boosting?

    A. Ritonavir is an effective booster because of its potent effects as a CYP inducer.
    B. When used as a booster, ritonavir should not be counted as a component of triple-drug ARV regimens.
    C. Ritonavir boosting is most often used to augment serum concentrations of reverse transcriptase inhibitors.
    D. When used as a booster, ritonavir doses are usually 200 mg twice daily.

18. A patient is to initiate an ARV regimen with emtricitabine/tenofovir DF/efavirenz (Atripla). Which adverse effect is best to monitor for?

    A. Anxiety, vivid dreams, gastrointestinal (GI) upset.
    B. Jaundice, nausea/vomiting, retinitis.
    C. Sedation, rash, erectile dysfunction.
    D. Hypersensitivity reaction, hypertension, malaise.

19. P.R. is a 45-year-old white man with a history of AIDS. His initial diagnosis was made 15 years earlier with an admission for PJP. The patient currently takes the following medications: Zidovudine, lamivudine, darunavir boosted with ritonavir, trimethoprim/sulfamethoxazole double strength (DS), omeprazole, and zolpidem. With his current ARV regimen, P.R.'s condition has remained stable with an undetectable viral load for more than 2 years, and his CD4$^+$ cell counts are 180–200 cells/mm^3. Recent laboratory tests show a viral load of 985 copies/mL and a CD4$^+$ cell count of 195 cells/mm^3. He reports that he is fully adherent, "never missing a dose of his medications." One week before his most recent laboratory tests, P.R. reports that he had a prolonged episode of otitis media requiring 14 days of oral antibiotics. Which is the most appropriate intervention now?

    A. Assess tympanic membranes and reinitiate oral antibiotics for another 14-day course.
    B. Order a genotypic resistance assay.
    C. Discontinue the current ARV regimen and initiate therapy with three new drugs.
    D. Repeat the viral load test and CD4$^+$ cell count at today's visit.

O. Vaccinations *(Domain 1, Task 5; Domain 5, Task 2)*
   1. Live vaccines must be given with caution to HIV-seropositive patients.
      a. Measles, mumps, rubella
         i. Recommended for adults with HIV infection having a CD4$^+$ cell count greater than 200 cells/mm^3 who lack immunity to measles
         ii. Contraindicated if CD4$^+$ cell count is less than 200 cells/mm^3

b. Varicella
   i. Recommended for adults with HIV infection having a CD4$^+$ cell count greater than 200 cells/mm^3 who lack immunity to VZV
   ii. Contraindicated if CD4$^+$ cell count is less than 200 cells/mm^3
c. Zoster
   i. Contains much higher titers of varicella virus than the varicella vaccine
   ii. The Advisory Committee on Immunization Practices (ACIP) guidelines do not recommend for or against this vaccine.
   iii. Contraindicated if CD4$^+$ cell count is less than 200 cells/mm^3
d. Live attenuated influenza vaccine (LAIV), nasal spray: LAIV is contraindicated in individuals with HIV infection but not in their household contacts.

2. Recommended inactivated vaccines
   a. Hepatitis A (chronic liver disease, intravenous drug users, or MSM)
   b. HBV
   c. Pneumococcal
      i. The ACIP guidelines changed in 2012 to recommend the conjugate 13-valent pneumococcal vaccine (PCV13) to certain high-risk adult patients (including patients with HIV infection). Of note, in 2014, ACIP began recommending one dose of PCV13 to all adults 65 years and older.
      ii. After one dose of PCV13, subsequent doses may be given with the 23-valent polysaccharide pneumococcal vaccine (PPSV23) at least 8 weeks after PCV13; a second dose of PPSV23 may be given 5 years after the first dose of PPSV23.
      iii. For patients who have previously received PPSV23, a one-time dose of PCV13 may be given no less than 1 year after the latest PPSV23 dose, and subsequent doses may be given with PPSV23.
      iv. In both situations, patients who have received PPSV23 before age 65 years should receive one additional dose of PPSV23 after age 65 years or if the latest PPSV23 was given within 5 years.
   d. Diphtheria, tetanus, and pertussis (Tdap) (once during adulthood and then tetanus and diphtheria [Td] every 10 years)
   e. Influenza (inactivated form yearly)
   f. HPV vaccine
      i. Recommended in 13- to 26-year-olds with HIV infection
      ii. Males – Quadrivalent or 9-valent
      iii. Females – Bivalent, quadrivalent, or 9-valent

Patient Case

20. You evaluate the condition of a new HIV-seropositive patient (risk factor: MSM) who refuses to consider the initiation of ARV drugs and does not meet the indications for opportunistic infection prophylaxis. His laboratory values are unremarkable. He is hepatitis A antibody negative, hepatitis B surface antigen negative and surface antibody positive, and hepatitis C antibody negative. The patient cannot recall his latest tetanus booster and is up-to-date on all childhood immunizations. The patient is allergic to penicillin (rash). Which set of vaccinations is best?

    A. Intranasal influenza, hepatitis B.
    B. Influenza (intramuscular), PPSV23 (Pneumovax).
    C. Hepatitis A; influenza (intramuscular); Tdap; PCV13 (Prevnar 13).
    D. Hepatitis A and B plus influenza (intramuscular), diphtheria and tetanus toxoids and acellular pertussis (DTaP), PPSV23 (Pneumovax).

P. TB Screening *(Domain 5, Task 2)*
1. Mantoux test (purified protein derivative ([PPD]) of tuberculin)
   a. Yearly screening
   b. Read in 48–72 hours.
   c. Positive test (greater than 5 mm) – Follow up with chest radiograph.
2. Blood-based assays: QuantiFERON-TB; T-SPOT may be used instead of PPD

Patient Case

21. A nurse places a PPD on a 26-year-old white man with AIDS. This test will serve as his yearly TB screen. Which statement best summarizes a correctly administered and read screening procedure?

A. Read the skin test reaction (induration) in 2 hours, and if positive, refer for pulmonary CT scan.
B. Boost the original PPD in 24 hours, and then read the infiltrate.
C. Read the induration in 48 hours, and if greater than 5 mm, refer for chest radiograph.
D. After PPD placement, administer an anergy panel and read in 72 hours; if greater than 15 mm, refer for pulmonary magnetic resonance imaging.

Q. Opportunistic Infections *(Domain 1, Task 6)*
1. Opportunistic infection prophylaxis
   a. Primary: Prevention of initial infection
   b. Secondary: Prevention of reinfection
   c. Discontinuation: Acceptable if patient's CD4$^+$ count is above threshold for at least 3 months with a sustained undetectable viral load (primary vs. secondary)
2. Common opportunistic infections
   a. PJP
      i. Symptoms: Cough, fever, hypoxia
      ii. Primary prophylaxis (CD4$^+$ cell count less than 200 cells/mm^3): Trimethoprim/sulfamethoxazole 1 DS tablet daily, 1 single-strength tablet daily, or 1 DS tablet three times weekly
      iii. Secondary prophylaxis: Trimethoprim/sulfamethoxazole (orally)
      iv. Treatment: Trimethoprim/sulfamethoxazole (intravenously; may change to oral formulation after clinical improvement) for 21 days; add prednisone taper if Pao2 less than 70 mm Hg
      v. Prophylaxis alternatives: Dapsone; atovaquone; pentamidine
      vi. Discontinuation: CD4$^+$ cell count greater than 200 cells/mm^3 for at least 3 months
   b. Toxoplasmosis (*Toxoplasma gondii*)
      i. Symptoms: Headache, confusion
      ii. Primary prophylaxis (CD4$^+$ cell count less than 100 cells/mm^3): Trimethoprim/sulfamethoxazole 1 DS tablet daily
      iii. Secondary prophylaxis: Sulfadiazine plus pyrimethamine (reduced treatment doses) plus leucovorin
      iv. Treatment: Sulfadiazine plus pyrimethamine plus leucovorin
      v. Prophylaxis alternatives: Dapsone plus pyrimethamine plus leucovorin: Atovaquone with or without pyrimethamine plus leucovorin
      vi. Discontinuation: CD4$^+$ cell count greater than 200 cells/mm^3 for at least 3 months (6 months in cases of secondary prophylaxis after a full treatment course)
   c. *Mycobacterium avium* complex
      i. Symptoms: Cough, fever, lymphadenopathy, disseminated infection (positive blood cultures)
      ii. Primary prophylaxis (CD4$^+$ cell count less than 50 cells/mm^3): Azithromycin 1200 mg weekly

  iii. Secondary prophylaxis: Clarithromycin plus ethambutol with or without rifabutin

  iv. Treatment: Clarithromycin plus ethambutol with or without rifabutin

  v. Prophylaxis alternative: Clarithromycin, rifabutin, pentamidine

  vi. Discontinuation: CD4$^+$ cell count greater than 100 cells/mm^3 for at least 3 months (6 months for secondary prophylaxis after a full treatment course)

 d. Candidiasis

  i. Treatment of oropharyngeal (thrush): Fluconazole

  ii. Treatment of esophageal: Fluconazole

 e. HSV-1 and HSV-2

  i. Acyclovir or similar analog

  ii. Treatment (high dose) versus suppressive therapy (ongoing low dose)

  iii. New recommendation: Consider initiating suppressive acyclovir for patients beginning ART with a CD4$^+$ count less than 250 cells/mm^3

Patient Cases

22. R.L. is a 22-year-old white man who acquired HIV from a blood transfusion when a child. His CD4$^+$ cell count is 210 cells/mm^3 with a viral load of 56,456 copies/mL. R.L. is to begin ART at today's clinic visit. His only concern is oral thrush, which he noticed while brushing his teeth this morning. Which intervention is most appropriate currently?

 A. Initiate 7–10 days of atovaquone therapy plus trimethoprim/sulfamethoxazole DS 1 tablet by mouth every day.

 B. Prescribe azithromycin 1200 mg by mouth once weekly.

 C. Suggest peroxide, have the patient rinse twice daily, and prescribe trimethoprim/sulfamethoxazole DS 1 tablet by mouth three times weekly.

 D. Initiate fluconazole therapy by mouth for 7–10 days.

23. C.C. is a 45-year-old HIV-seropositive woman who entered care after an episode of acute PJP that required intubation and intravenous therapy. During her PJP illness, a history of a sulfa allergy was discovered. C.C. currently receives ART for HIV plus dapsone, omeprazole, zolpidem as needed, fluconazole, and ondansetron as needed. Currently, the patient's viral load is 1000 copies/mL (down from 234,000 copies/mL 3 months earlier), and her CD4$^+$ cell count is 90 cells/mm^3. In reviewing her medication therapy, which intervention is most appropriate?

 A. The patient requires no alterations or additions to pharmacotherapy.

 B. Azithromycin 1200 mg by mouth once weekly should be added.

 C. If continued therapy is anticipated, dapsone should be administered intravenously.

 D. The current regimen provides insufficient prophylaxis against toxoplasmosis.

Patient Cases (*continued*)

24. A.A. is a 52-year-old African American man given a diagnosis of AIDS in 1994. The patient's viral load then was 150,000 copies/mL, and his CD4$^+$ cell count was 12 cells/mm^3. Throughout A.A.'s illness, he has received diagnoses of, and been treated for, PJP, zoster, and several episodes of community-acquired pneumonia. For the past 2 years, his viral load has been less than 48 copies/mL, and his CD4$^+$ cell count has been no lower than 300 cells/mm^3. Which statement regarding this patient is most consistent with current guidelines?
    A. He is probably not taking any opportunistic infection prophylaxis currently.
    B. He is likely receiving therapy with both azithromycin and trimethoprim/sulfamethoxazole DS.
    C. He is a candidate for immunization with varicella.
    D. He may initiate therapy with antibiotic prophylaxis for the prevention of recurrent community-acquired pneumonia.

R. Postexposure Prophylaxis (PEP) and Preexposure Prophylaxis (PrEP) (*Domain 1, Task 6, 7; Domain 5, Task 2*)
  1. Occupational PEP
     a. Principles
        i. Treatment should be immediately available.
        ii. Exposure should be confirmed.
        iii. A PEP regimen with the best chance of adherence should be selected.
        iv. Adverse effects should be anticipated, monitored, and treated.
     b. Risk of infection
        i. Percutaneous (risk: 0.3%)
        ii. Mucus membrane (risk: 0.09%)
        iii. Non-intact skin (risk: Less than 0.09%)
     c. Treatment
        i. Tenofovir DF plus emtricitabine plus raltegravir for 30 days
        ii. Baseline and follow-up testing
        iii. Safe sex
  2. Nonoccupational PEP (nPEP)
     a. Recommended for individuals exposed to blood, genital secretions, or other potentially infectious body fluids from a known individual with HIV infection within 72 hours of exposure
        i. ARVs should be initiated as soon as possible.
        ii. Preferred regimens include zidovudine or tenofovir DF plus lamivudine or emtricitabine plus efavirenz OR zidovudine plus lamivudine or emtricitabine plus lopinavir/ritonavir.
        iii. Clinicians may consider prescribing nPEP if patients present after 72 hours of exposure if the diminished potential benefit of nPEP outweighs the risks for transmission and adverse effects.
     b. If the HIV status is unknown, there is no formal recommendation. Clinicians must evaluate on a case-by-case basis.
  3. PrEP: Controversial public health intervention to reduce transmission among high-risk individuals
     a. May consider for any of the following populations deemed at substantial risk of HIV acquisition (risk based on the number of new partners, frequency of condom use, new STDs, sexual practices, sharing needles):
        i. Sexually active adult MSM
        ii. Heterosexually active adult men and women
        iii. Adult injection drug users
        iv. Adults with HIV-seropositive sexual partner (HIV discordant couples)

b. Confirm HIV status before PrEP initiation.

c. Screen for STDs/HBV/sufficient renal function (must be more than 60 mL/minute).

d. Tenofovir DF 300 mg plus emtricitabine 200 mg (Truvada) once daily x 90 days

e. Screen for incident HIV infection every 3 months.

f. Monitor renal function, and screen for STDs every 6 months.

g. Ongoing: Risk reduction, condoms, counseling

Patient Cases

25. You receive a frantic call from a registered nurse (RN) during your morning shift. She reports that in the past evening, she sustained a needlestick while performing a venipuncture in the emergency department. The patient's HIV status was unknown, but the patient did have a history of injection drug use. At home during the evening, the RN began searching the Internet for information on HIV transmission from needlesticks, and she became more concerned. Which recommendation is the best course of action?

A. Immediately consider initiating a three-drug ARV regimen.

B. The time at which the needlestick injury occurred is beyond the period during which it may be efficacious to begin PEP; refer the nurse for HIV rapid testing.

C. Immediately begin two-drug ART for the prevention of both HIV and HCV transmission.

D. Start administering hepatitis A and B immunizations.

26. T.T. is a 32-year-old homosexual man who regularly engages in unprotected anal intercourse. The patient sporadically uses condoms during sexual encounters, stating that they reduce sensations. He recently read an Internet article about the use of HIV drugs to prevent new infections and asks you about this practice. Which counseling point is most appropriate?

A. Atripla is commonly used to reduce transmission risk in high-risk seronegative patients.

B. Most PrEP protocols involving ARV drugs involve once-weekly dosing and increased HIV screening.

C. The use of PrEP will require more frequent HIV and HBV screening.

D. If PrEP is used, there is no need for condoms during sexual encounters.

S. Managing Adverse Effects and Comorbidities (*Domain 1, Task 3, 4, 5*)

1. Nausea and vomiting
   a. May respond to PPIs, histamine receptor blockers, antacids, prokinetics
   b. As-needed antiemetics such as prochlorperazine, promethazine, or ondansetron may be considered for patients with severe concerns.
   c. Avoid PPIs in combination with atazanavir and rilpivirine.
   d. Space doses of histamine-2 receptor blockers and antacids when they are combined with atazanavir and rilpivirine.

2. Diarrhea
   a. Consider loperamide.
   b. Nelfinavir-induced diarrhea is common and responds well to over-the-counter (OTC) products.

3. Depression
   a. Selective serotonin receptor inhibitors are often the preferred agents.
   b. Duloxetine and other selective serotonin and norepinephrine receptor blockers may be beneficial for patients with peripheral neuropathies.

4. Hyperlipidemia
   a. Treat it as you would in an HIV-seronegative patient.
   b. Counseling to promote diet and exercise

    c.   Certain ARV agents may be more commonly associated with lipid disturbances, whereas only atazanavir has been associated with reductions in serum lipids.

    d.   Preferred LDL-C–lowering agents include pravastatin, atorvastatin, and rosuvastatin. Other statins should be avoided because of their propensity to interact with various PIs.

5.   Anxiety: Avoid triazolam and midazolam.

6.   TB

    a.   Avoid rifampin; substitute with rifabutin, which decreases but does not avoid interaction.

    b.   Several drug-drug interactions; consult references and/or expert

7.   Erectile dysfunction

    a.   Common condition among men with HIV infection secondary to hypogonadism and/or depression

    b.   Use erectile dysfunction medications cautiously, especially when co-prescribed with ritonavir (dose reductions will be necessary).

        i.   Sildenafil: 25 mg every 48 hours

        ii.   Vardenafil: 2.5 mg every 72 hours

        iii.   Tadalafil: 10 mg every 72 hours

8.   Common recreational drugs of abuse

    a.   Methamphetamine

    b.   Methylenedioxymethamphetamine

    c. γ-Hydroxybutyric acid

    d.   Amyl and butyl nitrates and nitrite "poppers"

T. Patient Advocacy *(Domain 2, Task 5, 7; Domain 4, Task 7; Domain 5, Task 1)*

1.   HIV is a considerable financial burden for patients (clinic visits, consults, laboratory assays, ARV agents, antimicrobial medications, ancillary medications).

2.   Confidentiality: Critical when working with this population given the significant social stigma associated with HIV infection

3.   Healthy People 2020: Several HIV-related objectives, including the following: Reduce the number of U.S. HIV and AIDS cases; increase the percentage of Americans tested for HIV in the past 12 months and the number of Americans with HIV who are receiving standard-of-care treatment.

4.   Several national and local support, resource, and volunteer agencies

    a.   "The Body" (www.thebody.com)

    b.   UNAIDS (United Nations AIDS Service)

    c.   AIDS Treatment Data Network

    d.   AIDS Education and Training Centers

    e.   AIDS Info (aidsinfo.nih.gov)

U. Practice Management *(Domain 2, Task 6, 7; Domain 5, Task 2)*

1.   Comprehensive HIV care requires multidisciplinary teams that include physicians, pharmacists, nurses, social workers, and counselors.

2.   Pharmacist roles: Interaction monitoring, drug histories, drug selection, resistance testing analysis, medication acquisition, adherence counseling, therapeutic drug monitoring, safer-sex counseling, drug information

3.   Medication acquisition outlets: AIDS Drug Assistance Programs; patient assistance programs; manufacturer voucher programs as available

4.   Ryan White CARE Act (potential clinical funding source)

5. Credentialing programs: AAHIVP (American Academy of HIV Medicine Pharmacist), formerly AAHIVE (American Academy of HIV Medicine Subject Expert)
   a. Qualifications: Graduate of an accredited college of pharmacy, licensed pharmacist, required experience in HIV patient care (20 patients with HIV/AIDS in the past 24 months), 30 hours of HIV-related continuing education in the previous 24 months
   b. Examination (2-year renewal and recertification period)

III. NON-HIV VIRAL INFECTIONS

A. Influenza *(Domain 1, Task 2, 3, 4, 5, 6; Domain 5, Task 2)*
   1. Overview
      a. RNA viruses; influenza A and B are the most common serotypes
         i. Envelopes contain two surface proteins: hemagglutinin (H) and neuraminidase (N).
         ii. Influenza A viruses are further classified into subtypes according to the antigenicity of these surface proteins (i.e., H1N1 and H3N2).
            (a) Hemagglutinin (H), 17 subtypes
            (b) Neuraminidase (N), 10 subtypes
         iii. Influenza B is not divided into subtypes but can be further broken down into different strains on the basis of characteristics such as geographic origin and year of isolation.
      b. Genome is divided into eight segments.
      c. Influenza season is defined by when influenza viruses are circulating in the community, from about September to April in the Northern Hemisphere (typically peaks from December to March).
      d. Associated with high rates of morbidity and mortality in the United States annually
         i. Around 200,000 hospitalizations
         ii. Around 36,000 deaths
      e. Large impact on outpatient health services
      f. Transmission occurs by large-particle respiratory droplets that can be passed through personal contact and/or contact with contaminated surfaces.
      g. Incubation 1–4 days (average 2 days); adults shed viruses for 1 day before symptom onset and for 5–10 days after illness onset (children may be infectious for slightly longer)
      h. Most infections are self-limited and resolve without complications; however, severe disease can lead to hospitalization and even death, especially in high-risk patients.
         i. Older adults
         ii. Very young
         iii. Patients with chronic medical conditions (e.g., immunocompromised, diabetes, COPD, chronic renal dysfunction, cancer, neuromuscular diseases, sickle cell anemia, residence in long-term care facility, body mass index greater than 40 kg/m^2, women who are pregnant or within 2 weeks of delivery)
      i. Vaccination, the best means of prevention, should be administered to everyone, especially those who are at high risk of complications (see Prevention section below).
      j. Antigenic variation – Moving target for diagnostics and treatment
         i. Antigenic drift
            (a) Occurs in influenza A and B viruses
            (b) Minor antigenic change within H or N surface proteins caused by accumulation of point mutations
            (c) Allows spread of virus within a population, despite the presence of antibody to previous strains of the virus, which may result in small epidemics

      ii. Antigenic shift

          (a) Occurs in influenza A viruses only

          (b) Major antigenic change within H or N surface proteins resulting in a new subtype

          (c) These viruses enter an immunologically naive population and result in pandemics.

          (d) Animals may be a reservoir.

2. Presentation and diagnosis

    a. Signs and symptoms

        i. Sudden-onset fever and cough are the most characteristic signs/symptoms.

        ii. Myalgias

        iii. Headache

        iv. Fatigue

        v. Chest discomfort

        vi. Symptoms often seen, but are not as specific and may be more consistent with the common cold

          (a) Stuffy nose

          (b) Sneezing

          (c) Sore throat

        vii. Diarrhea

          (a) Up to 28% in infants and young children

          (b) Less common among adults

        viii. Presentation may vary by age, comorbidities, and immune status.

    b. Diagnosis

        i. Diagnosis is often made by clinical presentation only.

        ii. Nasopharyngeal aspirates and swabs taken within 5 days of illness onset; if taken after 5 days, may cause false-negative results because of decreased viral shedding

        iii. Diagnostic tests

          (a) Reverse transcriptase–polymerase chain reaction (RT-PCR)

             (1) Most sensitive and specific

             (2) Differentiate type of influenza (i.e., H1N1)

             (3) Results within 4–6 hours

             (4) May serve as a confirmatory test for negative results by other (less sensitive) methods

          (b) Immunofluorescence

             (1) Antigen detection

             (2) Less sensitivity and specificity, but results quickly available

             (3) Performance depends on laboratory expertise.

          (c) Commercial rapid influenza diagnostic tests

             (1) Decreased sensitivity compared with RT-PCR

             (2) Performance depends on patient age, illness duration, and sample type.

             (3) Results in 10–30 minutes

3. Treatment

    a. Treatment is recommended as soon as possible for any patient with confirmed or suspected influenza in the following circumstances:

        i. Requires hospitalization

        ii. Has severe, complicated, or progressive illness; or

        iii. Is at high risk of complications (see A.1.h. above)

    b. Consider treatment in the following instances:

        i. Patients at high risk of complications with persistent illness and a positive laboratory test result more than 48 hours after symptom onset

  ii. Patients with confirmed or highly suspected influenza within 48 hours of symptom onset who are not at high risk of complications but who wish to shorten duration of illness and/or who are in contact with individuals at high risk of complications from influenza infection

 c. Antiviral agents

  i. Antiviral susceptibility may vary from year to year depending on the predominant strain; current recommendations and viral susceptibility should be reviewed before initiating therapy. Information can be found on the CDC influenza website (www.cdc.gov/flu).

  ii. Adamantanes: Amantadine and rimantadine

   (a) Mechanism of action: Inhibit viral uncoating and release of viral nucleic acid

   (b) Active only against influenza A

   (c) Widespread resistance to H3N2 strain since 2006 and 2009 H1N1 strain; adamantanes currently not recommended

   (d) Adverse effects: CNS – Dizziness, confusion, headache; peripheral edema; orthostatic hypotension

   (e) Rimantadine tends to have a more favorable adverse effect profile and is preferred to amantadine in the 2009 Infectious Diseases Society of America (IDSA) influenza guidelines.

   (f) Rimantadine dose: 200 mg once daily or 100 mg twice daily for 3–7 days. Adjust in renal dysfunction; decrease to 100 mg once daily.

  iii. Oseltamivir

   (a) Mechanism of action: Inhibits neuraminidase, thus reducing viral shedding

   (b) Effective against influenza A and B

   (c) Adverse effects: Nausea/vomiting; transient neuropsychiatric events (self-injury and delirium) mainly reported among Japanese adolescents and adults

   (d) Dose

    (1) Adults and children weighing more than 40 kg: 75 mg orally twice daily for 5 days

    (2) A longer duration may be considered for patients who remain severely ill after 5 days of treatment.

    (3) Children 23–40 kg: 60 mg twice daily for 5 days

    (4) Children 15–23 kg: 45 mg twice daily for 5 days

    (5) Children older than 1 year and weighing less than 15 kg: 30 mg twice daily for 5 days

    (6) Children 2 weeks to 1 year of age: 3 mg/kg per dose twice daily for 5 days

  iv. Zanamivir

   (a) Mechanism of action: Inhibits neuraminidase, thus reducing viral shedding

   (b) Effective against influenza A and B

   (c) Adverse effects: Bronchospasm (use with caution in patients with asthma or COPD); cough; sore/dry throat; dizziness

   (d) Dose: Adults and children 7 years and older: 10 mg (2 inhalations) twice daily

Patient Case

27. B.M. is a 31-year-old first-grade teacher who presents to the clinic with a rising temperature and worsening cough, fatigue, and muscle aches for the past 24 hours. His symptoms are suggestive of influenza because 25% of his students have been sick with the flu. A rapid influenza test confirms the diagnosis of influenza A. The patient requests antiviral treatment so that he can return to the classroom as soon as possible. Which is the best course of management?

    A. No antiviral therapy is indicated because of the patient's low risk of complications from influenza.

    B. Give rimantadine 200 mg orally once daily for 5 days.

    C. Give oseltamivir 75 mg orally twice daily for 5 days.

    D. Give oseltamivir 75 mg orally twice daily until symptoms resolve.

4. Prevention: Annual vaccination is the best means of prevention.
    a. Influenza vaccination
        i. Indicated for everyone older than 6 months without contraindications to influenza vaccination
        ii. Timing of vaccination
            (a) Ideally, before onset of influenza in community
            (b) Begin offering to patients as soon as vaccine is available.
            (c) Continue to offer as long as influenza viruses are circulating in community.
            (d) Children 6 months to 8 years of age who have previously received two or more doses of influenza vaccine before July 1, 2015, require only one dose in 2015–2016. Children in this age group who have not previously received two doses require two doses in 2015–2016 given at least 4 weeks apart.
            (e) Vaccination should not be delayed to procure a specific formulation if an appropriate one is available.
    b. Inactivated influenza vaccine (IIV)
        i. Preferred for immunocompromised patients and close contacts of immunocompromised patients
        ii. High-dose vaccine is approved for patients 65 years and older.
        iii. Available in formulations for intramuscular and intradermal administration
        iv. Trivalent (IIV3) and quadrivalent (IIV4)
        v. Contraindications to IIV
            (a) Severe allergic reaction (e.g., anaphylaxis after previous influenza vaccine or vaccine component, including egg protein)
            (b) People with a history of hives only to egg exposure may receive the inactivated vaccine or the trivalent recombinant influenza vaccine (RIV3) with close monitoring.
    c. LAIV, quadrivalent
        i. Nasal spray
        ii. In 2014, ACIP recommended this formulation preferentially to IIV for children 2–8 years of age given data indicating increased efficacy. Subsequent data analyses are conflicting, so LAIV is no longer preferred in this age group; either IIV or LAIV is an appropriate option.
        iii. Contraindications to LAIV
            (a) Severe allergic reaction (e.g., anaphylaxis after previous influenza vaccine or vaccine component, including egg protein)
            (b) Individuals younger than 2 years or older than 49 years
            (c) Children 2–17 years of age who are receiving aspirin or aspirin-containing products
            (d) Not recommended by ACIP: Immunosuppressed people and their caregivers, pregnant women, people with chronic medical conditions such as asthma, diabetes, kidney or heart disease

  d. RIV3

    i. Indicated for patients 18 years and older

    ii. Egg-free

  e. Hand hygiene; avoidance of others with influenza

  f. For patients older than 1 year who cannot be vaccinated (severely immunocompromised, lack/shortage of vaccine), chemoprophylaxis is an option.

    i. See the CDC website for the most up-to-date recommendations (www.cdc.gov/flu).

    ii. Oseltamivir: 75 mg orally once daily (for adults and children weighing more than 40 kg)

    iii. Zanamivir: 10 mg (two inhalations) once daily (for adults and children 5 years and older)

    iv. Rimantadine: 200 mg orally once daily or 100 mg twice daily

    v. Duration

      (a) If vaccination is given, chemoprophylaxis may be discontinued at 2 weeks, which is sufficient time to allow an immune response.

      (b) If vaccination cannot be done, prophylaxis may be continued for as long as influenza viruses are circulating in the community.

Patient Case

28. V.T. is a 34-year-old woman with HIV infection who runs a day care out of her home. She currently receives therapy with abacavir/lamivudine/dolutegravir, with a CD4+ count of 389 cells/mm³ and a viral load of less than 48 copies/mL. V.T. reports no food or drug allergies. One of the children in her day care was just given a diagnosis of influenza B. Which is the optimal means of influenza prophylaxis for this patient?

  A. IIV.

  B. IIV and oseltamivir 75 mg orally once daily for 2 weeks.

  C. Oseltamivir 75 mg orally once daily for duration of influenza season.

  D. Rimantadine 200 mg orally once daily for duration of influenza season.

 B. Herpes Simplex Virus *(Domain 1, Task 1, 2, 6)*

  1. Overview

    a. HSV-1

      i. Most common HSV

      ii. Most develop the infection in childhood.

      iii. Adult seroprevalence greater than 90%

      iv. Latency in sensory neurons; reactivation results in viral shedding from mucosal and cutaneous tissues innervated by these neurons

    b. HSV-2

      i. Most often sexually transmitted

      ii. Adult seroprevalence: Around 20%–30%

      iii. Latency in sensory neurons; reactivation results in viral shedding from mucosal and cutaneous tissues innervated by these neurons

  2. Clinical presentation

    a. Mucocutaneous

      i. Genital herpes described in STD section above

      ii. Oral lesions

      iii. Finger lesions (herpetic whitlows)

      iv. Gingival stomatitis

      v.   Bell palsy: Paralysis or weakness of one side of the face caused by dysfunction of facial nerve (cranial nerve VII)

  b. Meningoencephalitis

    i.   Most common cause of community-acquired encephalitis

    ii. Estimated incidence: More than 2 million cases/year

    iii. More than 90% caused by HSV-1

  c. Neonatal herpes

    i.   90% perinatally acquired, 5%–8% congenitally acquired, 2% postnatally acquired

    ii. Risk of transmission to infant from mother with primary HSV-1 infection acquired late in pregnancy is about 30%–50% and is less than 1% among women who acquire genital HSV during the first half of pregnancy or earlier.

    iii. Prevent primary HSV infection late in pregnancy.

    iv. Cesarean section at the time of labor is recommended for all women with active lesions or early symptoms (i.e., vulvar pain, itching).

  d. Visceral disease (rare, but more common among immunocompromised patients)

    i.   Hepatic

    ii. Pulmonary

  e. Ophthalmologic complications: Retinitis or keratitis

3. Diagnosis

  a. Viral culture of tissue

  b. PCR testing on fluid

  c. Direct fluorescent antibody test (can distinguish between HSV-1 and HSV-2)

4. Treatment

  a. Acyclovir, valacyclovir, famciclovir, and penciclovir have activity against HSV-1 and HSV-2 (as do ganciclovir, valganciclovir, and foscarnet, which are rarely used).

  b. Treatment of genital herpes is discussed in the STD section.

  c. Intravenous therapy is preferred for disseminated infection or severe disease (e.g., encephalitis, visceral infections, ophthalmologic infections).

C. Varicella Zoster Virus (VZV) *(Domain 1, Task 1, 2, 5, 6)*

  1. Overview

    a. Transmitted by aerosolized droplets or direct contact

    b. Incubation period of about 2 weeks

    c. Infectivity begins 48 hours before onset of rash and ends when all skin lesions have fully crusted.

    d. Historically, 90% of infections have occurred in childhood; however, since routine use of the varicella vaccine began in 1996, the incidence of VZV has steadily declined.

    e. Latency in sensory neurons

  2. Clinical presentation

    a. Chickenpox

      i.   Fevers and rash; then vesicles

      ii. Vesicles become pustular; they then crust and scab.

      iii. Lesions on trunk, scalp

    b. Shingles

      i.   Reactivation of VZV from dorsal root ganglia

      ii. Affects about 20% of the population, typically older adults

      iii. Severe pain before the appearance of lesions, which often includes a prodrome of fever, malaise, dysesthesias, and headache preceding rash

      iv. Typically, a localized eruption in a single dermatome that becomes pustular/hemorrhagic within 3–4 days

     v.   In 7–10 days, lesions crust and are no longer infectious.

     vi.   Postherpetic neuralgia

       (a) 10%–15% of patients with shingles

       (b) Injury of peripheral nerves/altered CNS processing of pain signals

       (c) Increased risk in those older than 60 years and in those who have received immunosuppression

       (d) Consider gabapentin, pregabalin, lidocaine patches, or tricyclic antidepressants.

  c.   Visceral disease (rare, but more common among immunocompromised patients)

     i.   Pneumonia

     ii.   Hepatitis

     iii. Encephalitis

  d.   Ocular disease

     i.   Herpes zoster ophthalmicus

     ii.   Acute retinal necrosis

3. Diagnosis

  a.   Viral culture of tissue

  b.   PCR testing on fluid

  c.   Direct fluorescent antibody test

4. Treatment

  a.   Acyclovir is active but less so than for HSV; ganciclovir is active as well.

  b.   Chickenpox: Antiviral therapy is not indicated for primary varicella infection in most children, although it may be considered for treatment of primary infection in older children and adults because of increased risk of severe infection.

     i.   Acyclovir 800 mg orally five times daily (adult dose)

     ii.   Use intravenous acyclovir 10 mg/kg every 8 hours for immunocompromised or immunocompetent patients with serious complications.

  c.   Shingles: For uncomplicated herpes zoster infection, acyclovir 800 mg orally five times daily for 7–10 days should be initiated within 72 hours.

     i.   Treatment can expedite rash resolution.

     ii.   May decrease incidence of prolonged postherpetic neuralgia

     iii. Other options include valacyclovir 1 g orally three times daily for 7 days or famciclovir 500 mg orally three times daily for 7 days.

     iv. Intravenous therapy is preferred for disseminated infection or severe disease or in immunocompromised patients.

5. Prevention

  a.   VZV vaccine (Varivax)

     i.   Live vaccine – In general, not recommended for administration to immunocompromised or pregnant patients

     ii.   Routine childhood vaccine –Two doses

     iii. May be considered for certain immunocompromised patients (i.e., patients with HIV infection with CD4+ cell counts above 200 cells/mm^3, potential transplant recipients before transplantation) who are VZV seronegative

  b.   Zoster vaccine (Zostavax)

     i.   Live vaccine – In general, not recommended for administration to immunocompromised or pregnant patients

     ii.   U.S. Food and Drug Administration approved for individuals 50 years and older, although the ACIP recommends a one-time dose given at 60 years or older, regardless of herpes zoster history

    c.   Varicella zoster immune globulin (VariZIG)
        i.   PEP for patients at high risk of severe disease who also lack VZV immunity
       ii.   Recommended for the following populations:
           (a) Immunocompromised patients
           (b) Premature/newborn infants
           (c) Pregnant women
      iii.   Timing of VariZIG: As soon as possible after exposure and within 10 days
      iv.   Dose: 125 international units for every 10 kg of intramuscular body weight up to 625 international units

---

Patient Case

29. J.D. is a 68-year-old woman with hyperlipidemia and hypertension who presents to the clinic with a painful rash that wraps around the right side of her abdomen. She has noticed pain for a few days, but the rash appeared just yesterday. Which is the best treatment for this patient?

    A. Acyclovir 800 mg orally three times daily.
    B. Acyclovir 10 mg/kg intravenously three times daily.
    C. Valacyclovir 1 g orally three times daily.
    D. No antiviral therapy indicated.

    D.   Epstein-Barr Virus (EBV) *(Domain 1, Task 1, 2, 6)*
       1. Overview
          a. 90%–95% of adults EBV seropositive; 50% by 5 years of age
          b. Transmitted by close contact, perinatal, blood/tissue
          c. Latency in B lymphocytes, T lymphocytes, epithelial cells; no reactivation of disease with EBV in healthy hosts
       2. Clinical presentation
          a. Asymptomatic to mild illness (most common in young children)
          b. Infectious mononucleosis (more common in older children/young adults): Acute, self-limited infection consisting of fever, malaise, exudative pharyngitis, lymphadenopathy, and often splenomegaly
          c. EBV-related cancers
             i.   Nasopharyngeal carcinoma
            ii.   Lymphoma
           iii.   Posttransplant lymphoproliferative disorders: Wide spectrum of clinical conditions characterized by lymphoproliferation after transplantation, ranging from infectious mononucleosis to true malignancy
       3. Diagnosis: Primary infection
          a. Clinical presentation
          b. Lymphocytosis present in about 70% of cases
          c. Monospot test finding positive
          d. Serum/tissue PCR for EBV DNA (not used in healthy hosts; for immunocompromised hosts)
       4. Treatment
          a. Supportive therapy for those who are immunocompetent
          b. In vitro, ganciclovir is more active than acyclovir.

c. Role of antiviral agents in posttransplant lymphoproliferative disorders is unclear; may be considered in early disease with reduction in immunosuppression, but role in established malignancies is uncertain

d. After reduction in immunosuppression, may consider anti-CD20 therapy with rituximab for CD20⁺ B-cell posttransplant lymphoproliferative disorder

E. Cytomegalovirus (CMV) *(Domain 1, Task 1, 2, 6)*
1. Overview
   a. 60%–70% of adults CMV seropositive
   b. Transmitted by close contact, perinatal, blood/tissue
   c. Latency in monocytes, neutrophils
2. Clinical presentation
   a. Asymptomatic to mild illness
   b. Infectious mononucleosis: Acute, self-limited infection consisting of fever, lymphadenopathy, and relative lymphocytosis
   c. Immunocompromised hosts
      i. Primary infection or reactivation of latent infection
         (a) CMV IgG seronegative recipients can develop infection from CMV IgG–seropositive donors, blood products, or the community.
         (b) CMV IgG–seropositive recipients can also develop reactivation of latent infection.
         (c) The greatest risk of CMV infection is among CMV-seronegative recipients who receive an allograft from a CMV-seropositive donor.
      ii. CMV infection: Presence of CMV replication, regardless of symptoms
      iii. CMV disease: CMV replication and signs/symptoms
         (a) CMV syndrome: Malaise, cytopenias, fever
         (b) Tissue-invasive CMV disease: Pneumonitis, enteritis, hepatitis, encephalitis
3. Diagnosis
   a. Infectious mononucleosis
      i. Compatible clinical syndrome
      ii. Monospot test finding negative
      iii. Relative lymphocytosis
   b. CMV infection/disease
      i. Serum PCR for CMV or pp65 antigen assay
      ii. Viral culture
      iii. Histopathology
4. Treatment
   a. Ganciclovir 5 mg/kg intravenously twice daily or valganciclovir 900 mg orally twice daily
      i. Intravenous ganciclovir is preferred to valganciclovir in solid organ transplant recipients with severe or life-threatening disease, high viral load, or uncertain GI absorption.
      ii. Treatment should be continued until resolution of clinical symptoms, virologic clearance; for a minimum of 2 weeks
      iii. Consider 1–3 months of secondary prophylaxis (maintenance dosing) after completion of initial induction therapy.
      iv. Oral ganciclovir is not recommended for treatment because of its low bioavailability.
   b. Specific for CMV retinitis
      i. Surgically implanted ganciclovir implant is efficacious but no longer manufactured.
      ii. Intravitreal ganciclovir or foscarnet with oral valganciclovir
      iii. Systemic therapy reduces involvement of contralateral eye.

    c. For resistant virus or if intolerance, may consider intravenous foscarnet or cidofovir

  5. Prevention

    a. Antiviral prophylaxis

      i. Valganciclovir 900 mg orally once daily (preferred in adult transplant recipients) OR

      ii. Ganciclovir 1 g orally three times daily OR

      iii. Ganciclovir 5 mg/kg intravenously once daily

      iv. Duration depends on donor and recipient CMV serologic profile as well as type of allograft.

    b. Preemptive therapy

      i. Instead of routine antiviral prophylaxis, preemptive therapy requires close monitoring and the initiation of antiviral therapy at treatment doses based on specific viral cutoff values (vary by institution) until CMV is undetectable.

        (a) Ganciclovir 5 mg/kg intravenously twice daily OR

        (b) Valganciclovir 900 mg orally twice daily

      ii. Controversial whether this method can be used in high-risk patients (CMV-seronegative recipients who receive allografts from CMV-seropositive donors)

Patient Case

30. Which patient is at greatest risk of CMV infection?

    A. A 25-year-old woman with a renal transplant 13 years earlier has stable renal function and no recent complications; CMV donor positive and recipient negative; not taking antiviral drugs.

    B. A 32-year-old man with a liver transplant 1 week earlier develops postsurgical bleeding complications and biliary leak; CMV donor negative and recipient negative; taking acyclovir.

    C. A 44-year-old man with a renal transplant 1 month earlier is being treated for acute cellular rejection with high-dose methylprednisolone; CMV donor positive and recipient positive; taking valganciclovir.

    D. A 37-year-old woman with a renal transplant 8 months earlier is being treated for acute cellular rejection with high-dose methylprednisolone; CMV donor positive and recipient positive; not taking antiviral drugs.

IV. FUNGAL INFECTIONS

  A. Superficial Mycoses *(Domain 1, Task 1, 2, 5, 6)*

    1. Overview

      a. Infections limited to outermost layers of skin and hair on the trunk or proximal aspects of the limbs

      b. Usually mild with little to no inflammatory response

      c. Mainly cosmetic

      d. No physical discomfort

      e. Respond well to therapy

      f. Primary etiologic agent: *Malassezia* spp.

    2. *Malassezia* spp.

      a. Dimorphic fungi

      b. Normal skin flora (90% of adults); infection is not contagious

      c. Clinical infection associated with transformation from yeast to mycelial form, which may be triggered by the following:

        i. Hot, humid weather

        ii. Hyperhidrosis

        iii. Use of topical skin oils

      d. Usually causes tinea versicolor

   i. Hypopigmented, hyperpigmented, or erythematous macules

   ii. Usually during puberty

  e. Other clinical manifestations

   i. Seborrheic dermatitis

   ii. Folliculitis

  f. Diagnosis

   i. Clinical appearance

   ii. On potassium hydroxide preparation, round yeasts and short hyphae have "spaghetti and meatballs" appearance.

  g. Treatment

   i. Avoid oils on the skin.

   ii. Ketoconazole 2% cream once daily (also available as gel or foam)

   iii. Ketoconazole 2% shampoo

   iv. Terbinafine cream

   v. Selenium sulfide 2.5% lotion or shampoo (also available as a 2.25% foam)

B. Cutaneous Mycoses *(Domain 1, Task 1, 2, 5, 6)*

 1. Overview

  a. Infections slightly deeper in the epidermis

   i. Skin, hair, and nails

   ii. Keratinized layers

  b. Disease may be acute or chronic, depending on host immune status and etiologic agent.

  c. May be more common in tropical environments

  d. Infection may be transmitted from soil, from animals, or by person-to-person contact.

  e. Occupational risk to gardeners, florists

  f. In general, more difficult to treat than superficial infections

  g. Primary etiologic agent: Dermatophytes

 2. Dermatophytes

  a. *Trichophyton, Microsporum, Epidermophyton*

  b. Not part of normal skin flora

  c. Cause tinea or ringworm

   i. Classic lesion – Fungal mycelium in the stratum corneum

   ii. Presentation ranges from minimal signs of infection to inflammatory reaction in the dermis and epidermis.

   iii. Scaling may occur; may invade toe and fingernails

   iv. Dermatophyte lesions grow outwardly in a centrifugal pattern (ring).

   v. Easily transmitted; spread by close contact

    (a) Tinea capitis: Head

    (b) Tinea pedis: Feet (athlete's foot)

    (c) Tinea corporis: Body

    (d) Tinea cruris: Groin

    (e) Tinea barbae: Bearded area

    (f) Tinea unguium: Nails (dermatophytic onychomycosis; onychomycosis may be caused by non-dermatophytes as well)

  d. Diagnosis

   i. Clinical presentation

   ii. Potassium hydroxide preparation

e. Treatment
   i. Usually can be managed with topical antifungal agents
   ii. May use systemic therapy for severe or chronic infections and/or infections in immunocompromised patients
   iii. Adjunctive therapy includes keeping the area dry (e.g., use of talcum or desiccant powder for tinea cruris).
   iv. Therapies
       (a) Topical antifungal agents
           (1) Terbinafine
           (2) Naftifine
           (3) Topical azole
           (4) Ciclopirox nail lacquer: Apply once daily at bedtime for 48 weeks (tinea unguium).
       (b) Systemic antifungal agents
           (1) Terbinafine 250 mg orally once daily
           (2) Itraconazole 200 mg orally once daily
           (3) Fluconazole 150 mg orally once weekly
           (4) Griseofulvin 250 mg orally three times daily

C. Subcutaneous Mycoses *(Domain 1, Task 1, 2, 6)*
   1. Overview
      a. Infections in the dermis and subcutaneous tissue
      b. Caused by fungi typically isolated in the environment; entry by skin trauma
      c. May mimic infections caused by bacteria
      d. Surgical excision of lesion may be required.
      e. Primary etiologic agent: *Sporothrix schenckii*
   2. *S. schenckii*
      a. Dimorphic fungi
      b. Present worldwide, but areas of hyperendemicity (e.g., tropical regions of South America)
      c. Organism gains access by traumatic implantation.
         i. A small, hard nodule appears at the site of injury and enlarges into a fluctuant mass that eventually breaks down and ulcerates.
         ii. As the primary lesion enlarges, several other nodules may begin to develop along lymphatics that drain the site (may also become fluctuant and ulcerate).
         iii. Infection rarely extends beyond regional lymphatics.
         iv. Lymphocutaneous sporotrichosis (rose-handler's disease)
      d. Diagnosis: Culture or skin biopsy
      e. Treatment
         i. Lymphocutaneous and cutaneous sporotrichosis
            (a) Itraconazole 200 mg orally once daily for 2–4 weeks after resolution of all lesions; usually for a total of 3–6 months
            (b) For patients with refractory condition, may consider itraconazole 200 mg orally twice daily; terbinafine 500 mg orally twice daily; saturated solution of potassium iodide starting at a dose of five drops orally three times daily and increasing, as tolerated, to 40–50 drops three times daily; or fluconazole 400–800 mg orally once daily
         ii. Severe and/or life-threatening systemic sporotrichosis: Lipid formulation of amphotericin B 3–5 mg/kg intravenously once daily, followed by itraconazole 200 mg orally twice daily to complete at least 12 months of therapy

---

Patient Case

31. S.S. is a 66-year-old woman who comes to the clinic with an ulcerative lesion on her right hand. She explains that she noticed a scratch on her hand after gardening and that the area became red, but not painful. During the following days, a small compressible mass developed, which evolved into an ulcer. On examination, several nodules along her arm are noted, one of which has begun to ulcerate, similar to the original lesion. A biopsy of the lesion is performed, revealing *Sporothrix*. Which is the treatment of choice for this patient?

    A. Liposomal amphotericin B 3 mg/kg intravenously once daily.
    B. Terbinafine 500 mg orally twice daily.
    C. Saturated solution of potassium iodide five drops orally three times daily.
    D. Itraconazole 200 mg orally once daily.

    D. Systemic Mycoses *(Domain 1, Task 1, 2, 3, 4, 6; Domain 3, Task 2)*
       1. Overview
          a. Infections that enter the bloodstream and/or internal organs
          b. May be caused by primary pathogens or opportunistic pathogens (require debilitated host)
          c. Regardless of pathogen, infection tends to be more severe in immunocompromised hosts.
          d. The incidence of systemic mycoses is increasing because of HIV infection, bone marrow and solid organ transplantation, and immunomodulatory therapy.
          e. Infection may be caused by yeast, mold, or dimorphic fungal species.
             i. Yeasts: *Candida*, *Cryptococcus*
             ii. Molds: *Aspergillus*, Zygomycetes, many other molds
             iii. Dimorphic: *Histoplasma, Blastomyces, Coccidioides*
       2. *Candida* spp.
          a. Normal skin flora of GI tract, vagina, skin
          b. More than 200 *Candida* spp.; about 10 are medically significant
             i. *C. albicans*
                (a) Most common *Candida* spp.
                (b) Rapidly identified by germ-tube test
                (c) Usually susceptible to antifungal agents
             ii. *C. glabrata*
                (a) Second most common *Candida* spp.
                (b) Decreased antifungal susceptibility to azoles (especially fluconazole) and amphotericin B
             iii. *C. parapsilosis*
                (a) Often associated with foreign devices
                (b) Most common in neonatal intensive care units (ICUs)
                (c) Higher minimum inhibitory concentrations to echinocandins but generally still susceptible
             iv. *Candida tropicalis*: Usually susceptible to antifungal agents
             v. *Candida krusei*: Inherently resistant to fluconazole, retained susceptibility to voriconazole and posaconazole, decreased susceptibility to amphotericin B
             vi. *Candida lusitaniae*: Decreased susceptibility to amphotericin B but susceptible to other antifungal agents
             vii. Epidemiology of *Candida* spp.
                (a) Historically, *C. albicans* accounts for more than 50% of infections.
                (b) *C. albicans* is still the most prevalent species, but its relative prevalence has decreased.
                (c) As the prevalence of *C. albicans* has decreased, the prevalence of *C. glabrata* has doubled, making it the second most prevalent species.

    (d) *Candida* epidemiology is important because specific *Candida* spp. predicts antifungal susceptibility.

Table 3. General Patterns of Antifungal Susceptibility Among *Candida* spp.

Candida spp.	Fluconazole	Itraconazole	Voriconazole/ Posaconazole	Amphotericin B	Echinocandins
C. albicans	S	S	S	S	S
C. tropicalis	S	S	S	S	S
C. parapsilosis	S	S	S	S	S to R
C. glabrata	S-DD to R	S-DD to R	S to R	S to I	S
C. krusei	R	S-DD to R	S	S to I	S
C. lusitaniae	S	S	S	S to R	S

I = intermediately susceptible; R = resistant; S = susceptible; S-DD = susceptible dose-dependent.

  c. Clinical presentation
    i. Invasive candidiasis
      (a) *Candida* bloodstream infection
      (b) Intra-abdominal candidiasis
      (c) CNS candidiasis
      (d) May disseminate to other sites such as eye, heart, and kidney
      (e) Risk factors for invasive candidiasis
        (1) Receipt of broad-spectrum antibiotics
        (2) Prolonged hospital stay, especially in the ICU
        (3) Presence of central venous catheters
        (4) Receipt of immunosuppressive medications, including corticosteroids, chemotherapy
        (5) Surgery, especially intra-abdominal surgery
    ii. Urinary tract infection (UTI)
    iii. Oropharyngeal or esophageal candidiasis
    iv. Vulvovaginal candidiasis
  d. Diagnosis
    i. Isolation of *Candida* from sterile site such as bloodstream, CNS
    ii. Similar to UTIs caused by bacterial pathogens; determination of a UTI requires consideration of urinalysis and assessment for presence of signs/symptoms of infection
  e. Treatment of invasive candidiasis
    i. An echinocandin is favored for patients with invasive candidiasis because they have the broadest-spectrum anti-*Candida* activity.
      (a) Caspofungin 70 mg intravenously x 1 dose; then 50 mg intravenously once daily
      (b) Micafungin 100 mg intravenously once daily
      (c) Anidulafungin 200 mg intravenously x 1 dose; then 100 mg intravenously once daily
    ii. Fluconazole 800 mg (12 mg/kg) orally or intravenously x 1 dose; then 400 mg (6 mg/kg) orally or intravenously once daily is an acceptable alternative for patients who are not critically ill and are considered unlikely to have fluconazole-resistant *Candida* species
    iii. Change from echinocandin to fluconazole if the patient is stable, if the *Candida* isolate is fluconazole-susceptible, and once repeat blood cultures are negative.
    iv. Fluconazole is the drug of choice for fluconazole-susceptible *Candida* infections.

     v.   Itraconazole is rarely used for *Candida* infections.

     vi. Voriconazole and posaconazole have no advantage over fluconazole for fluconazole-susceptible infections, but they may be used for infections with decreased fluconazole susceptibility that retain activity to voriconazole or posaconazole.

     vii. Amphotericin B is infrequently used for *Candida* infections, but it is used in serious infections such as endocarditis.

   f. Treatment of noninvasive candidiasis

     i.   Oropharyngeal, esophageal candidiasis: Fluconazole 100–200 mg orally once daily or nystatin oral suspension four times daily

     ii. *Candida* UTI: Fluconazole 100–200 mg orally once daily

     iii. Vulvovaginal candidiasis: Fluconazole 150 mg orally once

     iv. May consider other azoles or echinocandins for fluconazole-refractory infections

---

Patient Cases

The following case pertains to questions 32 and 33.

D.M. is a 50-year-old woman who recently underwent a total gastrectomy for gastric cancer. She was unable to tolerate enteral feedings and was discharged to home with total parenteral nutrition. D.M. presents in the clinic with a temperature of 38.8°C, WBC count of 21.4 x 103 cells/mm³, and blood pressure of 85/50 mm Hg. Blood cultures are obtained, and intravenous fluids are given, as are one-time doses of piperacillin/tazobactam 3.375 g intravenously and vancomycin 1000 mg intravenously. As the patient is being transferred to the emergency department, the physician asks your opinion about empiric antifungal coverage.

32. Which is the best choice for this patient?

    A. Fluconazole 400 mg intravenously once daily.
    B. Micafungin 100 mg intravenously once daily.
    C. Posaconazole 200 mg orally four times daily.
    D. Amphotericin B lipid complex 3 mg/kg intravenously once daily.

33. One day later, D.M.'s blood cultures reveal the presence of *C. albicans*, and susceptibility tests later reveal a pan-susceptible isolate. Which is the drug of choice?

    A. Fluconazole 400 mg intravenously once daily.
    B. Micafungin 100 mg intravenously once daily.
    C. Posaconazole 200 mg orally four times daily.
    D. Amphotericin B lipid complex 3 mg/kg intravenously once daily.

Table 4. Systemic Antifungal Agents

Generic (Brand)	Antifungal Coverage	Dosing	Adverse Effects	Other
Amphotericin B deoxycholate (Fungizone)	Very broad spectrum; less active against *Candida lusitaniae*, *Aspergillus terreus*, *Scedosporium*	0.5–1.5 mg/kg intravenously QD	Nephrotoxicity, infusion-related reactions, electrolyte disturbances	Consider premedication with acetaminophen, diphenhydramine, hydrocortisone; slow infusion rate to minimize infusion reactions
Amphotericin B lipid complex (Abelcet)		3–5 mg/kg intravenously QD	The lipid formulations have improved tolerability compared with conventional amphotericin B	
Amphotericin B colloidal dispersion (Amphotec)				
Liposomal amphotericin B (AmBisome)				
Flucytosine (Ancobon)	Used primarily for *Cryptococcus* but active against *Candida* and *Aspergillus*	25 mg/kg PO q6hr	Bone marrow depression, GI upset, hepatotoxicity	Monitor serum concentrations; adjust dose in renal dysfunction
Fluconazole (Diflucan)	*Candida*, *Cryptococcus*, *Coccidioides*	100–800 mg QD; same dose IV or PO	Hepatotoxicity, rash, GI upset, QT prolongation	Only azole to concentrate in the urine; may give with or without food/acid suppression
Itraconazole (Sporanox)	Enhanced spectrum from fluconazole, including *Histoplasma*, *Blastomyces*, *Sporothrix*, *Aspergillus*; used primarily for *Histoplasma* and *Blastomyces*	Loading dose: 200 mg PO BID or TID Maintenance dose: 200 mg PO QD or BID	Hepatotoxicity, rash, GI upset (especially with the solution), poor taste (solution), QT prolongation	Capsules are best absorbed with food, whereas the solution is best absorbed in the fasting state (solutions better absorbed than capsules); measure serum concentrations of itraconazole and active metabolite
Voriconazole (Vfend)	Enhanced spectrum from itraconazole, including *Scedosporium*, *Fusarium*, and more reliable coverage against *Aspergillus*	Loading dose: 6 mg/kg q12hr x 2 doses followed by 4 mg/kg q12hr	Hepatotoxicity, rash, GI upset, QT prolongation, visual toxicity	Oral forms best absorbed on an empty stomach, regardless of acid suppression; saturable metabolism; potent CYP3A4 inhibitor; monitor serum trough concentrations

Table 4. Systemic Antifungal Agents *(continued)*

Generic (Brand)	Antifungal Coverage	Dosing	Adverse Effects	Other
Posaconazole (Noxafil)	Enhanced spectrum from voriconazole, including Zygomycetes	Treatment of invasive infections (off-label): 200 mg PO QID (oral suspension) Treatment of oropharyngeal candidiasis: 100 mg BID x 1 day; then 100 mg QD (oral suspension) Prophylaxis: 200 mg PO TID (oral suspension); 300 mg BID x 1 day; then 300 mg QD (delayed-release tablets and IV)	Hepatotoxicity, rash, GI upset, QT prolongation	Oral suspension: Best absorbed with food (ideally high in fat); carbonation may aid in absorption; avoid acid-suppressive therapy, if possible All formulations: Slightly less potent CYP3A4 inhibitor than voriconazole; monitor serum trough concentrations
Isavuconazonium sulfate (prodrug of isavuconazole; Cresemba)	Similar to posaconazole	Loading dose: 372 mg q8hr x 6 doses; maintenance dose: 372 mg QD (IV and PO)	Hepatotoxicity, GI upset, rash	372 mg of isavuconazonium sulfate is equivalent to 200 mg of isavuconazole; can be taken with or without food
Caspofungin (Cancidas)	Broad anti-*Candida* activity, though higher MICs to *Candida parapsilosis* (uncertain clinical significance); *Aspergillus*	Loading dose: 70 mg IV x 1; maintenance dose: 50 mg QD	Hepatotoxicity	Minimal drug interactions
Micafungin (Mycamine)		Invasive candidiasis: 100 mg IV QD		
Anidulafungin (Eraxis)		Loading dose: 200 mg IV x 1; maintenance dose: 100 mg IV QD		

BID = twice daily; IV = intravenous(ly); MIC = minimum inhibitory concentration; PO = orally; q = every; QD = once daily; QID = four times daily; TID = three times daily.

3. *Cryptococcus* spp.
   a. Epidemiology
      i. Encapsulated yeast found in the soil; often associated with pigeon droppings
      ii. Worldwide distribution; ubiquitous in the environment
      iii. Although exposure is common, clinical infections caused by *C. neoformans* were rare until the HIV epidemic, though they decreased with the introduction of ART.
      iv. Also observed among patients with cancer and in transplant recipients
      v. More recently, *Cryptococcus gattii* was implicated as the cause of an outbreak of cryptococcosis in immunocompetent humans and animals on Vancouver Island and in the Northwest United States; this section focuses on *C. neoformans*.
   b. Clinical presentation
      i. Most often manifests as meningitis
      ii. Infection may also involve the skin, lungs, prostate gland, urinary tract, eyes, heart, bone, and joints.
   c. Diagnosis
      i. Culture
      ii. Antigen detection (from blood, CSF)
      iii. Lumbar puncture
   d. Treatment of *C. neoformans*
      i. Treatment depends on host status, severity, and infection site.
      ii. Treatment consists of an initial induction period, followed by consolidation therapy and then maintenance therapy.
      iii. Meningoencephalitis
         (a) Induction therapy (minimum of 2 weeks)
            (1) Amphotericin B deoxycholate 0.7–1 mg/kg intravenously once daily plus flucytosine 25 mg/kg orally four times daily OR
            (2) Liposomal amphotericin B 3–4 mg/kg or amphotericin B lipid complex 5 mg/kg intravenously once daily plus flucytosine 25 mg/kg orally four times daily
            (3) The lipid formulation of amphotericin B may be selected for patients with renal dysfunction or at risk of renal dysfunction; preferred in transplant recipients
            (4) Patients intolerant of flucytosine require an extended period of induction with amphotericin B.
         (b) Consolidation therapy (8 weeks): Fluconazole 400–800 mg orally once daily
         (c) Maintenance therapy (minimum of 6–12 months): Fluconazole 200 mg orally once daily
      iv. Non-meningeal cryptococcosis
         (a) Severe infection – Treatment similar to that for CNS disease
         (b) Mild to moderate symptoms of infection – Fluconazole 400 mg orally once daily
4. *Aspergillus* spp.
   a. Epidemiology
      i. Septate mold found in the soil, food, water, and decaying vegetation
      ii. Worldwide distribution; ubiquitous in the environment
      iii. Exposure is common; clinical infections caused by *Aspergillus* are increasing because of the expanding immunocompromised population.
      iv. *A. fumigatus*
         (a) Most common species
         (b) Strongly angioinvasive
      v. *Aspergillus flavus*
      vi. *Aspergillus niger*
      vii. *Aspergillus terreus*: Decreased susceptibility to amphotericin B

b. Clinical presentation
  i. Exposure may lead to asymptomatic colonization, hypersensitivity reaction, life-threatening infection
  ii. Lungs are the most common infection site; characterized by progressive dry cough, fever, dyspnea, chest pain, and hemoptysis
  iii. Aspergillosis may involve any organ system such as sinuses, brain, skin, bone
  iv. Risk factors for aspergillosis
    (a) Prolonged neutropenia from chemotherapy lasting longer than 2 weeks
    (b) Stem cell transplantation (more common in allogeneic than in autologous)
    (c) Receipt of high-dose steroids
    (d) Graft-versus-host disease
    (e) Solid organ transplant recipients
    (f) HIV infection, especially with low CD4+ cell counts
    (g) Infection rare in immunocompetent individuals
c. Diagnosis
  i. A definitive diagnosis requires a tissue biopsy.
  ii. Tissue/sputum culture
  iii. Galactomannan assay
d. Treatment
  i. Voriconazole 6 mg/kg intravenously twice daily x 2 doses, followed by voriconazole 4 mg/kg intravenously twice daily
  ii. Oral voriconazole is approved at a dose of 200 mg orally twice daily, although given the drug's high bioavailability, some experts recommend dosing the oral formations in a weight-based fashion similar to the intravenous dose.
  iii. Alternative agents include amphotericin B and its lipid formulations, posaconazole, and the echinocandins.
  iv. Isavuconazole was approved for the treatment of invasive aspergillosis but after the guidelines were published. In a clinical study, isavuconazole was noninferior to voriconazole for aspergillosis.

Patient Case

34. S.C. is a 59-year-old man with acute myelogenous leukemia who underwent a matched unrelated donor stem cell transplant 4 months earlier and now comes to the clinic for a follow-up. He was recently discharged from the hospital after receiving high-dose steroids for the treatment of graft-versus-host disease. While the patient was in-house, voriconazole 200 mg orally twice daily was initiated for fungal prophylaxis. In addition, he currently takes prednisone 20 mg orally once daily, acyclovir 400 mg orally twice daily, mycophenolate mofetil 500 mg orally twice daily, lansoprazole, metoprolol, docusate, and a multivitamin. The decision is made to continue the prednisone taper to 15 mg orally once daily but to add tacrolimus. Which is the most appropriate consideration regarding tacrolimus for S.C.?

A. Voriconazole inhibits tacrolimus metabolism, so the tacrolimus dose should be empirically reduced.
B. Voriconazole induces tacrolimus metabolism, so the tacrolimus dose should be empirically increased.
C. Tacrolimus inhibits voriconazole metabolism, so the voriconazole dose should be empirically reduced.
D. Tacrolimus induces voriconazole metabolism, so the voriconazole dose should be empirically increased.

5. Zygomycetes
    a. Epidemiology
        i. Nonseptate mold found in decaying matter such as bread, vegetables, fruits, and seeds
        ii. Worldwide distribution; ubiquitous in the environment
        iii. Epidemiology difficult to characterize but, as with *Aspergillus*, infections are increasing because of expanding immunocompromised population
        iv. *Rhizopus*
        v. *Mucor*
        vi. *Rhizomucor*
    b. Clinical presentation
        i. Clinical hallmark – Rapid onset of tissue necrosis, with or without fever
        ii. Rhinocerebral is the most common infection site; characterized by facial pain, unilateral headache, sinus drainage, soft tissue swelling
        iii. Zygomycosis may involve any organ system such as the lungs, brain, skin, or GI tract.
        iv. Risk factors for zygomycosis
            (a) Prolonged neutropenia from chemotherapy lasting longer than 3 weeks
            (b) High-risk stem cell transplantation (i.e., matched unrelated donor)
            (c) Receipt of high-dose steroids
            (d) Graft-versus-host disease
            (e) Solid organ transplant recipients
            (f) HIV infection, especially with low CD4$^+$ cell counts
            (g) Iron overload
            (h) Uncontrolled diabetes mellitus
            (i) Infection rare in immunocompetent individuals
    c. Diagnosis
        i. Definitive diagnosis requires tissue biopsy.
        ii. Tissue/sputum culture
    d. Treatment
        i. Liposomal amphotericin B or amphotericin B lipid complex 5 mg/kg intravenously once daily. Some experts recommend a rapid dose escalation to 7.5–10 mg/kg intravenously once daily.
        ii. Posaconazole has activity against the Zygomycetes, and most experts consider it second line after amphotericin B for maintenance (with the exception of animal and in vitro data with amphotericin B and echinocandins). Posaconazole dose for zygomycosis (off-label): 200 mg orally four times daily (oral suspension) or 300 mg twice daily for 1 day; then 300 mg once daily (delayed-release tablet or intravenous formulation)
        iii. Isavuconazole was recently approved for the treatment of invasive mucormycosis according to the results of a non-comparative study before the publication of the most recent guidelines.
        iv. Reversal of predisposing factors
        v. Surgical debridement of infected and/or necrotic tissue

Patient Case

35. S.C. (from patient case 34) presents to the clinic 3 months later. In the interim, he was hospitalized for treatment of a presumed fungal pneumonia. During his hospitalization, S.C. received 10 days of therapy with amphotericin B lipid complex and posaconazole 200 mg suspension orally four times daily; he was recently discharged to home with instructions to continue the posaconazole dose. A posaconazole trough concentration was measured before discharge, but because it was a send-out laboratory test, the results are just now available. The trough concentration was subtherapeutic. S.C. tells you that he takes his posaconazole doses at the following times: early morning 1 hour before breakfast, with lunch, with dinner, and before bedtime on an empty stomach. Which intervention is most likely to increase S.C.'s posaconazole trough concentration?

A. Take all doses with food or snack (ideally high fat).
B. Take all doses with food or snack (ideally high fat) and carbonated beverage.
C. Take all doses with food or snack (ideally high fat) and carbonated beverage, and minimize (or eliminate) acid-suppressive therapy.
D. Change dose to 400 mg orally twice daily and take with high-fat breakfast and dinner.

6. Endemic fungal pathogens
   a. Epidemiology
      i. Dimorphic fungi that exist as a mold in the environment; yeast form associated with clinical infection
      ii. Reservoir is the soil; exposure through inhalation
      iii. Regionally geographic distribution
      iv. *Histoplasma capsulatum*: Exists worldwide, but the most endemic region is the Ohio/Mississippi river valleys
      v. *Blastomyces dermatitidis*
         (a) Native to North America, although cases reported worldwide
         (b) The most endemic regions are in the midwestern United States and in Canadian provinces that border the Great Lakes.
      vi. *Coccidioides* spp.
         (a) *C. immitis* found in California's San Joaquin valley
         (b) *C. posadasii* found in the desert southwest of the United States, Mexico, and South America
   b. Clinical presentation
      i. Histoplasmosis
         (a) Acute pulmonary infection
         (b) Chronic pulmonary infection
         (c) Disseminated infection (lymphadenopathy, oral ulcers)
      ii. Blastomycosis
         (a) Acute pulmonary infection
         (b) Chronic pulmonary infection
         (c) Disseminated infection (genitourinary or osteoarticular systems)
      iii. Coccidioidomycosis
         (a) The most common infection is a self-limited acute or subacute pneumonia, which occasionally leads to pulmonary nodules and/or cavities.
         (b) Rarely, infection spreads beyond lungs to skin, bones, joints, CNS

c. Diagnosis
   i. Tissue biopsy
   ii. Tissue/sputum culture
   iii. Antigen detection (urine) for *Histoplasma*, *Blastomyces*
   iv. Antibodies for *Coccidioides*

d. Treatment
   i. Severe or disseminated disease
      (a) Amphotericin B deoxycholate 0.7–1 mg/kg intravenously once daily OR
      (b) Lipid formulation of amphotericin B 3–5 mg/kg intravenously once daily
   ii. Mild to moderate disease
      (a) Itraconazole 200 mg orally three times daily for 3 days; then 200 mg orally twice daily for histoplasmosis and blastomycosis
      (b) Fluconazole 400–800 mg orally daily for coccidioidomycosis
   iii. Minimal disease does not require antifungal treatment.

Patient Case

36. J.F. is a 49-year-old renal transplant recipient who takes itraconazole 200-mg capsules orally twice daily for histoplasmosis. He reports taking the capsules twice daily, first thing in the morning 1 hour before breakfast and in the evening 1–2 hours after dinner. He presents in the clinic for a follow-up, and his itraconazole trough concentration is subtherapeutic. Which is the most appropriate recommendation in this patient?

   A. Continue with itraconazole 200-mg capsules orally twice daily, and encourage the patient to take the medication with food.
   B. Increase the itraconazole dose of 200-mg capsules from orally twice daily to orally three times daily, and encourage the patient to take the medication with food.
   C. Keep the current itraconazole dose, but change the formulation to an oral solution and encourage the patient to take the medication with food.
   D. Keep the current itraconazole dose, but change the formulation to an oral solution, and encourage the patient to continue his current administration schedule.

REFERENCES

Sexually Transmitted Infections

1. Centers for Disease Control and Prevention (CDC). FDA licensure of bivalent human papillomavirus vaccine (HPV2, Cervarix) for use in females and updated HPV vaccination recommendations from the Advisory Committee on Immunization Practices (ACIP). MMWR 2010;59:626-9.

2. Centers for Disease Control and Prevention (CDC). Primary and secondary syphilis – United States, 2005 – 2013. MMWR 2014;63:402-6.

3. Centers for Disease Control and Prevention (CDC). Quadrivalent human papillomavirus vaccine: recommendations of the Advisory Committee on Immunization Practices (ACIP). MMWR 2007;56(RR02):1-24.

4. Centers for Disease Control and Prevention (CDC). Recommendations on the use of quadrivalent human papillomavirus vaccine in males—Advisory Committee on Immunization Practices (ACIP). MMWR 2011;60:1705-8.

5. Centers for Disease Control and Prevention (CDC). Sexually Transmitted Disease Surveillance 2013. Atlanta: U.S. Department of Health and Human Services, 2014.

6. Corey L, Wald A, Patel R, et al. Once-daily valacyclovir to reduce the risk of transmission of genital herpes. N Engl J Med 2004;350:11-20.

7. Kirkcaldy RD, Weinstock HS, Moore PC, et al. The efficacy and safety of gemifloxacin plus azithromycin and gemifloxacin plus azithromycin as treatment of uncomplicated gonorrhea. Clin Infect Dis 2014;59:1083-91.

8. Mandell GL. Mandell, Douglas, and Bennett's Principles of Infectious Diseases, 5th ed. Edinburgh: Churchill Livingstone, 2000.

9. Romanowski B, Marina RB, Roberts JN. Patients' preference of valacyclovir once-daily suppressive therapy versus twice-daily episodic therapy for recurrent genital herpes: a randomized study. Sex Transm Dis 2003;30:226-31.

10. Wald A, Selke S, Warren T, et al. Comparative efficacy of famciclovir and valacyclovir for suppression of recurrent genital herpes and viral shedding. Sex Transm Dis 2006;33:529-33.

11. Workowski KA, Bolan GA. Sexually transmitted diseases treatment guidelines, 2015. MMWR Recomm Rep 2015;64(RR03):1-137.

Human Immunodeficiency Virus

1. ACIP Adult Immunization Work Group; Bridges CB, Woods L, Coyne-Beasley T; Centers for Disease Control and Prevention. Advisory Committee on Immunization Practices (ACIP) recommended immunization schedule for adults aged 19 years and older – United States, 2013. MMWR 2013;62(suppl 1):9-19.

2. Centers for Disease Control and Prevention (CDC). Use of 13-Valent Pneumococcal Conjugate Vaccine and 23-Valent Pneumococcal Polysaccharide Vaccine Among Adults Aged ≥65 Years: Recommendations of the Advisory Committee on Immunization Practices (ACIP). MMWR 2014;63:822-5.

3. Centers for Disease Control and Prevention (CDC). Intervals between PCV13 and PPSV23 vaccines: recommendations of the Advisory Committee on Immunization Practices (ACIP). MMWR 2015;64:944-7.

4. Centers for Disease Control and Prevention and Association of Public Health Libraries. Laboratory Testing for the Diagnosis of HIV Infection: Updated Recommendations. June 27, 2014. Available at http://stacks.cdc.gov/view/cdc/23447. Accessed September 20, 2014.

5. HIV InSite Database of Antiretroviral Interactions. Available at www.hivinsite.com. Accessed September 23, 2014.

6. Kuhar ET, Henderson DK, Struble KA, et al. Updated U.S. Public Health Service guidelines for the management of occupational exposures to human immunodeficiency virus and recommendations for postexposure prophylaxis. Infect Control Hosp Epidemiol 2013;34:875-92.

7. Panel on Antiretroviral Guidelines for Adults and Adolescents. Guidelines for the Use of Antiretroviral Agents in HIV-1-Infected Adults and Adolescents. Washington, DC: U.S. Department of Health and Human Services. January 28, 2016:1-277. Available at http://aidsinfo.nih.gov/ContentFiles/AdultandAdolescentGL.pdf. Accessed February 19, 2016.

8. Panel on Opportunistic Infections in HIV-Infected Adults and Adolescents. Guidelines for the Prevention and Treatment of Opportunistic Infections in HIV-Infected Adolescents and Adults: Recommendations from the Centers for Disease Control and Prevention, the National Institutes of Health, and the HIV Medicine Association of the

Infectious Diseases Society of America. September 17, 2015:1-411. Available at http://aidsinfo.nih.gov/contentfiles/lvguidelines/adult_oi.pdf. Accessed September 18, 2015.

9. Panel on Treatment of HIV-Infected Pregnant Women and Prevention of Perinatal Transmission. Recommendations for Use of Antiretroviral Drugs in Pregnant HIV-1-Infected Women for Maternal Health and Interventions to Reduce Perinatal HIV Transmission in the United States. August 6, 2015:1-236. Available at http://aidsinfo.nih.gov/contentfiles/PerinatalGL.pdf. Accessed September 18, 2015.

10. Smith DK, Grohskopf LA, Black RJ, et al. Antiretroviral postexposure prophylaxis after sexual, injection-drug use, or other nonoccupational exposure to HIV in the United States. MMWR Recomm Rep 2015;54:1-20.

11. U.S. Public Health Service; Centers for Disease Control and Prevention; National Center for HIV/AIDS, Viral Hepatitis, and TB Prevention. Preexposure prophylaxis for the prevention of HIV infection—2014: a clinical practice guideline. MMWR 2014;63:437.

Non-HIV Viral Infections

1. ACIP Adult Immunization Work Group; Bridges CB, Woods L, Coyne-Beasley T; Centers for Disease Control and Prevention. Advisory Committee on Immunization Practices (ACIP) recommended immunization schedule for adults aged 19 years and older – United States, 2013. MMWR 2013;62(suppl 1):9-19.

2. Allen UD, Preiksaitis JK; AST Infectious Diseases Community of Practice. Epstein-Barr virus and posttransplant lymphoproliferative disorder in solid organ transplantation. Am J Transplant 2013;13:107-20.

3. Centers for Disease Control and Prevention (CDC). Antiviral agents for the treatment and chemoprophylaxis of influenza: recommendations by the Advisory Committee on Immunization Practices–(ACIP). MMWR 2011;60(RR01):1-24.

4. Centers for Disease Control and Prevention (CDC). Prevention and control of influenza with vaccines: recommendations by the Advisory Committee on Immunization Practices–(ACIP)–United States, 2015-16. MMWR 2015;64:818-25.

5. Centers for Disease Control and Prevention (CDC). Sexually transmitted diseases treatment guidelines 2010. MMWR 2010;59(RR12):1-116.

6. Centers for Disease Control and Prevention (CDC). Updated recommendation for use of VariZIG – United States, 2013. MMWR 2013;62:574-6.

7. Danziger-Isakov L, Kumar D; AST Infectious Diseases Community of Practice. Vaccination in solid organ transplantation. Am J Transplant 2013;13:311-7.

8. Dworkin RH, Johnson RW, Breuer J, et al. Recommendations for the management of herpes zoster. Clin Infect Dis 2007;44(suppl 1):S1-26.

9. Harpaz R, Ortega-Sanchez IR, Seward F; Centers for Disease Control and Prevention. Prevention of herpes zoster – recommendations of the Advisory Committee on Immunization Practices (ACIP). MMWR 2008;57(RR05):1-30.

10. Harper SA, Bradley JS, Englund JA, et al. Seasonal influenza in adults and children—diagnosis, treatment, chemoprophylaxis, and institutional outbreak management: clinical practice guidelines of the Infectious Diseases Society of America. Clin Infect Dis 2009;48:1003-32.

11. Mandell GL. Mandell, Douglas, and Bennett's Principles of Infectious Diseases, 5th ed. Edinburgh: Churchill Livingstone, 2000.

12. Marin M, Guris D, Chaves SS, et al.; Centers for Disease Control and Prevention. Prevention of varicella – recommendations of the Advisory Committee on Immunization Practices (ACIP). MMWR 2007;56(RR04):1-40.

13. Panel on Opportunistic Infections in HIV-Infected Adults and Adolescents. Guidelines for the Prevention and Treatment of Opportunistic Infections in HIV-Infected Adolescents and Adults: Recommendations from the Centers for Disease Control and Prevention, the National Institutes of Health, and the HIV Medicine Association of the Infectious Diseases Society of America, July 8, 2013:1-417. Available at http://aidsinfo.nih.gov/contentfiles/lvguidelines/adult_oi.pdf. Accessed September 28, 2013.

14. Razonable RR. Antiviral drugs for viruses other than human immunodeficiency virus. Mayo Clin Proc 2011;86:1009-26.

15. Razonable RR, Humar A; AST Infectious Diseases Community of Practice. Cytomegalovirus in solid organ transplantation. Am J Transplant 2013;13:93-106.

Fungal Infections

1. Baddley JW, Forrest GN; AST Infectious Diseases Community of Practice. Cryptococcosis in solid organ transplantation. Am J Transplant 2013;13:242-9.

2. Chapman SW, Dismukes WE, Proia LA, et al. Clinical practice guidelines for the management of blastomycosis: 2008 update by the Infectious Diseases Society of America. Clin Infect Dis 2008;46:1801-12.

3. Dismukes WE, Pappas PG, Sobel JD. Clinical Mycology. New York: Oxford University Press, 2003.

4. Dodds-Ashley E. Management of drug and food interactions with azole antifungal agents in transplant recipients. Pharmacotherapy 2010;30:842-54.

5. Galgiani JN, Ampel NM, Blair JE, et al. Coccidioidomycosis. Clin Infect Dis 2005;41:1217-23.

6. Hu SW, Bigby M. Pityriasis versicolor. Arch Dermatol 2010;146:1132-40.

7. Kauffman CA, Bustamante B, Chapman SW, et al. Clinical practice guidelines for the management of sporotrichosis: 2007 update by the Infectious Diseases Society of America. Clin Infect Dis 2007;45:1255-65.

8. Kontoyiannis DP, Lewis RE. How I treat mucormycosis. Blood 2011;118:1216-24.

9. Lanternier F, Sun HY, Ribaud P, et al. Mucormycosis in organ and stem cell transplant recipients. Clin Infect Dis 2012;54:1629-36.

10. Lewis RE. Current concepts in antifungal pharmacology. Mayo Clin Proc 2011;86:805-17.

11. Mandell GL. Mandell, Douglas, and Bennett's Principles of Infectious Diseases, 5th ed. Edinburgh: Churchill Livingstone, 2000.

12. Pappas PG, Kauffman CA, Andes D, et al. Clinical practice guidelines for the management of candidiasis: 2016 update by the Infectious Diseases Society of America. Clin Infect Dis 2015 Dec 16 [epub ahead of print].

13. Perfect JR, Dismukes WE, Dromer F, et al. Clinical practice guidelines for the management of cryptococcal disease: 2010 update by the Infectious Diseases Society of America. Clin Infect Dis 2010;50:290-322.

14. Pfaller MA, Rhomberg PR, Messer SA, et al. Isavuconazole, micafungin, and 8 comparator antifungal agents' susceptibility profiles for common and uncommon opportunistic fungi collected in 2013: temporal analysis of antifungal drug resistance using CLSI species-specific clinical breakpoints and proposed epidemiological cutoff values. Diagn Microbiol Infect Dis 2015;82:303-13.

15. Smith J, Andes D. Therapeutic drug monitoring of antifungals: pharmacokinetic and pharmacodynamics considerations. Ther Drug Monit 2008;30:167-72.

16. Tragiannidis A, Tsoulas C, Kerl K, et al. Invasive candidiasis: update on current pharmacotherapy options and future perspectives. Expert Opin Pharmacother 2013;14:1515-28.

17. Walsh TJ, Anaissie EJ, Denning DW, et al. Treatment of aspergillosis: clinical practice guidelines of the Infectious Diseases Society of America. Clin Infect Dis 2008;46:327-60.

18. Wheat LJ, Freifeld AG, Kleiman MB, et al. Clinical practice guidelines for the management of patients with histoplasmosis: 2007 update by the Infectious Diseases Society of America. Clin Infect Dis 2007;45:807-25.

ANSWERS AND EXPLANATIONS TO PATIENT CASES

1. Answer: C

The patient's NAAT tests confirm both gonorrhea and chlamydia. Fluoroquinolones are not recommended because of resistance to the antibiotics, nor should the patient receive fluoroquinolones or tetracyclines because of her positive pregnancy test result (Answer A is incorrect). In addition to pregnancy, doxycycline is no longer recommended for gonorrhea due to increased tetracycline resistance and the convenience of single dose therapy with azithromycin (Answer D is incorrect). Cefixime is recommended only if ceftriaxone is not available (Answer B is incorrect). The most appropriate choice is ceftriaxone 250 mg intramuscularly once plus azithromycin 1 g orally once (Answer C is correct).

2. Answer: B

The patient's therapy for syphilis failed because his RPR titer did not decrease by 4-fold at follow-up. The FTA-ABS test result may remain positive after effective treatment. A lumbar puncture is indicated when the RPR does not decrease by 4-fold 6–12 months after appropriate treatment. This patient's lumbar puncture was negative for neurosyphilis, so intravenous penicillin is not indicated (Answer C is incorrect). Doxycycline is an alternative to penicillin for treatment of latent syphilis but is not recommended for this patient because he has no penicillin allergy (Answer D is incorrect). In this case, benzathine penicillin G 2.4 million units intramuscularly once weekly for 3 weeks is the optimal treatment for late latent syphilis (Answer B is correct; Answer A is incorrect).

3. Answer: D

The most effective means of preventing HSV transmission in a discordant relationship is the combination of suppressive antiviral therapy, consistent condom use, and refraining from sexual activity during recurrences (Answer D is correct; Answers A, B, and C are incorrect).

4. Answer: A

This patient has tested positive for HIV with both an HIV fourth-generation combination ELISA and HIV-1/HIV-2 antibody differentiation assay. The fourth-generation ELISA is the HIV screening test that detects antibodies to HIV-1 and HIV-2 as well as p24 antigen, whereas the antibody differentiation assay differentiates between HIV-1 and HIV-2 and confirms infection. The patient's condition does not meet the criteria for an AIDS diagnosis, which includes a CD4$^+$ cell count that is, or ever has been, less than 200 cells/mm^3 or infection with one of a long list of AIDS-defining illnesses. Episodic thrush infections are not considered AIDS-defining illnesses (Answer B is incorrect). There is no evidence to support Kaposi sarcoma or immune reconstitution syndrome (Answer A is correct; Answers C and C are incorrect).

5. Answer: A

The risk of acquiring HIV from oral sex is minimal (Answers B and D are incorrect). This is especially true for the insertive partner in an oral sex encounter (Answer A is correct). However, oral sex does carry the risk of efficient disease transmission of other STDs, including syphilis (Answer C is incorrect). Receptive anal intercourse carries the greatest risk of HIV transmission with respect to sexual practices.

6. Answer: B

The risk of HIV transmission perinatally in an untreated woman is about 26%. The use of zidovudine monotherapy reduces this risk to about 8%. Ideally, zidovudine should be initiated in pregnancy, as indicated, as part of a complete three-drug ARV regimen. When triple therapy is unwarranted or when patients refuse three-drug regimens, zidovudine monotherapy should be advised (Answer B is correct). Human immunodeficiency virus infection has not been associated with spontaneous abortion (Answer D is incorrect), and each ARV agent carries a differing level of risk-benefit with respect to fetal development, with some agents preferred to others (Answer C is incorrect). A cesarean section is recommended for women with viral loads greater than 1000 copies/mL, but ART is the first priority (Answer A is incorrect).

7. Answer: D

Latex or polyurethane condoms (in cases of latex allergies) are recommended to prevent exposure to sexual fluids and reduce the risk of HIV transmission (Answer D is correct). When condoms are used, water-based lubricants may also be used to reduce the extent of trauma and potential risk. Oil-based lubricants are not recommended because they may compromise the integrity of condoms and increase the potential for rupture (Answers A and C are incorrect). Serosorting is the practice of choosing a sexual partner with the same HIV serostatus (HIV-positive or HIV-negative). In this case, if T.P. has sex only with HIV-negative partners, his risk of HIV is reduced but not zero as partners could have seroconverted since their last HIV screening test. In addition, he would have no protection against other STDs (Answer B is incorrect).

8. Answer: B

Needle exchange programs have successfully reduced the extent of HIV transmission among injection drug users. The use of clean needles may also reduce the transmission of HBV and HCV (Answer B is correct; Answer D is incorrect). Hepatitis A is transmitted by the fecal-oral route; similarly, other STDs (e.g., gonorrhea, syphilis) are not transmitted percutaneously (Answers A and C are incorrect).

9. Answer: C

This patient presents with an HIV risk factor (MSM). His symptomatology (e.g., malaise, rash) may be consistent with acute HIV conversion syndrome. Given his presentation and risk factors, he is likely to have HIV infection with a high presenting viral load (Answer C is correct). If an OraQuick screening is indeed positive, it will need to be confirmed by fourth-generation combination ELISA and antibody differentiation assay (Answers B and D are incorrect). The patient's symptoms do not clearly establish infection with any of the more common opportunistic infections (Answer A is incorrect).

10. Answer: A

The CDC recommends HIV screening for all Americans 13–64 years of age and yearly screening for those at high risk of exposure. Screening is particularly advised if HIV prevalence in the local community exceeds 1%. Given this patient's locality (a large urban area with a seroprevalence of 1.3%), testing on a yearly basis would be advisable (Answer A is correct; Answers B, C, and D are incorrect).

11. Answer: C

OraQuick is an HIV ELISA test now available OTC. The OTC test kit is designed to assay oral fluids (Answer B is incorrect) with results available less than 1 hour (Answer D is incorrect). The test detects HIV antibodies that may not be present for up to 3 months after an initial HIV infection (Answer C is correct). Confirmation of a reactive test result should always be performed (Answer A is incorrect). Nonreactive or negative test results do not require confirmation, but it is commonly advised to retest in 6 months.

12. Answer: A

The revised U.S. Department of Health and Human Services guidelines in February 2013 recommend treating all HIV-seropositive individuals to reduce disease progression and HIV transmission. Previous guidelines recommended ART on the basis of CD4+ and HIV viral load cutoff values (Answers B, C, and D are incorrect). The recommendation changed to treat all patients, regardless of these values, because of the increased evidence suggesting the negative consequences of uncontrolled viral replication as well as the improved efficacy and tolerability of newer ART (Answer A is correct).

13. Answer: B

Genotypic resistance testing is recommended for all patients with HIV at the time of entry into care, regardless of treatment initiation (Answer B is correct). In addition, if therapy is deferred, repeated genotypic resistance testing is recommended when treatment is initiated because of the risk of acquiring a resistant virus in the interim. Phenotypic resistance testing is more costly and time-consuming and is generally reserved for patients with complex resistance mutations (Answer D is incorrect). The coreceptor tropism assay is recommended prior to initiation of maraviroc (Answer A is incorrect) and *HLA-B*5701* screening is recommended prior to initiation of abacavir (Answer C is incorrect).

14. Answer: C

Recommended first-line ARV regimens include emtricitabine/tenofovir DF/ritonavir-boosted daruna-vir, lamivudine/abacavir/dolutegravir, emtricitabine/tenofovir DF/dolutegravir, emtricitabine/tenofovir DF/cobicistat-boosted elvitegravir, emtricitabine/tenofovir DF/raltegravir, and emtricitabine/tenofovir AF/cobicistat-boosted elvitegravir because of their improved durability and tolerability and decreased pill burden compared with previously recommended regimens. Thus, only Answer C is a recommended first-line combination (Answer C is correct; Answers A, B, and D are incorrect). Answer A is an alternative regimen, but given the patient's history of substance abuse, an efavirenz-based regimen is not recommended.

15. Answer: B

The primary treatment goal is an undetectable viral load (below lowest quantifiable amount, varies by assay), with increased CD4+ cell counts as a secondary goal (Answer B is correct; Answer C is incorrect). Therapy is lifelong (Answer A is incorrect), and patients should seek medical attention before discontinuing ARV agents (Answer B is incorrect).

16. Answer: B

The combination product Epzicom (lamividuine/abacavir) contains the NRTI abacavir. Abacavir causes potentially life-threatening hypersensitivity reactions in certain patient subsets. The *HLA-B*5701* pharmacogenomic screening test can preemptively identify patients at risk of these reactions; therefore, this test should be prospectively done in all patients who are candidates for abacavir (Answer B is correct; Answers A, C, and D are incorrect).

17. Answer: B

Ritonavir boosting involves the concept of producing a favorable drug interaction by administering very low doses of the drug in combination with other substrate PIs. Ritonavir is a very potent inhibitor (Answer A is incorrect) of the CYP system and thus increases the serum concentrations of most other PIs (Answer C is incorrect), allowing reduced dosage and dosing frequency of the substrate drug. When used at low doses for boosting other PIs, ritonavir is not counted as one of the active agents in an ARV regimen (Answer B is correct). The normal ritonavir dose for boosting is 100 – 200 mg daily (Answer D is incorrect).

18. Answer: A

Atripla is a three-drug combination product consisting of tenofovir DF, emtricitabine, and efavirenz. Some degree of GI upset may occur with any of these three agents. Efavirenz is well known to cause CNS effects, which can include an increase in anxiety and the onset of vivid dreams that may be unpleasant. Rash may also occur, but the combination has not been associated with erectile dysfunction, sedation, jaundice, retinitis, or changes in blood pressure (Answer A is correct; answers B, C and D are incorrect).

19. Answer: D

This patient appears to adhere to his ARV regimen, and although inherent resistance and subsequent ART failure are possible, the effects of his recent illness should be ruled out initially. The acute episode of otitis media that required 14 days of antibiotic therapy may have resulted in a transient "blip" in the viral load. Therefore, it would be most appropriate to repeat a viral load test and CD4+ cell count before executing more costly and involved interventions (Answer D is correct; Answers A, B, and C are incorrect).

20. Answer: C

To prevent new-onset infections, close attention should be paid to the immunization histories of all patients with HIV infection. Patients with HIV may receive any "killed" vaccinations, whereas "live" vaccinations should be deferred in most cases. Given the overlap in risk factors associated with HIV and the hepatic diseases, immunizations against hepatitis A and B should be considered. For this patient, HBV immunization is unwarranted because he is hepatitis B antibody positive and antigen negative (indicating a history of vaccination; Answers A and D are incorrect). Consideration should be given to yearly influenza immunizations with the killed intramuscular formulation. Among patients with HIV infection, community-acquired pneumonia may be particularly serious; therefore, pneumococcal vaccination should be administered (ideally, first dose with PCV13 [Prevnar], followed by PPSV23 [Pneumovax]; Answer B is incorrect). Because this patient does not recall his latest tetanus vaccination, a booster dose using Tdap should be provided today and followed every 10 years thereafter with a Td booster (Answer C is correct). Of note, in studies of adults receiving concomitant Prevnar and IIV, the response of individuals to Prevnar was decreased compared with the response of those who received the two vaccines 1 month apart. Until further data are available, it may be prudent to separate Prevnar and IIVs by 1 month.

21. Answer: C

Patients with HIV infection should be screened once yearly for TB with an appropriately placed and read PPD skin test or a blood-based assay. After PPD placement, the infiltrate should be read within 48–72 hours (Answer A and B are incorrect). Infiltrates greater than 5 mm should be considered a cause for follow-up screening with a chest radiograph (Answer C is correct; Answer D is incorrect).

22. Answer: D

Nonrecurrent episodes of thrush may be managed with short-term courses of appropriate antifungal agents (e.g., fluconazole; Answer D is correct; Answers A and C are incorrect). For this patient, whose CD4+ cell count is 210 cells/mm³, no opportunistic infection prophylaxis is indicated (Answer B is incorrect). Single and nonrecurrent episodes of thrush are not considered AIDS-defining illnesses.

23. Answer: D

This patient has a CD4+ cell count of 90 cells/mm³, placing her at risk of reinfection (PJP) and new infection (toxoplasmosis) (less than 100 cells/mm³). Dapsone is being prescribed as prophylaxis in place of Bactrim DS, presumably to avoid a sulfa reaction. Although dapsone may itself induce sulfa reactions, this is less common than with Bactrim DS. Although Bactrim DS will provide prophylaxis against toxoplasmosis, dapsone will not; therefore, additional pharmacotherapy will be required to adequately avoid this infection while the CD4+ cell count remains less than 100 cells/mm³ (Answer D is correct; Answers A, B, and C are incorrect).

24. Answer: A

Despite this patient's history of PJP, prophylaxis is no longer required because the patient's CD4+ cell count has been above the threshold for prophylaxis (greater than 200 cells/mm³) with an undetectable viral load for several years. Secondary prophylaxis is indicated only if the patient's cell count is no greater than 200 cells/mm³ for at least 3–6 months in conjunction with an undetectable viral load (Answer A is correct; Answer B is incorrect). Varicella vaccine may be considered in varicella-nonimmune patients with a CD4+ count greater than 200 cells/mm³, but it is not indicated in this patient because of his history of VZV infection (Answer C is incorrect). Prophylaxis against community-acquired pneumonia with antibiotic therapy is not advised (Answer D is incorrect).

25. Answer: A

This needlestick case involves a source patient who is at an apparently high risk of HIV infection (injection drug user). The nurse is potentially within the window of opportunity for drug treatment (48–72 hours; Answer B is incorrect). Because of these factors, immediate administration of triple-drug PEP should be considered (Answer A is correct). Postexposure prophylaxis should be administered after baseline HIV testing of the nurse and then continued until the source patient is determined to be HIV seronegative for 4 weeks. Two-drug PEP is no longer recommended (Answer C is incorrect). Hepatitis B vaccination is recommended in healthcare workers, but would not be beneficial after the exposure in this scenario (Answer D is incorrect).

26. Answer: C

Preexposure prophylaxis may be undertaken in select high-risk HIV-seronegative individuals. Standard preexposure protocols involve the dispensing and administration of a 90-day supply of emtricitabine/tenofovir DF to be taken once daily (Answers A and B are incorrect). Use of PrEP will also require more frequent HIV and HBV screening to more quickly detect infection with either virus, should drug therapy fail (Answer C is correct). The use of PrEP is not completely protective against HIV and provides no protection against other STDs; therefore, it does not preclude the need for other risk reduction interventions such as condom use (Answer D is incorrect).

27. Answer: C

The use of antiviral therapy for a patient with a low risk of complications from influenza is a judgment call. The CDC guidelines recommend that treatment be considered in otherwise healthy, symptomatic patients within 48 hours of symptom onset. Given this patient's profession and request for antiviral treatment, it is reasonable to prescribe antiviral therapy (Answer A is incorrect). Although active against influenza, adamantanes are not currently recommended because of resistance in recent years (Answer B is incorrect). The standard treatment duration is 5 days, which is appropriate for this patient (Answer C is correct; Answer D is incorrect).

28. Answer: B

The influenza vaccine is the best means of prophylaxis, which is recommended for this patient. However, until she has full immunity from the vaccine, antiviral prophylaxis with oseltamivir or zanamivir is recommended (Answer B is correct; Answer A is incorrect). Alternatively, oseltamivir or zanamivir could be used as prophylaxis for the duration of the influenza (give for 7 days beyond last exposure), but the vaccine is preferred for patients without vaccine contraindications (Answer C is incorrect). Adamantanes are not active against influenza B, nor are they currently recommended for influenza A because of resistance (Answer D is incorrect).

29. Answer: C

This patient's rash is consistent with shingles caused by VZV. Treatment is reasonable to consider because it could expedite resolution of the rash and might decrease the incidence of postherpetic neuralgia (Answer D is incorrect). Intravenous acyclovir is appropriate for immunocompromised patients or other patients with serious infection (Answer B is incorrect). Oral therapy is sufficient in this patient; the acyclovir dose should be 800 mg orally five times daily (Answer A is incorrect), so the best answer is valacyclovir 1 g orally three times daily (Answer C is correct).

30. Answer: D

The patient in Answer B is at low risk of CMV infection or reactivation because of donor and recipient CMV seronegativity (Answer B is incorrect). The patient in Answer C is at moderate risk of CMV infection, but given his current receipt of valganciclovir, CMV infection is unlikely (Answer C is incorrect). The greatest risk of CMV infection in solid organ transplantation is among CMV-seronegative recipients who receive an organ from a CMV-seropositive donor. Even considering the CMV mismatch for the patient in Answer A, CMV infection is less likely to occur 13 years after transplantation given her stable allograft function and lack of recent complications (i.e., treatment of rejection) (Answer A is incorrect). The patient in Answer D has just received treatment for rejection, has a CMV mismatch, and is not currently receiving antiviral prophylaxis (Answer D is correct).

31. Answer: D

This patient has lymphocutaneous sporotrichosis, for which itraconazole 200 mg orally once daily is the first-line treatment (Answer D is correct). Amphotericin B is indicated for severe or life-threatening infections (Answer A is incorrect); terbinafine and saturated solution of potassium iodide are alternative agents for patients whose condition does not respond to itraconazole.

32. Answer: B

This patient is at risk of invasive candidiasis because of her recent hospitalization for GI surgery, presumed receipt of antibiotics for surgical prophylaxis, and current use of total parenteral nutrition. For initial empiric treatment of invasive candidiasis, the guidelines recommend any echinocandin as first-line therapy. Fluconazole is an alternative to an echinocandin for patients who are not critically ill and are unlikely to have fluconazole-resistant *Candida* species. This patient has no known risk factors for resistant *Candida* spp., but the guidelines recommend first-line therapy with an echinocandin over fluconazole (Answer B is correct; Answer A is incorrect). Posaconazole and amphotericin B are not recommended for initial treatment of invasive candidiasis (Answers C and D are incorrect).

33. Answer: A

This patient's *Candida* isolate is pan-susceptible, the patient is stable, and the blood has sterilized; thus, fluconazole is the appropriate choice (Answer A is correct). A loading dose is not required because fluconazole susceptibility has been confirmed. For this patient with questionable GI absorption, intravenous fluconazole is preferred, but if GI integrity were not an issue, oral fluconazole at the same dose would be sufficient. It is not necessary to continue the micafungin in this scenario or change to broader antifungal therapy (e.g., posaconazole or amphotericin B lipid complex) when fluconazole susceptibility is confirmed (Answers B, C, and D are incorrect).

34. Answer: A

Voriconazole is a potent CYP3A4 inhibitor; thus, the tacrolimus dose should be empirically reduced (Answer A is correct; Answer B is incorrect). For patients receiving tacrolimus (at goal concentrations), it is recommended to reduce the tacrolimus dose by 66% when concomitant voriconazole is initiated. Tacrolimus neither inhibits or induces the metabolism of voriconazole (Answers C and D are incorrect).

35. Answer: C

Posaconazole suspension is best absorbed with food, ideally food higher in fat. Moreover, in the fasted state, carbonation improves posaconazole absorption. Posaconazole requires an acidic environment for absorption; avoidance of acid-suppressive therapy is recommended, if possible (Answer C is correct; Answers A and B are incorrect). In addition, posaconazole has saturable absorption, so changing the dose from 200 mg orally four times daily to 400 mg twice daily would not improve drug exposure (Answer D is incorrect). Recently, a delayed-release tablet formulation of posaconazole was approved whose absorption is more reliable than that of the oral suspension. In addition, it may be given with concomitant acid-suppressive therapy. Like the oral suspension, it is recommended to give the oral tablet with food, although its absorption is less dependent on gastric state.

36. Answer: D

Itraconazole capsules are up to 55% bioavailable with food, whereas the oral solution is up to 100% absorbed in the fasting state. Because the patient has a demonstrated pattern of taking the medication on an empty stomach, it is most appropriate to change from the capsule to the oral solution, especially because the solution has more reliable absorption than the capsule (Answer D is correct; Answer A and C are incorrect). If a patient refuses to take the oral solution because of GI intolerance, it is recommended to optimize the administration of the capsule (with food) at the current dose before increasing the dose (Answer B is incorrect).

ANSWERS AND EXPLANATIONS TO SELF-ASSESSMENT QUESTIONS

1. Answer: C

The patient's clinical presentation and presence of gram-negative diplococci from a urethral smear are consistent with gonococcal infection. Ceftriaxone 250 mg intramuscularly is the drug of choice. Fluoroquinolones are not recommended because of high rates of resistance to these antibiotics. Because of high coinfection rates, a patient with gonorrhea should also be treated for chlamydia even if the test for chlamydia is negative. In addition, the treatment for chlamydia provides dual coverage against gonorrhea which may prevent development of drug resistance (Answer A is incorrect). The recommended regimen is ceftriaxone 250 mg intramuscularly once and azithromycin 1 g orally once (Answer C is correct). Tetracyclines may be used for chlamydia alone but are not recommended for treatment of gonococcal infections due to increased resistance (Answers B and D are incorrect). Although tetracyclines are not recommended for the treatment of gonorrhea, the correct dose of doxycycline is 100 mg orally twice daily for 7 days for the treatment of chlamydia.

2. Answer: D

For first episodes of herpes labialis, acyclovir 400 mg orally three times daily is a reasonable first-line option (Answer D is correct). Increasing the acyclovir dose to 800 mg is not necessary (Answer C is incorrect), and the correct valacyclovir dose for HSV is 1 g orally twice daily (Answer A is incorrect). Although valganciclovir is active against HSV, its spectrum is broader than necessary (Answer B is incorrect).

3. Answer: A

One of the most critical factors involved in the efficacy of PEP to prevent HIV infection is the time elapsed since the actual exposure. The earlier the PEP is administered, the greater the likelihood of efficacy (Answer A is correct). Most experts agree that the use of PEP beyond 72 hours of time zero is unlikely to reduce the risk of HIV transmission. The gender, medication history, CD4$^+$ cell count of the source patient do not impact the efficacy of PEP (Answers B, C, and D are incorrect).

4. Answer: A

It is recommended to obtain a genotype for all patients when they begin to receive HIV care, regardless of initiation of ART (Answer A is correct). A phenotypic resistance test is reserved for patients with known or suspected complex drug resistance mutations (Answer B is incorrect).

Vaccinations are also important but would not be the first priority (Answers C and D are incorrect).

5. Answer: A

Human immunodeficiency virus and certain ARV agents have been associated with a propensity to induce hyperlipidemia. Typically, the management of hyperlipidemia in patients with HIV infection is similar to that in uninfected patients, except for certain limitations in the selection of drug therapy with statins. Many of the statin agents will interact with PIs, increasing the risk of rhabdomyolysis. If statins are indicated to lower LDL-C, preferred agents include those with a lower propensity for CYP interactions (e.g., pravastatin, atorvastatin, rosuvastatin; Answer A is correct; Answer B is incorrect). Zidovudine and lamivudine are not associated with hyperlipidemia (Answers C and D are incorrect).

6. Answer: D

Of the listed options, emtricitabine/tenofovir DF/efavirenz, emtricitabine/tenofovir DF/rilpivirine, and emtricitabine/tenofovir DF/elvitegravir/cobistat represent once-daily treatment options that include three concurrent ARV agents. Emtricitabine/tenofovir DF/efavirenz and emtricitabine/tenofovir DF/rilpivirine are listed as alternative agents, not recommended agents in the current guidelines (Answers A and B are incorrect). In addition, the use of efavirenz is not recommended in this patient as it might further exacerbate this patient's difficulty sleeping; efavirenz has been associated with vivid dreams and CNS disengagement. Emtricitabine/tenofovir DF/elvitegravir/cobistat is a recommended treatment option for ARV-naïve patients and would be the best choice in this case (Answer D is correct). Emtricitabine/tenofovir DF/raltegravir is also a recommended option, but the raltegravir requires twice-daily dosing (Answer C is incorrect).

7. Answer: C

Vaccination is the most effective method for preventing influenza (Answer A is incorrect). The inactivated vaccine is preferred for this patient because she is a transplant recipient (Answer C is correct; Answer D is incorrect). The use of oseltamivir for 2 weeks at the time of influenza vaccination (to provide protection until immunity is established) may be considered if a patient has an influenza exposure (Answer B is incorrect because the patient did not report an influenza exposure).

8. Answer: C

The ACIP guidelines recommend a one-time dose of Zostavax to all individuals who are 60 years or older, regardless of herpes zoster history (Answer C is correct). It is thus unnecessary to obtain VZV serologic testing for this patient (Answer A is incorrect). Varivax is recommended as a routine childhood vaccine and may be given to certain immunocompromised patients who are VZV negative (Answer B is incorrect). The VariZIG vaccine is recommended only as PEP in high-risk VZV-negative patients (Answer D is incorrect).

9. Answer: B

This patient is at high risk of CMV infection because (1) the donor has a history of CMV infection and (2) the patient has no history of infection and thus lacks CMV-specific antibodies. Valganciclovir 900 mg orally once daily is preferred for adult transplant recipients (Answer B is correct); ganciclovir 1 g orally three times daily (Answer A is incorrect) or ganciclovir 5 mg/kg intravenously once daily are other options. Famciclovir has not been studied for CMV prophylaxis (Answer D is incorrect), and acyclovir may be an alternative but in doses higher than 800 mg/day (Answer C is incorrect).

10. Answer: B

Tinea pedis is a type of ringworm caused by the dermatophytes *Trichophyton*, *Microsporum*, and *Epidermophyton* (Answer B is correct). The other listed fungal pathogens are not dermatophytes (Answers A, C, and D are incorrect).

11. Answer: D

The finding of nonseptate hyphae is consistent with the Zygomycetes, such as *Mucor*, *Rhizopus*, or *Rhizomucor*. This patient's history of recent high-dose steroids and diabetes mellitus are risk factors for infections caused by the Zygomycetes. In addition, the most common infection site is rhinocerebral (Answer D is correct). *Aspergillus*, while also a mold, would have septate hyphae with acute-angle branching (Answer A is incorrect). *Blastomyces* and *Cryptococcus* would both be identified as yeast in culture or pathology (Answers B and C are incorrect).

12. Answer: B

Voriconazole is considered the drug of choice for the initial treatment of invasive aspergillosis (Answer B is correct). Itraconazole has anti-*Aspergillus* activity but is rarely used because voriconazole is more potent and has better data to support its use (Answer A is incorrect). The lipid formulations of amphotericin B and the echinocandins are considered alternatives to voriconazole if the patient experiences intolerance and/or lack of response (Answers C and D are incorrect). In addition, isavuconazole was recently approved for the treatment of invasive aspergillosis but after the guidelines were published. In a clinical study, isavuconazole was noninferior to voriconazole for aspergillosis.

13. Answer: B

H. capsulatum is endemic in the Ohio and Mississippi river valleys (Answer B is correct). *B. dermatitidis* is endemic around the Great Lakes (Answer A is incorrect), whereas *Coccidioides* spp. are endemic in the desert Southwest (Answers C and D are incorrect).

Infectious Diseases II

Adam Jackson, Pharm.D., BCACP

Kaiser Permanente Colorado
Denver, Colorado

Infectious Diseases II

Adam Jackson, Pharm.D., BCACP

Kaiser Permanente Colorado
Denver, Colorado

Learning Objectives

1. Design appropriate pharmacologic and nonpharmacologic treatment regimens for various patient populations with urinary tract infections, prostatitis, community-acquired pneumonia, sinusitis, pharyngitis, otitis media, skin and soft tissue infections, tuberculosis, ophthalmic infections, bone and joint infections, tickborne infections, infective endocarditis, central nervous system infections, antibiotic prophylaxis, infectious diarrhea, and *Clostridium difficile* infections.
2. Identify risk factors and clinical circumstances for antimicrobial resistance.
3. Design an antimicrobial therapeutic regimen to treat resistant infections and prevent future development.
4. Apply evidence-based medicine and patient-specific factors to design antimicrobial regimens that are appropriate and cost-effective for the patient.

Self-Assessment Questions

Answers and explanations to these questions may be found at the end of the chapter.

1. A female patient comes to the clinic with a urinary tract infection (UTI), and you are asked by the nursing student to explain the patient's urinary dipstick test because the student is confused by the results. The patient's results are positive for nitrite, leukocyte esterase, protein, and blood in the urine. Specifically, the nurse asks which urine dipstick result, if positive, is most indicative of a UTI?

    A. Nitrite positive.
    B. Leukocyte esterase positive.
    C. Positive for protein.
    D. Positive for blood.

2. R.T. is an 18-year-old woman who presents to the clinic with a 2-day history of urinary frequency and burning. She noticed this morning that her urine was dark red. She reports having unprotected sex with her boyfriend of 6 months. Her urinalysis comes back with the following results: urine hazy, white blood cell (WBC) count of 10 x 10^3 cells/mm^3, nitrite positive, leukocyte esterase positive, positive for protein, positive for blood,

and 10^3 CFU/mL gram-negative rods. Culture results are pending. Given her clinical and laboratory presentation, which is the best therapeutic decision for R.T.?

    A. Treat her for gonorrhea and chlamydia.
    B. Treat her for acute uncomplicated cystitis plus gonorrhea/chlamydia.
    C. Treatment is not needed because the bacterial inocula are less than 10^5 CFU/mL.
    D. Treat her for acute uncomplicated cystitis.

3. The Infectious Diseases Society of America (IDSA) and the American Thoracic Society (ATS) physicians recommend using guideline-based protocols for the management of community-acquired pneumonia (CAP). Which outcome has the most evidence to support the use of these guidelines?

    A. Decrease in mortality.
    B. Decrease in fluoroquinolone resistance.
    C. Increase in practitioner compliance.
    D. Decrease in intensive care unit (ICU) admissions.

4. A 7-year-old girl is brought to the clinic in October with a 1-day history of a red left eye. She says that she could barely take her test today at school because her eye is itchy and watery, and it feels like something is in it. On physical examination, she is afebrile, and her left conjunctiva is red and inflamed. No foreign objects or visual changes are noted. She is given a diagnosis of conjunctivitis. Which is the best treatment of her conjunctivitis?

    A. Supportive care only, with warm, moist compresses as needed.
    B. Azithromycin 1%, one drop in left eye twice daily for 2 days, followed by one drop twice daily for 5 days.
    C. Ofloxacin 0.3%, one or two drops in left eye once daily for 14 days.
    D. Ketotifen 0.025%, one drop in left eye twice daily for 7 days.

5. A 45-year-old man comes to the clinic with a red rash on his neck that started about a week ago, the day he flew back from his camping trip in Maine. He states that although he picked off a few ticks while he was there, he does not remember any ticks on his neck. On examination, he has an erythematous rash with a bull's-eye pattern on the right side of his neck. He has no other symptoms. His laboratory tests are positive for *Borrelia burgdorferi* antibodies, and he is given a diagnosis of Lyme disease. Which is the most appropriate management for his disease?

   A. Watch and wait to see if more symptoms develop.
   B. Give ceftriaxone 2 g intravenously daily for 14 days.
   C. Give doxycycline 200 mg orally once.
   D. Give doxycycline 100 mg orally twice daily for 14 days.

6. H.J. is a 19-year-old man who returns to the clinic with worsening nasal congestion, headache, and severe tooth pain. He has just completed a 10-day course of amoxicillin/clavulanate 2 g/125 mg orally twice daily. H.J. says that his symptoms got better for a few days but that they then continued to get worse during the past week. He states that he took his drugs as prescribed and has not skipped any days. He has no known drug allergies. Which regimen is the best recommendation for the treatment of H.J.'s sinusitis?

   A. Amoxicillin 1 g three times daily for 21 days.
   B. Azithromycin 500 mg daily for 21 days.
   C. Moxifloxacin 400 mg daily for 10 days.
   D. Linezolid 600 mg orally twice daily for 10 days.

7. R.T. is a 13-year-old boy who presents to the pediatrician's office with a 4-day history of severe sore throat and a temperature of 101°F. He states he can barely swallow because his throat hurts so badly. On physical examination, he weighs 41.2 kg, and his tonsils are erythematous and swollen. A throat swab is taken, and the rapid antigen detection test (RADT) comes back positive for *Streptococcus pyogenes*. R.T. has no known drug allergies. Which treatment recommendation is most appropriate for R.T.?

   A. No treatment necessary.
   B. Penicillin benzathine 0.6 million units intramuscularly once.
   C. Trimethoprim/sulfamethoxazole 1 double-strength tablet orally every 12 hours for 10 days.
   D. Penicillin benzathine 1.2 million units intramuscularly once.

8. J.K. is a 45-year-old man who presents to the clinic with a 48-hour history of severe diarrhea. J.K.'s medical history includes type 2 diabetes, hypertension, and recent surgical drainage of boils. He has two children younger than 4 years living at home. He is at day 12 of his 14-day amoxicillin/clavulanate therapy for the treatment of the carbuncles (boils) he had drained 12 days ago. Physical examination reveals significant improvement in the drained boils, and stool studies are positive for *Clostridium difficile* toxins A and B. Which risk factor is most likely responsible for J.K.'s development of *C. difficile* diarrhea?

   A. Type 2 diabetes.
   B. Recent surgery.
   C. Living with children younger than 5 years.
   D. Current amoxicillin/clavulanate treatment.

9. F.H. is a 62-year-old man who presents to the clinic with a weeklong history of a blister on the side of his right foot that has increased in redness and oozing for the past 24 hours. F.H.'s medical history includes type 2 diabetes for 25 years, coronary artery disease, hypertension, chronic kidney disease (creatinine clearance [CrCl] in the past week was 22 mL/minute/1.73 m²), and amputation of his right middle finger 3 years ago because of infection. He reports a rash to "sulfa drugs." Physical examination reveals a foul-smelling, pus-filled blister with surrounding erythema on the inside of the right foot with no necrosis. Radiographic study findings are negative for osteomyelitis, and cultures and sensitivities are pending. F.H. is being sent for wound debridement and outpatient antibiotic therapy. Which regimen is the best empiric coverage for F.H.'s diabetic foot infection?

   A. Trimethoprim/sulfamethoxazole 1 double-strength tablet orally twice daily for 14 days.
   B. Levofloxacin 250 mg orally daily for 14 days.
   C. Vancomycin 1 g intravenously every 12 hours for 14 days.
   D. Levofloxacin 750 mg orally daily for 14 days.

10. S.O. is an 18-year-old high-school senior who comes to the clinic worried she is going to get sick. Her best friend just received a diagnosis of meningitis caused by *Neisseria meningitidis*. S.O. is an otherwise healthy teenager with no known drug allergies, and she shows no signs of infection today. She has not yet received her meningococcal vaccination because she was going to wait until she went to college. Which would be the best recommendation for S.O. at this time?

   A. Ceftriaxone 1 g intramuscularly once daily for 14 days.
   B. Meningococcal conjugate vaccination only.
   C. Rifampin 600 mg orally twice daily for 4 days.
   D. Ciprofloxacin 500 mg orally once.

I. URINARY TRACT INFECTIONS

A. Introduction - *(Domain 5)*
1. UTIs are the most commonly occurring bacterial infections in women of childbearing age.
   a. 60% of women will develop a UTI in their lifetime.
   b. Occurrence is less, or very uncommon, in men until age 65 years.
2. UTIs are the presence of microorganisms in the urinary tract that cannot be accounted for by contamination; they may involve the upper and lower urinary tract.
   a. Lower UTIs involve the bladder and are called cystitis.
   b. Upper UTIs usually involve the kidney and are called pyelonephritis.
3. Infections are classified as complicated or uncomplicated, with uncomplicated infections more commonly seen in an ambulatory setting.
   a. Uncomplicated infections
      i. Occur in females with no functional or structural abnormalities
      ii. Usually occur in females 15–45 years of age
   b. Complicated infections
      i. Females with structural abnormalities or obstruction
         (a) Indwelling catheters, stents, or nephrostomy tubes
         (b) Renal calculi
         (c) History of renal transplantation
         (d) Functional or anatomic abnormality
         (e) Recent urinary tract instrumentation
      ii. Males
      iii. Pregnant women
      iv. Children
      v. Diabetes
      vi. Immunosuppression
      vii. Renal failure
      viii. Patients with indwelling catheters
      ix. Increased risk of infection with resistant pathogen
         (a) Acute pyelonephritis in the past year
         (b) Hospital-acquired infection or recent hospitalization
         (c) History of multidrug-resistant urinary pathogen

B. Etiology - *(Domain 1)*
1. Predominantly host bowel flora
2. Most common organisms in community-acquired UTIs
   a. Most are caused by *Escherichia coli* (80%–90%).
   b. Other organisms include *Staphylococcus saprophyticus, Proteus mirabilis,* and *Klebsiella pneumoniae.*
   c. The clinical relevance of organisms other than enteric gram-negative rods in uncomplicated UTIs in young females is likely minimal.
3. Usually caused by a single organism. Polymicrobial UTIs are possible, but these are more often seen in patients with complicated or recurrent UTIs.

C. Common Clinical Presentation - *(Domain 1)*
   1. Signs and symptoms
      a. Lower UTI: Dysuria, urgency, frequency, nocturia, suprapubic heaviness, gross hematuria
      b. Upper UTI: Flank pain, fever, nausea, vomiting, malaise
   2. Physical examination: Upper UTI: Costovertebral tenderness

D. Diagnosis - *(Domain 1)*
   1. Urinalysis
      a. Observing significant microorganisms in the urine specimen, in conjunction with clinical presentation consistent with infection, is key to diagnosing UTIs.
      b. Bacterial count
         i. Quantification of 10^5 CFU/mL or greater is indicative of a UTI.
         ii. 50% of symptomatic women can present with a lower bacterial count (10^3 CFU/mL).
         iii. Many patients have significant bacteriuria yet are asymptomatic: Older adults, children, pregnant patients, and patients with indwelling catheters
      c. Microscopic examination
         i. Pyuria: WBC count of 5000–10,000/mm^3: The presence of WBCs in the urine alone does not necessarily indicate infection; it does, however, indicate inflammation.
         ii. Hematuria is often present in patients with a UTI, but it is nonspecific.
         iii. Proteinuria is commonly found in the presence of infection.
      d. Chemistry: Done by a common dipstick test
         i. Nitrite
            (a) Formed by bacteria that reduce nitrate in the urine (e.g., *E. coli*, *Proteus* sp., *Klebsiella* sp.)
            (b) False negatives can be seen in UTIs caused by other organisms that do not produce nitrites (e.g., *Staphylococcus* sp. *Enterococcus* sp., *Pseudomonas aeruginosa*).
         ii. Leukocyte esterase indicates the presence of pyuria and detects a WBC count greater than 10,000/mm^3.
   2. Culture
      a. Most reliable method for confirmation of diagnosis
      b. Usually unnecessary and not routinely done in the outpatient setting for suspected uncomplicated cystitis but should always be done for suspected pyelonephritis

E. Treatment of Acute Uncomplicated Cystitis and Uncomplicated Pyelonephritis - *(Domain 1)*
   1. Therapy goals
      a. Eradicate the invading organism.
      b. Prevent and treat systemic consequences of infection.
      c. Prevent recurrence of infection.
   2. Antimicrobial selection
      a. Issues to consider
         i. Ability of antimicrobial to achieve adequate urinary concentrations
         ii. Most likely organisms
         iii. Local susceptibility patterns
         iv. Adverse effect and drug interaction potential (e.g., trimethoprim/sulfamethoxazole and warfarin)
         v. Cost
         vi. Adherence

    b. Common regimens for uncomplicated cystitis

      i. Evidence supports that 3-day courses of therapy are superior to single-dose therapy; recommended 3-day courses are as follows:

        (a) Trimethoprim/sulfamethoxazole

        (b) Fluoroquinolones (ciprofloxacin, levofloxacin) (NOT moxifloxacin)

      ii. Other regimens for uncomplicated UTIs

        (a) Nitrofurantoin (5- to 7-day course because 3-day courses are not as effective)

        (b) Fosfomycin (single dose)

        (c) Trimethoprim (3–5 days)

        (d) Alternatives (when other regimens cannot be used): β-Lactams

          (1) Amoxicillin/clavulanate x 5–7 days

          (2) Cefdinir, cefaclor, cefuroxime or cefpodoxime x 5–7 days

      iii. Because of collateral damage with the overuse of fluoroquinolones, the 2011 guidelines recommend using the fluoroquinolones only when trimethoprim/sulfamethoxazole, nitrofurantoin, or fosfomycin cannot be used as the first-line agent or if pyelonephritis or resistance is suspected.

    c. Uncomplicated acute pyelonephritis

      i. Fluoroquinolones or trimethoprim/sulfamethoxazole is the first-line therapy.

      ii. A longer therapy (7–14 days, depending on agent used) than in uncomplicated cystitis is required to achieve adequate penetration into tissues as well as to eradicate causative organisms.

Table 1. Outpatient Antimicrobial Therapy for UTIs in Adults

Indications	Antibiotic	Dose
Uncomplicated UTIs	Trimethoprim/sulfamethoxazole	1 double-strength tablet twice daily for 3 days
	Ciprofloxacin	250 mg twice daily for 3 days
	Levofloxacin	250 mg once daily for 3 days
	Amoxicillin/clavulanate	500/125 mg twice daily for 5–7 days
	Trimethoprim	100 mg twice daily for 3–5 days
	Nitrofurantoin monohydrate	100 mg twice daily for 5 days
	Fosfomycin	3-g single dose
Complicated UTIs in nonpregnant women	Trimethoprim/sulfamethoxazole	1 double-strength tablet twice daily for 7–10 days
	Ciprofloxacin	250–500 mg twice daily for 7–10 days
	Levofloxacin	250–500 mg/day for 7–10 days
Prophylaxis for recurrent infections	Nitrofurantoin	50 mg/day for 6 mo
	Trimethoprim/sulfamethoxazole	½ single-strength tablet daily for 6 mo
Acute pyelonephritis	Trimethoprim/sulfamethoxazole	1 double-strength tablet twice daily for 14 days
	Ciprofloxacin	500 mg twice daily for 7 days
	Levofloxacin	250 mg/day for 10 days 500 mg/day for 7 days (extrapolated from data with ciprofloxacin) 750 mg/day for 5 days

UTI = urinary tract infection.

F. Antimicrobial Resistance: Increasing Resistance to *E. coli* - *(Domain 5)*
  1. Amoxicillin resistance greater than 37%
  2. Trimethoprim/sulfamethoxazole resistance is as high as 27%. It is imperative to know local susceptibility when choosing treatment.
  3. Fluoroquinolone resistance is rapidly increasing, with rates as high as 9%.
     a. Increased use of fluoroquinolones for several types of infections
     b. Collateral damage important concern
  4. Recent antibiotic exposure is important to know before choosing an agent.

Patient Case

1. E.R. is a 22-year-old woman who calls the clinic today with the chief concern of dysuria, and she thinks she is getting another UTI. Although it has been 4 months since her most recent UTI, this is the third time she has had a UTI since she got married 15 months ago. She is tired of having to come to the office to be treated for such a simple infection, and she wants to know whether she can do anything to prevent this from occurring again. Which is the best recommendation to prevent E.R.'s having additional recurrent infections?

   A. Ciprofloxacin 500 mg orally twice daily for 14 days should be initiated for a resistant infection.
   B. Use prophylactic postcoital therapy with trimethoprim/sulfamethoxazole ½ single-strength tablet.
   C. Use prophylactic postcoital therapy with trimethoprim/sulfamethoxazole 1 double-strength tablet twice daily for 3 days.
   D. Use daily prophylaxis with trimethoprim/sulfamethoxazole 1 double-strength tablet daily for 6 months.

G. Recurrent Infections - *(Domain 1)*
  1. Reinfections
     a. Infections occurring more than 14 days after the original UTI
     b. 80% of recurrent infections
     c. Recurrence of infection by organism different from that in the preceding infection, but potentially of same genus and species
     d. Primarily in females
     e. Risk factors
        i. Sexual intercourse
        ii. Diaphragm use
        iii. Spermicide use
     f. Treatment options
        i. Self-administered/initiated therapy at symptom onset
        ii. Postcoital therapy if temporally related to intercourse
        iii. Continuous low-dose prophylaxis (see Table 1): In individuals with greater than three episodes per year, assess need for continued prophylaxis 6–12 months after starting. Some evidence indicates safety risk with chronic use of nitrofurantoin.
  2. Relapses
     a. Appears within 14 days of the original UTI
     b. Persistence of infection with same organism after treatment for a UTI
     c. Can indicate other factors
        i. Renal involvement
        ii. Urinary structural abnormality
        iii. Chronic bacterial prostatitis
        iv. Resistance
     d. May require longer treatment or use of an alternative agent

3. Possible prevention therapies
   a. Behavioral changes, although no firm evidence (e.g., avoid spermicides, urination after intercourse)
   b. Cranberry juice to acidify the urine; however, studies not consistent in showing benefit
   c. *Lactobacillus* may help decrease vaginal pH and *E. coli* colonization, but more studies are needed.
   d. Topical estrogen replacement in postmenopausal women is helpful in recurrent infections by decreasing *E. coli* colonization.

H. UTIs in Pregnancy - *(Domain 1)*
   1. Asymptomatic bacteriuria can occur in 4% 7% of pregnant patients.
   2. Pregnant women with asymptomatic bacteriuria are more likely to develop pyelonephritis as well as to have low birth weight infants and pre-term delivery.
      a. Routine screening for bacteriuria should be performed during prenatal visits.
      b. Treatment helps prevent pyelonephritis and other complications.
   3. Treatment
      a. 7 days of therapy is required for treatment of UTIs during pregnancy because the infections are considered complicated.
      b. Although the ideal therapy duration of asymptomatic bacteriuria is not known in pregnancy, 3–7 days is usually sufficient.
      c. Agent should be safe for mother and baby.
         i. Good options:
            (a) Penicillins and cephalosporins are considered safe in pregnancy and are preferred for this reason.
            (b) Broader-spectrum oral options such as amoxicillin/clavulanate, cefuroxime, cefpodoxime have better activity against the most likely pathogens when empirically treating UTIs.
            (c) Narrower-spectrum oral options such as amoxicillin and cephalexin are good choices when susceptibility to these agents is known.
            (d) Nitrofurantoin (some experts say to avoid)
            (e) Trimethoprim/sulfamethoxazole: Safe in the first and second trimesters but should be avoided in the third trimester because of the increased risk of kernicterus. Some experts recommend avoiding it in the first trimester; however, if used, administer with a supplemental multivitamin containing folic acid.
         ii. Avoid:
            (a) Tetracyclines
            (b) Fluoroquinolones
            (c) Sulfonamides (during third trimester)

Patient Case

2. W.A. is a 50-year-old woman who presents to the clinic with dysuria and increased urinary frequency in the past 2 days. This is her fifth UTI in the past 12 months since going through menopause. Otherwise, she is in good health, and her only drug is a multivitamin daily and loratadine as needed for seasonal allergies. She is very concerned about the frequency of her UTIs and would like to know whether there is any way she can prevent these. Which intervention is best for W.A.?

   A. Drinking a glass of cranberry juice daily.
   B. Using daily topical estrogen cream applied vaginally.
   C. Postcoital voiding after intercourse.
   D. Taking nitrofurantoin 100 mg orally twice daily for 6 months.

I. Bacterial Prostatitis - *(Domain 1)* and 5
    1. Inflammation infection of the prostate gland and surrounding tissue caused by infection
    2. Occurs mainly in men older than 30 years and affects up to 50% of men
    3. Assessment of possible prostatic source should be made in older men with UTIs.
    4. Symptoms
        a. Sudden onset of fever
        b. Genitourinary tenderness (perineal, rectal, sacrococcygeal)
        c. Urinary symptoms (frequency, urgency)
        d. Constitutional symptoms
    5. Physical examination
        a. Acute bacterial prostatitis—Swollen, tender, tense, or indurated gland
        b. Chronic bacterial prostatitis—Boggy, indurated/swollen prostate
    6. Laboratory tests
        a. Pyuria
        b. Bacteriuria
        c. Bacteria in expressed prostatic secretions
    7. Pathogens
        a. *E. coli* in 75% of cases
        b. Other gram-negative organisms: *K. pneumoniae, P. mirabilis,* and, less often, *P. aeruginosa, Enterobacter* spp., and *Serratia* spp.
        c. Occasionally
            i. *Neisseria gonorrhoeae*
            ii. *Staphylococcus* spp.
        d. Treatment
            i. Length of therapy for acute prostatitis should be 2–4 weeks.
            ii. May require intravenous treatment first (3–5 days) in severe cases
            iii. Antimicrobials
                (a) Fluoroquinolones (ciprofloxacin, levofloxacin) (NOT moxifloxacin)
                (b) Trimethoprim/sulfamethoxazole
                (c) Cephalosporins
            iv. Chronic bacterial prostatitis may require longer treatments—often, 6 weeks or more.

J. Pharmacoeconomic Considerations - *(Domain 5)*
    1. Cost-effective management is the best approach to the treatment of UTIs.
    2. Practitioners need to be aware of local susceptibility patterns.
        a. Trimethoprim/sulfamethoxazole is inexpensive, but resistance can lead to treatment failures.
        b. Fluoroquinolones are highly effective, but increased use can lead to resistance.
        c. Other alternatives should be considered (e.g., one-time dosing of fosfomycin, 5–7 days of nitrofurantoin).

II. COMMUNITY-ACQUIRED PNEUMONIA

A. Introduction - *(Domain 5)*
  1. CAP: Affects about 1.3 million Medicare patients annually in the United States
      a. One of the top 10 causes of mortality
      b. Most patients can be treated as outpatients.
  2. Annual total costs can be as high as $13 billion.
      a. Most costs can be attributed to patients admitted to the hospital.
      b. Major costs can be avoided by appropriate outpatient treatment.
  3. Most patients with CAP are treated in the outpatient setting by primary care physicians.

B. CAP Description - *(Domain 1)*
  1. CAP is a lower respiratory tract infection in patients who are not hospitalized, patients who are not on endotracheal intubation, or any individuals with recent contact with the health care setting (e.g., nursing home, dialysis, active chemotherapy) with infiltrates on chest radiographs or consistent with auscultatory findings.
  2. Risk factors
      a. Age older than 65 years
      b. Asthma
      c. Chronic obstructive pulmonary disease (COPD)
      d. Diabetes
      e. Smokers
      f. Congestive heart failure
      g. Chronic renal failure
      h. Patients with compromised immune systems/HIV infection
      i. Recent antibiotic therapy
      j. Alcohol abuse
  3. Pathogenesis: Organisms gain entry to the lower respiratory tract through the following routes:
      a. Inhalation or aspiration of aerosolized particles
      b. Entrance into the lung through the bloodstream from an extrapulmonary infection site
      c. Aspiration of oropharyngeal contents

C. Etiology - *(Domain 1)*
  1. *Streptococcus pneumoniae* – About 75% of CAP cases
  2. *Haemophilus influenzae*
  3. Atypical pneumonia pathogens
      a. *Mycoplasma pneumonia* – About 20% of CAP cases
      b. *Chlamydophila pneumoniae* (previously called *Chlamydia pneumoniae*) – 5%–15% of CAP cases
      c. *Legionella pneumophila* – 2%–15% of CAP cases; risk factors include COPD and hotel or cruise ship travel in previous 2 weeks
  4. Respiratory viruses: Influenza A and B, adenovirus, respiratory syncytial virus, and parainfluenza
  5. Less common: Methicillin-resistant *Staphylococcus aureus* (MRSA) and community-acquired MRSA (CA-MRSA), *Klebsiella* spp., *Pseudomonas*, *Acinetobacter*
      a. Mainly in older adults or in patients with severe comorbidities such as alcoholism, diabetes, and end-stage renal disease requiring dialysis
      b. Patients who have been recently hospitalized or in nursing homes; in these instances, it would be called health care–associated pneumonia

D. Diagnosis - *(Domain 1, 3, 5)*
   1. Signs and symptoms
      a. CAP diagnosis is largely based on clinical signs and symptoms, with the most common symptoms being fever (temperature greater than 100.4°F [38°C]) and cough with or without sputum, with confirmatory chest radiographs demonstrating infiltrates.
      b. Symptoms may be nonspecific in older patients.
      c. Other symptoms
         i. Dyspnea
         ii. Pleuritic chest pain
         iii. Wheezing
         iv. Myalgia, arthralgia, sweats, chills, rigors
         v. Malaise
   2. Diagnostic and laboratory tests
      a. Physical examination
         i. Rales, rhonchi, inspiratory crackles
         ii. Dullness to percussion
         iii. Increased tactile fremitus, egophony
      b. Positive chest radiograph findings: False negatives can be seen in severe dehydration, early pneumonia, neutropenia
      c. Microbiologic testing
         i. Not routinely done in outpatient practice
            (a) The IDSA/ATS 2007 guidelines recommend testing if the result is likely to change individual treatment.
            (b) May be indicated if previous antibiotic therapy has failed
         ii. Sputum Gram stain usually reveals many polymorphonuclear cells, with the predominance of a bacterial pathogen.
         iii. Blood cultures are more likely to be performed in more severe cases.
         iv. Sputum cultures rarely performed, difficult to obtain high-quality specimens
   3. Scoring systems/site-of-care decisions
      a. Important in determining whether patient can be treated in the outpatient setting or whether patient needs to be hospitalized, because inpatient costs can be as high as 25 times that of outpatient care
      b. CURB-65 (severity-of-illness scoring)
         i. Score of 0–5 is given, using 1 point for each of the following:
            (a) Confusion caused by pneumonia
            (b) Urea nitrogen concentration greater than 7 mmol/L (blood urea nitrogen [BUN] concentration greater than 19 mg/dL)
            (c) Respiratory rate of 30 breaths/minute or greater
            (d) Blood pressure less than 90 mm Hg systolic or 60 mm Hg or less diastolic
            (e) Age 65 years or older
         ii. Score of 2 or greater indicates a need for more intense treatment and hospitalization.
      c. Pneumonia severity index prognostic model
         i. Uses many demographic and historical findings, physical findings, and laboratory data to calculate a total score
         ii. On the basis of the score, patients are categorized into one of five classes, each with a different risk of mortality.
         iii. Tool was designed to predict mortality so that those with low risk of death from CAP could be treated in the outpatient setting.

Patient Case

3. M.J. is an 85-year-old woman whose daughter brings her to the physician's office because the family has noticed that she has been sleeping more lately and that she seems very confused. On physical examination, M.J. is lethargic and not alert and oriented. Her vital signs include temperature of 97.5°F, blood pressure 88/55 mm Hg, heart rate 90 beats/minute, and respiratory rate 27 breaths/minute. A chest radiograph taken in the office reveals a left lower lobe consolidation, and she is given a diagnosis of CAP. Using the CURB point-of-care patient scoring system, which statement is the best recommendation for continuing with the treatment of M.J.'s CAP?

   A. Treat her as an outpatient for 3 days and reassess.
   B. Treat her as an outpatient for 14 days and follow up.
   C. Transfer her to the emergency department (ED) at the local hospital to be admitted for treatment.
   D. Have her transferred to the ICU immediately.

E. Treatment - *(Domain 1, 3, 5)*
   1. Therapy goals: Eradicate infecting organism, prevent complications, and prevent resistance.
   2. The IDSA/ATS guidelines suggest treatment protocols because they decrease mortality.
   3. Initial treatment will be empiric and should target the most likely organisms. Although some debate remains, standard of care is usually to cover both typical pathogens (*S. pneumoniae, H. influenzae*) and atypical pathogens (*M. pneumoniae, C. pneumoniae,* and *Legionella*).
       a. β-Lactams do not cover atypical pathogens.
       b. Macrolides, doxycycline, and fluoroquinolones cover atypical pathogens.
   4. Antimicrobials should have the ability to reach adequate concentrations within the respiratory secretions.
   5. Risk factors for poor outcomes and drug-resistance, together with where patient is to be treated (outpatient or inpatient), should be considered in therapy decisions.
   6. Treatment duration should be 7–10 days unless otherwise noted (i.e., levofloxacin 750 mg and azithromycin package dosing of 5 days).
   7. Outpatient treatment based on IDSA/ATS guidelines
       a. Previously healthy and no antimicrobials in past 3 months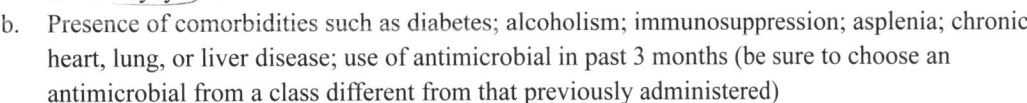
           i. Macrolide (azithromycin, clarithromycin)
           ii. Doxycycline
       b. Presence of comorbidities such as diabetes; alcoholism; immunosuppression; asplenia; chronic heart, lung, or liver disease; use of antimicrobial in past 3 months (be sure to choose an antimicrobial from a class different from that previously administered)
           i. Respiratory fluoroquinolone (levofloxacin 750 mg, moxifloxacin, gemifloxacin)
           ii. β-Lactam (high-dose amoxicillin 1 g three times daily, amoxicillin/clavulanate 2 g twice daily, or ceftriaxone 1 g once daily, cefpodoxime 200 mg twice daily, and cefuroxime 500 mg twice daily) plus a macrolide or doxycycline
       c. Suspected aspiration
           i. Amoxicillin/clavulanate
           ii. Clindamycin
       d. In regions with a high rate (greater than 25%) of macrolide-resistant *S. pneumoniae* (erythromycin minimum inhibitory concentration [MIC] of 16 mg/L or greater), use an alternative agent such as fluoroquinolone.
       e. If MRSA or CA-MRSA is suspected
           i. Add vancomycin or linezolid.
           ii. Patient may need to be hospitalized.

Patient Case

4. R.C. is a 60-year-old woman (height 66 inches, weight 90 kg) who presents to the clinic with a 4-day history of increasing productive cough, malaise, wheezing, and fever. Her medical history includes type 2 diabetes for 20 years, congestive heart failure, chronic kidney disease, and osteoarthritis. She states that her only medication allergy is a history of nausea with ciprofloxacin for a UTI several years ago. On examination, she has a temperature of 102.3°F, respiratory rate 22 breaths/minute, blood pressure 120/78 mm Hg, and heart rate 90 beats/minute. Her laboratory values are within normal limits except for serum creatinine concentration (SCr) 3.0 mg/dL and WBC count 18 x 10³ cells/mm³. A chest radiograph reveals consolidation in the right lower lobe. She is given a diagnosis of CAP. Which regimen is the best empiric option for managing this patient's CAP?

A. Levofloxacin 750 mg orally once daily for 10 days.
B. Azithromycin 500 mg orally once on day 1; then 250 mg orally daily for 4 days.
C. Linezolid 600 mg orally twice daily for 10 days.
D. Azithromycin 500 mg orally once on day 1; then 250 mg orally daily for 4 days plus amoxicillin 500 mg orally twice daily for 10 days.

F. Resistance - *(Domain 1, 5)*
   1. Resistance patterns vary geographically, and empiric antibiotic selections should consider local susceptibility patterns.
   2. Drug-resistant *S. pneumoniae*
      a. Penicillin
         i. Current breakpoints for non-meningeal infections set in 2008 by the Clinical and Laboratory Standards Institute (CLSI)
            (a) Susceptibility: 2 mg/L or less
            (b) Intermediate: 4 mg/L
            (c) Resistant: 8 mg/L or greater
         ii. Although MICs have risen for penicillin during the past 20 years, data suggest that the clinically relevant level of resistance is greater than 4 mg/L.
      b. Macrolides and fluoroquinolones
         i. Resistance continues to rise.
         ii. Resistance is more often associated with clinical failures.
      c. Multidrug resistant
         i. In the late 1990s, there was an increase in β-lactam plus macrolide-resistant *S. pneumoniae*.
         ii. A 2008 study found less than 5% multidrug resistance in Europe; the decreasing number is probably reflective of changes in CLSI susceptibility breakpoints for penicillin.
   3. Risk factors for resistance
      a. Age younger than 2 years or older than 65 years
      b. Previous β-lactam, macrolide, or fluoroquinolone exposure
      c. Alcoholism
      d. Medical comorbidities
      e. Immunosuppression
      f. Exposure to children in day care setting

III. TUBERCULOSIS

A. Overview - *(Domain 4, 5)*
   1. Tuberculosis (TB) is caused by the acid-fast, slow-growing, gram-positive bacilli *Mycobacterium tuberculosis*.
   2. 2 billion people worldwide are infected with TB.
   3. In 2010, the incidence in the United States was 3.2 cases/100,000 population, according to the Centers for Disease Control and Prevention (CDC).
   4. Large coordination efforts from national, state, and local resources in reporting and treatment have hastened the decline.
   5. All new cases are to be reported to the local health department.
   6. TB is a highly contagious bacterium spread through airborne transmission.
      a. Primary lung infection (80%–84%)
      b. Extrapulmonary sites include the central nervous system (CNS), bone and joints, and lymph nodes.
   7. Not everyone infected with TB develops active disease.
      a. Latent TB occurs when someone is infected and the organism becomes dormant.
      b. TB disease occurs when the bacteria continue to replicate and cause active symptomatic disease.
   8. Populations at risk of contracting or being exposed to TB are:
      a. Immigrants
      b. Medically underserved (i.e., homeless)
      c. Prison inmates
      d. Those residing in nursing homes and other long-term resident facilities
      e. Intravenous drug abusers
      f. Patients with HIV infection
      g. Other patients with compromised immune systems
      h. Health care workers
   9. It takes about 2–8 weeks after exposure for the immune system to respond.

B. TB Screening - *(Domain 1)*
   1. The key to containing TB is to identify those who have been exposed to *M. tuberculosis* through routine testing of the populations at risk of contracting TB.
      a. Tuberculin skin test/purified protein derivative (PPD)
      b. TB blood tests (interferon γ release assays)
         i. QuantiFERON-TB
         ii. T-SPOT
   2. Skin testing/PPD
      a. PPD is a noninfectious TB protein that causes a delayed hypersensitivity reaction to the bacteria in the exposed host 6–8 weeks after the initial exposure.
      b. A small amount of protein is injected intradermally into the patient's forearm and is evaluated for induration 48–72 hours later.
      c. Positive reactions are determined at 48–72 hours on the basis of induration and specific patient characteristics
         i. 5 mm or greater in individuals with HIV infection, those with recent TB contacts, patients with compromised immune systems, patients with a transplant history, and patients with fibrotic changes on radiography
         ii. 10 mm or greater in recent immigrants (having arrived in the United States less than 5 years from a country with a high rate of TB), intravenous drug abusers, residents and employees in high-risk settings, children younger than 4 years)
         iii. 15 mm or greater in all other patients outside the groups outlined above

      d.   Only individuals at high risk of contracting or being exposed to TB should be screened.

      e.   *Mycobacterium bovis* bacillus Calmette-Guérin (BCG) vaccination

           i.   Vaccine given worldwide (except in the United States) to provide protection for infants and children from meningeal and military TB

           ii. May cause false positives in PPD testing, so chest radiography or TB blood assays must be done for screening

  3. TB blood tests

      a.   Evaluates the immune reaction to *M. tuberculosis*

      b.   Results returned in 24 hours

      c.   QuantiFERON-TB and T-SPOT

      d.   Recommended only for certain patients

           i.   Patients who have received the BCG vaccination

           ii. Patients who have difficulty following up 48–72 hours after PPD

      e.   Not recommended to follow up PPD with blood test

  4. Latent TB diagnosed with positive PPD or blood test findings

  5. Chest radiography should be done to rule out any cavitary lung lesions in those with a positive PPD or blood test result before beginning treatment for latent TB infection. Possible findings include atelectasis, upper lobe cavitation in activation of latent disease

  C. Diagnosis of Active TB - *(Domain 1)*

    1. Signs and symptoms

      a.   Cough with or without hemoptysis

      b.   Pleuritic pain

      c.   Fever

      d.   Night sweats

      e.   Anorexia

      f.   Weight loss

      g.   Weakness

    2. Laboratory

      a.   Increased WBC count

      b.   Sputum culture

            i.   Positive for acid-fast bacilli

           ii. Positive culture results can take up to 2–4 weeks to come back.

      c.   Nucleic acid amplification assay, with results in 48 hours

      d.   Drug susceptibility testing is important for drug therapy, but it takes up to 4 weeks.

Patient Case

Questions 5 and 6 pertain to the following case.

E.C. is a 27-year-old male pharmacy resident (weight 70 kg) whose reaction to PPD is evaluated after being placed on his left forearm 48 hours ago. It is erythematous, with induration measured at 11 mm. E.C. denies any symptoms of active TB and has a negative chest radiograph.

>10mm
Health care worker.

5. Which is the best recommendation for E.C. at this time?

   A. Tell him to come back next year for an annual PPD test because his PPD test results are negative.
   B. Start therapy with isoniazid 300 mg orally daily plus vitamin B_6 for 9 months.
   C. Start therapy with rifampin 600 mg daily for 9 months.
   D. Start therapy with isoniazid 900 mg orally daily plus rifapentine 900 mg orally daily for 12 weeks.

6. E.C.'s physician asks you for the most important item to monitor after initiating therapy for E.C.'s latent TB infection. Which is the best answer?

   A. Monofilament testing.
   B. Cough.
   C. Chest radiograph.
   D. LFTs.

D. Treatment - *(Domain 1)*
   1. Baseline laboratory monitoring
      a. Liver function tests (LFTs): Aspartate aminotransferase (AST), alanine aminotransferase (ALT), alkaline phosphatase, prothrombin time, international normalized ratio, albumin, bilirubin
      b. Renal: SCr, BUN
      c. Complete blood cell count (CBC)
      d. Serum uric acid for patients taking pyrazinamide
      e. Visual red, green acuity testing for patients taking ethambutol
   2. Therapy can be given daily, several times per week, or weekly.
   3. Usually, directly observed therapy is preferred, and it is considered the responsibility of public health and TB facilities to ensure adherence to therapy.
   4. Treatment of latent TB infection
      a. Monotherapy is usually appropriate.
      b. Common regimens
         i. Isoniazid 300 mg daily or 900 mg two or three times weekly for 9 months (preferred adult treatment)
         ii. Isoniazid 300 mg daily or 900 mg two or three times weekly for 6 months (not to be used in HIV-positive patients, patients younger than 18 years, or those with fibrotic lesions)
         iii. Rifampin 600 mg daily for 4 months (in patients unable to tolerate isoniazid)
         iv. Isoniazid 15 mg/kg (maximum 900 mg) PLUS rifapentine 900 mg (for patients weighing 50 kg or more) weekly for 12 weeks administered by directly observed therapy (not recommended for children younger than 2 years, women who are pregnant or those who will become pregnant during therapy, or patients with HIV receiving antiretroviral therapy)
      c. Monitoring and considerations
         i. LFTs at baseline and periodically, with clinical monitoring of symptoms of hepatotoxicity (e.g., abdominal pain, nausea, vomiting) of paramount importance

      ii.   Discontinuation with LFTs <u>greater than 3 times the upper limit</u> of normal with symptoms OR greater than 5 times the upper limit of normal without symptoms

      iii.   Vitamin B$_6$ (pyridoxine) daily is usually added to isoniazid regimens to help prevent neuropathy.

      iv.   Patients taking rifampin should be warned that their body fluids will turn orange.

  5. Active TB infection treatment – Always in conjunction with public health authorities and physicians with experience in treating TB

    a. Treatment is for at least 6 months with combination therapy.

      i.   Helps eradicate actively replicating bacteria

      ii.   Prevents emergence of resistance

      iii. Continues bactericidal activity against persistent *M. tuberculosis* to prevent relapse

    b. Susceptibility is not known for at least 4 weeks, so therapy for active TB is empiric.

    c. Because of the potential for resistance, as well as the need for therapy with at least two active drugs, therapy is initiated with a four-drug regimen.

      i.   Isoniazid

      ii.   Rifampin

      iii. Pyrazinamide

      iv.   Ethambutol

    d. After 2 months (8 weeks) of the four-drug regimen (isoniazid, rifampin, pyrazinamide, and ethambutol), finish with 4 months (18 weeks) of isoniazid and rifampin if isolate is found susceptible to both agents.

    e. Other rifamycins

      i.   Rifabutin 300 mg sometimes replaces rifampin because drug interactions with rifampin are usually less severe than with rifampin.

      ii.   Rifapentine 10 mg/kg (maximum 600 mg) can be used in once-weekly regimens for rifampin in continuation phase.

    f. Second-line agents used in cases of resistance or intolerance

      i.   Streptomycin

      ii.   Amikacin

      iii. Fluoroquinolones (levofloxacin, moxifloxacin)

    g. For isoniazid-resistant infections, continue rifampin, pyrazinamide, and ethambutol for 6 months.

    h. For rifampin-resistant infections, continue isoniazid and pyrazinamide plus streptomycin for 9 months.

    i. For multidrug-resistant *M. tuberculosis* (isoniazid and rifampin), use second-line susceptible agents in combination.

Table 2. Adult Treatment of Active Tuberculosis Infection

Drug	Daily Dose (max)	Twice-Weekly Dose (max)	Thrice-Weekly Dose (max)
Isoniazid	5 mg/kg (300 mg)	15 mg/kg (900 mg)	15 mg/kg (900 mg)
Rifampin	10 mg/kg (600 mg)	10 mg/kg (600 mg)	10 mg/kg (600 mg)
Pyrazinamide	40–55 kg = 1.0 g 56–75 kg = 1.5 g > 75 kg = 2.0 g	40–55 kg = 2.0 g 56–75 kg = 3.0 g > 75 kg = 4.0 g	40–55 kg = 1.5 g 56–75 kg = 2.5 g > 75 kg = 3.0 g
Ethambutol	40–55 kg = 800 mg 56–75 kg = 1.2 g > 75 kg = 1.6 g	40–55 kg = 2.0 g 56–75 kg = 2.8 g > 75 kg = 4.0 g	40–55 kg = 1.2 g 56–75 kg = 2.0 g > 75 kg = 2.4 g

max = maximum.

E. Monitoring and Infection Control with Active TB - *(Domain 1)*, 4, 5
1. Considerations in care
   a. Adherence is of paramount importance.
   b. Observe the patient for clinical improvement.
      i. Signs and symptoms improving
      ii. Acid-fast bacilli smear is clear.
   c. Make sure close contacts are free of infection or have started latent TB therapy.
2. Laboratory monitoring
   a. Check sputum for acid-fast bacilli weekly until clear.
   b. Patients with positive acid-fast bacilli test results at 2 months: Recheck culture and sensitivity.
   c. Monitor for drug toxicities (e.g., LFTs, uric acid, eye examination).
   d. Repeat chest radiography periodically to evaluate fibrotic changes.

IV. UPPER RESPIRATORY TRACT INFECTIONS

A. Introduction - *(Domain 5)*
1. Upper respiratory tract infections are responsible for most antibiotics prescribed in ambulatory practice.
2. Most infections are self-limiting and caused by viral pathogens; this leads to unnecessary antibiotic use.
3. Unnecessary antibiotic use increases the risk of antimicrobial-resistant bacteria.
   a. Effect is greatest in the month immediately after exposure.
   b. The risk of resistance is usually defined as up to 90 days after antibiotic exposure, but infection can persist for up to 12 months.

B. Acute Sinusitis - *(Domain 1)*
1. Inflammation or infection of the paranasal and nasal mucosa
2. Viral respiratory infections usually precede sinusitis.
3. Primarily viral in origin, but differentiating between viral and bacterial causes is difficult
   a. Viral infections tend to resolve after 7–10 days.
   b. Persistence or worsening of sinus symptoms may indicate bacterial infection.
4. Other things that can present like sinusitis
   a. Allergies
   b. Trauma
   c. Environmental exposures
   d. Anatomic abnormalities
5. Very rare complications
   a. Orbital cellulitis
   b. Meningitis
   c. Brain abscess
6. Signs and symptoms
   a. Nasal discharge and congestion
   b. Facial, sinus, and maxillary tooth pain
7. Etiology
   a. Viruses in most cases
   b. Bacterial pathogens similar to those associated with otitis media
      i. *S. pneumoniae* and *H. influenzae* in about 70% of cases
      ii. *Moraxella catarrhalis* (often in children)
      iii. Less often—*S. pyogenes, S. aureus*, anaerobes, fungi

Patient Case

7. L.S. is a 35-year-old man who presents to the clinic with a 3-day history of headache, runny nose, nasal congestion, and tooth pain. He is an otherwise healthy man with no allergies or comorbidities. He is given a diagnosis of sinusitis. Which intervention is the best treatment recommendation for L.S.?

    A. Loratadine 10 mg daily for 10 days.
    B. Amoxicillin 1 g orally three times daily for 10 days.
    C. Azithromycin 500 mg orally once on day 1; then 250 mg orally daily for 3 days.
    D. Oxymetazoline two sprays in each nostril every 12 hours for 3 days.

8. Treatment
    a. Goals are to reduce the signs and symptoms, minimize the duration of symptoms, prevent complications, and reduce bacterial resistance by limiting antimicrobial treatment to those who need it.
    b. Most infections are self-limiting, and patients will recover on their own.
    c. Supportive therapy – Limited evidence of benefit
        i. Nasal decongestant sprays – Limit to the recommended duration.
        ii. Oral decongestants
        iii. Saline irrigations or steam inhalations
        iv. Mucolytics such as guaifenesin may decrease the viscosity of nasal secretions.
        v. Avoid antihistamines because they may dry out nasal secretions that need to drain from the sinuses.
    d. Antimicrobial therapy may be warranted with compatible syndrome unimproved after 10 days or more, severe symptoms for 3 days or more, or worsening after initial improvement over 3 days or more.
        i. First line – Amoxicillin/clavulanate
            (a) Proven efficacy and safety
            (b) Low cost
        ii. Penicillin-allergic patients
            (a) Doxycycline
            (b) Respiratory fluoroquinolones (levofloxacin, moxifloxacin)
        iii. Treatment failure
            (a) High-dose amoxicillin/clavulanate
            (b) Doxycycline
            (c) Respiratory fluoroquinolone
        iv. Resistant *S. pneumoniae*
            (a) High-dose amoxicillin
            (b) Respiratory fluoroquinolone
        v. Treatment is for 5–7 days unless otherwise noted or, if risk of resistance, treat for a longer period.
        vi. Because of penicillin resistance, macrolides and oral second- and third-generation cephalosporins are no longer recommended as empiric therapy for sinusitis.

Table 3. Antibiotics Used in Sinusitis

Antimicrobial	Adult Dose
Amoxicillin/clavulanate	500/125 mg three times daily or 875/125 mg twice daily (low dose) 2 g/125 mg twice daily (high dose)
Doxycycline	100 mg twice daily or 200 mg/day
Levofloxacin	500 mg/day
Moxifloxacin	400 mg/day

C. Pharyngitis - *(Domain 1, 5)*
1. Acute inflammation of the oropharynx or nasopharynx
2. Viruses cause most cases (rhinovirus, coronavirus, influenza, parainfluenza, Epstein-Barr).
3. Group A β-hemolytic *Streptococcus* (GABHS – *S. pyogenes*) is the most common bacterial etiology in 15%–30% of all cases.
   a. Not exclusive to, but more often seen in:
      i. Children 5–15 years of age
      ii. Parents of school-aged children
   b. The only common cause of pharyngitis that benefits from antibiotic therapy
4. Spread by direct contact with droplets of infected saliva or nasal secretions

D. Clinical Presentation - *(Domain 1, 4)*
1. Difficult to differentiate viral from bacterial etiology
2. Signs and symptoms
   a. Acute onset of sore throat
   b. Pain with swallowing
   c. Fever
   d. Erythema and inflammation of tonsils and pharynx with or without exudates
   e. Tender and swollen lymph nodes
3. Diagnosis
   a. Need to identify group A *Streptococcus* infection; definitive diagnosis cannot be made by clinical presentation alone
   b. Throat swab for culture or rapid antigen detection test (RADT)
      i. The RADT gives a very rapid result, and it can be performed in the clinic.
      ii. Culture usually takes 24–48 hours.
      iii. The RADT or culture should only be done for patients with a presentation consistent with GABHS pharyngitis.
      iv. In children and adolescents, negative RADT results should be backed up by a throat culture because of the risk of complications such as rheumatic fever.

Patient Case

8. T.R. is a 4-year-old female toddler who presents to the pediatric clinic with a 3-day history of runny nose, sore throat, and temperature of 102°F. She lives at home with her mother, father, and 11-year-old brother, and she attends preschool 3 days/week. On physical examination, she weighs 19 kg, and her tonsils are erythematous and inflamed. A throat swab is taken, and her RADT comes back negative for group A *Streptococcus*. Which is the most appropriate treatment recommendation for T.R.?

    A. Penicillin benzathine 0.6 million unit intramuscularly once.

    B. Ibuprofen 150 mg (7.5 mL of 100 mg/5 mL of elixir) every 4–6 hours as needed.

    C. Acyclovir 380 mg (20 mg/kg) orally four times daily for 10 days.

    D. Trimethoprim/sulfamethoxazole 76/380 mg (trimethoprim 4 mg/kg) orally every 12 hours for 10 days.

---

    4. Treatment

        a. Supportive care

            i. Resolve pain and fever with acetaminophen or nonsteroidal anti-inflammatory drugs (NSAIDs).

            ii. Topical analgesics/lozenges

            iii. Saltwater gargles

        b. Treatment goals:

            i. Relieve symptoms (rapid improvement often seen, complete resolution in 48–72 hours).

            ii. Prevent transmission (return to work or school after 24 hours of antibiotics and fever free).

            iii. Prevent rare but serious complications such as rheumatic fever.

        c. Antimicrobial therapy for group A *Streptococcus*

            i. Penicillin is the drug of choice because no group A *Streptococcus* resistance to penicillin exists.

                (a) Penicillin VK for 10 days: 500 mg twice daily for adults, 50 mg/kg/day in three doses for pediatric patients

                (b) Penicillin benzathine 1.2 million units intramuscularly once for adults and 0.6 million unit intramuscularly (for less than 27 kg) once for pediatric patients

                (c) Amoxicillin 500 mg two times daily for adults, 40–50 mg/kg/day (1000 mg maximum) for pediatric patients for 10 days

            ii. Other options include first-generation cephalosporins (i.e., cephalexin), clindamycin, and macrolides. Azithromycin should be used when no other options exist to help preserve utility in other disease states.

    E. Acute Otitis Media (AOM) - *(Domain 1, 5)*

        1. Most common reason for antimicrobial prescriptions in children

        2. Risk factors

            a. Siblings

            b. Attending day care

            c. Pacifier use

            d. Exposure to secondhand smoke (e.g., parents, caregivers)

        3. Breastfeeding may be protective.

        4. Diagnosis

            a. Abrupt onset of signs and symptoms of AOM (otalgia, fussiness, fever, inconsolability)

            b. Presence of middle-ear effusion

                i. Bulging of the tympanic membrane

                ii. Limited or absent mobility of the tympanic membrane

                iii. Air-fluid level behind the tympanic membrane

                iv. Otorrhea

c. Signs or symptoms of middle-ear inflammation as indicated by the following:
   i. Distinct erythema of the tympanic membrane OR
   ii. Distinct otalgia interfering with normal activities

5. Etiology
   a. Bacteria
      i. Primarily *S. pneumoniae*, *H. influenzae*, and *M. catarrhalis*
      ii. Others: *S. aureus*, *S. pyogenes*, anaerobes
   b. Viruses

6. Treatment
   a. Treatment goals
      i. Control pain.
      ii. Eradicate infection.
      iii. Prevent complications.
      iv. Avoid unnecessary antibiotics.
   b. Supportive care with acetaminophen or NSAIDs (avoid aspirin in children because of the risk of Reye syndrome)
   c. Treatment with antibiotics
      i. Otorrhea with AOM
      ii. AOM with severe symptoms (i.e., toxic appearing, temperature greater than 102.2°F, otalgia greater than 48 hours, uncertain access)
      iii. Bilateral AOM in children 6 months to 2 years of age
   d. Consider observation without antibiotics for 48–72 hours in:
      i. Bilateral AOM without otorrhea in children 2 years and older
      ii. Unilateral AOM without otorrhea in all children regardless of age
   e. Antimicrobial therapy
      i. Amoxicillin 80–90 mg/kg/day given in two divided doses if no amoxicillin treatment in the past 30 days
      ii. Amoxicillin/clavulanate 90 mg/kg/day (amoxicillin component) if amoxicillin in past 30 days or in patients with combined otitis/conjunctivitis presentation
      iii. Oral cephalosporins if non-anaphylactic allergy to penicillins (cefdinir, cefuroxime, cefpodoxime)
      iv. Ceftriaxone in severe presentation or in refractory disease
      v. Clindamycin alone for *S. pneumoniae* infections or in combination with cefdinir, cefuroxime, cefpodoxime, or cefixime for *H. influenzae* coverage
      vi. Macrolides are unreliable because of their high rates of resistance.
      vii. Treatment length is 5–10 days, with shorter courses in older children.
   f. Recurrent infections
      i. Recurrent infections are defined as three episodes in 6 months or four episodes in 1 year.
      ii. Prophylaxis with antibiotics is not recommended.
      iii. Consider tympanostomy tubes in recurrent AOM infections.

V. CONJUNCTIVITIS/OPHTHALMIC INFECTIONS

A. Overview - *(Domain 1)*
  1. Inflammation and/or infection of the conjunctiva
  2. Commonly called "pink eye"

B. Etiology - *(Domain 1)*
  1. Predominantly viruses (e.g., adenovirus, enterovirus, influenza)
  2. Bacteria
     a. *Streptococcus pneumoniae* and *H. influenzae* in children
     b. *S. aureus* in adults
  3. Allergens
  4. Irritants

C. Signs and Symptoms - *(Domain 1)*
  1. Red conjunctiva
  2. Foreign-body sensation in eye
  3. Mild photophobia
  4. Watery or purulent discharge from eyes
  5. Crusted
  6. Mild pruritus
  7. No visual changes

D. Treatment - *(Domain 1)*
  1. Can be self-limiting if viral infection, but difficult to tell viral from bacterial infection
  2. Bacterial infection is highly contagious.
  3. Topical antibiotics should be automatically prescribed for patients with certain risk factors.
     a. Health care workers
     b. Hospitalized patients or patients living in health care facilities
     c. Children in day care or school
     d. Patients with comorbidities such as those who are immunosuppressed, those with uncontrolled diabetes or recent ocular surgery, those who wear contact lenses
     e. All antibiotics are equally effective, so older, often less expensive options should be considered first.
  4. Children can usually return to school when therapy has been started unless direct contact cannot be avoided. Usually, symptoms begin to resolve within first 24 hours of treatment. Some day care facilities and schools may require a certain duration (e.g., 24 hours) of topical antibiotic therapy before child returns to school.
  5. Length of therapy is traditionally 1 week.
  6. Antibiotics can be delayed in patients with no risk factors.
  7. Conjunctivitis caused by allergies may require a topical antihistamine.
  8. Symptoms may be relieved with a warm, moist compress.

E. Prevention of Reinfection or Spread - *(Domain 1)*
  1. Frequent and correct hand washing
  2. Refrain from touching eyes.
  3. Change pillowcases often.
  4. Replace eye makeup.
  5. Refrain from wearing contact lenses.

Table 4. Conjunctivitis Treatment

Drug	Dose in Infected Eye(s)
Azithromycin 1% (AzaSite)	1 drop twice daily for 2 days; then 1 drop daily for 5 days
Fluoroquinolones	
Besifloxacin 0.6% (Besivance)	1 drop three times daily
Ciprofloxacin 0.3% (Ciloxan)	Ointment: ½-inch ribbon on conjunctival sac three times daily Solution: 1 or 2 drops four times daily
Gatifloxacin 0.3% (Zymar)	1 drop three times daily
Levofloxacin 0.5% (Quixin)	1 or 2 drops four times daily
Moxifloxacin 0.5% (Vigamox)	1 drop three times daily
Ofloxacin 0.3% (Ocuflox)	1 or 2 drops four times daily
Aminoglycosides	
Gentamicin 0.3%	Ointment: ½-inch ribbon on conjunctival sac four times daily Solution: 1 or 2 drops four times daily
Tobramycin 0.3% (Tobrex)	Ointment: ½-inch ribbon on conjunctival sac three times daily Solution: 1 or 2 drops four times daily
Sulfacetamide 10%	Ointment: ½-inch ribbon on conjunctival sac four times daily and at bedtime Solution: 1 or 2 drops four times daily
Trimethoprim/polymyxin B	1 or 2 drops four times daily

VI. UNCOMPLICATED SKIN AND SOFT TISSUE INFECTIONS

  A. Introduction - *(Domain 1)*
    1. Skin and soft tissue infections involve any of the skin layers.
      a. Epidermis
      b. Dermis
      c. Fascia
      d. Muscle
    2. Categorized as complicated or uncomplicated. Complicated infections are as follows:
      a. Involve deeper structures (fascia, muscle)
      b. Require surgical intervention
      c. May progress into severe, systemic infections
      d. Occur in patients with compromised immune systems
    3. Skin and soft tissue infections are among the most common infections seen in the community setting.
    4. Obtaining a detailed patient history is imperative for aiding in diagnosis.
      a. Patient's immune status
      b. Geographic locale
      c. Travel history
      d. Recent trauma or surgery
      e. Previous or current antimicrobial therapy
      f. Animal exposure or bites
    5. Issues with skin and soft tissue infections
      a. Diagnosis
      b. Severity of infection

    c.   Pathogen and antibiotic resistance – Especially CA-MRSA

        i.   MRSA is traditionally considered a nosocomial infection; however, in recent years, it has been isolated from patients without typical risk factors such as previous hospitalization or exposure to a long-term care facility.

        ii.   CA-MRSA differs genetically and in susceptibility from nosocomial MRSA.

            (a) Strains often carry genes for toxins such as Panton-Valentine leukocidin, which is responsible for tissue necrosis and increased virulence.

            (b) Usually susceptible to agents such as doxycycline and trimethoprim/sulfamethoxazole

            (c) May be susceptible to clindamycin, but clindamycin can induce its own resistance and often has lower susceptibility rates than doxycycline or trimethoprim/sulfamethoxazole

            (d) Health care providers need to be aware of geographic patterns and outbreaks of MRSA.

        iii. Empiric coverage against MRSA should be used if the infection is purulent (e.g., furuncles, carbuncles, abscesses) or if the patient has a compromised immune system.

B.   General Etiology - *(Domain 1)*

    1. Gram-positive organisms, many from skin surface

       a. *S. aureus* (methicillin-sensitive *S. aureus* [MSSA] predominantly, but can see MRSA)

       b. *S. pyogenes* (β-hemolytic *Streptococcus*)

       c. Coagulase-negative *Staphylococcus*

       d. *Corynebacterium* spp. (diphtheroids)

    2. Gram-negative organisms are not as common in community-acquired infections, but incidence increases with nosocomial exposure.

       a. *P. aeruginosa*

       b. *E. coli*

       c. *Acinetobacter*

    3. Yeast (*Candida* spp.)

    4. Likely etiology may vary with respect to skin and soft tissue infection type.

C.   Impetigo - *(Domain 1, 5)*

    1. Superficial skin infection with discrete purulent lesions

    2. Primarily seen in children 2–5 years of age, but can be seen in older children and adults

    3. Most common in hot, humid climates

    4. Readily spread with close contact, especially in schools and day care centers

    5. Most common organisms

       a. *S. pyogenes*

       b. *S. aureus* (usually MSSA, less commonly MRSA)

    6. Commonly infected sites are exposed areas of the body such as face and extremities.

    7. Signs and symptoms

       a. Lesions can be bullous or non-bullous; they initially appear as superficial vesicles and rapidly enlarge to bullae or pus-filled blisters that readily rupture to produce characteristic golden-yellow crusts.

       b. Systemic signs of infection are minimal.

       c. Regional lymph nodes may be enlarged.

    8. Diagnosis

       a. Diagnosis of uncomplicated presentation usually does not require culture and susceptibility testing.

       b. Cultures of vesicles or bullae should preferably be taken from crusted lesions and non–open draining pustules. Open pustules may be colonized with skin flora.

       c. CBC may show leukocytosis.

9. Treatment
   a. May be self-limiting, but antimicrobial treatment is preferred to prevent new lesions, alleviate symptoms, and prevent complications
   b. Oral antimicrobials
   c. Mupirocin ointment three times daily can be used for patients with only a few lesions or a small affected area.
   d. Therapy duration is usually 7 days.

Table 5. Antibiotics Used in Skin and Soft Tissue Infections

Antibiotic	Adults	Children
Amoxicillin/clavulanate	875/125 mg orally twice daily	25 mg/kg/day (amoxicillin component) orally divided in two doses
Cephalexin	250–500 mg orally four times daily	25–50 mg/kg/day orally divided in four doses
Clindamycin	300–450 mg orally three times daily	20–30 mg/kg/day orally divided in three doses
Dicloxacillin	250–500 mg orally four times daily	12 mg/kg/day orally divided in four doses
Doxycycline	100 mg orally twice daily	Not recommended for ages < 8 yr
Trimethoprim/ sulfamethoxazole	1 double-strength tablet orally twice daily	8–12 mg/kg/day (based on trimethoprim component) orally divided in two doses

D. Folliculitis, Furuncles, and Carbuncles - *(Domain 1)*
   1. Folliculitis is a superficial inflammation of the hair follicle caused by injury, chemical irritation, or infection.
   2. Furuncles (abscess or boil) and carbuncles occur when folliculitis extends from the hair shaft to deeper tissues.
   3. Etiology
      a. Usually caused by *S. aureus*, both MSSA and MRSA
      b. Outbreaks of *P. aeruginosa* infections are associated with inadequately chlorinated pools, hot tubs, and so forth.
   4. Signs and symptoms
      a. Folliculitis: Pruritic, erythematous papules within 48 hours of exposure to organisms – Systemic symptoms are rare.
      b. Furuncles: Usually occur in areas of friction or perspiration
         i. Lesion is usually a firm, tender, red nodule that becomes more painful and may drain pus.
         ii. MRSA furuncle can appear as spider bites, and it has a necrotic center and is usually purulent.
      c. Carbuncles: Broad, swollen, erythematous, deep, and painful masses, usually on the back of the neck
         i. Patients with diabetes or other immune compromising conditions more susceptible
         ii. Commonly associated with constitutional symptoms such as fever and chills
         iii. Bacteremia and spread of infection to deeper tissues is possible.

Patient Case

9. M.M. is a 16-year-old female adolescent (weight 55 kg) who presents to the clinic with a 24-hour history of a diffuse, itchy rash on her right calf. She went to a pool party yesterday and, about 10 hours afterward, noticed the development of the rash. She has no other symptoms. M.M. is an otherwise healthy teenager who takes loratadine as needed for allergies. On physical examination, significant findings are a diffuse erythematous papular follicular rash. She is given a diagnosis of folliculitis. Which recommendation is most appropriate for treatment of M.M.'s folliculitis?

A. Trimethoprim/sulfamethoxazole 1 double-strength tablet orally twice daily for 10 days.
B. Cephalexin 250 mg orally four times daily for 10 days.
C. Warm saline compresses.
D. Ciprofloxacin 500 mg orally twice daily for 10 days.

5. Treatment
   a. Folliculitis
      i. Antimicrobial treatment usually not necessary for smaller boils
      ii. Warm saline compresses to promote drainage
   b. Furuncles and carbuncles
      i. Incision and drainage may be required, especially for carbuncles.
      ii. Dicloxacillin (covers MSSA and *S. pyogenes*)
         (a) Adults: 250–500 mg orally every 6 hours
         (b) Pediatric patients: 25–50 mg/kg orally divided into four doses
      iii. Cephalexin (covers MSSA and *S. pyogenes*)
         (a) Adults: 250–500 mg orally every 6 hours
         (b) Pediatric patients: 25–50 mg/kg orally divided into four doses
      iv. Clindamycin (covers MSSA, some CA-MRSA strains, and *S. pyogenes*)
         (a) Adults: 300–600 mg orally every 6–8 hours
         (b) Pediatric patients: 10–30 mg/kg/day orally divided into three or four doses
         (c) Is an oral option for CA-MRSA but usually best used when susceptibility is confirmed, which requires D-test by microbiology laboratory, requiring additional time and labor
      v. Doxycycline (covers MSSA, MRSA)
         (a) Adults: 100 mg orally twice daily
         (b) Children: Not recommended for children younger than 8 years
      vi. Trimethoprim/sulfamethoxazole (covers MSSA and MRSA, but not good coverage against *S. pyogenes*)
         (a) Adults: 1 or 2 double-strength tablets twice daily (higher dosing may be necessary for CA-MRSA)
         (b) Pediatric patients: 8–12 mg/kg (based on trimethoprim component) orally divided into two doses
         (c) Is an oral option for MRSA
         (d) Because of trimethoprim/sulfamethoxazole's poor activity against *Streptococcus* organisms, clinicians recommend adding a penicillin, cephalosporin, or clindamycin to the patient's regimen until a definitive organism is identified when the patient's infection type (staphylococcal or streptococcal) is unknown.

vii. Severe MRSA infections may require intravenous antibiotics with good MRSA coverage such as the following:
   (a) Vancomycin
   (b) Linezolid (intravenous and oral formulations available)
   (c) Daptomycin
   (d) Ceftaroline
   (e) Dalbavancin
   (f) Oritavancin
c. Antimicrobial treatment should last 7–10 days.

E. Cellulitis - *(Domain 1)*
1. An acute, diffuse skin infection that initially affects the epidermis and dermis that can spread to deeper tissues
2. Ability to spread through the lymphatic tissue into the bloodstream
3. Etiology
   a. Most commonly
      i. *S. aureus* (MSSA, MRSA)
      ii. *S. pyogenes*
   b. Other pathogens
      i. Gram-negative bacilli
      ii. Anaerobes
      iii. Variety of gram-positive cocci
4. Signs and symptoms
   a. Usually preceded by some type of trauma to the skin (e.g., wound, abrasion, ulcer, surgery)
   b. Patients may have generalized symptoms of fever, chills, or malaise.
   c. Infected area is warm to the touch and painful and is characterized by erythema and edema.
   d. Inflammation generally is present with little or no necrosis or suppuration.
   e. Lesions are non-elevated with poorly defined margins.
   f. Tender lymphadenopathy may be present.
5. Diagnosis
   a. Usually made by clinical appearance
   b. Cultures should be collected, if possible.
   c. CBC usually shows leukocytosis.
   d. Blood culture results may be positive in as many as 30% of cases.
6. Treatment
   a. Directed against the most likely causative pathogen
      i. Empiric or directed therapy
      ii. See treatment options for furuncles and carbuncles.
      iii. Incision and drainage and intravenous antibiotics may be necessary if complicated cellulitis
      iv. Inpatient intravenous therapy may be necessary if the infection is rapidly spreading, if there is a pronounced systemic inflammatory response, or in the presence of significant comorbidities (e.g., neutropenia, cardiac or renal failure).
   b. Antimicrobial treatment should last 7–10 days.

Patient Case

10. K.M. is a 32-year-old woman who presents to the clinic with pain, redness, and swelling below her left knee-cap. It started about a week ago with what she describes as a bug bite that kept getting more sore, red, and swollen. She went to the emergency clinic 2 days ago, where she was given a prescription for cephalexin, but she states the area keeps getting more painful and red despite the antibiotics. K.M. is an otherwise healthy woman with no known drug allergies. She works as an elementary teacher and goes to the gym regularly. Physical examination reveals an erythematous and inflamed area with a necrotic center below the left knee-cap that is very warm to the touch. K.M.'s vital signs are normal, and she is afebrile. Incision and drainage are performed in the office, and 15 mL of purulent fluid is sent for culture and sensitivity testing. Which is the best recommendation for empiric coverage of K.M.'s cellulitis?

    A. Penicillin VK 500 mg orally every 6 hours for 10 days.

    B. Vancomycin 1 g intravenously every 12 hours for 10 days.

    C. Trimethoprim/sulfamethoxazole 2 double-strength tablets orally twice daily for 10 days.

    D. Dicloxacillin 250 mg orally four times daily for 10 days.

F. Erysipelas - *(Domain 1)*
   1. Infection of the upper dermis and superficial lymphatic system
      a. Clinically, looks very similar to cellulitis
      b. Differs from cellulitis because it affects the deeper dermis and subcutaneous fat
   2. More common among infants, young children, and older adults
   3. Etiology – Almost always β-hemolytic *Streptococcus* (*S. pyogenes*)
   4. Signs and symptoms
      a. Very bright red lesion with edema and possible lymphatic streaking
      b. Unlike cellulitis, the erysipelas lesion is raised with clearly demarcated margins.
      c. Patients usually have fever or flu-like symptoms.
   5. Diagnosis – May be able to culture by aspirating from the edge of the lesion
   6. Treatment
      a. Treatment is for 7–10 days.
      b. Penicillin is the treatment of choice because of the exquisite susceptibility of *S. pyogenes* to penicillin (intramuscularly or orally).
         i. Adult
            (a) Oral: Penicillin VK 250–500 mg orally every 6 hours
            (b) Intramuscular: Procaine penicillin G 600,000 units intramuscularly every 12 hours
         ii. Pediatric patients weighing less than 30 kg – Oral: Penicillin VK 25–50 mg/kg orally in three or four divided doses
      c. Clindamycin can be used for penicillin-allergic patients.

G. Diabetic Foot Infections (DFIs) - *(Domain 1, 5)*
   1. One of the most common complications of diabetes
      a. Cost of treating a patient can be up to $18,000 per year.
      b. 50% of non-traumatic low-extremity amputations in the United States are complications from DFIs.
   2. Etiology
      a. Usually polymicrobial with an average of two to six isolates per culture
      b. Includes gram-negative, gram-positive, and anaerobic organisms
      c. Staphylococci (coagulase-negative *Staphylococcus*, MSSA, MRSA) and streptococci are the most common.

d. Up to 50% can be caused by gram-negative bacilli.
   i. *E. coli*
   ii. *Klebsiella* spp.
   iii. *Proteus* spp.
   iv. *P. aeruginosa*
e. Anaerobes
   i. *Bacteroides fragilis*
   ii. *Peptostreptococcus* spp.

3. Pathophysiology:
  a. Peripheral neuropathy
  b. Ischemia caused by atherosclerosis
  c. Diabetic-associated immunologic defects

4. Clinical presentation and diagnosis
  a. Infections can be more extensive than they initially appear.
  b. Usual clinical signs of pain may be absent because of neuropathy.
  c. Fever may be present.
  d. Foul-smelling infection may be indicative of anaerobic infections.
  e. Diagnosis should include cultures and sensitivities for both aerobic and anaerobic organisms.
  f. Radiologic studies may be warranted to evaluate for osteomyelitis.

5. Treatment
  a. Should include wound care and antimicrobial therapy
  b. Goal is to preserve limb and limb function.
  c. Wounds must be kept clean and dressings changed often.
  d. Tight glycemic control is imperative for adequate wound healing.
  e. The severity of infection will determine the antimicrobial regimen used for empiric treatment.
  f. Most mild (not rapidly spreading or limited systemic response) infections can be treated with wound care and outpatient oral antimicrobial therapy similar to that of cellulitis in patients without diabetes.

Table 6. Antimicrobial Therapy for Diabetic Foot Infections

Severity	Description	Antibiotic Options
Mild	Local infection only without involvement of deeper skin structures, no signs of systemic inflammatory response	Dicloxacillin, cephalexin, amoxicillin/ clavulanate, clindamycin
Moderate	Local infection with involvement of deeper skin structures but without signs of systemic inflammatory response	Oral options: Amoxicillin/clavulanate, levofloxacin, moxifloxacin Parenteral options: Ampicillin/ sulbactam, ertapenem
Severe	Local or extensive infection with signs of systemic inflammatory response	Parenteral options: Vancomycin + antipseudomonal β-lactam (e.g., cefepime, ceftazidime, piperacillin/tazobactam, imipenem/ cilastatin, doripenem, meropenem)

g. Antimicrobials
   i. Amoxicillin/clavulanate 875 mg orally twice daily
   ii. Clindamycin 300–600 mg orally three times daily does not cover gram-negative organisms.
   iii. Fluoroquinolones (levofloxacin 500–750 mg orally daily, ciprofloxacin 500 mg orally twice daily, or moxifloxacin 400 mg orally daily)
      (a) Equivalent gram-negative coverage except moxifloxacin does not cover *P. aeruginosa*. Ciprofloxacin has poor activity against gram-positive organisms and requires combination therapy with clindamycin or appropriate penicillins or cephalosporins for adequate coverage.
      (b) Anaerobic coverage may be added if anaerobic infection is present or highly suspected; although moxifloxacin does have some coverage against anaerobic infections.
      (c) Metronidazole 500 mg orally three times daily or clindamycin 300–600 mg orally three times daily reasonable additions for anaerobic coverage
   iv. Coverage against MRSA should be added in severe infections, patients with a history of MRSA infections, or patients with other risk factors for MRSA infection (e.g., indwelling catheter, dialysis).
h. Treatment usually lasts 1–2 weeks but may last longer, depending on the response and severity of the infection.

VII. TICKBORNE INFECTIONS/LYME DISEASE

A. Introduction - *(Domain 5)*
   1. Lyme disease is the most common tickborne infection in North America and Europe.
   2. The causative pathogen of Lyme disease is *B. burgdorferi*, which is transmitted by deer tick bites from two predominant tick species.
      a. *Ixodes scapularis*
      b. *Ixodes pacificus*
   3. New England, the Mid-Atlantic, and parts of Minnesota and Wisconsin have a greater than 20% incidence of *B. burgdorferi*.
   4. *I. scapularis* also can transmit *Ehrlichia phagocytophila* and *Babesia microti* (babesiosis).

B. Signs and Symptoms - *(Domain 1)*
   1. Early manifestations include cutaneous erythema migrans ("bull's-eye" rash), which may be accompanied by flu-like symptoms (fever, chills, fatigue, body aches).
   2. Later Lyme disease signs and symptoms
      a. Joint pain
      b. Neurologic problems (e.g., numbness, weakness, Bell's palsy)
      c. Heart problems such as arrhythmias

C. Diagnosis - *(Domain 1)*
   1. Difficult to diagnose early unless the tick or characteristic Lyme disease rash is observed by a health care professional
   2. Most signs and symptoms go unrecognized or are nonspecific.
   3. Laboratory tests
      a. Enzyme-linked immunosorbent assay to detect the most common *B. burgdorferi* antibodies
      b. Polymerase chain reaction (PCR) can be done on joints to detect the organism.

D. Treatment: - *(Domain 1)*
   1. Prophylaxis
      a. When attached tick is identified as adult or nymphal *I. scapularis* and has been attached for 36 hours or more
      b. Prophylaxis should be started within 72 hours of tick removal.
      c. Ecologic local rate of ticks infected with *B. burgdorferi* is greater than 20%.
      d. Doxycycline if not contraindicated (pregnancy, children younger than 8 years)
      e. Give doxycycline 200 mg orally once in adults and 4 mg/kg (up to 200 mg) orally once in children 8 years or older.
      f. Monitor for at least 30 days after tick bite for signs and symptoms of Lyme disease.
         i. Expanding skin lesion
         ii. Viral-like illness
   2. Early Lyme disease (absence of neurologic or cardiac disease)
      a. Adults
         i. Doxycycline 100 mg orally twice daily for 14 days
         ii. Amoxicillin 500 mg orally three times daily for 14 days
         iii. Cefuroxime axetil 500 mg orally twice daily for 14 days
      b. Children
         i. Amoxicillin 50 mg/kg/day in three divided doses for 14 days
         ii. Cefuroxime axetil 30 mg/kg/day in two divided doses for 14 days
         iii. Age 8 years or older: Doxycycline 4 mg/kg/day in two divided doses for 14 days
   3. Lyme meningitis/neurologic disease
      a. Adults
         i. Ceftriaxone 2 g intravenously daily for 14 days
         ii. Cefotaxime 2 g intravenously three times daily for 14 days
         iii. Penicillin G 18–24 million units intravenously divided six times daily for 14 days
         iv. Doxycycline 200–400 mg orally divided twice daily for 10–28 days is adequate, especially for those who are β-lactam intolerant.
      b. Children
         i. Ceftriaxone 50–75 mg/kg/day (maximum 2 g) intravenously for 14 days
         ii. Cefotaxime 150–200 mg/kg/day intravenously in three or four divided doses for 14 days
         iii. Penicillin G 200,000–400,000 units/kg/day (maximum 24 million units) intravenously in six divided doses for 14 days
         iv. In children 8 years and older, doxycycline 4–8 mg/kg/day orally in two divided doses (maximum 200 mg per dose)
   4. Lyme carditis
      a. For atrioventricular heart block and/or myopericarditis, use effective oral or parenteral therapy for Lyme disease infection for 14–21 days.
      b. Hospitalization is recommended for continuous monitoring if the patient is symptomatic.
         i. Syncope
         ii. Dyspnea
         iii. Chest pain
   5. Lyme arthritis
      a. Oral antibiotics for 28 days
      b. For consistent joint pain or recurrent swelling, re-treat with oral antibiotics for 4 weeks or with intravenous ceftriaxone for 2–4 weeks.

E. 2014 International Lyme and Associated Diseases Society Guideline Recommendations - *(Domain 3)*
    1. Goal is to prevent the illness when possible and cure illness if it occurs.
        a. Evidence base for treating Lyme disease is sparse.
        b. These guidelines placed high value on clinician judgment.
    2. Prophylaxis for known *Ixodes* tick bites: 100–200 mg doxycycline twice daily for 20 days
    3. Erythema migrans rash
        a. Amoxicillin 500 mg orally three or four times daily for 4–6 weeks
        b. Cefuroxime 500 mg orally twice daily for a minimum of 21 days
        c. Doxycycline 100–200 mg orally twice daily for a minimum of 21 days
    4. Clinicians should continue antibiotic therapy for patients who have not recovered after set therapy.

F. Prevention of Tick Bites - *(Domain 1)*
    1. Wear protective clothing when outdoors in areas with ticks.
    2. Use tick repellents.
    3. Check for ticks daily and promptly remove them when found.
    4. Routine use of antimicrobial prophylaxis for tick bites is not recommended.

Patient Case

11. J.T. is a 23-year-old man who goes for a morning walk in the woods. On returning home, he notices a tick attached to his right lower leg. He is very worried about Lyme disease because there are many cases of this disease in Wisconsin, where he is currently visiting. He calls the clinic to ask what he should do. Which is the most appropriate recommendation for this patient according to the guidelines?

A. Remove the tick and watch to make sure no rash develops.
B. Go to the ED to have the tick removed and examined.
C. Immediately initiate doxycycline 100 mg orally twice daily for 14 days.
D. Remove the tick and bring it to the clinic to be identified for species.

VIII. INFECTIVE ENDOCARDITIS

A. Introduction - *(Domain 5)*
    1. Endocarditis is an infection of the endocardium and heart valves and is associated with high morbidity and mortality.
    2. Mean onset occurs in individuals 50–60 years of age, but different age of onset is seen in intravenous drug abusers and patients with central venous catheters.
    3. Incidence is around four cases/100,000 population.

B. Risk Factors - *(Domain 1)*
    1. Cardiac valve abnormalities
    2. Prosthetic valves
    3. Mitral valve prolapse with regurgitation
    4. Intravenous drug abusers
    5. Poor dental hygiene
    6. Central venous catheters
    7. Chronic hemodialysis

C. Etiology - *(Domain 1)*
   1. *Streptococcus* spp. (*Streptococcus viridans*, *Streptococcus bovis*)
   2. *Staphylococcus* spp. (MSSA, MRSA, *Staphylococcus epidermidis*)
   3. Enterococci (*Enterococcus faecalis*, *Enterococcus faecium*, vancomycin-resistant enterococci)
   4. HACEK (*Haemophilus* spp., *Aggregatibacter*, *Cardiobacterium hominis*, *Eikenella corrodens*, *Kingella* spp.)

D. Complications - *(Domain 1)*
   1. Destruction of heart valves
   2. Heart failure
   3. Septic embolism
   4. Metastatic infection
   5. Immune-related glomerulonephritis

E. Presentation/Diagnosis - *(Domain 1)*
   1. Signs and symptoms
      a. Fever: Low grade and remittent
      b. Cutaneous signs: Petechiae, Janeway lesions, splinter hemorrhages
      c. Cardiac murmur
      d. Arthralgias, myalgias, Osler nodes
   2. Laboratory findings
      a. Positive blood culture results
      b. Anemia (normochromic, normocytic)
      c. Leukocytosis
      d. Increased erythrocyte sedimentation rate (ESR) and C-reactive protein (CRP) concentration
      e. Positive for vegetation noted on echocardiogram

F. Treatment - *(Domain 1)*
   1. Treatment difficulties
      a. Antibiotics have poor penetration into the vegetation.
      b. Large bacterial inocula inside vegetation
      c. Bacteria are in stationary/dormant growth in vegetation.
      d. Resistant pathogens
   2. General approach
      a. Prolonged treatment courses: Duration should start from the last positive blood culture finding.
      b. Intravenous antibiotics are needed.
      c. Combination therapies and bactericidal agents are best.
      d. Know the MIC of the organism.

Table 7. Treatment of Infective Endocarditis

Organism	Therapy	Duration, wk
Streptococcus viridans (penicillin MIC ≤ 0.12 mcg/mL)	Penicillin G	4
	Ceftriaxone	4
	Penicillin G + gentamicin	2
	Ceftriaxone + gentamicin	2
	Vancomycin (severe β-lactam allergy)	4
S. viridans (penicillin MIC > 0.12 mcg/mL)	Penicillin G + gentamicin	4
	Ceftriaxone + gentamicin	4
	Vancomycin (severe β-lactam allergy)	4
Staphylococcus aureus – MSSA	Nafcillin or oxacillin ± gentamicin for 3–5 days	6
	Cefazolin ± gentamicin for 3–5 days	6
	Vancomycin (severe β-lactam allergy)	6
S. aureus – MRSA	Vancomycin	6
	Daptomycin	6
Enterococcus	Penicillin G or ampicillin + gentamicin	4–6
	Vancomycin + gentamicin	6
Enterococcus (penicillin resistant)	Ampicillin/sulbactam or vancomycin + gentamicin	6
	Daptomycin	6
VRE	Linezolid	≥ 8
	Quinupristin/dalfopristin	≥ 8
	Daptomycin	≥ 8
HACEK	Ceftriaxone	4
	Ampicillin/sulbactam	4
	Fluoroquinolones (cipro, levo, moxi)	4

HACEK = *Haemophilus* spp., *Aggregatibacter, Cardiobacterium hominis, Eikenella corrodens, Kingella* spp.; MIC = minimum inhibitory concentration; MRSA = methicillin-resistant *Staphylococcus aureus*; MSSA = methicillin-sensitive *S. aureus;* VRE = vancomycin-resistant enterococci.

3. Outpatient therapy
   a. Most patients can receive the bulk of their therapy in the outpatient setting after bacteremia has cleared.
   b. Contraindications for outpatient therapy:
      i. Severe congestive heart failure
      ii. Severe cardiac arrhythmias
      iii. Persistent bacteremia
      iv. Fulminant staphylococcal infections
      v. Lack of reliable intravenous access

G. Endocarditis Prophylaxis - *(Domain 1, 3)*
   1. Prophylaxis is warranted in patients at increased risk of infective endocarditis (IE), and bacteremia known to cause IE are associated with dental, gastrointestinal, and genitourinary procedures.
   2. Patients or conditions needing prophylaxis
      a. Prosthetic heart valves
      b. Previous IE

    c. Congenital heart disease (CHD)
-      i. Unrepaired cyanotic CHD
-     ii. Completely repaired CHD with prosthetic material or device for 6 months after the procedure
-    iii. Repaired CHD with residual defects near the site of prosthesis

    d. Cardiac transplantation with cardiac valvulopathy

3. Procedures requiring antibiotic prophylaxis
-    a. Tonsillectomy and/or adenoidectomy
-    b. Surgical operations that involve the respiratory mucosa
-    c. Dental procedures involving gingival or periapical tissue of teeth
-    d. Perforation of oral mucosa

4. Prophylaxis is not needed in the following situations:
-    a. Dental radiographs
-    b. Placement, removal, or adjustment of orthodontia
-    c. Shedding of deciduous teeth
-    d. Bleeding from trauma to lips or oral mucosa

Table 8. Infective Endocarditis Prophylaxis for Dental and/or Respiratory Procedures

Situation	Antibiotic	Adult Regimen	Pediatric Regimen
Standard prophylaxis	Amoxicillin	2 g orally 1 hr before procedure	50 mg/kg orally 1 hr before procedure
Unable to take oral agent IM or IV therapy	Ampicillin	2 g IM/IV within 30 min of procedure	50 mg/kg IM/IV within 30 min of procedure
	Cefazolin or ceftriaxone	1 g IM/IV within 30 min of procedure	50 mg/kg IM/IV within 30 min of procedure
Penicillin allergy	Clindamycin	600 mg orally 1 hr before procedure	20 mg/kg orally 1 hr before procedure
	Cephalexin	2 g orally 1 hr before procedure	50 mg/kg orally 1 hr before procedure
	Azithromycin or clarithromycin	500 mg orally 1 hr before procedure	15 mg/kg orally 1 hr before procedure
Penicillin allergy, unable to take oral agent	Cefazolin or ceftriaxone	1 g IM/IV within 30 min of procedure	50 mg/kg within 30 min of procedure
	Clindamycin	600 mg IV within 30 min of procedure	20 mg/kg within 30 min of procedure

IM = intramuscular(ly); IV = intravenous(ly).

Patient Case

12. J.K. is a 68-year-old man who recently underwent surgery for placement of an artificial aortic valve. During the admission, the attending physician recommended that he receive antibiotics before any dental work. He has not seen a dentist in several years, which has resulted in poor dental hygiene. His dentist states that he will need have several teeth extracted as well have work done on his gums. J.K. states that when he received penicillin earlier in life, his tongue became swollen and he had difficulty breathing. Which is the best choice for antibiotic prophylaxis before his dental visit?

  A. Clindamycin 600 mg orally 1 hour prior.
  B. Ceftriaxone 1 g intravenously 30 minutes prior.
  C. Levofloxacin 750 mg orally 1 hour prior.
  D. Amoxicillin 2 g orally 1 hour prior.

IX. INFECTIOUS DIARRHEA/GASTROINTESTINAL INFECTIONS

A. Introduction - *(Domain 1, 5)*
1. Infectious diarrhea is a major cause of morbidity and mortality worldwide and is the most common illness among individuals traveling from industrialized to developing countries.
2. There are 200–375 million cases of acute diarrheal illness each year.
   a. 900,000 hospitalizations
   b. 6000 deaths
3. Infectious diarrhea is a major public health problem because of its etiology and risk of spread.
4. Prompt diagnosis is necessary to alleviate symptoms and prevent secondary transmission; public health officials can determine the source, prevent its spread, and promote public awareness.

B. Etiology - *(Domain 1)*
1. Infectious diarrhea is caused by a variety of enteric pathogens (bacteria, viruses, and parasites).
   a. Bacteria: *E. coli, Salmonella, Shigella, Campylobacter jejuni*, enterohemorrhagic *E. coli/Shigella* toxin *E. coli, C. difficile*
   b. Parasites: *Cyclospora, Cryptosporidium, Giardia*
   c. Viruses: Enterovirus, rotavirus
2. Severity of diarrhea can range from self-limiting disease to hemorrhagic and persistent diarrhea.

C. Transmission and Exposure - *(Domain 1, 5)*
1. Ingestion of raw or undercooked meat
2. Contaminated produce and milk
3. Ill contacts (e.g., food handlers, family)
4. Day care centers
5. Institutional exposures
6. Water exposures

D. Signs and Symptoms - *(Domain 1)*
1. Diarrhea: 3 or more stools a day that are a change in normal bowel movements
2. Nausea and vomiting
3. Abdominal cramping
4. Fever
5. Blood or pus in stool

E. Diagnosis - *(Domain 1)*
1. Patient history
   a. Timeline of diarrhea and illness
   b. Stool characteristics (e.g., bloody, water, quantity, frequency)
   c. Other symptoms (e.g., fever, abdominal cramping, nausea, vomiting, tenesmus)
2. Social history
   a. Recent travel
   b. Ingestion of high-risk foods such as undercooked or raw meat
   c. Exposure to farm animals, petting zoos, reptiles
   d. Exposure to ill contacts
   e. Recent antibiotics or other medications
   f. Comorbidities

3. Laboratory tests
    a. Should be done if unknown cause and in severe cases, outbreaks, persistent cases
    b. Etiology
        i. Stool culture
        ii. Assays and subtyping
    c. Importance of laboratory diagnosis
        i. Identifies the specific etiology
        ii. Decreases relapse and resistance with appropriate therapy
        iii. Prevents transmission to others
        iv. Aids public health authorities in ensuring appropriate follow-up

F. Treatment - *(Domain 1)*
    1. Goals
        a. Rule out other causes of diarrhea to avoid unnecessary antimicrobial exposure.
        b. Eliminate symptoms.
        c. Determine which tests to order and if any public health measures need to be taken.
        d. Prevent future transmission.
        e. Prevent resistance.
    2. Rehydrate the patient orally or, if needed, intravenously.
    3. Determine the most likely cause of infectious diarrhea.
        a. Community-acquired or traveler's diarrhea
            i. *Salmonella*
            ii. *Shigella*
            iii. *Campylobacter*
            iv. *E. coli* (consider *Shigella* toxin *E. coli* such as O157:H7 if bloody diarrhea)
            v. Enterovirus
            vi. Rotavirus (specifically in day care settings)
        b. Nosocomial and/or recent antibiotics: *C. difficile*
        c. Persistent diarrhea for more than 7 days
            i. *Giardia*
            ii. *Cryptosporidium*
            iii. *Cyclospora*
    4. Antimicrobials
        a. *E. coli*
            i. Trimethoprim/sulfamethoxazole 160/800 mg orally twice daily for 3 days
            ii. Fluoroquinolone orally (levofloxacin, ciprofloxacin) for 3 days
        b. Enterohemorrhagic *E. coli* such as O157:H7
            i. Because the role of antibiotics is unclear and may be harmful, they should be avoided.
            ii. Avoid antimotility drugs.
            iii. Supportive care and hospitalization
        c. *Shigella* spp.
            i. Trimethoprim/sulfamethoxazole 160/800 mg orally twice daily for 3 days
            ii. Fluoroquinolone orally (levofloxacin, ciprofloxacin) for 3 days
            iii. Other options: Ceftriaxone or azithromycin

d. *Salmonella* spp.: Use antibiotics only in severe cases; if the patient is younger than 6 months or older than 50 years; or if the patient has prostheses, valvular heart disease, severe atherosclerosis, malignancy, or uremia.
  i. Trimethoprim/sulfamethoxazole 160/800 mg orally twice daily for 5–7 days
  ii. Fluoroquinolone orally (levofloxacin, ciprofloxacin) for 5–7 days
e. *C. difficile* (see section X)
f. *Giardia*: Metronidazole 250–750 mg orally three times daily for 7–10 days or tinidazole 2 g orally once
g. *Cryptosporidium*: If severe, paromomycin 500 mg orally three times daily for 7 days or nitazoxanide 500 mg orally three times daily for 3 days
h. Enterovirus: Supportive care
i. Rotavirus: Supportive care or vaccination (RotaTeq, Rotarix)
j. Newer therapies
  i. Rifaximin (traveler's diarrhea, noninvasive/hemorrhagic strains of *E. coli*)
  ii. Nitazoxanide (*Giardia, Cryptosporidium*)

X. *CLOSTRIDIUM DIFFICILE*

A. Introduction - *(Domain 1, 5)*
  1. *C. difficile* is an anaerobic, spore-forming, gram-positive bacillus and a known toxin producer.
  2. *C. difficile* infection (CDI) is the most common cause of antibiotic-associated diarrhea and colitis.
      a. Antibiotic-associated diarrhea: 20%–25%
      b. Antibiotic-associated colitis: 90%–100%
      c. Pseudomembranous colitis: 90%–100%
  3. Incidence has increased through the years from 30–40 cases/100,000 population in the mid-1990s to 50 cases/100,000 population in the 2000s, including increases in fatal cases and outbreaks.
  4. Epidemiologic shift: CDI is a problem not only a hospital or health care facility, but also in the community setting.
  5. Increased hospital costs for patients with CDI can be greater than $4000 per case.

B. Risk Factors for CDI - *(Domain 1)*
  1. Host factors
      a. Older than 65 years
      b. Compromised immune system
  2. Pharmacology
      a. Exposure to broad-spectrum antibiotics
          i. Affects the balance of intestinal flora
          ii. Can occur weeks after finishing antimicrobial therapy
          iii. Any antibiotic may cause CDI; the most common culprits are clindamycin, the fluoroquinolones, and the β-lactams.
      b. Chemotherapy
      c. Proton pump inhibitors
  3. Infection control
      a. Must use soap and water for hand washing because alcohol gels/foams do not kill *C. difficile* spores
      b. Spores are easily spread from patient to patient.

4. *C. difficile* pathogenicity/toxins
   a. Toxins A and B are produced on the pathogenicity locus (PaLoc) of *C. difficile*
      i. *tcdA* codes for toxin A
      ii. *tcdB* codes for toxin B
   b. Hypervirulent strain *C. difficile* NAP1/BI/027
      i. Associated with severe CDI; sometimes called different names depending on typing method
      ii. Ribotype 027: European typing method
      iii. Group BI "bee eye": U.S. typing method
      iv. Nap-1: CDC typing method

C. Diagnosis - *(Domain 1)*
   1. Signs and symptoms
      a. Some patients may be asymptomatic carriers.
      b. Mild to severe watery diarrhea in the presence of CDI risk factors
      c. Dehydration
   2. General laboratory findings
      a. Leukocytosis
      b. Hypoalbuminemia may be present.
      c. Electrolyte imbalances may be present.
   3. Testing for *C. difficile* and toxins
      a. Stool culture
         i. Tested only on unformed stool
         ii. Most sensitive
         iii. Many false positives because it can also detect non-toxigenic *C. difficile*
         iv. Labor-intensive and long turnaround time, so not clinically practical
         v. Toxin testing is considered the gold standard.
      b. Toxin A and B testing for *C. difficile*
         i. Tissue culture cytotoxicity assay
         ii. Enzyme immunoassay
         iii. PCR

D. Treatment - *(Domain 1)*
   1. Discontinue offending antibiotic, if possible.
   2. Use good infection control in both inpatients and outpatients.
   3. Give supportive care.
   4. Avoid antiperistaltics.
   5. Determine disease severity.
      a. Mild to moderate: WBC count of 15×10^3 cells/mm^3 or less, SCr 1.5 times or less the premorbid concentration
      b. Severe: WBC count greater than 15×10^3 cells/mm^3, SCr greater than 1.5 times the premorbid concentration
   6. Begin antimicrobial therapy (see Table 8).
      a. Metronidazole
      b. Vancomycin

Table 8. Treatment of CDI

CDI Severity	Recommended Agent	Dosing Regimen
Mild to moderate	Metronidazole	500 mg orally three times daily for 10–14 days
Severe	Vancomycin	125 mg orally four times daily for 10–14 days
Severe with complications (e.g., hypotension, shock, ileus)	Vancomycin + metronidazole	Vancomycin 500 mg orally four times daily plus metronidazole 500 mg intravenously every 8 hr, consider rectal vancomycin if ileus

CDI = *C. difficile* infection.

7. Recurrence
    a. First recurrence: Treat with the same drug as in the initial episode.
    b. Second recurrence: Vancomycin in tapered and/or pulsed regimen
        i.   Oral taper
             (a) 125 mg four times daily for 10–14 days
             (b) 125 mg twice daily for 1 week
             (c) 125 mg daily for 1 week
        ii. Followed by vancomycin pulse dosing 125 mg every 2 or 3 days for 2–8 weeks
    c. Metronidazole use is not recommended beyond the first recurrent episode because of possible neurotoxicity.
    d. Other options
        i.   Fidaxomicin 200 mg orally twice daily (U.S. Food and Drug Administration [FDA] approved for CDI)
        ii. Rifaximin (not FDA approved for CDI)
        iii. Nitazoxanide (not FDA approved for CDI)
        iv. Biotherapy with *Lactobacillus* or *Saccharomyces*
        v.   Fecal transplant

Patient Case

13. A.T. is a 55-year-man who was treated for his first recurrent CDI 3 weeks ago with another treatment course of metronidazole 500 mg orally three times daily for 10 days. He has not taken antibiotics or any other medications in the past 3 weeks, and he now comes to the clinic with severe abdominal pain and frequent loose stools for the past few days. The *C. difficile* toxin immunoassay comes back positive, and he is given a diagnosis of recurrent CDI. Which is the best recommendation for his recurrent infection?

   A. Metronidazole 500 mg orally three times daily for 4 weeks.
   B. Vancomycin orally tapered during 4 weeks, followed by 4 weeks of pulse dosing.
   C. Fidaxomicin 200 mg twice daily for 10 days.
   D. Vancomycin 125 mg orally four times daily for 10 days.

XI. CENTRAL NERVOUS SYSTEM INFECTIONS

A. Introduction - *(Domain 1, 5)*
1. Central nervous system infections can be caused by a variety of pathogens and have a high rate of mortality (2%–30%), with most patients dying within the first 24–48 hours of presentation.
2. Incidence is about 8.6 cases/100,000 population.
3. Prompt diagnosis and management is imperative to decrease and prevent complications.

B. Etiology - *(Domain 1)*
1. Usually caused by bacteria, but also can be caused by viruses, fungi, drugs, etc.
2. Specific bacterial organisms are age-specific.
3. Age younger than 1 month
    a. *S. agalactiae*
    b. *E. coli*
    c. *Klebsiella* spp.
    d. *Enterobacter* spp.
4. Age 1–23 months
    a. *S. pneumoniae*
    b. *N. meningitidis*
    c. *S. agalactiae*
    d. *H. influenzae*
    e. *E. coli*
5. Age 2–50 years
    a. *N. meningitidis*
    b. *S. pneumoniae*
6. Older than 50 years
    a. *S. pneumoniae*
    b. *N. meningitidis*
    c. *Listeria monocytogenes*
    d. Aerobic gram-negative bacilli
7. Risk factors for specific organisms
    a. *S. pneumoniae* – Compromised immune system (e.g., HIV, asplenia), alcoholism, chronic liver or renal disease, malignancy
    b. Aerobic gram-negative bacilli – Head trauma, neurosurgical procedures
    c. *L. monocytogenes* – Consumption of contaminated foods, diabetes mellitus

C. Signs and Symptoms - *(Domain 1)*
1. Fever, chills
2. Headache, altered mental status, nuchal rigidity, photophobia
3. Nausea, vomiting
4. Brudzinski sign, Kernig sign
5. Purpuric rash on extremities, disseminated intravascular coagulation, rhabdomyolysis (*N. meningitidis*)
6. Rhinorrhea or otorrhea secondary to cerebrospinal fluid (CSF) leak (*S. pneumoniae*)

D. Diagnosis - *(Domain 1)*
1. Lumbar puncture
2. Simultaneous blood glucose testing and CBC
3. Predictors of bacterial meningitis (Table 9)

Table 9. CSF in Meningitis

	Normal CSF	**Bacterial Meningitis**
WBC count	$< 5 \times 10^3$ cells/mm^3	$> 12 \times 10^3$ cells/mm^3
Glucose	2/3 serum values (30–70 mg/dL)	$< 1/2$ serum values
Protein	< 50 mg/dL	> 150 mg/dL

CSF = cerebrospinal fluid; WBC = white blood cell.

    4. CSF studies
        a. Gram stain of CSF is a rapid and accurate means of identifying the pathogen.
        b. Latex agglutination test for encapsulated bacteria: *S. pneumoniae, N. meningitidis, H. influenzae*
        c. PCR, especially if culture negative
        d. Probability of isolating an organism decreases with prior antibiotic use.

  E. Empiric Therapy - *(Domain 1)*
    1. Newborns younger than 1 month
        a. Ampicillin plus aminoglycoside
        b. Ampicillin plus cefotaxime
    2. Age 1–23 months: Vancomycin plus ceftriaxone or cefotaxime
    3. Age 2–50 years: Vancomycin plus ceftriaxone or cefotaxime
    4. Age 50 years or older: Vancomycin plus ampicillin plus ceftriaxone or cefotaxime

  F. Prophylaxis - *(Domain 1, 3, 5)*
    1. Rationale is to prevent meningitis in those who are colonized and to prevent its spread to young children by eradicating nasopharyngeal colonization.
    2. Vaccination is protective before exposure to *S. pneumoniae* and *N. meningitidis* (see Vaccine chapter).
    3. Prophylaxis is determined by the specific organism the patient is exposed to.
    4. *H. influenzae*
        a. Prophylaxis of close contacts
        b. Give to all individuals if a child younger than 48 months is in the home.
        c. Not recommended for day care contacts older than 2 years unless more than two cases are reported
        d. Children: Rifampin 20 mg/kg/day orally for 4 days (infants younger than 1 month: 10 mg/kg)
        e. Adults: Rifampin 600 mg/day orally for 4 days
    5. *N. meningitidis*
        a. All close contacts (i.e., household, school, day care, military, dormitories)
        b. Adults: Rifampin 600 mg orally twice daily for 2 days or ciprofloxacin 500 mg orally once
        c. Children: Rifampin 10 mg/kg orally twice daily for 2 days (infants younger than 1 month: 5 mg/kg)
        d. Pregnancy: Ceftriaxone 250 mg intramuscularly once

XII. BONE AND JOINT INFECTIONS

  A. Introduction - *(Domain 1, 5)*
    1. Osteomyelitis is an inflammatory process with bone destruction caused by an infecting organism.
    2. Incidence: 20 cases/100,000 population
    3. Affects both children and adults
    4. Types
        a. Acute (56% of cases): Caused by infections of recent onset, lasts several days to 1 week
        b. Chronic (44% of cases): Long-standing infections that evolve for months to years with persistence of microorganisms and dead bone

B. Risk Factors - *(Domain 1)*
   1. Diabetes mellitus
   2. Decubitus ulcers
   3. Surgery
   4. Trauma
   5. Intravenous drug use
   6. Compromised immune system

C. Osteomyelitis Characteristics - *(Domain 1)*
   1. Contiguous spread: Spread of bacteria from an adjacent tissue infection or by direct inoculation
      a. Follows trauma, bone surgery, joint replacement, open wounds, soft tissue infections, etc.
      b. Can occur in any bone and at any age
   2. Hematogenous spread: Seeding of the bacteria from the bloodstream
      a. Children and older adults are most often affected.
      b. Bones affected are long bones (tibia, femur) in children and vertebral bones in adults.
      c. Increased risk of bacteremia because of intravenous catheters, skin infections, respiratory tract infections, etc.
   3. Vascular insufficiency refers to insufficient blood supply to the affected area resulting in impaired healing and immune response.
      a. Adults, especially those with diabetes and peripheral vascular disease
      b. In many cases, it follows a soft tissue infection that spreads to the bone.

D. Etiology - *(Domain 1)*
   1. *S. aureus* most common, both MSSA and MRSA
   2. *Staphylococcus epidermidis*
   3. *S. pyogenes*
   4. Nosocomial exposure: Enterobacteriaceae, *Pseudomonas* spp.
   5. Patients with sickle cell anemia: *Salmonella, S. pneumoniae*
   6. Diabetic foot/decubitus ulcers: *Streptococcus* spp., anaerobes
   7. HIV: *Bartonella* spp.
   8. Intravenous drug abusers: *Pseudomonas* spp.
   9. Immunocompromised: *Aspergillus* spp., *Candida* spp., *Mycobacterium*

E. Diagnosis - *(Domain 1)*
   1. Signs and symptoms
      a. Fever, chills, malaise
      b. Tenderness; pain and swelling of the affected area
      c. Decreased motion
   2. Laboratory values
      a. Elevated ESR
      b. Elevated WBC count
      c. Elevated CRP concentration
      d. Positive blood culture findings
   3. Diagnostics
      a. Bone changes seen on radiography about 10–14 days after infection onset
      b. Technetium and gallium scans positive as early as 1 day after infection onset
      c. Computed tomography and magnetic resonance imaging scans

F. Treatment - *(Domain 1)*
   1. Newborns (1 month or younger)
      a. Likely organisms: *S. aureus*, streptococci, *E. coli*
      b. Nafcillin or oxacillin plus cefotaxime
   2. Children (younger than 5 years)
      a. Likely organisms: *S. aureus*, streptococci, *H. influenzae* type B (if not vaccinated)
      b. Nafcillin, cefazolin, or cefuroxime (especially if unvaccinated)
   3. Children (5 years and older)
      a. Likely organism: *S. aureus*
      b. Nafcillin, cefazolin, or clindamycin
   4. Adults
      a. Likely organisms: MSSA or MRSA
      b. MSSA: Nafcillin or cefazolin
      c. MRSA: Vancomycin
   5. Intravenous drug abusers
      a. Likely organisms: *Pseudomonas* spp.
      b. Ciprofloxacin or ceftazidime plus aminoglycoside
   6. Vascular insufficiency
      a. Polymicrobial (gram positive, gram negative, and/or anaerobes)
      b. Ceftazidime plus clindamycin
   7. Prosthetic joint
      a. Likely organisms: MSSA or MRSA
      b. Vancomycin plus rifampin or nafcillin plus rifampin
   8. Other options for MRSA
      a. Trimethoprim/sulfamethoxazole plus rifampin
      b. Daptomycin
      c. Linezolid
      d. Clindamycin
   9. Treatment length is usually 4–6 weeks with acute osteomyelitis and 6–8 weeks for chronic osteomyelitis. Therapy will start with intravenous antibiotics, followed by oral therapy if warranted.
   10. Antibiotic therapy is often given together with drainage and debridement of infected tissue or removal of hardware and prosthetics.

G. Intravenous to oral therapy - *(Domain 1, 4)*
   1. Organism susceptibility
   2. Initial clinical response to intravenous antibiotics
   3. Patient adherence ensured
   4. Common options depend on the infectious organism: Trimethoprim/sulfamethoxazole, clindamycin, fluoroquinolone (ciprofloxacin, levofloxacin, moxifloxacin), amoxicillin, linezolid

H. Recommended monitoring - *(Domain 1)*
   1. WBC count weekly until normalized
   2. ESR or CRP weekly
   3. Clinical signs of inflammation daily
   4. Antimicrobial adherence

Patient Case

14. B.S. is a 23-year-old woman who comes to the clinic with a fever, severe right knee pain, and swelling that started about 3 days ago. She has no memory of any injuries or trauma to her knee. B.S. is an otherwise healthy, sexually active woman with no known drug allergies. On physical examination, she has a temperature of 100°F; her right knee has limited mobility, with inflammation and erythema, and it is tender and warm. Laboratory findings reveal a WBC count of 15 x 103 cells/mm3 and elevated ESR and CRP concentration. Needle aspiration of the right knee joint shows a WBC count of 180 x 10^3 cells/mm^3 and gram-negative diplococci. Which treatment choice would be best for this patient?

A. Ceftriaxone 1 g intramuscularly daily for 10 days plus doxycycline 100 mg orally twice daily for 7 days.

B. Ceftazidime 2 g intravenously every 8 hours for 4 weeks.

C. Ciprofloxacin 750 mg orally twice daily for 4 weeks.

D. Ceftriaxone 1 g intramuscularly daily for 10 days.

I. Septic Arthritis - *(Domain 1)*
1. Inflammatory reaction within the joint space leading to persistent purulent effusion within the joint
2. Risk factors
   a. Systemic corticosteroid use
   b. Preexisting arthritis
   c. Arthrocentesis
   d. Diabetes mellitus
   e. Trauma
3. Spread by hematogenous dissemination (most cases), adjacent bone infection, direct contamination
4. Etiology
   a. *S. aureus* (MSSA and MRSA)
   b. *Streptococcus* spp.
   c. Gram-negative organisms (*E. coli*, *Pseudomonas* spp.)
   d. *N. gonorrhoeae* most common in adults 18–30 years old
5. Diagnosis
   a. Signs and symptoms
      i. Joints: Painful, swollen, tender, warm, with decreased motion
      ii. Laboratory values
         (a) Elevated ESR, CRP concentration, WBC count
         (b) Blood culture results positive
   b. Diagnostic studies
      i. Needle aspiration of synovial fluid
         (a) WBC count: 5–20 x 10^3 cells/mm^3
         (b) Gram stain positive
         (c) Glucose decreased relative to serum glucose concentration (less than 40 mg/dL)
      ii. Imaging shows distention of joint capsule with soft tissue swelling.
6. Management
   a. Appropriate antibiotics immediately for 3–4 weeks
   b. Joint drainage and rest
   c. Antibiotic choices are the same as for osteomyelitis unless gonococcal infection.
   d. *N. gonorrhoeae*: Treat with ceftriaxone for 7–10 days, and provide presumptive concomitant treatment for *Chlamydia trachomatis* infection for 7 days.

XIII. COLLATERAL DAMAGE

A. Overuse or Inappropriate Use of Antimicrobial Therapy: Can lead to the selection of drug-resistant organisms or unwanted colonization or infection with *C. difficile* diarrhea or multidrug-resistant organisms - *(Domain 1, 3, 5)*

    1. Broad-spectrum antibiotics and resistance

        a. Broad-spectrum antimicrobials are convenient for a "one-size-fits-all" approach to treatment of infections, especially if the agent has good efficacy and convenient dosing.

        b. Several studies have shown a parallel increase in resistance with increased use of fluoroquinolones and third-generation cephalosporins.

            i. Third-generation cephalosporin-associated resistance

                (a) Vancomycin-resistant enterococci

                (b) Extended-spectrum β-lactamase–producing *E. coli* and *Klebsiella* spp.

            ii. Fluoroquinolone use and increased resistance

                (a) Methicillin-resistant *S. aureus*

                (b) Fluoroquinolone-resistant gram-negative bacilli such as *E. coli* and *P. aeruginosa*

            iii. Fluoroquinolones are the most-prescribed antimicrobials for adults in ambulatory care settings and emergency departments.

                (a) A study in a single institution showed that 50% of levofloxacin prescribing for CAP in an emergency department was inappropriate according to practice guidelines.

                (b) Fluoroquinolone-resistant *E. coli* present in patients with cancer previously exposed to levofloxacin

B. Antimicrobial Stewardship - *(Domain 2, 3, 4, 5)*

    1. Key to combating and preventing antimicrobial resistance

    2. Emphasis of most stewardship programs and examples come from institutional practices; however, most prescribing of antimicrobials is in outpatient settings.

    3. Appropriate antimicrobial prescribing is imperative.

        a. Avoid the prescribing/use of antibiotics when they are not warranted (viral infections).

        b. Avoid the prolonged use of antimicrobials.

        c. Use practice guidelines and/or protocols when feasible.

        d. Educate practitioners on the risks of antimicrobial resistance and appropriate antimicrobial prescribing.

REFERENCES

Urinary Tract Infections

1. Bergman M, Nyberg ST, Huovinen P, et al. Association between antimicrobial consumption and resistance in *Escherichia coli*. Antimicrob Agents Chemother 2009;53:912-7.

2. Grigoryan L, Trautner BW, Gupta K. Diagnosis and management of urinary tract infections in the outpatient setting – a review. JAMA 2014;312:1677-84.

3. Gupta K, Hooton TM, Naber KG, et al. International clinical practice guidelines for the treatment of acute uncomplicated cystitis and pyelonephritis in women: a 2010 update by Infectious Diseases Society of America and European Society for Microbiology and Infectious Diseases. Clin Infect Dis 2011;52:e103-20.

4. Hooton TM. Uncomplicated urinary tract infection. N Engl J Med 2012;366:1028-37.

5. Hooton TM, Roberts PL, Cox ME, et al. Voided midstream urine culture and acute cystitis in premenopausal women. N Engl J Med 2013;369:1883-91.

6. Hooton TM, Roberts PL, Stapleton AE. Cefpodoxime vs ciprofloxacin for short-course treatment of acute uncomplicated cystitis – a randomized trial. JAMA 2012;307:583-9.

7. Johnson L, Sabel A, Burman WJ, et al. Emergence of fluoroquinolone resistance in outpatient urinary *Escherichia coli* isolates. Am J Med 2008;121:876-84.

8. Murphy AB, Macejko A, Taylor A, et al. Chronic prostatitis management strategies. Drugs 2009;69:71-84.

9. Nicolle LE, Bradley S, Colgan R, et al. Infectious Diseases Society of America guidelines for the diagnosis and treatment of asymptomatic bacteriuria in adults. Clin Infect Dis 2005;40:643-54.

10. Olson RP, Harrell LJ, Kaye KS. Antibiotic resistance in urinary isolates of *Escherichia coli* from college women with urinary tract infections. Antimicrob Agents Chemother 2009;53:1285-6.

Community-Acquired Pneumonia

1. Malcolm C, Marrie TJ. Antibiotic therapy for ambulatory patients with community-acquired pneumonia in an emergency department setting. Arch Intern Med 2003;163:797-802.

2. Mandell LA, Wunderink RG, Anzueto A, et al. Infectious Diseases Society of America/American Thoracic Society consensus guidelines on the management of community-acquired pneumonia in adults. Clin Infect Dis 2007;44(suppl 2):S27-72.

3. Musher DM, Thorner AR. Community-acquired pneumonia. N Engl J Med 2014;371:1619-28.

4. Niederman MS. Making sense of scoring systems in community acquired pneumonia. Respirology 2009;14:327-35.

5. Wunderink RG, Waterer GW. Community-acquired pneumonia. N Engl J Med 2014;370:543-51.

6. Yu H, Rubin J, Dunning S, et al. Clinical and economic burden of community-acquired pneumonia in Medicare fee-for-service population. J Am Geriatr Soc 2012;60:2137-43.

Tuberculosis

1. American Thoracic Society; Centers for Disease Control and Prevention; Infectious Diseases Society of America. American Thoracic Society/Centers for Disease Control and Prevention/Infectious Diseases Society of America: controlling tuberculosis in the United States. Am J Respir Crit Care Med 2005;172:1169-227.

2. Centers for Disease Control and Prevention. Tuberculosis: Treatment. Available at www.cdc.gov/tb/topic/treatment/default.htm. Accessed November 13, 2013.

3. Getahun H, Matteelli A, Chaisson RE, et al. Latent *Mycobacterium tuberculosis* infection. N Engl J Med 2015;372:2127-35.

4. Sterling TR, Villarino ME, Borisov AS, et al. Three months of rifapentine and isoniazid for latent tuberculosis infection. N Engl J Med 2011;364:2155-66.

5. Zumla A, Raviglione M, Hafner R, et al. Tuberculosis. N Engl J Med 2013;368:745-55.

Upper Respiratory Tract Infections

1. Chan TV. The patient with sore throat. Med Clin North Am 2010;94:923-43.

2. Chow AW, Benninger MS, Brook I, et al. IDSA clinical practice guideline for acute bacterial rhinosinusitis in children and adults [published online ahead of print March 20, 2012]. Clin Infect Dis 2012;54:e72-112.

3. Costelloe C, Metcalfe C, Lovering A, et al. Effect of antibiotic prescribing in primary care on antimicrobial resistance in individual patients: systematic review and meta-analysis. BMJ 2010;340:c2096.

4. Gonzales R, Bartlett JG, Besser RE, et al. Principles of appropriate antibiotic use for treatment of nonspecific upper respiratory tract infections in adults: background. Ann Intern Med 2001;134:490-4.

5. Lieberthal AS, Caroll AE, Chonmaitree T, et al. The diagnosis and management of acute otitis media. Pediatrics 2013;131:e964-99.

6. Ryan MW. Evaluation and management of the patient with "sinus." Med Clin North Am 2010;94:881-90.

7. Shulman ST, Bisno AL, Clegg HW, et al. Clinical practice guideline for the diagnosis and management of group A streptococcal pharyngitis: 2012 update by the Infectious Diseases Society of America [published online ahead of print September 9, 2012]. Clin Infect Dis 2012;55:e86-102.

8. Wald ER, Applegate KE, Bordley C, et al. Clinical practice guideline for the diagnosis and management of acute bacterial sinusitis in children aged 1 to 18 years. Pediatrics 2013;132:e262-80.

Ophthalmic Infections/Conjunctivitis

1. Cronau H, Kankanala RR, Mauger T. Diagnosis and management of red eye in primary care. Am Fam Physician 2010;81:137-44.

2. Visscher KL, Hutnik CM, Thomas M. Evidence-based treatment of acute infective conjunctivitis. Can Fam Physician 2009;55:1071-5.

Skin and Soft Tissue Infections

1. Bisno AL, Stevens DL. Streptococcal infections of skin and soft tissues. N Engl J Med 1996;334:240-5.

2. Lipsky BA, Berendt AR, Cornia PB, et al. 2012 Infectious Diseases Society of America clinical practice guidelines for the diagnosis and treatment of diabetic foot infections. Clin Infect Dis 2012;54:132-73.

3. Lipsky BA, Berendt AR, Deery HG, et al. Diagnosis and treatment of diabetic foot infections. Clin Infect Dis 2004;39:885-910.

4. Liu C, Bayer A, Cosgrove E, et al. Clinical practice guidelines by the Infectious Diseases Society of America for treatment of methicillin-resistant *Staphylococcus aureus* infections in adults and children. Clin Infect Dis 2011;52:1-38.

5. Stevens DL, Bisno AL, Chambers HF, et al. Practice guidelines for the diagnosis and management of skin and soft-tissue infections: 2014 update by the Infectious Diseases Society of America. Clin Infect Dis 2014;59:147-59.

Tickborne Infections/Lyme Disease

1. Cameron DJ, Johnson LB, Maloney EL. Evidence assessments and guideline recommendations in Lyme disease: the clinical management of known tick bites, erythema migrans rashes and persistent disease. Expert Rev Anti Infect Ther 2014;12:1103-35.

2. Wormser GP, Dattwyler RJ, Shapiro ED, et al. The clinical assessment, treatment, and prevention of Lyme disease, human granulocytic anaplasmosis, and babesiosis: clinical practice guidelines by the Infectious Diseases Society of America. Clin Infect Dis 2006;43:1089-134.

Infective Endocarditis

1. Baddour LM, Wilson W, Bayer AS, et al. Infective endocarditis: diagnosis, antimicrobial therapy, and management of complications: a statement for healthcare professionals from the Committee on Rheumatic Fever, Endocarditis, and Kawasaki Disease, Council on Cardiovascular Disease in the Young, and the Councils on Clinical Cardiology, Stroke and Cardiovascular Surgery and Anesthesia, American Heart Association: endorsed by the Infectious Diseases Society of America. Circulation 2005;111:e394-434.

2. Hoen B, Duval X. Infective endocarditis. N Engl J Med 2013;368:1425-33.

3. Wilson W, Taubert KA, Gewitz M, et al. Prevention of infective endocarditis: guidelines from the American Heart Association: a guideline from the American Heart Association Rheumatic Fever, Endocarditis, and Kawasaki Disease Committee, Council on Cardiovascular Disease in the Young, and the Council on Clinical Cardiology, Council on Cardiovascular Surgery and anesthesia, and the Quality of Care and Outcomes Research Interdisciplinary Working Group. Circulation 2007;116:1736-54.

Infectious Diarrhea/Gastrointestinal Infections

1. Cottreau JM, Baker SF, DuPont HL, et al. Rifaximin: a non-systemic rifamycin antibiotic for gastrointestinal infections. Expert Rev Anti Infect Ther 2010;8:747-60.

2. Guerrant RL, Gilder TV, Steiner TS, et al. Practice guidelines for the management of infectious diarrhea. Clin Infect Dis 2001;32:331-50.

3. Thielman NM, Guerrant RL. Acute infectious diarrhea. N Engl J Med 2004;350:38-47.

Clostridium difficile

1. Cohen SH, Gerding DN, Johnson S, et al. Clinical practice guidelines for *Clostridium difficile* infection in adults: 2010 update by the Society for Healthcare Epidemiology of America (SHEA) and the Infectious Diseases Society of America (IDSA). Infect Control Hosp Epidemiol 2010;31:431-55.

2. Leffler DA, Lamont JT. *Clostridium difficile* infection. N Engl J Med 2015;372:1539-48.

3. Louie TJ, Miller MA, Mullane KM, et al. Fidaxomicin versus vancomycin for *Clostridium difficile* infection. N Engl J Med 2011;364:422-31.

4. McDonald EG, Milligan J, Frenette C, et al. Continuous proton pump inhibitor therapy and the associated risk of recurrent *Clostridium difficile* infection. JAMA Intern Med 2015;175:784-91.

5. McDonald LC, Kilgore GE, Thompson A, et al. An epidemic toxin gene-variant strain of *Clostridium difficile*. N Engl J Med 2005;353:2433-41.

Central Nervous System Infections

1. Thigpen MC, Whitney CG, Messonnier NE, et al. Bacterial meningitis in the United States, 1998-2007. N Engl J Med 2011;364:2016-25.

2. Tunkel AR, Hartman BJ, Kaplan SL, et al. Practice guidelines for the management of bacterial meningitis. Clin Infect Dis 2004;39:1267-84.

Bone and Joint Infections

1. Berendt T, Byren I. Bone and joint infection. Clin Med 2004;4:510-8.

2. Lew DP, Waldrvogel FA. Osteomyelitis. Lancet 2004;364:369-79.

3. Liu C, Bayer A, Cosgrove SE, et al. Clinical practice guidelines by the Infectious Diseases Society of America for the treatment of methicillin resistant *Staphylococcus aureus* infections in adults and children. Clin Infect Dis 2011;52:1-38.

4. Osmon DR, Berbari EF, Berendt AR, et al. Diagnosis and management of prosthetic joint infection: clinical practice guidelines by the Infectious Diseases Society of America. Clin Infect Dis 2013;56:e1-25.

5. Smith JW, Chalupa P, Hasan MS. Infectious arthritis: clinical features, laboratory findings and treatment. Clin Microbiol Infect 2006;12:309-14.

Collateral Damage

1. Chalmers JD, Al-Khairalla M, Short PM, et al. Proposed changes to management of lower respiratory tract infections in response to the *Clostridium difficile* epidemic. J Antimicrob Chemother 2010;65:608-18.

2. Dellit TH, Owens RC, McGowan JE Jr, et al. Infectious Diseases Society of America and the Society for Healthcare Epidemiology of America guidelines for developing an institutional program to enhance antimicrobial stewardship. Clin Infect Dis 2007;44:159-77.

3. Paterson DL. "Collateral damage" from cephalosporin or quinolone antibiotic therapy. Clin Infect Dis 2004;38(suppl 4):S341-5.

4. Rangaraj G, Granwehr BP, Jiang Y, et al. Perils of quinolone exposure in cancer patients. Cancer 2010;116:967-73.

5. Wong-Beringer A, Nguyen LH, Lee M, et al. An antimicrobial stewardship program with a focus on reducing fluoroquinolone overuse. Pharmacotherapy 2009;29:736-43.

ANSWERS AND EXPLANATIONS TO PATIENT CASES

1. Answer: B

Recurrence develops in about 20% of women with cystitis. If it has been more than 2 weeks since the last infection, it is considered a reinfection and should be treated with an appropriate course of therapy; therefore, ciprofloxacin for 14 days would not be appropriate. In women who experience symptomatic reinfections in association with sexual activity, voiding after intercourse may help prevent infection. In addition, single-dose prophylactic therapy with trimethoprim/sulfamethoxazole (½ single-strength tablet) taken after intercourse considerably reduces the incidence of recurrent infection. Self-initiated UTI treatment is also an option in recurrent infections. Long-term prophylaxis is usually not initiated until the frequency of UTIs is more than three per year.

2. Answer: B

Clinical benefits of cranberry juice in sexually active adult women with recurrent UTIs have been suggested. However, the consistency of study results has varied, as have the types of cranberry products tested, leading to inconclusive evidence. Postcoital voiding after intercourse may be helpful, but sexual intercourse is probably not the primary reason for this patient's recurrent UTIs. Menopause can cause a change in vaginal flora and increase the risk of recurrent UTIs in postmenopausal women. In a randomized, double-blind, placebo-controlled study, postmenopausal women receiving topical estriol vaginal cream had considerably fewer UTIs than did those receiving placebo. Estrogens are only recommended in topical formulation for postmenopausal women who have three or more recurrent UTIs per year and are not taking oral estrogens. Nitrofurantoin prophylaxis therapy would be an option, but at a dose of 50 mg daily for 6 months. In addition, some evidence indicates safety risks with chronic use of nitrofurantoin.

3. Answer: C

The CURB scoring system is based on a scale of 0–5, giving 1 point for each of the following: confusion caused by pneumonia, urea nitrogen concentration greater than 7 mmol/L, respiratory rate 30 breaths/minute or greater, blood pressure less than 90 mm Hg systolic or 60 mm Hg or less diastolic, and age 65 or older. A score of 2 or greater indicates a need for more intense treatment and hospitalization. This patient, whose score is 3, should be admitted to the hospital for treatment. The CURB score does not determine whether the patient should be admitted to the ICU.

4. Answer: D

According to the IDSA/ATS guidelines, patients with co-morbidities such as diabetes, immunosuppression, renal failure, and heart failure should be given a respiratory fluoroquinolone (levofloxacin, moxifloxacin, gemifloxacin) or azithromycin or clarithromycin PLUS high-dose amoxicillin or amoxicillin/clavulanate because of the risk of drug-resistant *S. pneumoniae*. Although this patient describes nausea with ciprofloxacin, such a history is not a contraindication to use of levofloxacin. This patient has a calculated CrCl less than 30 mL/minute/1.73 m^2; therefore, levofloxacin 750 mg daily would not be the appropriate dose.

5. Answer: B

This patient is a health care worker with a PPD reading greater than 10 mm; therefore, initiation of latent TB therapy is warranted. Rifampin 600 mg daily would be good except the duration is only 4 months. The combination of isoniazid 900 mg and rifapentine 900 mg is a new option for latent treatment, but it is given at the stated doses by DOT weekly, not daily. Isoniazid 300 mg orally daily plus vitamin B6 for neuropathy prevention is the best choice.

6. Answer: D

Monitoring for hepatotoxicity is the primary monitoring parameter in patients being treated for latent TB infection, regardless of the regimen chosen. Monofilament testing for neuropathy is unnecessary. This patient does not have cough or a positive chest radiograph indicative of active TB so follow up monitoring of those items is unnecessary during therapy for latent TB.

7. Answer: D

The primary cause of sinusitis is viral pathogens, and differentiating between viral and bacterial causes can be difficult. However, viral infections usually precede bacterial sinusitis infections, and viral infections are self-limiting. This patient has had symptoms for only 3 days, so the diagnosis is most likely viral sinusitis. Therefore, antibiotic use should be avoided at this time to decrease the amount of unnecessary antibiotic use and the risk of resistance. Antihistamines should be avoided in sinusitis because they can dry out the nasal mucosa. Use of topical nasal decongestants such as oxymetazoline will help with the symptoms.

8. Answer: B

This patient probably has viral pharyngitis, given the negative rapid strep test result. Treatment should be supportive care (e.g., acetaminophen or ibuprofen for pain and fever as well as plenty of fluids). Antiviral therapy is not indicated for viral pharyngitis because viral pharyngitis is a self-limiting infection, and antibiotic use would not be prudent at this time.

9. Answer: C

This patient has a simple folliculitis that has not progressed. Folliculitis is usually a self-limiting infection that seldom requires antimicrobial treatment, especially with small lesions. Warm saline compresses to the infected area can help promote drainage. Although outbreaks of CA-MRSA can occur, the best approach for this patient is supportive care; also, watch to make sure the infection does not progress. Folliculitis caused by *P. aeruginosa* is possible after exposure in hot tubs or other moist environments but empiric coverage of this organism in uncomplicated folliculitis is usually not necessary.

10. Answer: C

In this case, CA-MRSA should be highly considered. Community-acquired MRSA is commonly described as an infection that begins as a bug bite and then develops into a progressive cellulitis. This patient received appropriate coverage with cephalexin for common cellulitis, which would cover the most common and even the most virulent organisms except for MRSA, and the infection has continued to progress. The patient is exposed to environments in which CA-MRSA can be a risk (elementary school, gym); therefore, coverage for CA-MRSA is warranted. Penicillin and dicloxacillin would not be appropriate choices for MRSA. Although vancomycin would offer appropriate coverage, other, more convenient, oral options are available. Trimethoprim/sulfamethoxazole would be the best choice in this case, but at a dose twice that used for uncomplicated UTIs.

11. Answer: A

Although the patient is in an area where there is a prevalence of ticks that can transmit Lyme disease, the tick has not been attached for more than 36 hours; therefore, the possibility that *B. burgdorferi* was transmitted by the tick is decreased. The patient does not need to go to the emergency department for tick removal or to the clinic to have it identified. Routine prophylaxis for tick bites is not recommended. Having the patient remove the tick and watch for signs of the bull's eye rash is the best recommendation.

12. Answer: A

This patient requires antibiotic prophylaxis for a procedure that will clearly involve dental bleeding and also because of his history of an artificial heart valve. The description of the patient's penicillin allergy precludes the use of amoxicillin and is severe enough to preclude the use of cephalosporins. Levofloxacin is not a recommended antibiotic for endocarditis prophylaxis, so the best choice is clindamycin.

13. Answer: B

Because of the potential for neurotoxicity, metronidazole use is not recommended after the first recurrence of CDI. Although fidaxomicin may work, there is less experience supporting its use in recurrent infections than for a vancomycin taper and pulse. Vancomycin is the best choice, but because this is the patient's second recurrent infection, a tapered regimen followed by pulse dosing would be the recommended dosing, not 125 mg four times daily for 10 days.

14. Answer: A

This 23-year-old patient has disseminated gonococcal septic arthritis. Ceftazidime is not the best agent for *N. gonorrhoeae*, and treatment would be for 7–10 days, making this agent incorrect. *N. gonorrhoeae* resistance to fluoroquinolones continues to rise; therefore, ciprofloxacin would not be a good choice. Ceftriaxone is the drug of choice for 7–10 days, with oral doxycycline for 7 days for presumed concomitant chlamydial infection.

ANSWERS AND EXPLANATIONS TO SELF-ASSESSMENT QUESTIONS

1. Answer: A

Leukocyte esterase, proteinuria, and hematuria are not specific for a UTI. Although leukocyte esterase indicates the presence of WBCs in the urine, it could be a sign of inflammation in the urinary tract. Proteinuria and hematuria could also be present in other disease states. A positive nitrite test result indicates the presence of nitrate-reducing bacteria such as *E. coli*; therefore, it would be most indicative of a UTI.

2. Answer: D

Although the patient could be at risk of gonorrhea and/or chlamydia because of having unprotected sex, she does not have vaginal discharge, and her symptom onset is within 3 days of sexual contact; the usual symptom onset in women takes up to 10 days. A Gram stain and NAAT would need to be performed by a clinician using a vaginal swab to determine whether she has gonorrhea or chlamydia before treatment is initiated. Significant bacteriuria traditionally has been defined as bacterial counts greater than 100,000 (10^5) CFU/mL of urine. Many clinicians, however, have challenged this statement as too general. Indeed, significant bacteriuria in patients with symptoms of a UTI may be defined as greater than 10^2 organisms per milliliter.

3. Answer: A

Several studies have shown a decrease in mortality with the introduction of guideline-based protocols. A 5-year study of 28,700 patients with pneumonia admitted with a guideline protocol showed a 30-day mortality rate that was 3.2% lower with the guideline than for patients treated concurrently with non–guideline-based treatment (Am J Med 2001;110:451-7). Other studies have shown a decrease in hospitalizations with guideline protocols, but not specifically on ICU admission.

4. Answer: B

Although conjunctivitis can be caused by many things such as allergens, bacteria, and, more predominantly, viruses, this 7-year-old girl goes to school; therefore, she should be automatically treated with topical antibiotics. Supportive care would be good in addition to antibiotics, but this should not be the only treatment. Antihistamines might help, but again, topical antibiotics are warranted in this case. Ofloxacin would be a good choice, but it should be given four times daily and for only 7 days unless there is reinfection or persistence.

Azithromycin would cover the most likely organisms of *S. pneumoniae* and *H. influenzae*; thus, it would be a good choice.

5. Answer: D

This patient presents to the clinic with early Lyme disease, a classic bull's-eye rash, and positive *B. burgdorferi* antibodies. Treatment is imperative to prevent the development of late Lyme disease. Ceftriaxone intravenously would not be used for early disease, but for cardiac or neurologic disease. Treatment for 14 days with doxycycline would be the treatment of choice.

6. Answer: C

This patient is not responding to his current regimen of high-dose amoxicillin/clavulanate. According to the new guidelines, his medication should be switched to a respiratory fluoroquinolone such as moxifloxacin, and because the patient's first-line therapy has failed, treatment would be extended to 7–10 days. Amoxicillin is no longer recommended for sinusitis. Linezolid would not cover the possibility of infections with gram-negative pathogens such as *H. influenzae* or *M. catarrhalis,* and its adverse effects and cost would be problems.

7. Answer: D

This patient has a positive strep antigen test result, so treatment with antimicrobial therapy is necessary. Penicillin is the treatment of choice for group A *Streptococcus*, so an intramuscular shot of benzathine penicillin would be appropriate. The patient weighs more than 27 kg, so the adult dose of 1.2 million units would be needed. Group A *Streptococcus* has a high rate of resistance to trimethoprim/sulfamethoxazole and would not be a good choice.

8. Answer: D

One of the most modifiable risk factors for *C. difficile* diarrhea is the exposure to antimicrobial agents. Although some antimicrobials may give the impression of being more associated with *C. difficile*, almost all antimicrobials can be potential risks because of the changes they can produce on the gut flora. Changes in gut flora will increase the risk of toxin-producing *C. difficile*. Health care exposure (e.g., recent surgery) can be a risk, as can immunosuppression or exposure to other individuals with *C. difficile* diarrhea, but these would not be the most likely causes in this case.

9. Answer: B

Diabetic foot infections are usually polymicrobial, so empiric antimicrobial therapy should cover gram-negative organisms, gram-positive organisms, and anaerobes. Levofloxacin has coverage against most of these organisms and would be the best choice. The patient has a CrCl of 22 mL/minute/1.73 m²; therefore, levofloxacin at 750 mg daily would be too high. Vancomycin has mainly gram-positive coverage, and the 1-g dose every 12 hours might be too aggressive because of this patient's renal function. Trimethoprim/sulfamethoxazole does not offer adequate coverage for polymicrobial infections, and the patient reports a past allergic reaction to sulfa drugs. More severe infections may require broader coverage and/or hospitalization; however, this patient has a mild infection.

10. Answer: D

This patient has had close contact with someone who has meningococcal meningitis, and she is unvaccinated; therefore, she requires prophylaxis. Ceftriaxone could be used, but the dose should be 125–250 mg intramuscularly once. This patient will require the vaccine at some point, but not without receiving prophylaxis. Rifampin is a good choice, but the dose should be 600 mg twice daily for 2 days. Ciprofloxacin 500 mg orally once is fine for adult prophylaxis and the patient is 18 years old, so she could receive this regimen.

Nephrology

Katie E. Cardone, Pharm.D., BCACP, FNKF, FASN

Albany College of Pharmacy
and Health Sciences

Nephrology

Katie E. Cardone, Pharm.D., BCACP, FNKF, FASN

Albany College of Pharmacy
and Health Sciences

Learning Objectives

1. Identify a patient at risk of, or presenting with, acute kidney injury and formulate an appropriate recommendation.
2. Identify a patient at risk of, or presenting with, drug-induced kidney disease and formulate an appropriate recommendation.
3. Compare and contrast the available methods to assess kidney function. Using appropriate data, assess kidney function in a patient.
4. Formulate an evidence-based treatment plan for managing the most common medical problems in patients with chronic kidney disease (CKD), including anemia and CKD-related mineral and bone disorder.
5. Construct a treatment plan to slow the progression of CKD in patients with hypertension and diabetes.
6. Describe the pharmacokinetic effects of peritoneal and hemodialysis on drug disposition.
7. List the most common nephrolithiasis prevention measures and treatment options.
8. List the multidisciplinary dialysis team members and their roles in patient care.
9. Describe Medicare Part B policies related to end-stage renal disease (ESRD) and dialysis care (i.e., ESRD Prospective Payment System, Quality Incentive Program, Conditions for Coverage).
10. Describe the CMS (Centers for Medicare & Medicaid Services) Comprehensive ESRD Care Model (ESCO).
11. Explain relevant Medicare Part D policies and issues for patients with ESRD.

Self-Assessment Questions

Answers and explanations to these questions can be found at the end of the chapter.

Questions 1–3 pertain to the following case.

A.B. is a 50-year-old woman on hemodialysis (HD) for 9 years. Her medical history includes ESRD secondary to type 2 diabetes mellitus (DM), diabetic neuropathy, hypertension and gastroesophageal reflux disease. AB is generally adherent with her dialysis prescription. Current medications include: calcium acetate 667 mg one capsule with meals TID, insulin glargine 10 units every morning and insulin apart 3-5 units with meals, ranitidine 150 mg once daily, aspirin 81 mg once daily, renal multivitamin one tablet daily, gabapentin 600 mg QHS and atorvastatin 20 mg once daily. She receives epoetin alfa 8,000 units

intravenously and paricalcitol 2 mcg intravenously at each dialysis session. AB has received dietary counseling and states that she adheres to her diet as closely as possible. Her serum albumin concentration is 4.0 g/dL. Her most recent laboratory values reveal intact parathyroid hormone (iPTH) 700 pg/mL, calcium 10.4 mg/dL, and phosphorus 6.8 mg/dL.

1. Which is the best recommendation with respect to controlling the phosphorus concentration in this patient?

    A. Increase calcium acetate to 2 capsules TID.
    B. Discontinue calcium acetate and initiate calcium carbonate 1000 mg with meals and 500 mg with snacks.
    C. Discontinue calcium acetate and begin aluminum hydroxide 1 g with meals and snacks.
    D. Discontinue calcium acetate and begin sevelamer carbonate 1600 mg with meals TID.

2. For this patient, the nephrology team considers the addition of cinacalcet to directly reduce the PTH concentration. Which laboratory value is most important to monitor for safety?

    A. Liver function.
    B. Calcium.
    C. PTH.
    D. Creatinine.

AB's epoetin dose has been unchanged for 6 months. Most recently, her laboratory values were as follows: hemoglobin 8.8 g/dL, transferrin saturation (TSAT) 14%, and serum ferritin 90 ng/mL. In the past month, her hemoglobin concentration was 9.4 g/dL. There are no obvious signs of infection or bleeding.

3. Which therapeutic changes would be most appropriate to manage this patient's anemia?

    A. Administer intravenous iron sucrose 100 mg with each dialysis session for 10 dialysis sessions.
    B. Counsel the patient to take ferrous sulfate 325 mg twice daily with meals.
    C. Initiate folic acid 1 mg orally once daily.
    D. Increase the epoetin dose to 10,000 units intravenously with each HD session.

4. Which drug is most likely to be removed by high-flux HD?

	Water Solubility	Molecular Weight (Daltons)	Volume of Distribution (L/kg)
Drug A	Moderate	180	1
Drug B	High	1400	7
Drug C	High	250	0.3
Drug D	Low	300	2

A. Drug A.
B. Drug B.
C. Drug C.
D. Drug D.

handwritten annotation: - Water soluble - Low VD. molecular weight ≤ all drugs ≤ 20,000

5. An adult patient with stage 5 CKD who is receiving maintenance automated peritoneal dialysis is experiencing abdominal pain, fever, and cloudy dialysate bags. The nephrology team suspects peritonitis and wants to initiate empiric antibiotic therapy. Which is the best empiric antibiotic therapy for this patient?

A. Oral ciprofloxacin and metronidazole.
B. Intraperitoneal vancomycin alone.
C. Intravenous gentamicin alone.
D. Intraperitoneal cefazolin and ceftazidime.

handwritten annotation: gram ⊕ and gram ⊖ (pseudomonas)

Questions 6 and 7 pertain to the following case.
C.D. is a 54-year-old African American man who presents with diagnosed type 2 DM. His serum creatinine concentration (SCr) is 1.6 mg/dL, and a spot albumin to creatinine ratio (ACR) is 410 mg/g. His blood pressure is 145/89 mm Hg and A1C is 7.1%.

6. Which would provide the best therapeutic intervention at this time to slow diabetic kidney disease progression?

A. Metformin.
B. Lisinopril.
C. Metoprolol.
D. Amlodipine.

7. Which dietary intervention is best to reduce albuminuria in patients such as CD?

A. Protein-restricted diet.
B. Omega-3 fatty acid administration.
C. Low-carbohydrate (Atkins) diet.
D. Low-potassium diet.

8. A 76-year-old woman presents with an acute febrile illness that includes some diarrhea and generalized aches. She has been taking ibuprofen for pain for the past 48 hours and presents to the emergency department feeling "awful." Her laboratory tests and physical examination suggest she is not volume depleted. Her SCr has doubled since her past visit 1 year ago. Her physician believes she has acute kidney injury (AKI). A urinalysis does not reveal red blood cells (RBCs) or white blood cells (WBCs) or cellular casts. Which is the most likely diagnosis in this case?

A. Prerenal AKI.
B. Hemodynamically mediated AKI.
C. Intrinsic AKI.
D. Postrenal AKI.

handwritten annotations:

$$CC = \frac{SCa + 0.8(4 - a.5)}{}$$

$$CC = 10.7 + 0.8(4 - 4)$$

$$= 10.4 + 0.8$$

$$\frac{11.2}{}$$

prerenal - blood flow

NSAID - inhibit - vasodilatory prostaglandin in afferent artery

I. ACUTE KIDNEY INJURY (AKI) *(Domain 1: Patient-Centered Care: Ambulatory Care Pharmacotherapy and Domain 2: Patient-Centered Care: Collaboration and Patient Advocacy)*

A. Definitions and Background
   1. AKI is defined as an acute decrease in kidney function or glomerular filtration rate (GFR) over a period of hours, days, or even weeks and is associated with an accumulation of waste products and (usually) volume.
      a. Definitions vary. There have been recent efforts to standardize the criteria for AKI.
      b. Kidney Disease: Improving Global Outcomes (KDIGO 2012) diagnostic criteria must meet at least **one** of the following:
         i. Absolute increase in serum creatinine concentration (SCr) of at least 0.3 mg/dL within a 48-hour period
         ii. Increase in baseline SCr by at least 1.5 times
         iii. Urine output less than 0.5 mL/kg/hour for at least 6 hours
   2. Community-acquired AKI
      a. Low incidence in otherwise healthy patients
      b. Risk increases substantially among patients with CKD
      c. Usually has a very high survival rate
      d. Single insult to the kidney, often drug induced
      e. Often reversible, but may contribute to faster decline in function in patients with CKD
   3. Hospital-acquired AKI
      a. Has a moderate incidence and moderate survival rate
      b. Single or multifocal insults to the kidney
      c. Can still be reversible
      d. Intensive care unit–acquired AKI: It is estimated that up to 60% of patients in intensive care develop AKI during unit stay, and patients who develop this condition in the intensive care unit have a low survival rate (10%–30%).

B. Risk Factors Associated with AKI
   1. Preexisting CKD (estimated glomerular filtration rate [eGFR] less than 60 mL/minute/1.73 m^2
   2. Volume depletion (e.g., vomiting, diarrhea, poor fluid intake, fever, diuretic use)
   3. Effective (intravascular) volume depletion (e.g., congestive heart failure [CHF], liver disease with ascites)
   4. Use of nephrotoxic agents/medications: Intravenous radiographic contrast, aminoglycosides, amphotericin, nonsteroidal anti-inflammatory drugs (NSAIDs) and cyclooxygenase-2 (COX-2) inhibitors, angiotensin-converting enzyme inhibitors (ACEIs) and angiotensin II receptor blockers (ARBs), cyclosporine, and tacrolimus
   5. Obstruction of the urinary tract

C. Classifications of AKI
   1. Prerenal AKI
      a. Initially, the kidney is undamaged.
      b. Characterized by hypoperfusion to the kidney
         i. Systemic hypoperfusion: Hemorrhage, volume depletion, drugs, CHF
         ii. Isolated kidney hypoperfusion: Renal artery stenosis, emboli
      c. Urinalysis will initially be normal (no sediment) but urine will be concentrated.
      d. Physical examination: Hypotension, volume depletion

    2.   Functional (also called *hemodynamically mediated*) AKI—Often seen in ambulatory care; sometimes classified as prerenal

        a.   Similar to prerenal AKI, kidney is undamaged.

        b.   Caused by reduced glomerular hydrostatic pressure

        c.   Most often medication related (cyclosporine, ACEIs and ARBs, and NSAIDs)

        d.   Patients present with a concentrated urine and elevated SCr. Note that small increases (under 30%) in SCr are acceptable.

    3.   Intrinsic AKI

        a.   Kidney is damaged, and damage can be linked to structure involved: Small blood vessels, glomeruli, renal tubules, or interstitium.

        b.   Most common cause is acute tubular necrosis (ATN); other causes include acute interstitial nephritis, vasculitis, and acute glomerulonephritis.

        c.   Urinalysis will reflect damage; urine is generally not concentrated.

        d.   Physical examination: Normotensive, euvolemic, or hypervolemic depending on the cause. Check for signs of allergic reactions or embolic phenomenon.

        e.   History: Identifiable insult, drug use, infections

    4.   Postrenal AKI

        a.   Kidney is initially undamaged. Bladder outlet obstruction is the most common cause of postrenal AKI. Lower urinary tract obstruction may be caused by calculi. Ureteric obstructions may be caused by clots or intraluminal obstructions. Extrarenal compression can also cause postrenal disease. Increased intraluminal pressure upstream of the obstruction will result in damage if obstruction is not relieved.

        b.   Urinalysis may be nonspecific.

        c.   Physical examination: Distended bladder, enlarged prostate

        d.   History: Trauma, benign prostatic hypertrophy, cancers

D. Prevention of AKI

    1.   Avoid nephrotoxic drugs when possible.

    2.   Ensure adequate hydration unless otherwise contraindicated (e.g., CHF, liver cirrhosis).

    3.   Patient education

    4.   Drug therapies to decrease incidence of contrast-induced nephropathy—See Drug-Induced Kidney Damage section.

E. Treatment and Management of Established AKI

    1.   Prerenal azotemia: Correct primary hemodynamics.

        a.   Normal saline if volume depleted

        b.   Pressure management if needed

        c.   Blood products if needed

    2.   Functional AKI—Remove offending agent.

    3.   Intrinsic: No specific therapy universally effective

        a.   Eliminate the causative hemodynamic abnormality or toxin.

        b.   Avoid additional insults.

        c.   Fluid and electrolyte management to prevent volume depletion or overload and electrolyte imbalances

        d.   Medical therapy: Vasculitis may be treated on an outpatient basis.

    4.   Postrenal AKI: Relieve obstruction. Early diagnosis is important. Consult urology and/or radiology specialists.

II. DRUG-INDUCED KIDNEY DAMAGE *(Domain 1: Patient-Centered Care: Ambulatory Care Pharmacotherapy and Domain 2: Patient-Centered Care: Collaboration and Patient Advocacy)*

A. Introduction
1. Drugs are responsible for kidney damage through many mechanisms. Kidney damage can occur in both outpatient and inpatient settings. Evaluate potential drug-induced nephropathy on the basis of the period of ingestion, patient risk factors, and the propensity of the suspected agent to cause kidney damage.
2. Common risk factors
   a. History of CKD
   b. Increased age
   c. Other nephrotoxins

B. Hemodynamically Mediated (Functional) AKI
1. Caused by an abrupt decrease in intraglomerular pressure through the vasoconstriction of afferent arterioles or the vasodilation of efferent arterioles
2. ACEIs and ARBs
   a. Pathogenesis: Caused by vasodilation of the efferent arteriole. This leads to a decrease in glomerular hydrostatic pressure and a resultant decrease in GFR.
   b. Presentation: Note that a relatively small increase in SCr (less than 30%) is normal. Elevation usually occurs within 2–5 days and stabilizes within 2–3 weeks. Usually reversible on drug discontinuation
   c. Risk factors: Patients with bilateral (unilateral with a solitary kidney) renal artery stenosis, decreased effective kidney blood flow (CHF, cirrhosis), preexisting kidney disease, and volume depletion
   d. Prevention: Initiate therapy with low doses of short-acting agents and gradually titrate. Switch to long-acting agents once tolerance is established. Initially, monitor kidney function and SCr often: Daily for inpatients, weekly for outpatients. Avoid use of concomitant diuretics, if possible, during therapy initiation.
   e. Treatment: Discontinue agent.
3. Nonsteroidal anti-inflammatory drugs
   a. Pathogenesis: Vasodilatory prostaglandins help maintain glomerular hydrostatic pressure by afferent arteriolar dilation, especially in times of decreased kidney blood flow. Administering an NSAID in the setting of decreased kidney perfusion reduces this compensatory mechanism by decreasing the production of prostaglandins, resulting in afferent vasoconstriction and reduced glomerular blood flow.
   b. Presentation: Can occur within days of starting therapy. Patients generally have low urine volume and low urine sodium concentration. In addition, there are increases in blood urea nitrogen (BUN), SCr, potassium, edema, and weight.
   c. Risk factors: Preexisting kidney disease, systemic lupus erythematosus, high plasma renin activity (e.g., CHF, hepatic disease), diuretic therapy, atherosclerotic disease, and advanced age
   d. Prevention: Use therapies other than NSAIDs when appropriate (e.g., acetaminophen for osteoarthritis). Sulindac is a potent NSAID that may affect prostaglandin synthesis in the kidney to a lesser extent than other NSAIDs.
   e. Treatment: If NSAID-induced AKI is suspected, discontinue drug and provide supportive care. Recovery is usually rapid.

4. Cyclosporine and tacrolimus
   a. Pathogenesis: Causes vasoconstriction of afferent arterioles through possible increased activity of various vasoconstrictors (thromboxane A_2, endothelin, sympathetic nervous system) or decreased activity of vasodilators (nitric oxide, prostacyclin). Increased vasoconstriction from angiotensin II may also contribute.
   b. Presentation: Can occur within days of starting therapy. Patients often present with hypertension, hyperkalemia, and hypomagnesemia. A biopsy is often needed for kidney transplant patients to distinguish drug-induced nephrotoxicity from acute allograft rejection.
   c. Risk factors for toxicity: Increased age, high initial cyclosporine dose, kidney graft rejection, hypotension, infection, and concomitant nephrotoxins
   d. Prevention
      i. Monitor serum cyclosporine and tacrolimus concentrations closely.
      ii. Use lower doses in combination with other non-nephrotoxic immunosuppressants.
      iii. Calcium channel blockers may help antagonize the vasoconstrictor effects of cyclosporine by dilating afferent arterioles.
   e. Treatment: Lower dose and/or discontinue agent.

C. Intrinsic AKI
   1. ATN: Most common drug-induced kidney disease in the inpatient setting
      a. Aminoglycoside nephrotoxicity
      b. Radiographic contrast media nephrotoxicity related to intravenous contrast use. Prevention: Mainstay is hydration. Acetylcysteine is widely used and may be initiated on an outpatient basis. Other medications have been tried, but there are no well-documented outcomes.
      c. Cisplatin and carboplatin nephrotoxicity
      d. Amphotericin B nephrotoxicity
   2. Tubulointerstitial disease
      a. Involves the renal tubules and the surrounding interstitium
      b. Onset can be acute or chronic. Acute onset generally involves interstitial inflammatory cell infiltrates, rapid loss of kidney function, and systemic symptoms (i.e., fever and rash). Chronic onset shows interstitial fibrosis, slow decline in kidney function, and no systemic symptoms.
      c. Acute allergic interstitial nephritis
         i. Cause of up to 3% of all AKI cases. Caused by an allergic hypersensitivity reaction that affects the interstitium of the kidney
         ii. Many medications and medication classes can cause this type of kidney failure. The most commonly implicated are the β-lactams and the NSAIDs (although the presentations are different).
            (a) Penicillins: Classic presentation of acute allergic interstitial nephritis. Signs/symptoms occur about 1–2 weeks after therapy initiation and include fever, maculopapular rash, eosinophilia, pyuria, hematuria, and proteinuria. Eosinophiluria may also be present.
            (b) NSAIDs: Onset, much more delayed, typically begins about 6 months into therapy. Usually occurs in elderly patients receiving chronic NSAID therapy. Patients usually do not have systemic symptoms.
         iii. Kidney biopsy may be needed to confirm diagnosis.
         iv. Treatment includes discontinuing the offending agent and possibly initiating steroid therapy.

D. Chronic Interstitial Nephritis
1. Lithium
   a. Lithium: Develops insidiously over a period of years. Associated with elevated SCr, polydipsia, polyuria. Major risk factor is duration of therapy. Prevent by maintaining lithium concentrations as low as possible and avoiding dehydration. Symptoms may resolve with discontinuation.
   b. Cyclosporine: Presents later in therapy (about 6–12 months) than hemodynamically mediated toxicity. Progressive and often irreversible
2. Papillary necrosis
   a. Form of chronic interstitial nephritis affecting the papillae, causing necrosis of the collecting ducts. Associated with diabetes, sickle cell disease, and other conditions but most commonly associated with analgesic use
   b. Results from the long-term use of analgesics
      i. "Classic" example was with products that contained phenacetin.
      ii. Occurs more often with combination products (acetaminophen + NSAID)
      iii. Products containing caffeine may also pose an increased risk.
   c. Evolves slowly as time progresses
   d. Affects women more often than men
   e. Difficult to diagnose, and much controversy remains regarding risk, prevention, and cause

E. Postrenal (Obstructive) Nephropathy
1. Results from obstruction of urine flow after glomerular filtration
2. Renal tubular obstruction
   a. Caused by intratubular precipitation of tissue degradation products (uric acid, drug-induced rhabdomyolysis) or precipitation of drugs or their metabolites (sulfonamides, methotrexate, acyclovir, ascorbic acid)
   b. Prevention includes pretreatment hydration, maintenance of high urinary volume, and alkalinization of the urine.
3. Nephrolithiasis
   a. Usually does not affect GFR, so does not have the classic signs/symptoms of nephrotoxicity
   b. Some medications contribute to the formation of kidney stones: Triamterene, sulfadiazine, indinavir, and ephedrine derivatives.

F. Glomerular Disease
1. Proteinuria is the hallmark sign of glomerular disease and may occur with or without a decrease in GFR.
2. A few distinct drugs can cause glomerular disease:
   a. NSAIDs: Associated with acute allergic interstitial nephritis
   b. Heroin: Can be caused by direct toxicity or toxicity from additives or infection from injection, and end-stage renal disease (ESRD) develops in most cases.
   c. Parenteral gold: Results from immune complex formation along glomerular capillary loops

III. CKD – OVERVIEW *(Domain 1: Patient-Centered Care: Ambulatory Care Pharmacotherapy and Domain 2: Patient-Centered Care: Collaboration and Patient Advocacy)*

Patient Cases

Questions 1 and 2 pertain to the following case.

A 62-year-old man presents with a history of hypertension and newly diagnosed type 2 diabetes mellitus (DM). He reports occasional alcohol use and smokes 1 pack/day. His medications include hydrochlorothiazide and valsartan. At your pharmacy, his blood pressure (BP) is 130/80 mm Hg. A spot urine dipstick reveals albumin/creatinine ratio (ACR) 350 mg/g. A recent SCr is 2.3 mg/dL (SCr was 2.4 mg/dL 6 months ago). His eGFR is 29 mL/minute/1.73 m².

1. Which category best classifies the GFR for this patient?

    A. Stage G3a.
    B. Stage G3b.
    C. Stage G4.
    D. Stage G5.

2. Which best represents the albuminuria category for this patient?

    A. Category A1.
    B. Category A2.
    C. Category A3
    D. Category A4

3. A 72-year-old white woman (height 63 inches, weight 48 kg) (ideal body weight 52.4 kg) presents to the clinic. She is visibly small and frail. The SCr, unchanged from the past year, is 0.4 mg/dL. Which is the best method to assess kidney function in this patient?

    A. Cockcroft-Gault.
    B. Modification of Diet in Renal Disease (MDRD).
    C. Chronic Kidney Disease Epidemiology Collaboration (CKD-EPI).
    D. 24-Hour urine collection for creatinine clearance (CrCl).

A. Epidemiology, Definition, and Staging
    1. Prevalence: About 14% of the general population has CKD, and more than 660,000 individuals have ESRD. The incidence of ESRD cases in the United States has slightly declined in recent years, yet the prevalence continues to increase. Definition of CKD according to National Kidney Foundation Kidney Disease Outcomes Quality Initiative (KDOQI): Kidney damage for more than 3 months, as defined by structural or functional abnormality of the kidney, with or without decreased GFR, manifested by either pathologic abnormalities or markers of kidney damage, including abnormalities in the composition of blood or urine or abnormalities in imaging tests **or** GFR less than 60 mL/minute/1.73 m² for 3 months, with or without kidney damage
    2. Albuminuria: Marker of kidney damage suggesting increased glomerular permeability. Can be assessed by timed urine collection, dipsticks, or ACR in a spot urine sample (most common). Normal ACR is less than 10 mg/g.

3. Stages of CKD (KDIGO 2012)
   a. GFR (G-categories):
      i.   G1 – GFR greater than 90 mL/minute/1.73 m^2
      ii. G2 – GFR 60–89 mL/minute/1.73 m^2
      iii. G3a – GFR 45–59 mL/minute/1.73 m^2
      iv. G3b – GFR 30–44 mL/minute/1.73 m^2
      v.   G4 – GFR 15–29 mL/minute/1.73 m^2
      vi. G5 – GFR less than 15 mL/minute/1.73 m^2 or treatment by dialysis (5D if undergoing dialysis)
   b. Staging of albuminuria by ACR (A-categories). The absolute number of ACR is equivalent to the albumin excretion rate.
      i.   A1 – ACR less than 30 mg/g (normal to high normal)
      ii. A2 – ACR 30–300 mg/g (high)
      iii. A3 – ACR greater than 300 mg/g (very high)
4. Etiology
   a. Diabetes (~40% of new ESRD cases in the United States)
   b. Hypertension (~25% of new cases)
   c. Glomerulonephritis (~10%)
   d. Others

B. Risk Factors
   1. Susceptibility factors
      a. Associated with increased risk of CKD, but not proven to cause CKD
      b. Mostly unmodifiable
      c. Advanced age, reduced kidney mass, low birth weight, racial/ethnic minority, family history, low income or education, systemic inflammation, dyslipidemia
   2. Initiation factors
      a. Cause CKD
      b. May be modifiable
      c. Diabetes, hypertension, autoimmune disease, polycystic kidney diseases, nephrotoxic drugs
   3. Progression factors
      a. Result in faster decline in kidney function
      b. Modifiable
      c. Hyperglycemia, elevated BP, proteinuria, smoking

C. Assessment of Kidney Function
   1. Use GFR to approximate function of entire kidney.
   2. Ideal marker of GFR: Freely filtered, not secreted or reabsorbed
   3. Measurement of GFR: Insulin, iothalamate, and others. Not routinely used in clinical practice
   4. Serum creatinine and creatinine-based equations
      a. SCr derived from the metabolism of creatine in skeletal muscle and from dietary intake (meats, dietary supplements)
      b. Creatinine is freely filtered at the glomerulus, making it a good marker for kidney function; also undergoes some tubular secretion, so CrCl always overestimates GFR.
      c. SCr varies inversely with kidney function, and small changes in SCr represent more significant alterations in kidney function in patients with higher baseline function.
      d. SCr concentration depends on age, sex, weight, diet, and muscle mass, so avoid use as the sole assessment of kidney function. Certain medications (cimetidine, trimethoprim) interfere with renal tubular secretion and will raise SCr values without a change in GFR (clinically evident in patients with reduced kidney function).

e. Most laboratories now use "standardized" cases of creatinine traceable to isotope dilution mass spectrometry, which will decrease the variability in results between laboratories. The MDRD and CKD-EPI equations have been adjusted for this.

f. Measurement of CrCl by timed/24-hour urine collection

    i. Overestimates GFR by 10%–20% because of the tubular secretion of creatinine

    ii. Reserve for vegetarians, patients with low (or unusually high) muscle mass, patients with amputations, and patients needing dietary assessment, as well as when documenting need to start dialysis.

    iii. Urine collection will give a better estimate of CrCl in patients with very low muscle mass. Limited use because of the logistics of collecting urine and blood samples

g. Estimated CrCl (eCrCl) using the Cockcroft-Gault equation

    i. Original equation: $[(140 - \text{Age}) \times \text{Actual Body Weight}]/[\text{SCr} \times 72] \times (0.85 \text{ for women})$

    ii. Commonly used for drug dosing

    iii. Requires stable kidney function

    iv. Body size estimates

        (a) Actual/total body weight

        (b) Ideal body weight

        (c) Lean body weight

        (d) Adjusted body weight

    x. "Rounding up"

        (a) In frail/elderly patients with very low SCr, eCrCl will be falsely high (overestimated)

        (b) Rounding SCr to 1 in patients with low SCr may *underestimate* kidney function.

    xi. Cockcroft-Gault formula has not been revised to accommodate for standardized creatinine assays, which may result in a 10%–40% overestimation of CrCl.

h. Other creatinine-based equations

    i. Modification of Diet in Renal Disease

    (a) Estimates GFR in patients with CKD (mL/minute/1.73 m^2)

    (b) Abbreviated MDRD: Considers age, SCr, sex, and race (African American) in estimation equation

    ii. Chronic Kidney Disease Epidemiology Collaboration (CKD-EPI)

        (a) Relatively new formula to estimate GFR

        (b) More accurate than MDRD for patients with an eGFR greater than 60 mL/minute/1.73 m^2.

    iii. Schwartz equation – For children

    iv. Salazar-Corcoran equation – For obese patients; not widely used in clinical practice (most use Cockcroft-Gault formula with lean or adjusted body weight)

5. Cystatin-C

a. Endogenous substance less influenced by age, sex, and size

b. May be particularly useful in patients with alterations in creatinine production (e.g., the elderly).

c. CKD-EPI equations available, based on the following:

    i. Serum creatinine concentration

    ii. Cystatin C

    iii. Cystatin C + SCr

IV. CKD – MANAGEMENT *(Domain 1: Patient-Centered Care: Ambulatory Care Pharmacotherapy and Domain 2: Patient-Centered Care: Collaboration and Patient Advocacy)*

Patient Case

4. A 60-year-old Asian American man presents with a medical history of hypertension and newly diagnosed type 2 DM at the clinic. He reports neither alcohol consumption nor smoking. His only medication is atenolol 25 mg daily. At your pharmacy, his BP is 155/96 mm Hg and heart rate is 76 beats/minute. A 24-hour urine collection reveals 0.4 g of albumin. A recent SCr is 1.9 mg/dL. His eGFR is 37 mL/minute/1.73 m². Enalapril is added to this patient's regimen. Two weeks later, he presents back to his physician. His BP is 145/93 mm Hg. A repeated SCr measurement is 2.3 mg/dL, and his serum potassium is 5.2 mEq/L. Which is the best recommendation for this patient?

    A. Change enalapril to diltiazem (Cardizem CD). Monitor BP, SCr, and potassium concentration in 2 weeks.
    B. Add chlorthalidone 50 mg daily. Monitor BP, SCr, and potassium concentration in 2 weeks.
    C. Change enalapril to valsartan.
    D. Increase atenolol.

A. General Management of CKD
    1. Treatment of reversible causes of kidney failure
    2. Preventing or slowing the progression of kidney disease
    3. Treatment of the complications of kidney disease
    4. Adjusting drug dosages, when appropriate, for the eGFR level
    5. Identification and adequate preparation of the patient for whom renal replacement therapy will be required

B. Diabetic Nephropathy
    1. Pathogenesis
        a. Hypertension (systemic and intraglomerular)
        b. Glycosylation of glomerular proteins
        c. Genetic links
    2. Diagnosis
        a. Long history of diabetes
        b. Proteinuria
        c. Retinopathy (suggests microvascular disease)
    3. Monitoring
        a. Type 1—Begin annual monitoring for albuminuria 5 years after diagnosis.
        b. Type 2—Begin annual monitoring for proteinuria immediately (do not know how long patients have had DM).
    4. Management/slowing progression – KDOQI 2012 (DM), KDIGO 2012 (CKD, BP)
        a. Aggressive BP management
            i. In patients with diabetes and CKD with a urine albumin excretion rate of less than 30 mg/24 hours or an ACR less than 30 mg/g, the target BP is 140/90 mm Hg or less. If the urine albumin excretion rate is at least 30 mg/24 hours or ACR is at least 30 mg/g, the goal BP is 130/80 mm Hg or less (KDIGO). The Eight Joint National Committee (JNC 8) recommends a BP goal of less than 140/90 mm Hg.

    ii. ACEIs and ARBs are preferred when albuminuria is present (ACR at least 30 mg/g, even if the patient is normotensive).

        (a) Recommendation is to titrate to the maximal recommended dose (as tolerated).

        (b) Monitor serum creatinine and potassium values after 1 week for development of increased creatinine and hyperkalemia if using ACE inhibitors, ARBs, or diuretics.

        (c) Hold ACEI/ARB if serum potassium concentration is greater than 5.6 mEq/L or if rises in SCr are greater than 30% after initiation.

    iii. Most patients will also require a diuretic. (Thiazide in stages 1–3 and loop in stages 4–5). If BP is greater than 160/100 mm Hg, start with two-drug regimen. *< 30mL/min*

    iv. Calcium channel blockers (non-dihydropyridine) are second line to ACEIs/ARBs for proteinuria.

    v. According to JNC 8, ACEI and ARB combination is not recommended.

    vi. Dietary sodium consumption should be less than 2 g daily. Modify DASH (Dietary Approaches to Stop Hypertension) diet to limit potassium intake.

    vii. Spironolactone or eplerenone may reduce albuminuria but there is no meaningful clinical outcomes data.

    viii. Aliskirin added to ACEI or ARB may reduce proteinuria but data are limited and it is not recommended. (Per package insert – Contraindicated in patients with DM; warning to use combination, especially with CrCl below 60 mL/minute.)

  b. Blood glucose control: Glycosylated hemoglobin

    i. Target A1C: Approximately 7% for most patients

    ii. A1C less than 7% not recommended for patients at risk of hypoglycemia

    iii. Less aggressive with more advanced CKD/limited life expectancy/risk of hypoglycemia/comorbidities

  c. Protein restriction: There may be a modest reduction in the decline of GFR in patients with CKD with a diet of 0.6–0.8 g/kg/day of protein. KDIGO recommends target dietary protein intake of 0.8 g/kg/day in patients with CKD stages G4–G5; KDIG recommends avoidance of high-protein diets (above 1.3 g/kg/day) for patients with CKD (all stages). The American Diabetes Association does not recommend protein restriction.

C. Nondiabetic Nephropathy

  1. Manage hypertension.

    a. If urine albumin excretion rate is less than 30 mg/24 hours, maintain a BP of 140/90 mm Hg or less. If urine albumin excretion rate is at least 30 mg/24 hours, target BP of 130/80 mm Hg or less.

    b. If proteinuric and hypertensive, use an ACEI or an ARB. Often need to add (or start with) combination agents. Diuretic is usually the second drug. Monitor serum potassium concentration.

  2. Minimize protein in diet. Controversial. May slow progression according to MDRD study but may also impair nutrition. Very low protein diet may increase mortality.

D. Other Interventions

  1. Manage hyperlipidemia. There are conflicting data on the benefit of HMG CoA reductase inhibitor ("statin") therapy solely for renal protection. However, statin therapy has shown cardiovascular prevention benefit in patients with CKD who are not yet receiving dialysis (Lancet 2011;377:2181-92). A reasonable goal is a low-density lipoprotein cholesterol concentration less than 100 mg/dL. Do not initiate statin therapy for patients with diabetes who are treated by dialysis because of the lack of a cardiovascular benefit (4D and AURORA trials) (KDOQI diabetes guidelines 2012). The 2013 American College of Cardiology/American Heart Association (ACC/AHA) Guideline on Blood Cholesterol does not recommend the routine use of statins for patients undergoing hemodialysis.

2. Stop smoking.
3. Avoid nephrotoxins especially NSAIDs.
4. Maintain healthy diet, with moderate alcohol consumption.

V. COMPLICATIONS OF CKD (*Domain 1: Patient-Centered Care: Ambulatory Care Pharmacotherapy and Domain 2: Patient-Centered Care: Collaboration and Patient Advocacy*)

Patient Cases

Questions 5 and 6 pertain to the following case.

A 73-year-old man presents with a 20-year history of type 2 DM, CKD stage G5, and is not receiving dialysis. He presents with dyspnea on exertion and fatigue. His BP is 157/70 mm Hg. Fecal occult blood findings are negative. Medications include enalapril 10 mg daily, amlodipine 10 mg daily, rosuvastatin 10 mg daily, furosemide 40 mg daily, insulin glargine 12 units at bedtime, insulin aspart 4–6 units before meals and calcium acetate 667 mg three times daily with meals. His BUN and SCr values are 75 mg/dL and 6.5 mg/dL, respectively. One year ago, SCr was 4.9 mg/dL. Other pertinent laboratory values include serum potassium 6.2 mEq/L, CO_2 18 mEq/L, phosphorus 4.2 mg/dL, glucose 150 mg/dL, hemoglobin 8.9 g/dL, and eGFR 8 mL/minute/1.73 m². Serum ferritin is 259 ng/mL, serum iron 30 mcg/dL, and transferrin saturation (TSAT) 28%.

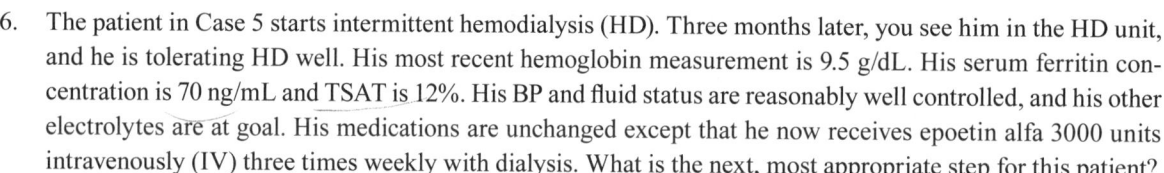

5. What is the most likely cause of anemia in this patient?
   - A. Absolute iron deficiency.
   - B. Dietary deficiency.
   - C. Epoetin (EPO) deficiency.
   - D. Enalapril.

6. The patient in Case 5 starts intermittent hemodialysis (HD). Three months later, you see him in the HD unit, and he is tolerating HD well. His most recent hemoglobin measurement is 9.5 g/dL. His serum ferritin concentration is 70 ng/mL and TSAT is 12%. His BP and fluid status are reasonably well controlled, and his other electrolytes are at goal. His medications are unchanged except that he now receives epoetin alfa 3000 units intravenously (IV) three times weekly with dialysis. What is the next, most appropriate step for this patient?
   - A. Add oral iron.
   - B. Add intravenous iron.
   - C. Increase the epoetin alfa dose.
   - D. Maintain therapy because the patient is at goal.

A. Uremia: Group of symptoms associated with CKD or AKI. Symptoms are caused by accumulation of nitrogenous waste products normally removed by the kidneys. Clinicians monitor BUN to assess presence of uremia, although urea is not likely the cause of uremic symptoms. Dialysis reduces the signs and symptoms of uremia by removing these waste products. Signs and symptoms of uremia include the following:
   1. Cardiovascular (CV)—Pericarditis, sodium and water retention, hyperlipidemia or dyslipidemia
   2. Gastrointestinal (GI)—Anorexia, taste changes, uremic fetor, constipation, nausea and vomiting
   3. Blood—Anemia, impaired platelet function
   4. Skin—Dry skin, uremic pruritus and uremic frost
   5. Restless legs syndrome, leg cramps
   6. Reduced reproductive function, erectile dysfunction
   7. Encephalopathy

B. Anemia (KDIGO 2012)
   1. Several factors are responsible for anemia in CKD: Decreased EPO production (most important), iron deficiency (very common), shorter life span of red blood cells (RBCs), blood loss during dialysis, GI blood loss, anemia of chronic disease, and renal osteodystrophy.
   2. Prevalence: Twenty-six percent of patients with a GFR greater than 60 mL/minute/1.73 m^2 have anemia versus 75% of patients with a GFR less than 15 mL/minute/1.73 m^2.
   3. Signs and symptoms—Similar to anemia associated with other causes. Anemia contributes to fatigue, cold intolerance, depression, reduced exercise capacity, dyspnea, and cardiac complications. Associated with increased morbidity and mortality, decreased quality of life, increased hospitalizations
   4. Testing for anemia
      a. For patients with CKD without anemia, measure hemoglobin concentrations when clinically indicated and at least annually in patients with CKD stage 3; twice yearly in patients with non-dialysis (ND) CKD stages 4–5; and at least every 3 months in patients with CKD stage 5D.
      b. For patients with CKD and anemia not being treated with an erythropoiesis-stimulating agent (ESA), measure hemoglobin concentration when clinically indicated—At least every 3 months in patients with ND CKD stages 3–5 and at least monthly in patients with CKD stage 5 HD.
   5. Diagnosis of anemia in adults and children older than 15 years who have CKD when the hemoglobin concentration is less than 13 g/dL in men and less than 12 g/dL in women
   6. Anemia workup: For patients with anemia and CKD, include the following in the initial evaluation of anemia:
      a. Complete blood cell count to include hemoglobin, RBC indices, white blood cell (WBC) counts with differential, and platelet count
      b. Reticulocyte count
      c. Serum ferritin (to measure stored iron)
      d. Serum TSAT calculated as iron/total iron-binding capacity to measure available iron
      e. Serum vitamin B$_{12}$ and folate
      f. Stool guaiac to rule out GI bleed
   7. Treatment—Treatment of anemia of CKD can decrease morbidity/mortality, reduce left ventricular hypertrophy, increase exercise tolerance, and improve quality of life. These benefits need to be weighed carefully with the risks of treatment, which generally consists of iron therapy (orally or IV) and ESAs. Most patients with CKD who are receiving EPO therapy require iron therapy to meet their needs (increased requirements, decreased oral absorption).
      a. Oral iron
         i. For patients with CKD, may consider a 1- to 3-month trial of oral iron
         ii. Not recommended for patients with CKD undergoing HD; however, it can be used for patients with CKD who are undergoing peritoneal dialysis (PD) and those not yet receiving dialysis.
         iii. 200-mg elemental iron per day is recommended (divided doses) if oral iron is used.
      b. Intravenous iron
         i. Use in patients with HD-dependent CKD and anemia (regardless of ESA use) if TSAT is below 30% and ferritin concentration is above 500 ng/mL. (For pediatric patients, administer iron when TSAT is 20% or less and ferritin concentration is 100 ng/mL or less.) (KDIGO 2012)
         ii. For adults with iron deficiency, an empiric cumulative or total dose of 1000 mg is usually given, and equations are rarely used. Maintenance therapy is often required. Dosing strategies vary but include weekly to monthly administration of intravenous iron.
         iii. Monitor TSAT and ferritin values as noted during EPO therapy.

    iv. Commercial intravenous iron preparations are available in the United States.
- (a) Iron dextran (InFeD, Dexferrum)
  - (1) Test dose required before starting therapy
  - (2) Black box warning (BBW): anaphylaxis
- (b) Sodium ferric gluconate (Ferrlecit, Sodium Ferric Gluconate Complex)
  - (1) Lower risk of anaphylaxis than with dextran, higher rate of free iron reactions (hypotension)
  - (2) Typical repletion doses 125 mg IV x 8 doses
- (c) Iron sucrose (Venofer)
  - (1) Lower risk of anaphylaxis than with dextran, higher rate of free iron reactions (hypotension)
  - (2) Typical repletion doses 100 mg IV x 10 doses (if on HD) or 200 mg x 5 doses
- (d) Ferumoxytol (Feraheme)
  - (1) BBW anaphylaxis
  - (2) No IV push per labeling changes in 2015 (initially FDA approved as 510-mg IV push over 17 seconds); now 510-mg IV infusion over 15 minutes with repeat in 3–8 days
- (e) Injectofer (Ferric Carboxymaltose)
  - (1) Not approved for patients on dialysis
  - (2) Infusion or slow IV push (100 mg/minute), up to 750 mg per dose

    v. Monitor for 60 minutes post infusion for serious adverse reactions. Highest risk with dextran formulations and ferumoxytol (BBW)

    vi. Avoid intravenous iron in patients with systemic infection (KDIGO 2012).

    vii. Intravenous irons are nonbiological complex drugs – Interchangeability concerns exist, because similar agents are not identical molecules.

c. ESAs: (Note: ESAs are under the FDA's Risk Evaluation and Mitigation Strategy [REMS] program.) Use REMS and modified dosing because of data showing increased risks of CV events with ESAs in patients with higher hemoglobin concentrations or at relatively rapid rises in hemoglobin concentration.

    i. ESA risks
- (a) The Normal Hematocrit Study evaluated the benefit of raising hemoglobin to target values of approximately 14 g/dL versus 10 g/dL using epoetin in patients with CV disease who are receiving hemodialysis. The study was stopped early: Higher mortality in group with higher-target hematocrit values (N Engl J Med 1998;339:584-90).
- (b) The CHOIR (Correction of Hemoglobin and Outcomes in Renal Insufficiency) trial enrolled ND-dependent patients with CKD and GFR 15–50 mL/minute/1.73 m^2. Study found that treatment to high hemoglobin concentrations (greater than 13 g/dL) using epoetin increases cardiovascular events (N Engl J Med 2006;355:2085-98).
- (c) The TREAT (Trial to Reduce Cardiovascular Events with Darbepoetin alfa Therapy) study failed to show a benefit in outcomes of death, CV event, or renal event but was associated with an increased risk of stroke in patients with ND CKD, diabetes, and moderate anemia (N Engl J Med 2009;361:2019-32).

    ii. Epoetin alfa (Epogen, Procrit)
- (a) Same molecular structure as human EPO (recombinant DNA technology)
- (b) Binds to and activates EPO receptor
- (c) Administered subcutaneously or intravenously

      iii. Darbepoetin alfa (Aranesp)

        (a) Molecular structure of human EPO has been modified from three N-linked carbohydrate chains to five N-linked carbohydrate chains; increased duration of activity

        (b) The advantage is less frequent dosing (FDA approved every 1–2 weeks, has been used monthly off-label).

        (c) Binds to and activates EPO receptor

        (d) May be administered subcutaneously or intravenously. Conversion (epoetin to darbepoetin) recommendations are widely available.

      iv. Methoxy polyethylene glycol–epoetin beta (Mircera)

        (a) Long-acting continuous erythropoietin receptor activator (CERA)

        (b) Initially approved by the FDA in 2007 but had not been marketed because of patent infringement issues. Genentech recently entered into an exclusive distribution agreement with Fresenius Medical Care (FMC) dialysis company to distribute. FMC is the largest dialysis company in the United States so the use of this drug will be widespread.

        (c) Same black box warnings as ESAs

        (d) Dosed every 2 weeks. Administered by using prefilled syringes

      v. Availability of biosimilar ESA's may be alternative to brand-name ESAs in the near future.

  d. KDIGO recommendations (2012) for ESAs

    i. For adult patients with ND CKD and hemoglobin concentration of 10 g/dL or greater, suggest that ESA therapy not be initiated. The decision to initiate ESAs with hemoglobin concentration of less than 10 g/dL should be individualized, and benefits should be weighed against risk.

    ii. For adult patients with CKD 5D, ESA therapy should be used to avoid hemoglobin concentrations of 9 g/dL by initiating an ESA when hemoglobin concentration is between 9 and 10 g/dL. The guidelines state that individualization is reasonable, and some patients may benefit from having ESAs initiated with hemoglobin concentration greater than 10 g/dL.

    iii. Recommend that ESAs not be used to maintain hemoglobin concentration above 11.5 g/dL; individualized patients may benefit from hemoglobin concentration less than 11.5 g/dL. The ESA should not be used to intentionally increase hemoglobin concentrations above 13 g/dL.

  e. Modified dosing recommendations of ESAs from the FDA (June 2011): For patients with CKD, consider initiating ESA treatment when the hemoglobin concentration is less than 10 g/dL; does not define how far below 10 g/dL and does not recommend a goal hemoglobin concentration. Individualize dosing, use the lowest dose of ESAs sufficient to reduce the need for RBC transfusions; adjust dosing as appropriate. Because of more recent studies and updated labeling information, most units use a goal of 10–11 g/dL.

  f. ESA dose adjustment is based on hemoglobin response.

    i. Adjustment variables are the same for epoetin alfa and darbepoetin alfa.

    ii. Upward dosage adjustments should not be made more often than every 4 weeks. Downward adjustment, at any time

    iii. In general, dose adjustments are made in 25% increments (i.e., dosages adjusted upward or downward by 25% according to current dose).

  g. ESA monitoring

    i. Monitor hemoglobin concentrations initially every 1–2 weeks and then every 2–4 weeks when stable.

    ii. Iron stores should be monitored every 1–3 months.

    iii. Monitor for adverse drug reactions such as hypertension (treat as necessary), pure red cell aplasia (rare), and allergic reactions.

Patient Case

7. A 60-year-old patient undergoing HD presents with a 10-year history of ESRD. His HD access is a left arteriovenous fistula. He has a history of hypertension, coronary artery disease, mild CHF, type 2 DM, and a seizure disorder. His medications are as follows: epoetin 14,000 units IV three times weekly at dialysis; a multivitamin (Nephrocaps) once daily; atorvastatin 20 mg daily; insulin glargine 8 units HS; calcium acetate two capsules three times daily with meals; phenytoin 300 mg daily; and intravenous iron sucrose 100 mg monthly. Laboratory values are as follows: hemoglobin 10.2 g/dL; intact parathyroid hormone (iPTH) 800 pg/mL; sodium 140 mEq/L; potassium 4.9 mEq/L; SCr 7.0 mg/dL; calcium 9 mg/dL; albumin 2.5 g/dL; and phosphorus 7.8 mg/dL. Serum ferritin is 300 ng/mL, and TSAT is 32%. The patient's RBC indices are normal. His WBC count is normal. He is afebrile. What is most likely contributing to relative epoetin resistance in this patient?

   A. Iron deficiency.
   B. Hyperparathyroidism.
   C. Phenytoin therapy.
   D. Infection.

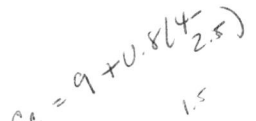

$$Ca = 9 + 0.8(4 - 2.5)$$
$$1.5$$

   h. Common causes of inadequate response to ESA therapy
      i. Before the widespread use of intravenous iron, iron deficiency was the most common cause of EPO resistance in patients undergoing dialysis. Iron deficiency is still quite common in patients with CKD.
      ii. Infection and inflammation are very common causes of EPO resistance, particularly in patients with CKD who are receiving dialysis. Associated with elevated values of hepcidin, which inhibits iron absorption in the GI tract and reduces iron release from the reticuloendothelial system
      iii. Other causes include chronic blood loss, renal bone disease/hyperparathyroidism, aluminum toxicity, folate or vitamin B_{12} deficiency, inadequate dialysis, hospitalization, autoimmune disease, malignancies, malnutrition, hemolysis, and vitamin C deficiency. Medications that cause anemia in other patient populations should also be considered.

Patient Case

8. A 45-year-old patient has hypertension, type 2 DM (diet controlled), and CKD (eGFR 40 mL/minute/1.73 m²). Medications include atenolol, valsartan, and hydrochlorothiazide. He has no health insurance. His most recent laboratory values were within limits except for serum phosphorus, which, for the second month in a row, was 5.1 mg/dL. Serum calcium concentration is 9.0 mg/dL, and iPTH concentration is 40 pg/mL. He tells you that he is following a low-salt, low-potassium, and low-phosphate diet. Which is the most appropriate intervention at this point?

   A. Add calcium carbonate with meals.
   B. Add calcium acetate with meals.
   C. Add sevelamer with meals.
   D. Add calcitriol.

C. CKD Mineral and Bone Disorders
  1. Chronic kidney disease–mineral and bone disorder (CKD-MBD) is a syndrome encompassing bone disease, mineral abnormalities and extraskeletal calcifications. Primary types of bone diseases include osteitis fibrosa cystica (from secondary hyperparathyroidism), adynamic bone disease (excessive suppression of parathyroid gland), osteomalacia (rare), and mixed disorder.
  2. Pathophysiology of secondary hyperparathyroidism and osteitis fibrosa: High-turnover bone disease caused by secondary hyperparathyroidism. Calcium and phosphorus homeostasis is complex, involving the interplay of hormones affecting the bone, GI tract, kidneys, and PTH. This process may begin as early GFR of 60 mL/minute/1.73m^2. The main abnormalities that contribute to hyperparathyroidism include the following:
      a. Phosphate retention: May be the most important cause of hyperparathyroidism. Hyperphosphatemia caused by decreased renal excretion of phosphorus. Hyperphosphatemia induces hypocalcemia, decreases formation of activated vitamin D, and increases *PTH* gene expression.
      b. Decreased free calcium concentrations
      c. Decreased 1,25-dihydroxyvitamin D values
      d. Reduced expression of vitamin D receptors and calcium-sensing receptors
      e. Fibroblast growth factor-23 (FGF-23) elevation. FGF-23 reduces renal phosphate reabsorption and increases urinary phosphate excretion in healthy individuals, so values are increased in CKD because of hyperphosphatemia. Contributes to decreased vitamin D synthesis
  3. Pathophysiology of adynamic bone disease is related to over-suppression of the parathyroid gland, most likely because of the excessive use of calcium-based phosphate binders and vitamin D products. Diabetes and increasing age are also risk factors.
  4. Prevalence
      a. Major cause of morbidity and mortality in patients undergoing dialysis
      b. Very common. Greater than 80% of patients with CKD stage 5 have secondary hyperparathyroidism.
  5. Signs and symptoms
      a. Insidious onset: Patients may experience fatigue and musculoskeletal and GI pain; calcification may be visible on radiography; bone pain and fractures can occur if progression is left untreated.
      b. Laboratory abnormalities
          i.   Phosphorus
          ii. Corrected calcium
          iii. Intact parathyroid hormone
  6. Treatment
      a. Therapy goals (KDIGO 2009)
          i.   Serum phosphorus: For patients with stage 3–5 CKD (not receiving dialysis), phosphorus should be maintained in the normal range. Among patients receiving dialysis, phosphorus should be lowered "toward the normal range."
          ii. Serum calcium: Concentrations in CKD 3–5, including for patients undergoing dialysis, should be maintained in the normal range. *Note: Serum calcium concentrations should be corrected for low serum albumin.
          iii. PTH: The optimal PTH concentration in patients with CKD (not receiving dialysis) is unknown. In patients with CKD 5D, PTH concentration should be maintained at 2–9 times the upper limit of normal.
      b. Nondrug therapy
          i.   Dietary phosphorus restriction 800–1200 mg daily in stage 3 CKD or higher
          ii. Dialysis removes various amounts of phosphorus, depending on treatment modalities, but, by itself, is insufficient to maintain phosphorus balances in most patients.
          iii. Parathyroidectomy—Reserved for patients with unresponsive hyperparathyroidism

c. Drug therapy
   i. Phosphate binders: Take with meals to bind phosphorus in the gut; products may be used together for additive effect.
      (a) Aluminum-containing phosphate binders (aluminum hydroxide): Effectively lower phosphorus concentrations. In general, avoid except for very short-term use (2–4 weeks) if serum phosphorus values are greater than 7 mg/dL (KDOQI guidelines). Avoided because of aluminum toxicity (adynamic bone disease, encephalopathy, and EPO resistance) and other effective options available.
      (b) Calcium-containing phosphate binders (calcium carbonate and calcium acetate)
         (1) Calcium carbonate is a widely used phosphate binder because of its low cost, efficacy, and multiple dosage forms.
         (2) Calcium acetate: 667-mg capsule contains 167 mg of elemental calcium. Better binder than carbonate, so less calcium given. Unlike calcium carbonate, soluble with achlorhydria. Liquid formulation also available.
         (3) Use of calcium salts may be limited by the development of hypercalcemia and overall positive calcium balance, which may increase the risk of vascular calcification and arterial disease. Particularly problematic when vitamin D analogs are used
         (4) To prevent positive calcium balance, recommendations now limit total elemental calcium intake to 2000 mg daily (e.g., 1500-mg binder; 500-mg diet).
      (c) Sevelamer: Nonabsorbable binding resin
         (1) Effectively binds phosphorus
         (2) As with calcium, considered primary therapy in stage 5 CKD. Sevelamer use is also suggested for patients with corrected calcium concentration greater than 9.5 mg/dL.
         (3) Decreases low-density lipoprotein cholesterol and increases high-density lipoprotein cholesterol
         (4) Available as sevelamer hydrochloride (Renagel tablet) and sevelamer carbonate (Renvela tablet and powder). Carbonate salt is the preferred agent because it provides a base load (carbonate). Worsening acidosis has been reported with the use of sevelamer HCl. May reduce absorption of quinolone antibiotics, levothyroxine, and mycophenolate – Separate dosing.
      (d) Lanthanum carbonate (Fosrenol)
         (1) As effective as aluminum in phosphate-binding capacity
         (2) Tasteless, chewable/crushable tablet
         (3) Indications basically the same as those for sevelamer
      (e) Sucroferric oxyhydroxide chewable tablets (Velphoro)
         (1) Iron-based (calcium-free); no iron absorption from gut
         (2) One tablet per meal as starting dose may be advantageous.
         (3) Must be chewed (not swallowed whole). Can crush (disadvantage)
         (4) Can cause black stools.
         (5) Potential iron-drug interactions with other orally administered drugs
      (f) Ferric citrate (Auryxia)
         (1) Iron based (calcium-free)
         (2) Iron is absorbed from gut: May require dosage reductions for intravenous iron; do not use in patients with iron overload.
         (3) Monitor ferritin and TSAT in addition to CKD-MBD laboratory test results.

(g) General

    (1) A recent meta-analysis revealed a 22% decrease in all-cause mortality among patients randomly assigned to receive non–calcium-based binders versus calcium-based binders.

    (2) Binders should be taken before meals. Between-meal calcium will result in more calcium absorption (which may be desired in some cases).

    (3) Avoid calcium binders for patients who have both hyperphosphatemia and hypercalcemia because of the risk of calcification. In addition, avoid for patients with low PTH concentration (adynamic bone disease).

    (4) May see calcium and sevelamer/lanthanum used in combination

    (5) Intensive dialysis may also reduce phosphate values. This would include daily dialysis and nocturnal dialysis, both of which are relatively uncommon in the United States.

ii. Vitamin D and vitamin D analogs: Suppress PTH synthesis and reduce PTH concentrations; therapy is limited by resultant hypercalcemia and hyperphosphatemia. Products include 25-hydroxyvitamin D (25-OH vitamin D) products (ergocalciferol and cholecalciferol) and 1,25-$(OH)_2$ vitamin D product and analogs (calcitriol, doxercalciferol, and paricalcitol).

    (a) Ergocalciferol: Recommended for CKD stages 3–5 in the presence of an elevated PTH concentration and documented vitamin D deficiency (25-hydroxyvitamin D concentration less than 30 ng/mL). Cholecalciferol has been used as well. Ergocalciferol is also being used for dialysis patients with a documented vitamin D deficiency (weak evidence).

    (b) Calcitriol (Calcijex, Rocaltrol): The pharmacologically active form of 1,25-dihydroxyvitamin D_3 is FDA approved for the management of hypocalcemia and the prevention and treatment of secondary hyperparathyroidism.

        (1) Oral and parenteral formulations

        (2) Does not require hepatic or renal activation

        (3) High incidence of hypercalcemia, limiting PTH suppression

        (4) Dose adjustment at 4-week intervals

    (c) Paricalcitol (Zemplar): Active vitamin D analog; FDA approved for the treatment and prevention of secondary hyperparathyroidism

        (1) Parenteral and oral formulations

        (2) Does not require hepatic or renal activation

        (3) Lower incidence of hypercalcemia than calcitriol (decreased mobilization of calcium from the bone and decreased absorption from the gut)

    (d) Doxercalciferol (Hectorol): Vitamin D analog; FDA approved for treatment and prevention of secondary hyperparathyroidism

        (1) Parenteral and oral formulations

        (2) Prodrug, requires hepatic activation; may have more physiologic values

        (3) Lower incidence of hypercalcemia than calcitriol (decreased mobilization of calcium from the bone and decreased absorption of calcium from the gut)

iii. Calcimimetic agent (cinacalcet HCl [Sensipar]): Attaches to the calcium receptor on the parathyroid gland and increases the sensitivity of receptors to serum calcium concentrations, thus reducing PTH values. Especially useful in patients with high calcium/phosphate concentrations and high PTH concentrations when vitamin D analogs cannot be used

    (a) The initial dose is 30 mg orally daily, irrespective of patient PTH concentration.

    (b) Monitor serum calcium concentration every 1–2 weeks (risk of hypocalcemia is about 5%); do not initiate therapy if serum calcium concentration is less than 8.4 mg/dL.

    (c) Lowers PTH, calcium, and phosphorus concentrations

    (d) Can be used in patients irrespective of phosphate binder or vitamin D analog use

    (e) Caution in patients with a seizure disorder (hypocalcemia may exacerbate)

(f) Adverse effects are nausea (30%) and diarrhea (20%).

(g) Cinacalcet inhibits cytochrome P450 (CYP) 2D6 metabolism, thereby inhibiting the metabolism of CYP2D6 substrates, such that dose reductions in drugs with narrow therapeutic indexes may be required (e.g., flecainide, tricyclic antidepressants, thioridazine).

(h) Cinacalcet is primarily metabolized by CYP3A, so drugs that are potent inhibitors of CYP3A (ketoconazole) may increase cinacalcet concentrations by up to 2-fold.

(i) Cinacalcet does not lower the risk of death or major cardiovascular events in patients with CKD undergoing hemodialysis (N Engl J Med 2012;367:2482-94).

D. Immunization: Vaccinations that may be needed include yearly influenza vaccine, pneumococcal vaccines (PCV13 and PPSV23), and hepatitis B vaccine.

VI. RENAL REPLACEMENT THERAPY (Domain 1: Patient-Centered Care: Ambulatory Care Pharmacotherapy and Domain 2: Patient-Centered Care: Collaboration and Patient Advocacy)

Patient Case

9. A 70-year-old man is being assessed for HD access. He has a history of DM and hypertension. Which dialysis access has the lowest rate of complications and the longest life span and is thus the best access to use?
   A. Subclavian catheter.
   B. Tenckhoff catheter.
   C. Arteriovenous graft.
   D. Arteriovenous fistula.

A. Indications for Renal Replacement Therapy

A – Acidosis (not responsive to bicarbonate)

E – Electrolyte abnormality (hyperkalemia; hyperphosphatemia)

I – Intoxication (boric acid; ethylene glycol; lithium; methanol; phenobarbital; salicylate; theophylline)

O – Fluid overload

U – Uremia (pericarditis and weight loss)

B. Two Primary Modes of Dialysis
   1. Hemodialysis—Most common modality
   2. Peritoneal dialysis

C. Hemodialysis: Most Common Form of HD in the United States: In-center intermittent HD (usually three times weekly). Home-based HD (daily and nocturnal) is also used – Less common.
   1. Vascular access
      a. Arteriovenous fistula—Preferred access!
         i. Natural, formed by anastomosis of artery and vein
         ii. Lowest incidence of infection and thrombosis, lowest cost, longest survival
         iii. Takes weeks/months to "mature"
      b. Arteriovenous graft
         i. Synthetic (polytetrafluoroethylene)
         ii. Often used for patients with vascular disease

    c. Central venous catheters
       i. Commonly used if permanent access unavailable or if dialysis is an emergency situation
      ii. Problems include high infection and thrombosis rates. Low blood flow leads to inadequate dialysis.
  2. Dialysis membranes
    a. Conventional—Not used much anymore. Small pores. Made of cuprophane
    b. High flux (large pores) and high efficiency (large surface area). Can remove drugs that were impermeable to standard membranes (e.g., vancomycin); large amount of fluid removal (ultrafiltrate)
  3. Adequacy
    a. Kt/V—Unitless variable. K = clearance, t = time on dialysis, and V = volume of distribution of urea. KDOQI set goal of 1.2 or more.
    b. Urea reduction ratio (URR)
     URR = [(PreBUN – PostBUN)/PreBUN] • 100%
  4. Common complications of HD
    a. Intradialytic
       i. Hypotension—Primarily related to fluid removal. Common in elderly people and in people with DM. Treatment: Limit fluid gains between sessions; give normal or hypertonic saline. Less well-studied agents include fludrocortisone, selective serotonin reuptake inhibitors, levocarnitine, and midodrine.
      ii. Cramps—Vitamin E 400 international units daily (oral) has shown some benefit. Quinine was used widely in the past but is no longer recommended.
     iii. Nausea/vomiting
     iv. Headache/chest pain/back pain
     v. Pruritus
     vi. Restless legs syndrome. Treating iron deficiency and optimizing dialysis may help. Pharmacologic treatment is similar to that in the general population.
    vii. Steal syndrome
    b. Vascular access complications—Most common with catheters
       i. Infection—*Staphylococcus aureus*. Need to treat aggressively. May need to remove catheter. Antimicrobial locks may be beneficial.
      ii. Thrombosis—Suspected with low blood flow. Antiplatelet treatment may protect fistula from thrombosis or loss of patency, but has little or no effect on graft patency. Increased risk of bleeding. Can treat with alteplase in catheter lumen
  5. Factors that affect the efficiency of HD
    a. Type of dialyzer used (changes in membrane surface area and pore size)
    b. Length of therapy
    c. Dialysis flow rate
    d. Blood flow rate

D. Peritoneal Dialysis
  1. The peritoneal membrane is 1–2 m² (approximates the body surface area) and consists of the vascular wall, the interstitium, the mesothelium, and the adjacent fluid films. Between 1.5 and 3 L of peritoneal dialysate may be instilled in the peritoneum (fill), allowed to dwell for a specified time, and then drained.
  2. Solutes and fluid diffuse across the peritoneal membrane. Glucose is the most commonly used osmotic agent in peritoneal dialysate. Glucose can be problematic in DM control, and it contributes to weight gain. Icodextrin (Extraneal) is a non-glucose, high-molecular-weight substance that can be used as an alternative for patients with diabetes. Of note, icodextrin can interfere with and cause falsely elevated glucose results, possibly leading to inappropriate therapy (specific glucometers must be used [www.glucosesafety.com]).

3. PD is usually not used to treat AKI in adults.
4. Types of PD
   a. Continuous ambulatory PD: Oldest form of PD; requires many manual changes throughout the day. Can be interruptive to daytime routine
   b. Automated PD: Many variants exist, but continuous cycling PD is the most common. Patient undergoes many exchanges during sleep by a cycling machine. May have one or two dwells during day. Minimizes potential contamination; lowest incidence of peritonitis
5. Peritonitis
   a. Infection of the peritoneal cavity. Patient technique and population variables influence the infection rate. Elderly patients or those with diabetes have a higher infection rate. Peritonitis is a primary cause of the failure of PD.
   b. Clinical presentation
      i. Patients undergoing PD who present with cloudy effluent should be presumed to have peritonitis. Usually accompanied by abdominal pain
      ii. This is confirmed by obtaining effluent cell count, WBC with differential, and culture.
   c. Treatment
      i. The most common gram-positive organisms include *Staphylococcus epidermis, S. aureus,* and *Streptococcus*. The most common gram-negative organisms include *Escherichia coli* and *Pseudomonas aeruginosa*.
      ii. The 2010 guidelines from the International Society of Peritoneal Dialysis state that empiric therapy must cover both gram-positive and gram-negative bacteria. Gram-positive organisms may be covered by vancomycin or a first-generation cephalosporin, and gram-negative organisms may be covered by a third-generation cephalosporin or aminoglycoside. Other combinations of medications have been studied and may be used according to local sensitivities. Intraperitoneal administration of antibiotics is preferred.
      iii. Adjust antimicrobials according to culture and sensitivities.

VII. DOSAGE ADJUSTMENTS IN KIDNEY DISEASE *(Domain 1: Patient-Centered Care: Ambulatory Care Pharmacotherapy and Domain 2: Patient-Centered Care: Collaboration and Patient Advocacy)*

Patient Case

10. A 40-year-old patient receiving hemodialysis has a history of grand mal seizures. He takes phenytoin 300 mg daily. His albumin concentration is 3.0 g/dL. His total phenytoin concentration is 5.0 mg/dL. Which is the best interpretation of this patient's phenytoin concentrations?

    A. The concentration is subtherapeutic, and a dose increase is warranted.
    B. The concentration is therapeutic, and no dosage adjustment is needed.
    C. The concentration is toxic, and a dose reduction is needed.
    D. The concentration result is uninterpretable.

A. Overview
   1. Dosing guidelines in package inserts are usually based on the Cockcroft-Gault equation, and most studies were done before the creatinine assay was standardized. Thus, there is controversy regarding which method (Cockcroft-Gault, MDRD) should be used when adjusting doses.
   2. The National Kidney Disease Education Program of the National Institutes of Health/National Institute of Diabetes and Digestive and Kidney Diseases suggests that either GFR or CrCl be used for drug dosing. If using GFR in very large or small patients, the GFR should be multiplied by the actual body surface area to obtain GFR in milliliters per minute (rarely done in practice).

B. Pharmacokinetic Principles Can Guide Therapy Adjustments

    1. Absorption—Oral absorption can be altered (more commonly decreased than increased).

        a. Nausea and vomiting

        b. Increased gastric pH (uremia)

        c. Edema

        d. Physical binding of drugs to phosphate binders

    2. Distribution

        a. Changes in concentrations in highly water-soluble drugs occur as extracellular fluid status changes (i.e., volume of distribution [Vd] is increased).

        b. Acidic and neutral protein-bound drugs are displaced by toxin buildup. Other mechanisms include conformational changes of the plasma protein–binding site.

        c. Phenytoin – Classical and clinically important example. The "normal" free fraction of phenytoin is 10%. Therapeutic range of phenytoin is 10–20 mg/L (1–2 mg/L free concentration). Free fraction can be as high as 25%–30% in patients with ESRD and hypoalbuminemia. So in a patient with ESRD with a free phenytoin concentration of 1.5 mg/L the laboratory may report a total phenytoin concentration of 6 mg/L. Incorrectly, some clinicians make dose adjustments to increase the total phenytoin concentration. Can assume a free faction of 25% with these patients when evaluating total phenytoin concentrations. Alternatively, may check a measured free phenytoin concentration

        Normal Concentration = [Observed Concentration in Patient with ESRD] ÷ [0.1 x Albumin + 0.1]

    3. Metabolism—Variable changes can occur with uremia. Metabolites can accumulate.

    4. Excretion—Decreased

C. General Recommendations

    1. Patient history and clinical data

    2. Estimate CrCl.

    3. Identify medications that require modification (Table 1).

    4. Monitor for efficacy and safety.

    5. Revise regimen as needed.

Table 1 . Dose Adjustments in Decreased Kidney Function

Agent	Dose Adjustment
Antimicrobials	Almost all antibiotics will require dosage adjustment (some exceptions include cloxacillin, clindamycin, linezolid, metronidazole, erythromycin, azithromycin) Antiretrovirals: Individualize therapy. Monitor CD4 counts, viral load, and adverse effects (agents requiring dose adjustment: Lamivudine, adefovir, didanosine, stavudine, tenofovir, zalcitabine, emtricitabine, and zidovudine) Others: Acyclovir, valacyclovir, foscarnet, fluconazole, amantadine
Cardiac medications	Atenolol, ACEIs, digoxin, nadolol, sotalol; avoid potassium-sparing diuretics if CrCl < 30 mL/minute, higher-dose loop diuretics needed as CrCl declines; avoid thiazides at CrCl < 30 mL/minute (controversial); dabigatran, enoxaparin
Lipid-lowering therapy	Clofibrate, fenofibrate, most statins (monitor adverse events)
Pain medications	Caution with codeine, morphine, and tramadol because of accumulation; other agents may also accumulate; avoid meperidine because of seizure risk

Table 1. Dose Adjustments in Decreased Kidney Function *(continued)*

Agent	Dose Adjustment
Antipsychotic/ antiepileptic agents	Chloral hydrate, gabapentin, pregabalin, lithium, paroxetine, primidone, topiramate, trazodone, vigabatrin
Hypoglycemic agents	Acarbose, chlorpropamide, glyburide, insulins, and metformin (risk of lactic acidosis); (insulin is commonly used in CKD; monitor blood glucose and adjust accordingly); SGLT2 inhibitors (ineffective); incretin mimetics; DPP4 inhibitors (exception liraglutide)
Miscellaneous	Allopurinol, colchicine, bisphosphonates, histamine-2 receptor antagonists, terbutaline; try to avoid all NSAIDs in CKD

ACEIs = angiotensin-converting enzyme inhibitors; CKD = chronic kidney disease; DPP4 = dipeptidyl peptidase-4; CrCl = creatinine clearance; NSAIDs = nonsteroidal anti-inflammatory drugs; SGLT2 = sodium glucose cotransporter 2

6. Identify or calculate drug doses individualized for the patient.
    a. Tertiary sources (e.g., Micromedex) are a good first place to look. Sometimes different sources have different recommendations so in critical medication issues, may need to be diligent.
    b. Published data or may need to call company for dosing information
7. Monitor patient (e.g., kidney function, clinical values, response and adverse events) and drug concentration (if applicable).
8. Revise regimen as appropriate.

D. Drug Dosing in HD
    1. Dosing changes for patients receiving HD may be necessary because of accumulation caused by kidney failure AND/OR because the procedure may remove the drug from the circulation.
    2. The following drug-related factors affect drug removal during dialysis:
        a. Molecular weight (MW)—With conventional dialysis membranes, larger-molecule drugs (greater than 500 Da MW) do not pass through the membranes; thus, they are not removed. With high-flux membranes, molecules of up to 20,000 Da MW are removed. So with high-flux HD, vancomycin (1480 Da MW) is removed. Because albumin has an MW of 50,000, it would not be removed by any type of hemodialysis membrane.
        b. Water solubility—Non–water-soluble drugs not likely removed
        c. Protein binding—Because albumin cannot pass through membranes, protein-bound drugs cannot pass either.
        d. Volume of distribution—Drugs with a small *Vd* (less than 1 L/kg) are present in the central circulation/compartment for removal. Drugs with large *Vd* (e.g., tricyclic antidepressants) are not effectively removed by dialysis.
    3. Dialysis procedure–related factors affecting drug removal
        a. Type of dialyzer—High flux widely used now
        b. Blood flow rate: Increased rates will increase delivery and maintain the gradient across membranes.
        c. Duration of dialysis session
        d. Dialysate flow rate: High flow rates will increase removal by maintaining the gradient across membranes.

VIII. KIDNEY STONES (NEPHROLITHIASIS) *(Domain 1: Patient-Centered Care: Ambulatory Care Pharmacotherapy and Domain 2: Patient-Centered Care: Collaboration and Patient Advocacy)*

A. Reported Annual Incidence: 100 per 100,000 men and 36 per 100,000 women; 12% of men and 5% of women will develop a symptomatic stone by age 70 years

B. Rates of Nephrolithiasis
    1. Prevalence is higher in men than in women and in white than in African American people.
    2. Recurrence rate is high after lithotripsy.

C. Eighty Percent of Stones Contain Calcium (oxalate most common, phosphate less common). Other stones are often caused by metabolic disorders; they contain uric acid, struvite (magnesium ammonium phosphate), cystine.

D. Prevention of Idiopathic Calcium Kidney Stones
    1. Low-calcium and low-oxalate diet—Reduces substrate to form the stone
    2. Hydration—Dilutes calcium so that stones are less likely to precipitate
    3. Potassium citrate—Citrate moiety combines with calcium in the urine, preventing the formation of crystals. Citrate also raises urinary pH, preventing uric acid or cystine kidney stones from forming.
    4. Thiazide diuretics—Reduce urinary calcium excretion
    5. Allopurinol—Reduces uric acid production but may also be useful in preventing the formation of some calcium-containing stones

E. Treatment of Existing Kidney Stones
    1. Guidelines published by the American Urological Association (www.auanet.org)
    2. Stones less than 5 mm likely to pass within 1 month; lithotripsy commonly used otherwise
    3. Pain can be severe. Treat with NSAIDs as medications of choice. Opioids for severe pain. Thiazides may be used to reduce stone formation in patients with hypercalciuria.

IX. ESRD PRACTICE MANAGEMENT *(Domain 4: Practice Models and Policy)*

A. Patients with ESRD Qualify for Medicare Benefits, Regardless of Age.
    1. Medicare Part A hospital
    2. Part B outpatient care (including dialysis)
    3. Part D (prescription drugs)
    4. Patients with ESRD not eligible for Part C unless they were enrolled before ESRD

B. ESRD Prospective Payment System (PPS, a.k.a. "the bundle"): Began January 1, 2011; bundled payment (includes dialysis treatment, laboratory tests, some medications) Parenteral medications related to ESRD (e.g., ESAs, IV irons, vitamin D analogs) AND oral medications with an IV equivalent (e.g., vitamin D analogs) included in the bundle. Eventually all ESRD medications to be included in the bundle (in 2024)

C. ESRD Quality Incentive Program (QIP): First federal pay-for-performance system. Initially only included dialysis adequacy and anemia management; now includes many measures (clinical and reporting measures)

D. ESRD Facilities Conditions for Coverage
   1. Explains requirements for CMS to pay for treatments at dialysis facilities
   2. Personnel: Medical director, nurse, dietitian, social worker mandated
   3. No requirement for pharmacists

E. Part D: Although Not Mandatory, 74% of ESRD Medicare Beneficiaries Enroll in a Medicare Part D prescription drug plan.
   1. Prescription drug coverage
      a. Some oral medications covered in the bundle (Part B) –for example, vitamin D analogs
      b. Some medications MAY be covered under Part B OR Part D, depending on indication (ESRD related or not); could lead to patient access problems if plan requires prior authorization for patients on dialysis.
         i. Antiemetics
         i. Anti-infectives
         ii. Antipruritics
         iii. Anxiolytics
         iv. Fluid management (for fluid overload)
         v. Pain management
         vi. Fluid and electrolyte management/volume expanders

   2. Medication Therapy Management (MTM) Services
      a. Criteria for high-risk beneficiary to qualify for MTM services – Varies by plan
         i. Number of medications: Set threshold at no more than 8.
         ii. Number of conditions: 2 or 3 disease states
         iii. Cost threshold
      b. ESRD is one of the core disease states plans may choose in development of MTM program.
   3. Comprehensive ESRD Care Model (ESCO)

REFERENCES

Acute Kidney Injury

1. Himmelfarb J, Ikizler TA. Acute kidney injury: changing lexicography, definitions, and epidemiology. Kidney Int 2007;71:971-6.

2. Kidney Disease: Improving Global Outcomes (KDIGO) Acute Kidney Injury Work Group. KDIGO clinical practice guideline for acute kidney injury. Kidney Int Suppl 2012;2:1-138.

Drug-Induced Kidney Damage

1. Alsady M, Baumgarten R, Deen PM, et al. Lithium in the kidney: friend and foe? J Am Soc Nephrol 2015 Nov 17. pii: ASN.2015080907. [Epub ahead of print]

2. Aurelio A, Durante A. Contrast-induced nephropathy in percutaneous coronary interventions: pathogenesis, risk factors, outcome, prevention and treatment. Cardiology 2014;128:62-72.

3. Besarab A, Bolton WK, Browne JK, et al. The effects of normal as compared with low hematocrit values in patients with cardiac disease who are receiving hemodialysis and epoetin. N Engl J Med 1998;339:584-90.

4. Elseviers MM, DeBroe ME. Analgesic nephropathy: is it caused by multi-analgesic abuse or single substance use? Drug Saf 1999;20:15-24.

5. McCullough PA. Contrast-induced acute kidney injury. J Am Coll Cardiol 2008;51:1419-28.

6. Naesens M, Kuypers DR, Sarwal M. Calcineurin inhibitor nephrotoxicity. Clin J Am Soc Nephrol 2009;4:481-508.

7. National Kidney Disease Education Program (NKDEP). Renal Hemodynamics Animation. Available at https://www.youtube.com/watch?v=J2YaULhMx5g. Published September 23, 2014. Accessed February 24, 2016.

8. Pannu N, Nadim MK. An overview of drug-induced acute kidney injury. Crit Care Med 2008;36:S216–23.

9. Perazella MA, Markowitz GS. Drug-induced acute interstitial nephritis. Nat Rev Nephrol 2010;6:461-70.

10. Whelton A. Nephrotoxicity of nonsteroidal anti-inflammatory drugs: physiologic foundations and clinical implications. Am J Med 1999;106(5B):13S-24S.

Chronic Kidney Disease

1. Aranesp (darbepoetin alfa) [package insert]. Thousand Oaks, CA: Amgen, July 2015.

2. Dexferrum (iron dextran) [package insert]. Shirley, NY: American Regent, April 2014.

3. Epogen (epoetin alfa) [package insert]. Thousand Oaks, CA: Amgen, June 2014.

4. Feraheme (ferumoxytol) [package insert]. Waltham, MA: AMAG, March 2015.

5. Food and Drug Administration (FDA). Biosimilars. Available at www.fda.gov/Drugs/DevelopmentApprovalProcess/HowDrugsareDevelopedandApproved/ApprovalApplications/TherapeuticBiologicApplications/Biosimilars/default.htm. Accessed February 24, 2016.

6. InFeD (iron dextran) [package insert]. Parsippany, NJ: Actavis, January 2014.

7. Injectafer (ferric carboxymaltose) [package insert]. Shirley, NY: American Regent, July 2013.

8. Kidney Disease: Improving Global Outcomes (KDIGO) Anemia Work Group. KDIGO clinical practice guideline for anemia in chronic kidney disease. Kidney Int Suppl 2012;2:279-335.

9. Kidney Disease: Improving Global Outcomes (KDIGO) Blood Pressure Work Group. KDIGO clinical practice guideline for the management of blood pressure in chronic kidney disease. Kidney Int Suppl 2012;2:337-414.

10. Kidney Disease: Improving Global Outcomes (KDIGO) CKD-MBD Work Group. KDIGO clinical practice guideline for the diagnosis, evaluation, prevention, and treatment of chronic kidney disease-mineral and bone disorder (CKD-MBD). Kidney Int 2009;76 (suppl 113):S1-130.

11. Mircera (methoxy polyethylene glycol-epoetin beta) [package insert]. South San Francisco, CA: Roche, August 2015.

12. National Kidney Foundation. KDOQI clinical practice guidelines for diabetes and CKD: 2012 update. Am J Kidney Dis 2012;60:850-86.

13. Pfeffer MA, Burdmann EA, Chen CY, et al. A trial of darbepoetin alfa in type 2 diabetes and chronic kidney disease. N Engl J Med 2009;361:2019-32.

14. Procrit (epoetin alfa) [package insert]. Thousand Oaks, CA: Amgen, December 2013.

15. Schellekens H, Stegemann S, Weinstein V, et al. How to regulate nonbiological complex drugs (NBCD) and their follow-on versions: points to consider. AAPS J. 2014;16:15-21.

16. Sensipar (cinacalcet) [package insert]. Thousand Oaks, CA: Amgen, November 2014.

17. Singh AK, Szczech L, Tang KL, et al. Correction of anemia with epoetin alfa in chronic kidney disease. N Engl J Med 2006;355:2085-98.

18. Wang C, Graham DJ, Kane RC, et al. Comparative risk of anaphylactic reactions associated with intravenous iron products. JAMA 2015;314:2062-8.

Renal Replacement Therapy

1. Li PK, Szeto CC, Piraino B, et al. Peritoneal dialysis-related infections recommendations: 2010 update. Perit Dial Int 2010;30:393-423.

2. National Kidney Foundation. KDOQI Clinical Practice Guidelines and Clinical Practice Recommendations for 2006 Updates: Hemodialysis Adequacy, Peritoneal Dialysis Adequacy and Vascular Access. Am J Kidney Dis 2006;48(suppl 1):S1-S322.

Drug Therapy Adjustment in CKD

1. Matzke GR, Arnoff GR, Atkinson AJ, et al. Drug dosing consideration in patients with acute and chronic kidney disease: a clinical update from Kidney Disease: Improving Global Outcomes (KDIGO). Kidney Int 2011;80:1122-3.

Nephrolithiasis

1. Goldfarb DS. In the clinic: nephrolithiasis. Ann Intern Med 2009;151:ITC2.

2. Worcester EM, Coe FL. Calcium kidney stones. N Engl J Med 2010;363:954-63.

ESRD Practice Management

1. Centers for Medicare & Medicaid Services. End-Stage Renal Disease Prospective Payment System; final rule. Regulation CMS-1418-F. Federal Register 2010;75:49029-214.

2. Centers for Medicare & Medicaid Services. End-Stage Renal Disease Quality Incentive Program; final rule. Regulation CMS-3206-F. Federal Register 2011;76:628-46.

3. Centers for Medicare & Medicaid Services. ESRD Quality Incentive Program. Available at https://www.cms.gov/medicare/quality-initiatives-patient-assessment-instruments/esrdqip/index.html. Accessed February 24, 2016.

4. Centers for Medicare & Medicaid Services. Medicare and Medicaid Programs; conditions for coverage for end-stage renal disease facilities; final rule (42 CFR 405, 410, 413, et al.). Federal Register 2008;73:20370-484.

5. Centers for Medicare & Medicaid Services. Medicare Coverage of Kidney Dialysis and Kidney Transplant Services; August 2015. Available at www.medicare.gov/Pubs/pdf/10128.pdf. Accessed month day, year.

6. Centers for Medicare & Medicaid Services. Medication Therapy Management. Available at https://www.cms.gov/medicare/prescription-drug-coverage/prescriptiondrugcovcontra/mtm.html. Accessed month day, year.

7. Pai AB, Cardone KE, Manley HJ, et al. Medication reconciliation and therapy management in dialysis-dependent patients: need for a systematic approach. Clin J Am Soc Nephrol 2013;8:1988-99.

8. Watnick S, Weiner DE, Shaffer R, et al.; Dialysis Advisory Group of the American Society of Nephrology. Comparing mandated health care reforms: the Affordable Care Act, accountable care organizations, and the Medicare ESRD program. Clin J Am Soc Nephrol 2012;7:1535-43.

ANSWERS AND EXPLANATIONS TO PATIENT CASES

1. Answer: C

The patient has stage G4 CKD (GFR 15–29 mL/minute/1.73 m²), which can be calculated by the MDRD or CKD-EPI equations, provided in the eGFR. The patient has had stable function for greater than 3 months.

2. Answer C

The patient has an ACR greater than 300 mg/g, classifying this patient's albuminuria as A3.

3. Answer: D

Clinicians should be aware that all creatinine-based equations to estimate kidney function will provide overestimations if the SCr is low because the patient has low muscle mass. Some clinicians "round up" the SCr in these patients to 0.8 or 1.0 mg/dL, but few data support this approach and rounding up can underestimate kidney function. If an accurate measure of kidney function is needed, a 24-hour urine collection for CrCl assessment should be ordered.

4. Answer: B

The patient's BP is not at goal (should be less than 130/80 mm Hg). To improve BP control and enhance the effect of the ACEI, chlorthalidone should be added to the regimen (Answer B). Adding chlorthalidone will also counter the tendency for hyperkalemia. Monitoring of SCr and serum potassium concentration is appropriate for this patient. There is less than a 30% increase in SCr, so enalapril should be continued, making Option A and Option C inappropriate. Increasing atenolol (Option D) would probably lower BP but is not the preferred route because renal protection would likely not be enhanced.

5. Answer: C

This patient has stage 5 CKD, so anemia caused by EPO deficiency should be high on the differential diagnosis (Answer C). Although iron deficiency (Option A) can be quite common in patients with CKD, this patient's iron study results are in the normal range. A dietary deficiency causing anemia (Option B) is usually linked to iron deficiency. Angiotensin-converting enzyme inhibitors (Option D) have been linked to epoetin resistance, but the effect is unlikely to be this dramatic.

6. Answer: B

From the laboratory values, this patient has iron deficiency, making Option D incorrect. Oral iron (Option A) is not recommended for patients undergoing dialysis because it is generally ineffective and has significant GI adverse effects and drug interactions. Increasing the epoetin dose (Option C) might increase the hemoglobin concentration, but excessive doses of epoetin would be needed, which would not be cost-effective. Intravenous iron (Answer B) should be administered.

7. Answer: B

Hyperparathyroidism is associated with epoetin resistance in patients receiving HD (Answer B). Although iron deficiency is the most common cause of epoetin resistance, the laboratory results for this patient do not indicate iron deficiency (Option A). Phenytoin therapy (Option C) has been associated with folate deficiency in other patient populations but is not likely the primary issue when receiving HD. Infection (Option D) and inflammation are very common causes of epoetin deficiency in patients undergoing HD, but there is nothing in this patient's presentation to suggest an infectious or inflammatory process.

8. Answer: A

This patient has hyperphosphatemia. Other than serum phosphorus, his laboratory values are normal. Because dietary restrictions of phosphorus have been insufficient, a phosphate binder is required. The medications in choices A, B, and C are all phosphate binders and would work. However, calcium acetate and sevelamer are very expensive (Option B and Option C), and this patient is without health insurance. Therefore, calcium carbonate (Answer A) is correct. Calcitriol (Option D) is sometimes used for patients with CKD to raise serum calcium concentration; however, this patient's calcium concentration is not low.

9. Answer: D

A native arteriovenous fistula is the preferred access for chronic HD (Answer D). If an arteriovenous fistula cannot be constructed, a synthetic arteriovenous graft (Option C) is considered second line. A subclavian catheter (Option A) is a poor choice because of the increased risk of infection and thrombosis and because of the poor blood flow obtained through a catheter. Catheter use should be limited to emergency and short-term situations as well as when all other access options have been exhausted. A Tenckhoff catheter (Option B) is incorrect because it is used for PD.

10. Answer: B

The presence of kidney failure and low albumin concentration results in an increased free fraction of phenytoin. Using the correction equation gives a corrected concentration of 12.5 mg/L, which is therapeutic (range 10–20 mg/L). A free phenytoin concentration can also be obtained.

ANSWERS AND EXPLANATIONS TO SELF-ASSESSMENT QUESTIONS

1. Answer: D

This patient's PTH, calcium, and phosphorus values are not at goal. Answer A is not the best choice because it would add more calcium load. Answer B similarly gives a calcium product to someone whose calcium concentration is too high already. Aluminum (Answer C) should be avoided in patients with CKD because of the risk of aluminum intoxication. Answer D, sevelamer, is the best choice because it lowers phosphorus while avoiding additional calcium administration. Sevelamer dosage may need to be adjusted to reduce phosphate concentrations to goal.

2. Answer: B

Cinacalcet is a good choice for this patient because both the high calcium and phosphorus values limit the use of vitamin D analogs. However, serum calcium values (Answer B) should be monitored closely because hypocalcemia can occur. Hypocalcemia may lead to seizures (most likely in patients with a history of them), and/or QT prolongation. Parathyroid hormone (Answer C) should also be monitored because its concentration should decrease, but this is a sign of efficacy. Liver function tests may be performed, but serious liver problems are rare. Creatinine need not be monitored in a patient already receiving dialysis.

3. Answer: A

This patient's anemia has worsened while receiving epoetin therapy, most likely because of iron deficiency. Answer A is a recommended iron-loading regimen. Patients undergoing dialysis universally require parenteral iron to maintain iron stores. Oral iron (Answer B) is not recommended in patients receiving HD. It is unlikely to provide sufficient iron to overcome the anemia and replenish body stores. Folic acid (Answer C) is already being administered to this patient with her renal multivitamin, and it does not address the primary problem of iron deficiency. Although increasing the epoetin dose (Answer D) might increase the patient's hemoglobin concentration minimally, it is not appropriate without first addressing the patient's iron deficiency. In addition, it will increase dialysis-related costs with very little benefit to the patient.

4. Answer: C

For a drug to be dialyzed, it should be water soluble, ruling out Answer A and Answer D. In addition, drugs with relatively large volumes of distribution (Answer B) are not effectively removed by dialysis because the drug is in the tissues. With high-flux membranes, molecules of up to 20,000 Da MW are removed, so MW is not an issue with any of these drugs. Consequently, drug C is most likely to be removed by dialysis.

5. Answer: D

This patient shows the classic signs and symptoms of PD-associated peritonitis. Immediate treatment is indicated. Empiric therapy must cover both gram-positive species (*Staphylococcus* spp. and *Streptococcus* spp.) and gram-negative species (including *Pseudomonas* spp.). Answer D is best at covering both, and the drugs are administered by the preferred, intraperitoneal route. Answer A uses oral medications and provides insufficient gram-positive coverage. In addition, the anaerobic coverage provided by metronidazole is not recommended for empiric treatment of PD-related peritonitis. Answer B provides only gram-positive coverage. Answer C is incorrect because it has inadequate gram-positive coverage and uses the intravenous route.

6. Answer: B

Although this patient might require treatment for hyperglycemia (Answer A), metformin is contraindicated in a man with a SCr greater than 1.5 mg/dL. The presence of albuminuria category A2 or greater indicates that an ACEI or ARB (Answer B) is beneficial to reduce intraglomerular pressure and slow kidney disease progression. Because this patient's BP is above goal, lowering it would be beneficial. However, neither metoprolol nor amlodipine (Answer C and Answer D) decrease proteinuria significantly.

7. Answer: A

Protein restriction (Answer A) to 0.8 g/kg/day or less will likely reduce albuminuria and is the best choice. Omega-3 fatty acids (Answer B) have not been studied in diabetic kidney disease. Atkins diet (Answer C) is not recommended because it tends to be a high-protein diet. Low-potassium diets (Answer D) would be appropriate for a patient with advanced kidney disease (not this patient) to prevent hyperkalemia but would not affect disease progression.

8. Answer: B

This is a fairly classic presentation of hemodynamically mediated AKI (Answer B). In this case, the NSAID is inhibiting vasodilating prostaglandins in the afferent arteriole. Prerenal kidney injury (Answer A) refers to abrupt changes in kidney function caused by low-flow states to the kidney (e.g., hypotension). Intrinsic AKI (Answer C) includes ATN and AIN. The presentation and a urinalysis confirming absence of cellular casts rule out this option. Postrenal failure (Answer D) is usually caused by obstruction, and there is no reason to suspect obstruction in this patient.

Bone/Joint and Rheumatology

Daniel S. Longyhore, Pharm.D., M.Ed., BCACP

Wilkes University
Wilkes-Barre, Pennsylvania

Bone/Joint and Rheumatology

Daniel S. Longyhore, Pharm.D., M.Ed., BCACP

Wilkes University
Wilkes-Barre, Pennsylvania

Learning Objectives

1. Systematically identify patients to screen for osteoporosis and use the screening results to guide the decision on how to treat the patient.
2. Use a STEPS-wise approach for comparing, recommending, and justifying a drug therapy regimen for osteoporosis.
3. Evaluate the severity and prognostic indicators of rheumatoid arthritis to choose the most appropriate initial regimen with disease-modifying antirheumatic drugs (DMARDs).
4. Identify appropriate health maintenance interventions when caring for a patient receiving biologic and nonbiologic DMARD therapy.
5. Select the most appropriate treatment regimen for psoriatic arthritis on the basis of patient limitations because of the disease.
6. Create an algorithm or a stepwise approach to minimize pain and maximize functionality in patients with osteoarthritis.
7. Choose a drug therapy for treating fibromyalgia syndrome, based on drug efficacy and a patient's comorbid conditions.
8. Select follow-up screenings or laboratory tests at correct intervals for patients with systemic lupus erythematous treated with hydroxychloroquine.
9. Formulate a care plan to help patients decrease their uric acid concentrations, gout symptoms, and gouty attacks by using nonpharmacologic and pharmacologic interventions.

Self-Assessment Questions

Answers and explanations to these questions can be found at the end of the chapter.

1. J.T. is a 68-year-old Cuban American woman returning to her primary care practitioner's office to review the results of her most recent dual-energy x-ray absorptiometry (DEXA) scan. Her physician reports that her L1–L4 T-score is −2.1 standard deviations (SDs) (Z-score: −1.1). The physician also reports that J.T. has a WHO (World Health Organization) Fracture Risk Assessment Tool (FRAX) score of 12% for major osteoporotic fracture and 4% for hip fracture. Which is the best action for J.T.'s physician to take in helping preserve her bone density?

   A. Start high-dose vitamin D (50,000 international units) weekly for 8 weeks and then 2000 units daily thereafter.
   B. Start calcium carbonate plus vitamin D (600 mg elemental plus 400 international units) twice daily.
   C. Start alendronate 35 mg weekly plus calcium/vitamin D supplementation.
   D. Start alendronate 70 mg weekly plus calcium/vitamin D supplementation.

2. M.Z. is a 71-year-old Hispanic woman, discharged from the local hospital 2 months ago after a right hip replacement secondary to a fall and fracture. She was prescribed alendronate 70 mg weekly, which she has been taking every Monday morning since discharge, as instructed. At this visit, she reports new symptoms of gastroesophageal reflux that persist for about 48 hours after each dose. Her provider confirmed that she was taking the drug properly, remaining upright for at least 30 minutes after each dose. She discontinues alendronate, and her symptoms subside. Which is the most appropriate way to continue treating M.Z.?

   A. Reinitiate alendronate 70 mg once weekly.
   B. Decrease alendronate to 35 mg once weekly.
   C. Start risedronate 35 mg once weekly.
   D. Start raloxifene 60 mg once daily.

3. C.A. is a 69-year-old woman with rheumatoid arthritis (RA). She is treated with oral methotrexate 15 mg once weekly, prednisone 10 mg once daily, and naproxen 500 mg twice daily as needed. On returning for a follow-up visit with her rheumatologist, she is instructed to continue prednisone 10 mg once daily for another 6 months. A recent DEXA report shows her lumbar spine T-score to be −0.6. According to the American College of Rheumatology (ACR), which approach is best to prevent osteoporosis?

   A. No intervention is required because the patient is premenopausal.
   B. Administer calcium carbonate 500 mg PLUS cholecalciferol 400 units twice daily.
   C. Administer risedronate 150 mg monthly PLUS calcium and cholecalciferol supplementation.
   D. Administer raloxifene 60 mg once daily PLUS calcium and cholecalciferol supplementation.

4. In which situation would the risk of an adverse event most outweigh the benefit of raloxifene to treat postmenopausal osteoporosis?

    A. 56-year-old woman with invasive breast cancer 3 years earlier.

    B. 62-year-old woman with lower extremity venous insufficiency and edema for 6 years.

    C. 58-year-old postmenopausal woman with an intact uterus and ovaries.

    D. 61-year-old woman with a history of an above-the-knee, idiopathic, deep venous thromboembolism 18 months earlier.

5. F.R. is a 62-year-old woman with RA. She is currently using etanercept 50 mg subcutaneously once weekly and ibuprofen 600 mg every 6 hours as needed for pain. At her latest visit to her primary care physician's office, she requested that her immunization history be reviewed and her immunizations be updated. If F.R. requires immunization today, which vaccine is *least* acceptable because of her RA therapy?

    A. Seasonal influenza vaccine (intramuscular).

    B. 23-Valent pneumococcal vaccine.

    C. Tetanus, diphtheria, pertussis (Tdap).

    D. Varicella zoster.

6. Which is the optimal time after diagnosis to start disease-modifying antirheumatic drug (DMARD) therapy?

    A. Less than 12 months.

    B. Less than 9 months.

    C. Less than 6 months.

    D. Less than 3 months.

7. Which agent for treating RA, although not free of risk, is most safe with respect to teratogenicity?

    A. Methotrexate.

    B. Leflunomide.

    C. Sulfasalazine.

    D. Minocycline.

8. G.S. is a 29-year-old unemployed and uninsured man (height 74 inches, weight 85 kg) with a diagnosis of RA and hypertension. His RA was diagnosed 7 months ago. Although he has been treated with methotrexate 20 mg orally once weekly for the past 5 months, he has not achieved low disease activity. His pain has been controlled with systemic corticosteroids and nonsteroidal anti-inflammatory drugs (NSAIDs), but he requires additional treatment. Before starting methotrexate, he was classified as having high disease activity and had many factors indicative of a poor prognosis. According to the ACR, which is the most appropriate next step for this therapy?

    A. Increase methotrexate weekly dose.

    B. Change to methotrexate injection.

    C. Recommend rituximab now, 2 weeks later, and then every 24 weeks

    D. Recommend rituximab now, 2 weeks later, and then every 24 weeks plus hydroxychloroquine daily.

9. J.P. is a 34-year-old man with a medical history significant for psoriasis. For the past 15 years, he has been treated successfully with hydrocortisone cream and moisturizers, rarely requiring oral systemic corticosteroids. Today, he presents to his primary care physician's office with a worsening joint pain in his hands and hips. He says the pain is minimal (2/10), but annoying. He has been receiving sufficient pain relief from naproxen 500 mg twice daily as needed, but he wonders if he could be doing more. His physician performs some radiographic evaluations and determines that J.P. has symptoms of psoriatic arthritis. Given the patient's presentation, which is the best regimen to treat his arthritic symptoms?

    A. Continue naproxen 500 mg twice daily as needed.

    B. Begin sulfasalazine 1000 mg three times daily.

    C. Begin etanercept 50 mcg twice weekly.

    D. Begin etanercept 50 mcg twice weekly plus sulfasalazine 1000 mg three times daily.

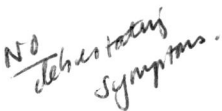

10. J.O. is a 76-year-old woman with bilateral knee osteoarthritis pain that has not been sufficiently controlled with physical therapy, simple analgesics, systemic NSAIDs, or a short trial of opioid combination analgesics. She is unable to perform many activities of daily living because she requires a walker, which considerably impairs her mobility. Which regimen is best to help alleviate the patient's chronic pain?

    A. Glucosamine 1500 mg and chondroitin 1200 mg/day.
    B. Topical diclofenac 1% gel.
    C. Ketorolac 10 mg every 6 hours.
    D. Morphine sulfate extended release 15 mg twice daily.

11. T.Q. is a 29-year-old nonobese woman being treated with hydroxychloroquine for systemic lupus erythematosus (SLE) for the past 3 years. Her current dose is 400 mg once daily (about 5.4 mg/kg). She is speaking with her pharmacist, who asks her whether she has been receiving regular ophthalmologic screenings for patients chronically treated with hydroxychloroquine. The patient reports that she has never had her eyes checked. Which would be the best recommendation for current and future ophthalmologic screening for this patient?

    A. Initial screening now and then every 5 years.
    B. Initial screening now and then annually thereafter.
    C. Initial screening now and then annually starting at year 5.
    D. Initial screening now and then every 6 months starting at year 5.

12. R.V. is a 42-year-old woman with a significant history of depression and schizophrenia. Her current drug regimen is ziprasidone 40 mg twice daily and selegiline transdermal 6 mg/24 hours. She has symptoms consistent with fibromyalgia syndrome, but she has been reluctant to start treatment until now because she was afraid it would interfere with her other mental health medications. However, the symptoms have worsened during the past 6 months, and now she is requesting to start therapy. Which medication would be the best for R.V. to begin taking?

    A. Nortriptyline 25 mg once daily in the evening.
    B. Gabapentin 100 mg twice daily.
    C. Pregabalin 75 mg twice daily.
    D. Duloxetine 60 mg once daily.

13. L.L. is a 58-year-old man with chronic tophaceous gout and chronic renal insufficiency (creatinine clearance [CrCl] 32 mL/minute). The patient has 10–12 alcoholic drinks a day and regularly consumes a large amount of meat proteins. In addition to dietary counseling, which therapy below is best to initiate to decrease tophi and prevent gouty attacks in this patient?

    A. No therapy required until he experiences two or more gouty attacks in a 12-month period.
    B. Administer allopurinol 100 mg once daily.
    C. Administer allopurinol 300 mg once daily.
    D. Administer colchicine 0.6 mg three times weekly.

I. EVIDENCE AT THE POINT-OF-CARE
(Domain 3, Task 1, Knowledge 1/2) (Domain 3, Task 3, Knowledge 2/3)

A. Pharmacists in an Ambulatory Care or Community Pharmacy setting are faced with needing to make informed decisions for patients in a relatively short period of time (to avoid delays and backups).
   1. Most clinicians will allow 60 seconds to search for an answer to a question before allowing the question to go unanswered.
   2. Clinicians will develop 1–2 patient care questions for every 2–3 patient encounters, but will only be able to answer 10%–20% of these questions.
   3. Pharmacists should have an information network in place that provides them with quick access to high-quality resources to quickly summarize information to answer patient care questions at the point-of-care.
   4. Extensive searches of databases such as the National Library of Medicine (PubMed) and reading full-text journal articles are important, but not feasible at the point-of-care.

B. Evaluating Point-of-Care Resources
   1. Professional treatment guidelines
      a. Usefulness determined by:
         i. Relevance: The applicability of the information in the guideline. The guideline should address the applicable
            population, outcomes that are important to the clinician and the patient, and information that influences how a condition is managed.
         ii. Validity: The quality of the information based on the justification of recommendations (strength of recommendations) and the quality of the evidence to support these recommendations (level of evidence).
         iii. Work: The speed and ease at which information is accessed for use at the point-of-care
      b. If a resource/guideline fails to meet an acceptable level for any of these three categories (practitioner-dependent), then consider the guideline as NOT good for use at the point-of-care.
   2. Hunting tools
      a. Online or print resources that allow providers to easily search out and access to information at the point-of-care.
      b. Usefulness determine by:
         i. Relevance: The database or print tool addresses patient conditions that are common in the pharmacist's area of practice (e.g., family medicine office, anticoagulation clinic, diabetes clinic, community pharmacy).
         ii. Validity: The database or tool describes the process for updating its information; to what extent it searched for new information, and the frequency at which it is updated. It also provides a key for determining the quality of the evidence and strength of recommendations it provides.
         iii. Work: The database or tool can be used quickly on a computer or through portable electronic device while caring for a patient.
         iv. If a tool fails to meet an acceptable level for any of these three categories (practitioner-dependent), then consider the guideline as NOT good for use at the point-of-care.
      c. Example hunting tools include the following:
         i. Ebscohost Dynamed
         ii. Up-to-Date
         iii. Essential Evidence Plus
         iv. The NNT

3. Foraging tools
   a. Online or print resources that act as an early alert system of useful information for practitioners, which may change their practice.
   b. Usefulness is determined by:
      i. Relevance: The early alert system addresses patient conditions that are common in the pharmacist's area of practice (e.g., internal medicine clinic, hypertension management, health screenings, community pharmacy programs).
      ii. Validity: The early alert system describes the process for searching and acquiring its information; to what extent it searched for new information, and the frequency at which it is updated. It also provides a key for determining the quality of the evidence it provides.
      iii. Work: The early alert system uses a notification and access system that providers can easily review and access to search for historical alerts.
      iv. If a tool fails to meet an acceptable level for any of these three categories (practitioner-dependent), then consider the guideline as NOT good for use at the point-of-care.
   c. Example foraging tools include the following:
      i. BMJ Evidence Updates
      ii. Essential Evidence Plus
      iii. NTK (Need to Know) Institute
      iv. Pharmacist's Letter
4. Worksheets for evaluating the usefulness of point-of-care tools are available at http://medicine.tufts.edu/Education/Academic-Departments/Clinical-Departments/Family-Medicine/Center-for-Information-Mastery.

II. OSTEOPOROSIS

A. Clinical Guidelines *(Domain 1; Tasks 3, 6, 7; Knowledge 2/1/2)*
   1. 2011 U.S. Preventive Services Task Force (USPSTF)
   2. 2014 National Osteoporosis Foundation (NOF)
   3. 2010 American College of Rheumatology (ACR) (glucocorticoid-induced osteoporosis)
   4. 2013 National Institute for Health and Care Excellence (NICE)

Table 1. Factors Associated with Decreased BMD and/or Osteoporotic Fractures

Age	Women > 65 years Men > 70 years	
Hormone deficiency	Estrogen deficiency in women Androgen deficiency in men	
Body habitus	Decreased BMI Calorie-restricted weight loss	
Social history	Smoking Alcohol use (>2 drinks per day) 120 mL of wine, 30 mL of liquor, 260 mL of beer High caffeine intake	
Medical history	Rheumatoid arthritis Cardiovascular disease Type 2 diabetes mellitus Celiac disease	Asthma/COPD Autoimmune disorders Hepatic disease History of falls
Drug-induced causes	Antiepileptic agents Immunosuppressants Lithium Proton pump inhibitors Systemic corticosteroids (>5 mg daily of prednisone or equivalent for 3 months or more) Selective serotonin reuptake inhibitors Excessive thyroid hormone supplementation Tricyclic antidepressants Warfarin or heparin (long-term use)	

Sex-specific factors	Women
	  Anorexia nervosa
	  Medroxyprogesterone depot use
	  Excessive vitamin A intake
	  Gastrointestinal malabsorption syndromes
	  Parental history of osteoporosis
	Men
	  Loop diuretic use
	  Gonadotropin-releasing hormone agonists (prostate cancer)
	  Psoriasis	

BMD = bone mineral density; BMI = body mass index; COPD = chronic obstructive pulmonary disease.

Abbreviated from: Cosman F, de Beur SJ, LeBoff MS, et al. Clinician's guide to preventions and treatment of osteoporosis. Osteoporosis Int 2014;25:2359-81.

Patient Case

1. F.R. is a 74-year-old woman with a history of a right hip replacement after a fall and fracture. In addition to her hip fracture, she has a history of type 2 diabetes mellitus (most recent hemoglobin A1C reading 7.3%) and hypothyroidism (current thyroid-stimulating hormone concentration [TSH] 0.1 mIU/L), for which she receives treatment. A dual-energy x-ray absorptiometry (DEXA) finding revealed F.R.'s T-score at her femoral neck to be −2.7. The Z-score associated with her femoral neck T-score was −2.1. Her physician believes this was a fracture secondary to drug-induced bone density loss. Which medication most likely contributed to her bone mineral density (BMD) loss and fracture?

   A. Metformin.
   B. Glipizide.
   C. Levothyroxine.
   D. Lovastatin.

Table 2. Fracture Prevention Counseling (all individuals older than 50 years) *(Domain 1, Task 1, Knowledge 1)* *(Domain 1, Task 6, Knowledge 3)*

Calcium intake	*NOF*: Calcium 1000–1200 mg (elemental)/day from diet or supplementation *USPSTF*: 1000 mg (elemental)/day from diet or supplementation Milk, nonfat (1 cup): 300 mg Orange juice, fortified: 350 mg Cereal, fortified: 20–400 mg/serving Cheese (1 oz): 150–300 mg/serving
Vitamin D intake	*NOF*: 800 to 1000 units/day *USPSTF*: 400 units/day Cereals, fortified: 40 units Milk, nonfat (1 cup): 100 units Salmon (3 oz): 530 units Sunlight exposure (bare arms and legs for 15 minutes/day)
Exercise and physical activity	Walking Aerobics (low impact) Strength training
Social habit changes	Smoking cessation/avoidance Limited to moderate alcohol intake (<2 drinks/day) 120 mL of wine, 30 mL of liquor, or 260 mL of beer

NOF = National Osteoporosis Foundation; USPSTF = United States Preventive Services Task Force.

Table 3. Screening Recommendations *(Domain 5, Task 2, Knowledge 1)*

National Osteoporosis Foundation (2014)	U.S. Preventive Services Task Force (2011)	American Association of Clinical Endocrinologists (2010)

Women:
 	
BMD testing
  >65 years
  Postmenopausal (age 50–69 years) with clinical risk factors
Vertebral imaging
  Age >70 years if BMD at any location is greater than −1 SD
  Age 65–69 years if BMD at any location is greater than −1.5 SD
  Postmenopausal woman: Age > 50 years with risk factors (low BMI, previous low-trauma fracture, high-risk medication use, height loss)
	Women:
	≥65 years without known fractures or secondary causes of osteoporosis
	Age 50–65 years with 10-year major osteoporotic risk (FRAX)
	> 9.3%
		Women:
		≥65 years
		≤65 years at an increased risk of fracture, based on risk factors

Men:
BMD testing
  >70 years
  Age 50–69 years with clinical risk factors
Vertebral imaging
  Age >80 years if BMD at any location is greater than −1 SD
  Age 70–79 if BMD at any location is greater than −1.5 SD
  Men: Age >50 years with risk factors (low BMI, previous low-trauma fracture, high-risk medication use, height loss)
	Men:
	No recommendation
		Men:
		No recommendation

Any adult: Fracture after age 50 years Condition associated with bone loss		

BMD = bone mineral density; BMI = body mass index; FRAX = Fracture Risk Assessment Tool; SD = standard deviation.

Table 4. Fracture Risk Assessment Tools *(Domain 1; Tasks 2, 3; Knowledge 1)*

WHO FRAX	Available online at www.sheffield.ac.uk/FRAX
	Developed to assess a 10-year probability for hip or other major osteoporotic fracture
	For screening, results may be used to identify patients who require diagnostic evaluation with a DEXA scan, but it is not a definitive tool for deciding to treat a patient
	For treatment, results may be used to determine whether patients with osteopenia require pharmacologic treatment (see Figure 1)
ClinRisk QFracture	Available at http://qfracture.org
	Developed by ClinRisk Ltd. to assess the 10-year risk of developing an osteoporosis-related fracture in patients from the United Kingdom
	Consider diagnostic evaluation with a DEXA scan in the following situations:
	Women's 10-year risk calculated to be ≥8.75%
	Men's 10-year risk calculated to be ≥2.11%
Peripheral (Calcaneal) DEXA	Useful tool found in many community screenings
	This method of screening/assessment is useful for identifying individuals with a low BMD, but it should not be used as a diagnostic tool to quantify the severity of bone loss
	Pharmacies using this form of outpatient DEXA should develop a policy and/or protocol for referral of patients to a physician if the test results are abnormal and require additional investigation

BMD = bone mineral density; DEXA = dual-energy x-ray absorptiometry; FRAX = Fracture Risk Assessment Tool; WHO = World Health Organization.

B. Diagnostic Criteria
1. Dual-energy x-ray absorptiometry
   a. Definitions
      i. T-score: Reports how many standard deviations (SDs) separate a patient's BMD compared with the BMD of a young, healthy adult of the same sex
      ii. Z-score: Reports how many SDs separate a patient's BMD compared with the BMD of another patient matched for age, sex, and ethnicity
   b. Measures the lumbar spine (1–4) and femoral neck of nondominant hip
   c. T-scores are based on the mean BMD for a healthy young man or woman.
      i. "Normal": 0–1 SDs below the mean value
      ii. Osteopenia: 1–2.5 SDs below the mean value
      iii. Osteoporosis: Greater than 2.5 SDs below the mean value
   d. The lumbar spine T-score is reported as the average of L1–L4. Consider a diagnosis of osteoporosis if two individual lumbar spine measurements are greater than 2.5 SDs below the mean, regardless of the lumbar spine average.
   e. If a patient's Z-scores are greater than 2 SDs below the mean, the result is usually indicative of accelerated bone loss unrelated to menopause and/or aging.
2. Quantitative ultrasonography
   a. Does not measure BMD, but assesses fracture risk by using speed of sound and broadband ultrasound attenuation
   b. Not associated with radiation exposure
3. Quantitative computed tomography: Able to predict fracture risk, but with greater radiation exposure than DEXA

Table 5. Additional Tests to Consider When Evaluating for Secondary Causes of Osteoporosis

25-Hydroxy-vitamin D	Alkaline phosphatase	Calcium, serum
Creatinine	Phosphate	Thyroid-stimulating hormone
Estradiol	Free testosterone	PTH (PTH intact)
Serum protein electrophoresis		

PTH = parathyroid hormone.

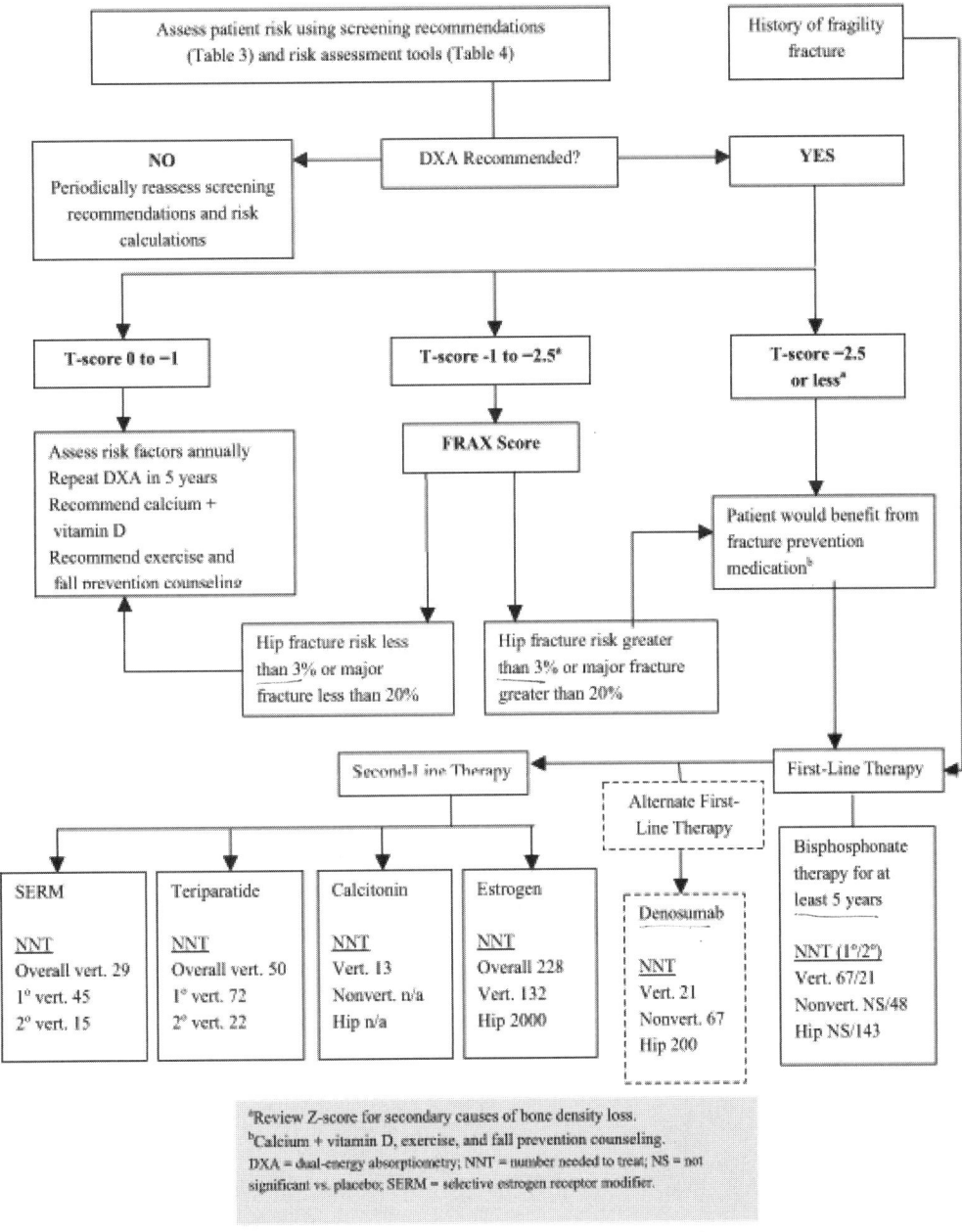

Figure 1. Osteoporosis evaluation and treatment algorithm.

Patient Cases

2. M.J. is a 71-year-old white woman consulting with her pharmacist about the best means to preserve her bone density and prevent a fracture. During the consultation, the pharmacist uses the Fracture Risk Assessment Tool (FRAX) to determine the patient's 10-year risk of a fracture. The patient weighs 68 kg (150 lb) and is 65 inches tall; her medical history is significant for a maternal hip fracture (age 71 years). Her 10-year risk of a major osteoporotic fracture is estimated at 19% and, for the hip, 6.3%. From these results, which is the best course of action for the pharmacist to take?

    A. Recommend that the patient contact her primary care provider to request a DEXA scan.

    B. Recommend that the patient contact her primary care provider to request a DEXA scan and start calcium plus vitamin D supplementation.

    C. Recommend that the patient contact her primary care provider to request a DEXA scan, start calcium plus vitamin D supplementation, and start taking a bisphosphonate.

    D. Recommend that the patient NOT have a DEXA scan and that she begin calcium plus vitamin D supplementation and start taking a bisphosphonate.

3. O.T. is a 65-year-old woman given a diagnosis of osteopenia after a scheduled DEXA scan. Her other medical conditions include type 2 diabetes mellitus, irritable bowel syndrome, gastroesophageal reflux disease, and migraine headaches. Her medications include metformin, pantoprazole, amitriptyline, and sumatriptan. She is an active woman who regularly participates in aqua aerobics and walking, and she uses laundry detergent bottles to strengthen her upper body. Her dietary calcium intake is limited to one glass of milk (8 oz each) per day. She has not yet started calcium, but she would like to add it to her medications and daily supplements. Which over-the-counter calcium regimen is best to recommend for her?

    A. Calcium carbonate 600 mg one tablet twice daily with food.

    B. Calcium carbonate 600 mg two tablets twice daily with food.

    C. Calcium citrate 315 mg one tablet twice daily.

    D. Calcium citrate 315 mg two tablets twice daily.

4. E.U. is a 58-year-old woman with a medical history significant for primary progressive multiple sclerosis with severe limitation, for which she spends most of her time in bed or lying on a couch. She attempts to ambulate but is unable to do so without a walker and/or assistance. Her DEXA scan results show that she has osteoporosis of the lumbar spine, and she now requires treatment. She already takes 1200 mg of calcium carbonate daily (600 mg twice daily) and 800 units of vitamin D (400 units twice daily). Which agent is best for E.U. to prevent vertebral fracture?

    A. Zoledronic acid 5-mg infusion once yearly.

    B. Risedronate 150-mg tablet once monthly.

    C. Raloxifene 60-mg tablet once daily.

    D. Calcitonin nasal spray, 1 spray per nostril each day.

Table 6. Nonpharmacologic Interventions[a]

Dietary Changes	Physical Activity	Other Interventions

Adequate intake of calcium-containing foods
Adequate intake of vitamin D and exposure to sunlight
	Aerobic exercise
	  Low impact
	  Weight bearing
	  Muscle strengthening
	  Balance training
		Fall assessments
		  TUG
		Vision correction
		Medication review
		Fall prevention counseling
		Smoking cessation

[a]See Table 2.

TUG = Timed Up and Go.

    C.   Pharmacologic Interventions *(Domain 1, Task 2, Knowledge 5) (Domain 1, Task 3, Knowledge 7)*
        1.   Calcium supplementation: Available formulations (be aware of whether calcium supplement labels list calcium content as elemental or compound)
            a.   Calcium carbonate (40% elemental)
            b.   Calcium citrate (21% elemental)

Table 7. Calcium STEPS Analysis

Safety	May increase in risk of myocardial infarction Nephrolithiasis risk slightly increased with calcium carbonate Hypercalcemia in patients with later-stage chronic kidney disease
Tolerability	Constipation GI discomfort
Efficacy	Improves and/or sustains bone mineral density With or without vitamin D, evidence that calcium supplementation reduces fracture risk is not robust; some isolated studies show benefit, but systematic reviews and meta-analyses do not agree whether there is a significant impact

Preference (Pearls)	Calcium citrate preferred in following instances:
	  Chronic gastric acid-suppressive therapy
	  Intolerance of calcium carbonate formulations
	Should be used (at a minimum) in patients receiving chronic systemic corticosteroid therapy
	Should be administered with an appropriate dose of vitamin D

Simplicity	Various formulations available to meet the needs of patients:
	  Tablets (varying sizes)
	  Chewable tablets
	  Soft chews and "gummy" formulations
	  Liquid

GI = gastrointestinal; STEPS = Safety, Tolerability, Efficacy, Preference (Pearls), Simplicity.

2. Vitamin D: Available formulations
   a. Vitamin D$_2$ (ergocalciferol)
   b. Vitamin D$_3$ (cholecalciferol)

Table 8. Vitamin D STEPS

Safety	Annual dosing alternatives (500,000 units) may result in higher rates of falls and fractures in older patients
Tolerability	Hypercalcemia Constipation
Efficacy	Increases BMD May reduce risk of falls in elderly population with low serum vitamin D concentrations
Preference (Pearls)	Unclear whether vitamin D without calcium is effective for improvement in bone mineral density or fracture prevention In elderly patients with low vitamin D concentrations, daily administration of vitamin D may be associated with a reduced fall risk
Simplicity	Coformulated with calcium supplements (200–400 units per dose) Administered daily as 400- to 1000-unit tablets/capsules Option for quarterly dosing (100,000 units every 3 months) is available

BMD = bone mineral density; STEPS = Safety, Tolerability, Efficacy, Preference (Pearls), Simplicity.

3. Bisphosphonates: Available agents
   a. Alendronate (Fosamax)
   b. Ibandronate (Boniva)
   c. Risedronate (Actonel, Atelvia [delayed release])
   d. Zoledronic acid (Reclast)

Table 9. Bisphosphonates STEPS

Safety	Concerns regarding osteonecrosis of the jaw with bisphosphonate use are still in question FDA issued warning regarding increased incidence of atypical femur fractures in patients using bisphosphonates (October 2010) More prevalent in patients receiving therapy for >5 years Cautious use in patients with impaired renal function (<30 mL/minute for risedronate and ibandronate or <35 mL/minute for alendronate and zoledronic acid) or low serum calcium concentration In patients with hypocalcemia, resolve low calcium values before starting therapy
Tolerability	Abdominal pain Acute-phase reaction (zoledronic acid and ibandronate infusions) Arthralgias Dyspepsia Cautious use in patients with severe esophageal reflux disease, Barrett esophagus, or esophageal strictures Scleritis and/or uveitis

Table 9. Bisphosphonates STEPS *(continued)*

Efficacy	All bisphosphonates have evidence to support use for preventing vertebral fractures Alendronate, risedronate, and zoledronic acid have proved efficacious for preventing nonvertebral and hip fractures Used in patients taking chronic systemic corticosteroids to prevent BMD loss and subsequent fracture (see Rheumatoid Arthritis, Figure 5 and Figure 6, for assistance when deciding to use a bisphosphonate for corticosteroid-induced BMD loss)
Preference (Pearls)	Most oral doses should be taken with 6–8 oz of water at least 30–60 minutes before food, drink, or other medications (risedronate delayed release should be taken with 4 oz of water right after breakfast) Patients should remain upright for at least 30 minutes after being administered an oral dose (60 minutes with ibandronate) *(Domain 1, Task 6, Knowledge 5)* If a patient is unable to tolerate one bisphosphonate, discontinue the agent until the adverse effect resolves, and offer the patient the option to try another available bisphosphonate Questionable efficacy beyond 5 years; may warrant reevaluation and possible discontinuance of therapy
Simplicity	Once-daily, once-weekly, and once-monthly tablets; quarterly and yearly infusions Alendronate: Prevention (5 mg/day or 35 mg/week) and treatment (10 mg daily or 70 mg weekly) Risedronate: Prevention and treatment (5 mg daily, 35 mg weekly, or 150 mg monthly) Ibandronate: Prevention (150 mg monthly) and treatment (150 mg monthly OR 3 mg intravenously every 3 months) Zoledronic acid: Prevention (5 mg intravenously every 2 years) and treatment (5 mg intravenously every year) All dosage forms and intervals are equally effective, so consider the patient's prescription drug coverage (or lack of) when choosing a medication

BMD = bone mineral density; FDA = U.S. Food and Drug Administration; STEPS = Safety, Tolerability, Efficacy, Preference (Pearls), Simplicity.

4. RANKL antagonist – Denosumab (Prolia)

Table 10. RANKL Antagonist STEPS

Safety	Cellulitis was the most common serious adverse event in clinical trials Osteonecrosis of the jaw Infections
Tolerability	Eczema Flatulence
Efficacy	Decreased incidence of vertebral, nonvertebral, and hip fractures in patients with osteoporosis Increases bone mineral density in the hip and lumbar spine Comparable in efficacy to the bisphosphonates, but with much less frequent dosing
Preference (Pearls)	NICE in the United Kingdom recommends denosumab for patients at risk of an osteoporotic fracture and unable to adhere to the dosing recommendations or tolerate an oral bisphosphonate Must be administered by a health professional, either in a physician's office practice or a by a pharmacist
Simplicity	Subcutaneous injection every 6 months

NICE = National Institute for Health and Clinical Excellence; STEPS = Safety, Tolerability, Efficacy, Preference (Pearls), Simplicity.

Table 11. NICE Recommendations for T-Score at Which to Recommend Denosumab as an Alternative to Bisphosphonates *(Domain 1; Tasks 2, 3; Knowledge 1)*

Age, years	Number of Independent Clinical Risk Factors for Fracture[a]		
	0	1	2
65–69	Not recommended	−4.5	−4.0
70–74	−4.5	−4.0	−3.5
75 and older	−4.0	−4.0	−3.0

[a]Independent clinical risk factors include parental history of hip fracture, more than four alcoholic drinks per day, and rheumatoid arthritis.
NICE = National Institute for Health and Clinical Excellence.

5. Estrogen replacement therapy

Table 12. Estrogen Replacement STEPS

Safety	Based on information from the WHI trial, the risk of adverse events with hormone replacement therapy exceeds the fracture prevention benefits Hormone replacement therapy is more likely to be associated with the following: Coronary heart disease (estrogen/progesterone only) Stroke Invasive breast cancer (estrogen/progesterone only) Venous thromboembolic event
Tolerability	Breast discomfort GI symptoms Headache disorders Vaginal bleeding Venous thromboembolism
Efficacy	Reduced risk of vertebral fractures Reduced risk of nonvertebral fractures
Preference (Pearls)	Results from the WHI trial showed the benefit of fracture prevention to be similar to or less than the patient's risk of heart disease, stroke, venous embolism, and breast cancer Acts in conjunction with a bisphosphonate to increase BMD more than either agent alone
Simplicity	Once-daily oral dosing Transdermal patch is approved for the prevention of postmenopausal osteoporosis

BMD = bone mineral density; GI = gastrointestinal; STEPS = Safety, Tolerability, Efficacy, Preference (Pearls), Simplicity; WHI = Women's Health Initiative (trial).

6. Selective estrogen receptor modulator (SERM): Available agents: Raloxifene (Evista)

Table 13. Selective Estrogen Receptor Modulator STEPS

Safety	Increased risk of fatal stroke in women with a history of coronary heart disease Increased risk of venous thromboembolism
Tolerability	Arthralgias Hot flashes/flushes Peripheral edema Sweating
Efficacy	Increased BMD Reduced incidence of clinical vertebral fractures, but not nonvertebral fractures
Preference (Pearls)	The rates of preventing clinical vertebral fractures are similar to rates of venous throboembolisms Evidence to support its use to prevent invasive breast cancer (5-year risk >3%)
Simplicity	Fixed-dose, once-daily dosing

BMD = bone mineral density; STEPS = Safety, Tolerability, Efficacy, Preference (Pearls), Simplicity.

7. Parathyroid hormone: Available agent: Teriparatide (biosynthetic parathyroid hormone 1–34) (Forteo)

Table 14. Parathyroid Hormone STEPS

Safety	Avoid use in patients with the following: Alkaline phosphatase elevation (unexplained) Open epiphyses Paget disease Prior skeletal radiation Associated with osteosarcoma (in rats) after about 24 months of therapy (3–60 times the human dose)
Tolerability	Influenza-like symptoms Hypercalcemia Injection site pain and/or rash Urolithiasis
Efficacy	Increases vertebral and total hip BMD Decreased incidence of new or worsening vertebral and nonvertebral fractures Prevents BMD loss and vertebral fractures in patients receiving chronic systemic corticosteroid therapy
Preference (Pearls)	Diminished efficacy if used concurrently with a bisphosphonate After discontinuing teriparatide, adding a bisphosphonate preserves BMD benefits Dropout and discontinuance rates in clinical studies are almost double those of alendronate
Simplicity	Once-daily injection Available as a prefilled (3 mL) pen

BMD = bone mineral density; STEPS = Safety, Tolerability, Efficacy, Preference (Pearls), Simplicity.

Table 15. NICE Recommendations for When to Use Teriparatide as an Alternative to Bisphosphonates for Secondary Prevention of Fragility Fractures *(Domain 1; Tasks 2, 3; Knowledge 1)*

Column 1[a]	Column 2[a]
Unable to take a bisphosphonate	65 years or older with a T-score of −4.0 or below
Have an intolerance or contraindication to bisphosphonates or strontium (United Kingdom only)[b]	65 years or older with a T-score of −3.5 or below with more than two fractures
Unsatisfactory response to treatment with a bisphosphonate[c]	55–64 years old with a T-score of −4.0 or below with more than two fractures

[a]Patient must meet one criteria from both Column 1 and Column 2.

[b]Intolerance to bisphosphonates is defined as persistent gastrointestinal irritation, severe enough to warrant a change in therapy, despite administering correctly.

[c]Unsatisfactory response is defined as a fracture or decline in BMD to below baseline despite adherence to treatment for at least 12 months.

BMD = bone mineral density; NICE = National Institute for Health and Care Excellence.

8. Calcitonin (Miacalcin, Fortical)

Table 16. Calcitonin STEPS

Safety	Anaphylactoid and anaphylaxis reactions associated with injection	
Tolerability	Injection GI symptoms Injection site reaction Flushing	Nasal spray Rhinitis Nasal congestion Mucosal irritation
Efficacy	Reduced incidence of recurrent vertebral fractures Beneficial effects on BMD in patients treated with steroid-induced disease	
Preference (Pearls)	Inferior to alendronate for preventing BMD loss May help relieve bone pain associated with fractures but is not an indication to choose as the primary treatment FDA (2013) stated that the lack of effectiveness combined with the increased risk of cancer (oral calcitonin) raises concerns about the overall utility of calcitonin	
Simplicity	Nasal administration in only ONE nostril per day, alternating nostrils each day	

BMD = bone mineral density; FDA = U.S. Food and Drug Administration; GI = gastrointestinal; STEPS = Safety, Tolerability, Efficacy, Preference (Pearls), Simplicity.

D. Follow-up
1. Dual-energy x-ray absorptiometry
a. Recheck at about 24 months to evaluate for changes: Do not consider treatment failure if initial, solitary evaluation shows net bone loss.
b. In patients NOT receiving drug therapy, may recheck DEXA findings every 5 years unless the patient has developed risk factors for osteoporotic fracture
2. Medication adherence
a. Review adherence at least every 6 months.
b. As many as one-half of patients being treated with a bisphosphonate will self-discontinue therapy within the first 6 months, so pharmacists should continually assess for medication adherence.

3. Patient resources
   a. Various handouts available from the American Family Physician Web site
   b. National Library of Medicine MedlinePlus has patient-oriented educational materials at no cost to provider or patient.
   c. National Osteoporosis Awareness and Prevention Campaign examination room booklets and posters

E. Cost-effectiveness Evaluation
   (Domain 4, Task 6, Knowledge 1)
   1. The World Health Organization (WHO) defines cost-effectiveness at three levels.
      a. Highly cost-effective: Less than the gross domestic product (GDP) per capita of a WHO region
      b. Cost-effective: Between one and three times the GDP per capita of a WHO region
      c. Not cost-effective: Greater than three times the GDP per capita of a WHO region
   2. For the region of North America (Amro A), the GDP per capita per WHO is $39,950.
      a. Highly cost-effective: Less than $39,950
      b. Cost-effective: $39,950 to $119, 849
      c. Not cost-effective: Greater than $119,849
   3. The available evidence for cost-effectiveness of antiresorptive and other agents for osteoporosis is as follows:
      a. Bisphosphonates (~$11,600/quality-adjusted life-year [QALY])
      b. RANKL inhibitors (~$31,600/QALY, but possibly less with more recent reviews)
      c. Estrogen-receptor agonist/antagonist (~$26,100/QALY for breast cancer prevention, ~$164,200/QALY for fracture prevention)
      d. Biosynthetic parathyroid hormone (~$264,500/QALY)

F. Physician Quality Reporting System 2015 Quality Measures (physician-reported quality of care to the Centers for Medicare & Medicaid Services)

Table 17. 2015 Physician Quality Reporting System Quality Measures *(Domain 5, Task 1, Knowledge 3)*

No.	Category	Criteria
24	Osteoporosis: Communication with the physician managing ongoing care after fracture	Percentage of patients aged 50 years who were treated for a hip, spine, or distal radial fracture with documentation of communication with the physician managing the patient's ongoing care that a fracture occurred and that the patient was or should be tested or treated for osteoporosis
39	Screening or therapy for osteoporosis for women 65 years and older	Percentage of female patients aged 65 years who have had a central DEXA measurement ordered or performed at least once since age 60 years or pharmacologic therapy prescribed within 12 months
40	Osteoporosis: Management after fracture	Percentage of patients aged 50 years with fracture of the hip, spine, or distal radius with a central DEXA measurement ordered or performed or pharmacologic therapy prescribed
41	Osteoporosis: Pharmacologic therapy	Percentage of patients aged 50 years with a diagnosis of osteoporosis who were prescribed pharmacologic therapy within 12 months

DEXA = dual-energy x-ray absorptiometry.

Table 18. Drugs and Doses Reference Table

Medication Name	Brand Name	Dosing
Calcium plus vitamin D	Several OTC formulations	500 mg of elemental calcium PLUS vitamin D 400 international units twice daily
Alendronate	Fosamax	5–10 mg by mouth once daily 35–70 mg by mouth once weekly
Risedronate	Actonel	5 mg by mouth once daily 35 mg by mouth once weekly 150 mg by mouth once monthly
Ibandronate	Boniva	150 mg by mouth once monthly 3 mg intravenously every 3 months
Zoledronic acid	Reclast	5 mg intravenously every 1–2 years
Denosumab	Prolia	60 mg subcutaneously every 6 months
Raloxifene	Evista	60 mg by mouth once daily
Teriparatide	Forteo	20 mcg subcutaneously once daily
Calcitonin	Miacalcin	100 units intramuscularly every other day 200 units sprayed into one nostril each day

OTC = over-the-counter.

III. RHEUMATOID ARTHRITIS

A. Clinical Guidelines *(Domain 1; Tasks 3, 6, 7; Knowledge 2/1/2)*
   1. 2010 rheumatoid arthritis (RA) classification criteria: An ACR/European League Against Rheumatism (EULAR) collaborative initiative
   2. The EULAR 2013 recommendations for the management of RA with synthetic and biologic disease-modifying drugs
   3. 2012 update of the 2008 ACR recommendations for the use of disease-modifying antirheumatic drugs (DMARDs) and biologic agents in the treatment of RA

B. Patient Symptom Presentation
   1. Diffuse pain (myalgias, arthralgias, arthritis)
   2. Variable time to symptom onset
   3. Morning joint stiffness (gelling) lasting more than 1 hour
   4. Affected joints are swollen and inflamed.
      a. Elbow
      b. Foot and ankle
      c. Hands and wrists (proximal interphalangeal and metacarpophalangeal joints)
      d. Hip
      e. Knee
      f. Shoulder

C. Other Contributing Factors
1. Family history of other inflammatory disorders such as the following:
    a. Autoimmune thyroid disease
    b. Multiple sclerosis
    c. Myasthenia gravis
    d. Rheumatoid arthritis
    e. Systemic lupus erythematosus
2. Smoking is associated with increased disease activity.

D. Evaluation and Diagnosis: 2010 ACR/EULAR Classification Criteria for RA
1. Test patients who have at least one joint with clinical synovitis not otherwise explained by another disease (e.g., systemic lupus erythematosus [SLE], gout, psoriatic arthritis).
2. Although this tool (Table 19) is not intended to be diagnostic, a score of at least 6 of 10 points classifies patients as having definite RA. (Note: Use the highest score from each category.)
3. Classification criteria score of at least 6 may also be a good guide for identifying individuals with the highest probability of persistent or erosive disease who would benefit from enrolling in clinical trials or DMARD intervention.

Table 19. 2010 ACR/EULAR Classification Criteria for Rheumatoid Arthritis

Classification Criteria	Scoring (points)
Joint involvement	
>10 joints, including at least 1 small joint	5
4–10 small joints	3
1–3 small joints	2
2–10 large joints	1
1 large joint	0
Serology	
Positive RF or positive ACPA test results > 3 times the upper limit of normal	3
Positive RF or positive ACPA test results up to 3 times the upper limit of normal	2
Negative RF and ACPA test results	0
Acute-phase reactants	
Abnormal CRP or ESR test results	1
Normal CRP and ESR test results	0
Duration of symptoms	
At least 6 weeks	1
<6 weeks	0
Total points	

ACPA = anti–citrullinated protein antibody; ACR = American College of Rheumatology; CRP = C-reactive protein; ESR = erythrocyte sedimentation rate; EULAR = European League Against Rheumatism; RF = rheumatoid factor.

Patient Case

5.   F.T. is a 38-year-old man recently referred by his primary care provider to a rheumatologist for assessment and treatment of RA. During the initial interview, the rheumatologist assesses the patient for various subjective and objective markers of disease activity. Of the four markers used to assess disease activity, which is the most clinically relevant prognostic marker?

   A.   Joint involvement (quantity).
   B.   Erythrocyte sedimentation rate (ESR).
   C.   Rheumatoid factor (RF).
   D.   C-reactive protein (CRP).

4.   Laboratory and radiographic testing in RA

Table 20. Testing to Consider for Diagnosis and Treatment Decisions in RA

Diagnosing RA	ACR-Suggested Baseline Evaluation	ACR Recommendations for Initiating or Titrating Pharmacotherapy
Laboratory	Laboratory	Laboratory
ACPA	CBC	CBC
CBC with differential	Creatinine	Creatinine
CRP	CRP	Hepatitis B and C[b]
ESR	ESR	(nonbiologic and biologic DMARDs)
Liver function tests	Liver function tests	Liver function tests
RF[a]	Metabolic (Chem) panel	Retinal examination[c]
Radiographic	Stool guaiac	(hydroxychloroquine)
Radiography, ultrasonography, or magnetic resonance imaging of affected joints	Synovial fluid (to rule out other diseases)	Tuberculosis screening[d] (biologic DMARDs)
	Urinalysis	
	Radiographic	
	Radiography, ultrasonography, or magnetic resonance imaging of affected joints	

[a]May repeat at 6–12 months if the initial value is low or negative.

[b]If patient has a high-risk history.

[c]Every 5 years for low-risk patients and annually for high-risk patients.

[d]Screen regardless of history of BCG vaccination.

ACPA = anti–citrullinated protein antibody; ACR = American College of Rheumatology; BCG = bacillus Calmette-Guerin; CBC = complete blood cell count; CRP = C-reactive protein; DMARD = disease-modifying antirheumatic drug; ESR = erythrocyte sedimentation rate; RA = rheumatoid arthritis; RF = rheumatoid factor.

Table 21. Disease Prognosis

Clinically important markers (ACR)	Functional limitations Positive RF or ACPA test results Radiographic evidence of bony erosions Extra-articular disease (Felty syndrome, RA lung disease, RA vasculitis, rheumatoid nodules, secondary Sjögren syndrome)
Disease activity during first 3–6 months of treatment	Lower disease activity (tender or swollen joints) for up to 6 months increases the likelihood of 12-month disease remission Higher disease activity (tender or swollen joints) in first 3 months increases likelihood of presence of symptoms at 12 months

ACPA = anti–citrullinated protein antibody; ACR = American College of Rheumatology; RA = rheumatoid arthritis; RF = rheumatoid factor.

E. Before Initiating Pharmacologic Therapy
   1. Address the entire scope of patient needs with respect to RA.
      a. Discuss potential functional limitations and strategies to overcome and/or compensate.
      b. Involve other health professionals to care for and educate the patient.
         i. Physical therapy
         ii. Occupational therapy
         iii. Social workers and counseling/cognitive services
   2. Educate the patient regarding physical conditioning.
      a. Energy conservation
      b. Joint protection
      c. Range-of-motion exercises
      d. Strengthening exercises
   3. Tuberculosis screening
   4. Immunizations

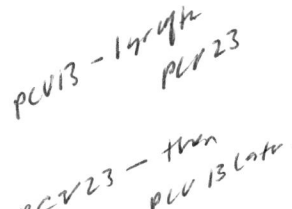

Table 22. Vaccinations to Consider in Patients Receiving Rheumatoid Arthritis Immunosuppressive Therapy
(Domain 1, Task 5, Knowledge 6) (Domain 5, Task 2, Knowledge 2)

Vaccination	Recommendations	Before Starting DMARDs	During DMARD Therapy
Influenza vaccine (trivalent, inactivated)	Administer annually to all patients	Yes	Yes
PCV13[a]	Administer to all patients receiving biologic DMARDs, methotrexate, leflunomide, and/or sulfazalazine before PPSV23 or at least 1 year after administering PPSV23	Yes	Yes
PPSV23	Administer to all patients receiving biologic DMARDs, methotrexate, leflunomide, and/or sulfasalazine at least 8 weeks after administering PCV13	Yes	Yes

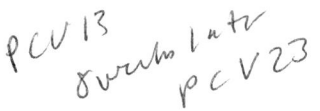

Table 22. Vaccinations to Consider in Patients Receiving Rheumatoid Arthritis Immunosuppressive Therapy (Domain 1, Task 5, Knowledge 6) (Domain 5, Task 2, Knowledge 2) *(continued)*

Hepatitis B vaccine series	Administer to all patients with risk factors and receiving biologic DMARDs, methotrexate, and/or leflunomide	Yes	Yes
Human papillomavirus	Administer to all patients who meet the recommendations from the CDC	Yes	Yes
Herpes zoster	Administer to all patients who meet the recommendations from the CDC	Yes	Yes/no[b]

[a]PCV13 is not included in the ACR 2012 update, but the CDC/ACIP recommendations for iatrogenic immunosuppression apply.

[b]Yes: Patients who are actively being treated with DMARD monotherapy or combination therapy; No: Patients who are actively being treated with an anti-TNF or non-TNF biologic agent.

ACIP = Advisory Committee on Immunization Practices; ACR = American College of Rheumatology; CDC = Centers for Disease Control and Prevention; DMARD = disease-modifying antirheumatic drug; PCV13 = pneumococcal vaccine (13-valent conjugate); PPSV23 = pneumococcal vaccine (23-valent polysaccharide); TNF = tumor necrosis factor.

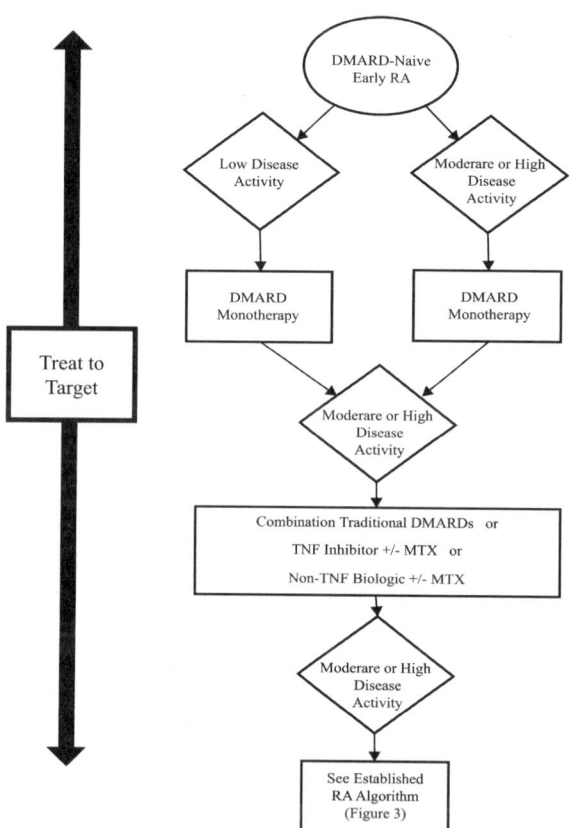

Figure 2. 2015 ACR recommendations for the treatment of RA in patients with disease duration of less than 6 months.

ACR = American College of Rheumatology; DMARD: Disease-modifying anti-rheumatic drug; MTX: methotrexate; RA = rheumatoid arthritis; TNF: Tunor Necrosis Factor

Reprinted with permission from: Singh JA, Saag KG, Bridges SL, et al. 2015 American College of Rheumatology Guideline for the Treatment of Rheumatoid Arthritis. Available online at: http://www.rheumatology.org/Portals/0/Files/ACR%202015%20RA%20Guideline.pdf. Accessed February 1, 2016.

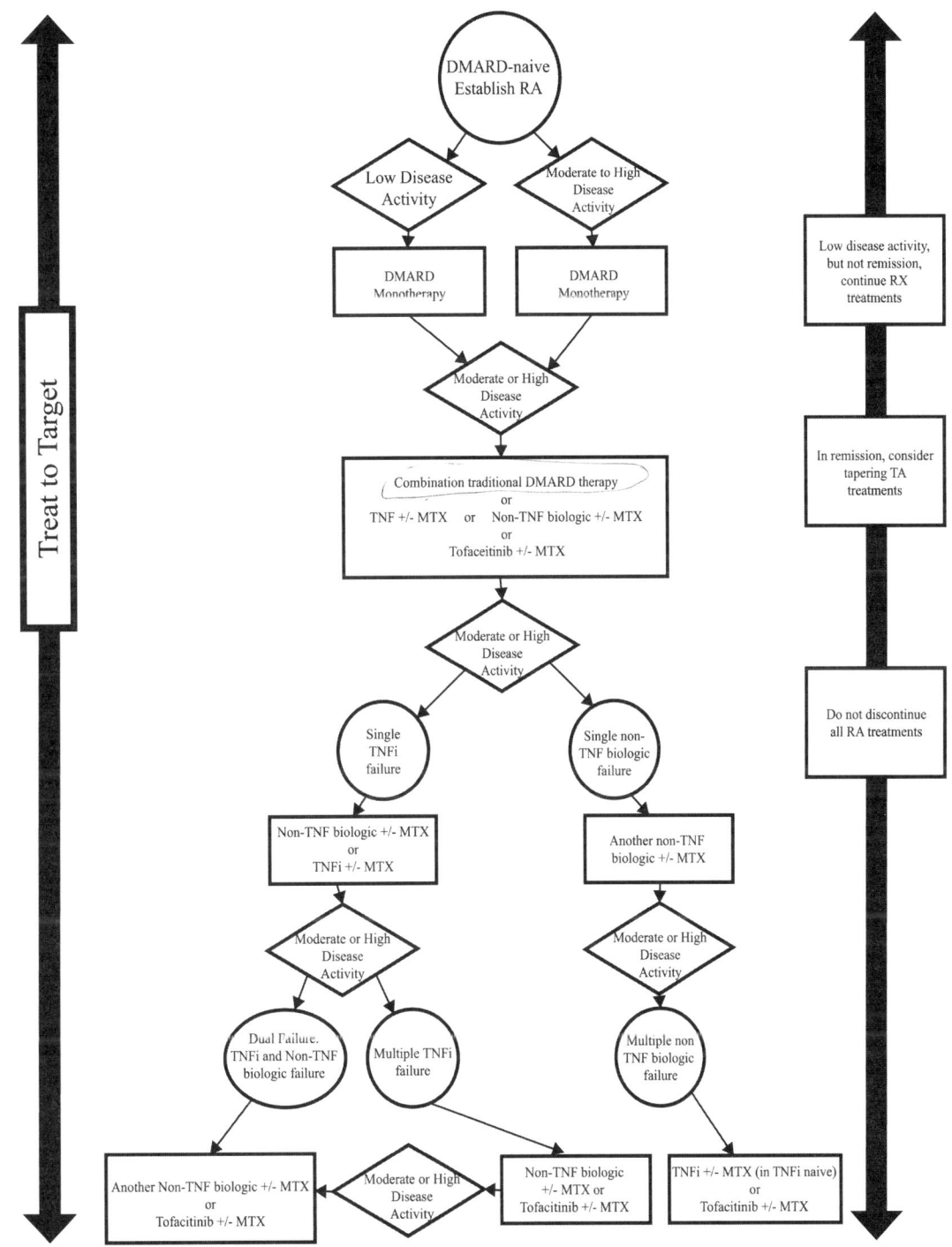

Figure 3. 2015 ACR recommendations for the treatment of RA in patients with disease duration of greater than 6 months.

ACR = American College of Rheumatology; RA = rheumatoid arthritis.

Reprinted with permission from: Singh JA, Saag KG, Bridges SL, et al. 2015 American College of Rheumatology Guideline for the Treatment of Rheumatoid Arthritis. Available online at: http://www.rheumatology.org/Portals/0/Files/ACR%202015%20RA%20Guideline.pdf. Accessed February 1, 2016.

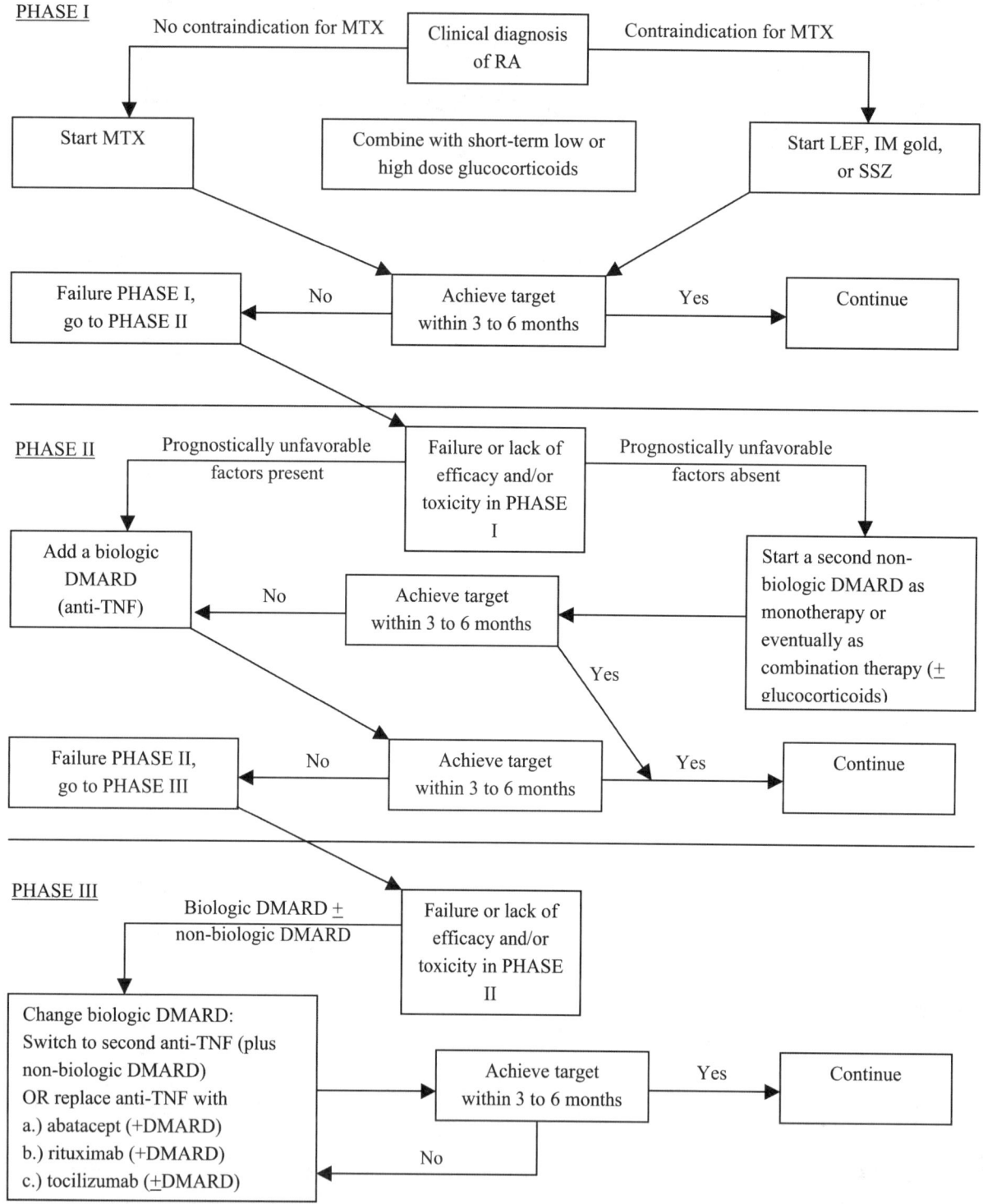

Figure 4. EULAR-recommended use of nonbiologic and biologic DMARDs.

DMARD = disease-modifying antirheumatic drug; EULAR = European League Against Rheumatism.

Reprinted with permission from: Smolen JS, Landewé R, Breedveld FC, et al. EULAR recommendations for the management of rheumatoid arthritis with synthetic and biological disease-modifying antirheumatic drugs: 2013 update. Ann Rheum Dis 2014;73:492-509.

F. Guideline Recommendations *(Domain 1; Tasks 2, 6, 7; Knowledge 2/1/2)*
    1. American College of Rheumatology (2012 update)
        a. Symptomatic pain control achieved with the following:
            i.   Nonsteroidal anti-inflammatory drugs
            ii. Low-dose systemic steroids (ACR defines as 10 mg of prednisone per day or less)
            iii. Local steroid injections (not more frequent than every 3 months)
        b. DMARDs should be initiated within the first 3 months of diagnosis as monotherapy or combination therapy, depending on the patient's prognosis and disease activity.
        c. ACR recommendations consider a patient's ability to pay for therapy as self or through a third party.
    2. European League Against Rheumatism (2014 update)
        a. Initiate synthetic DMARDs early as soon as the patient's condition is diagnosed (see Figure 4 for EULAR's recommended treatment algorithm).
            i.   Methotrexate is preferred.
            ii. Consider leflunomide, sulfasalazine, or injectable gold (gold sodium thiomalate) when methotrexate is contraindicated for or not tolerated by the patient.
            iii. Initiate DMARD with a systemic corticosteroid.
                (a) Begin to taper the corticosteroid to the lowest effective dose with target of discontinuing at or before 6 months.
                (b) If the patient is unable to discontinue systemic corticosteroids, modify DMARDs to better control symptoms.
        b. In treatment-naive patients with a poor prognosis or for patients who have not achieved response to synthetic DMARDs, adding a biologic DMARD (tumor necrosis factor [TNF] antagonist or selective T-cell antagonist) is appropriate.
        c. Consider changing synthetic and biologic DMARDs if patient has an inadequate response to therapy.
        d. In patients who show evidence of persistent remission, consider the following:
            i.   Tapering the dose of corticosteroids
            ii. Tapering biologic DMARDs
            iii. Decreasing the dose of nonbiologic DMARDS to the lowest efficacious dose

G. Supportive Care Medications
    1. NSAIDs: Systemic and/or topical

Table 23. NSAID STEPS

Safety	In patients at risk of or with existing cardiovascular disease, NSAIDs may increase the risk of a fatal or nonfatal event All NSAIDs carry the risk of causing changes in renal function Patients at greater risk of GI toxicity include the following: Elderly patients Patients with a history of GI bleed Patients concurrently using anticoagulants, antiplatelet drugs, and/or systemic corticosteroids
Tolerability	Dyspepsia Prolonged bleeding Dermatologic reactions
Efficacy	Available NSAIDs are equally effective, but individuals' responses to agents will vary NSAIDs will reduce joint pain and swelling to some degree, but they will not modify the destruction or progression of RA

Table 23. NSAID STEPS *(continued)*

Preference (Pearls)	Celecoxib has fewer GI adverse events than other NSAIDs; however, it is no more effective at reducing pain and inflammation
	Adding misoprostol to an NSAID will decrease the risk of GI ulceration
	Adding a proton pump inhibitor to an NSAID will decrease nonulcerative symptoms
	If a patient does not achieve response to NSAID therapy (after an appropriate 14- to 28-day trial), providers should consider trying other NSAIDs before concluding therapeutic failure
Simplicity	Widely available prescription and over-the-counter agents
	Once-daily formulations allow continuous analgesia

GI = gastrointestinal; NSAID = nonsteroidal anti-inflammatory drug; RA = rheumatoid arthritis; STEPS = Safety, Tolerability, Efficacy, Preference (Pearls), Simplicity.

2. Corticosteroids: Oral or intra-articular injections

Table 24. Corticosteroid STEPS

Safety	Increased risk of osteoporosis and fracture	
	Risk of symptoms of a psychiatric disturbance with increasing doses of corticosteroids	
	<40 mg of prednisone per day (1%–2% incidence)	
	>40 mg of prednisone per day (5% incidence)	
	>80 mg of prednisone per day (20% incidence)	
Tolerability	Cataracts	Hypertension (high dose)
	Dyslipidemia (high dose)	Hypothalamic-pituitary-adrenal axis suppression
	Glaucoma	Osteoporosis
	Hirsutism	Pancreatitis (high dose)
	Hyperglycemia	Weight gain
Efficacy	Short-term (weeks), low-dose (<10 mg of prednisone daily) corticosteroids are effective for symptoms flare	
	Early initiation of corticosteroids and continuance at a low dose reduce joint destruction and increase likelihood of clinical remission	
	Higher corticosteroid doses may be warranted to treat symptoms of severe or advanced disease (e.g., presence of vasculitis)	
	Intra-articular injections may be beneficial, but limit injections in joint to no more often than every 3–4 months	
Preference (Pearls)	Start appropriate calcium and vitamin D supplementation in all patients taking corticosteroid therapy	
	See Figure 5 and Figure 6 for recommendations for using bisphosphonates in patients receiving chronic corticosteroid therapy	
Simplicity	Once-daily fixed dose appears to be effective for symptom control and possibly slowing disease progression	

STEPS = Safety, Tolerability, Efficacy, Preference (Pearls), Simplicity.

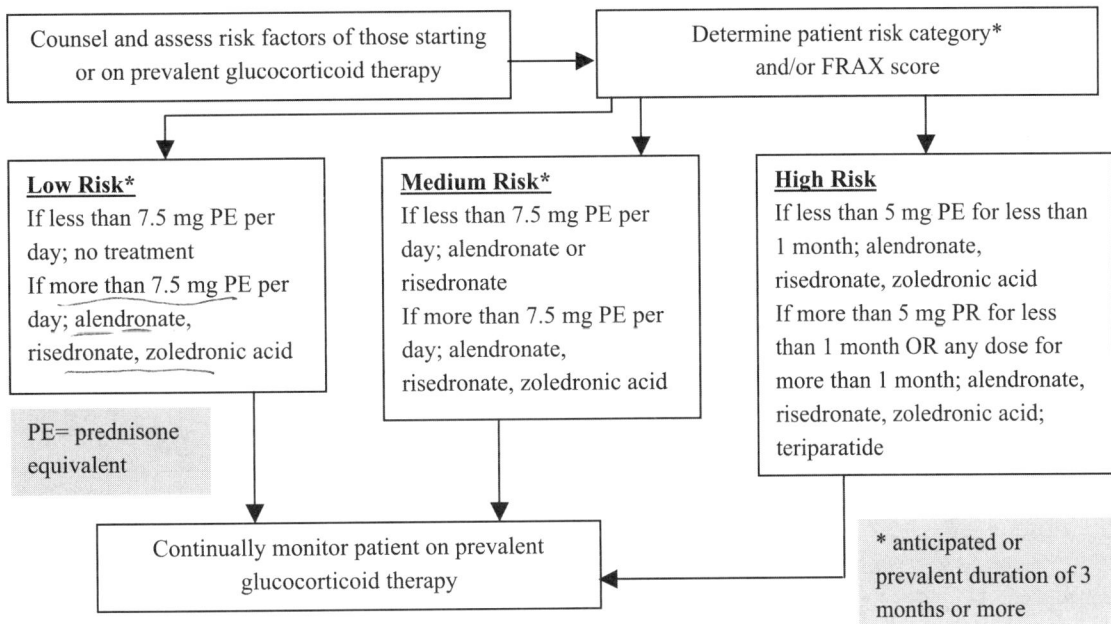

Figure 5. Preventing corticosteroid-induced BMD loss in postmenopausal women and men older than 50 years.

*Risk is defined in Figure 2 of the ACR guidelines as follows: Low risk (<10%), medium risk (10%–20%), or high risk (>20%).

ACR = American College of Rheumatology; BMD = bone mineral density.

Reprinted with permission from: Grossman JM, Gordon R, Ranganath VK, et al. American College of Rheumatology 2010 recommendations for the prevention and treatment of glucocorticoid-induced osteoporosis. Arthritis Care Res 2010;62:1515-26.

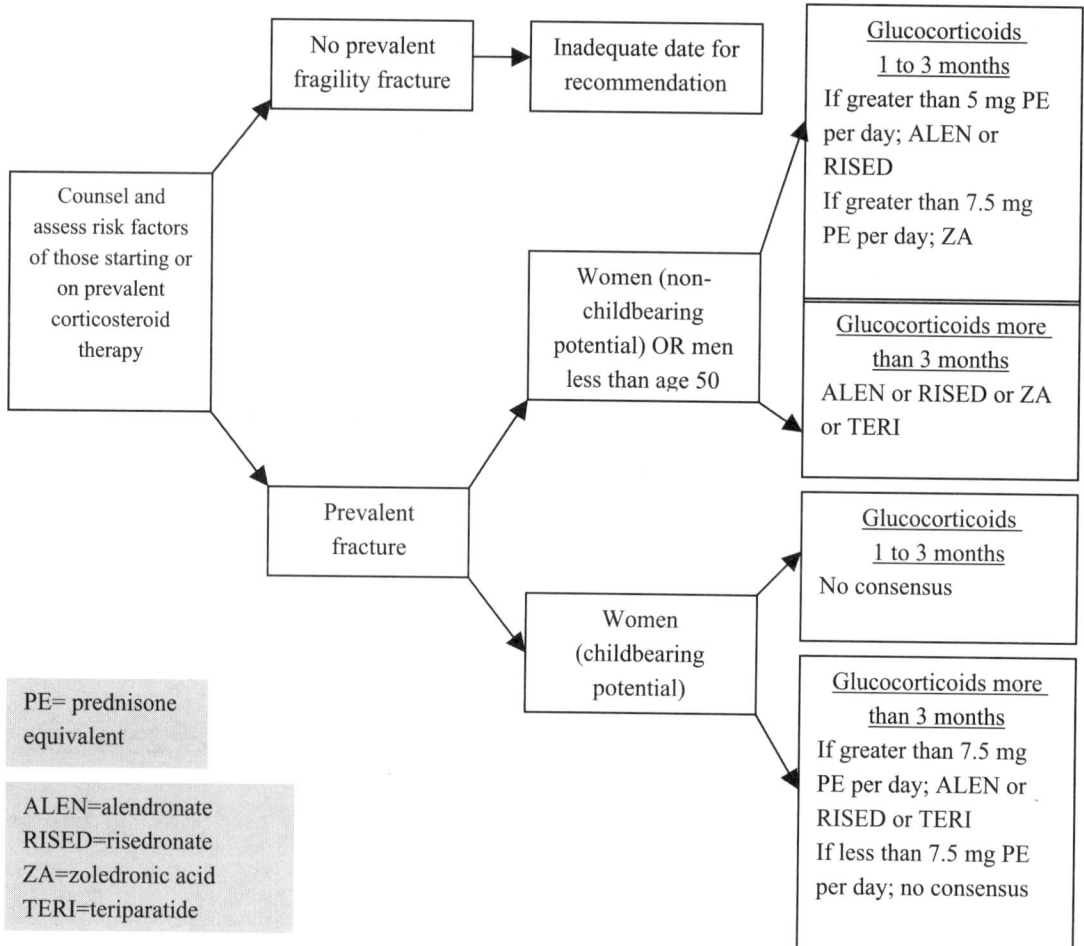

Figure 6. Preventing corticosteroid-induced BMD loss in premenopausal women and men younger than 50 years.

BMD = bone mineral density.

Reprinted with permission from: Grossman JM, Gordon R, Ranganath VK, et al. American College of Rheumatology 2010 recommendations for the prevention and treatment of glucocorticoid-induced osteoporosis. Arthritis Care Res 2010;62:1515-26.

Patient Case

6. K.W. is a 27-year-old female executive with RA (diagnosed 3 months ago), type 2 diabetes mellitus, and hypertension who smokes cigarettes. Her basic metabolic profile and complete blood cell count (CBC) are all within normal limits. Her RF is about 4 times the upper limit of normal; she has elevated anticyclic citrullinated peptide antibody values and ESR (high disease activity). Her radiographs show evidence of bony erosions. During the 2 months before her diagnosis, she experienced severe functional limitation, sometimes missing work because she was unable to prepare herself in a timely fashion. According to the ACR recommendations, which medication regimen is best for K.W.?

A. Hydroxychloroquine 400 mg once daily.

B. Methotrexate 10 mg once weekly.

C. Methotrexate 10 mg once weekly plus infliximab 3 mg/kg every 8 weeks.

D. Methotrexate 10 mg once weekly plus anakinra 100 mg daily.

H. Synthetic DMARDs
   1. Methotrexate

Table 25. Methotrexate STEPS

Safety	Contraindicated in pregnancy and breastfeeding; pregnancy should be avoided for at least 3 months with men and at least one ovulatory cycle for women after discontinuing methotrexate Significantly diminishes ability to generate an immune response Increased incidence of the following: Any malignancy Lung cancer Melanoma Non-Hodgkin lymphoma Avoid in patients with the following: CrCl < 30 mL/minute Platelet count < 50,000/mm^3 White blood cell count < 3 x 10^3 cells/mm^3 Liver transaminase concentrations > 2 times the upper limit of normal Avoid concurrent use of NSAIDs in patients before or actively using high-dose methotrexate
Tolerability	Abdominal cramping / Increased aminotransferases Anorexia / Infections Bone marrow suppression / Nausea Hypersensitivity pneumonitis / Stomatitis
Efficacy	Intense treatment strategy and dose may result in an increased chance of disease remission, but also an increased likelihood of having an adverse event or discontinuing therapy Consider changing to subcutaneous methotrexate in patients with an inadequate response to oral therapy (secondary to increased bioavailability of the injectable formulation) and unable to use biologic DMARDs Proposed benefit of decreased risk of cardiovascular mortality
Preference (Pearls)	Considered first choice for nonbiologic DMARD therapy in both ACR and EULAR recommendations Adding a folic acid supplement decreases adverse events (folic acid daily or folic acid weekly) Emerging evidence that coadministration of omega-3 fatty acids with triple DMARD therapy (methotrexate, sulfasalazine, and hydroxychloroquine) significantly reduced disease progression
Simplicity	Dosed as one subcutaneous injection or one oral dose weekly (5–20 mg)

ACR = American College of Rheumatology; CrCl = creatinine clearance; DMARD = disease-modifying antirheumatic drug; EULAR = European League Against Rheumatism; NSAID = nonsteroidal anti-inflammatory drug; STEPS = Safety, Tolerability, Efficacy, Preference (Pearls), Simplicity.

2. Leflunomide (Arava)

Table 26. Leflunomide STEPS

Safety	Stevens-Johnson syndrome and toxic epidermal necrolysis May decrease defenses against malignancy Women who wish to become pregnant or men who wish to father children should discontinue leflunomide use and use cholestyramine to achieve plasma (leflunomide) active metabolite concentrations < 0.02 mg/L Patients with preexisting liver disease or aspartate aminotransferase/alanine aminotransferase values > 2 times the upper limit of normal should not receive leflunomide

Tolerability	Alopecia Debilitating diarrhea	Rash Severe hepatotoxicity

Efficacy	Available evidence shows leflunomide is comparable to methotrexate therapy May be added to methotrexate therapy to further improve symptoms, but at risk of hepatic toxicity
Preference (Pearls)	An alternative for patients unable to tolerate or who do not achieve response to methotrexate therapy
Simplicity	100 mg by mouth daily for 3 days (loading dose) and then 20 mg by mouth once daily Dosage may be reduced (10 mg daily) for patients unable to tolerate full dose Loading dose can be omitted for patients at high risk of hepatic or hematologic toxicities

STEPS = Safety, Tolerability, Efficacy, Preference (Pearls), Simplicity.

3. Sulfasalazine (Azulfidine)

Table 27. Sulfasalazine STEPS

Safety	"Probably" safe for use in pregnancy; has not demonstrated abnormal/adverse fetal outcomes Avoid use in patients with the following: Platelet count < 50,000/mm^3 Liver transaminase concentrations > 2 times the upper limit of normal Acute hepatitis B/C Chronic hepatitis B, not receiving therapy Chronic hepatitis B, Child-Pugh class C Chronic hepatitis C, Child-Pugh class B or C
Tolerability	GI effects (may be lessened with enteric-coated tablets) A lupus-like syndrome has been reported in patients taking sulfasalazine
Efficacy	Available data suggest that sulfasalazine is effective at modifying rheumatic disease activity, but data are less supportive of its effects on radiologic progression
Preference (Pearls)	May be an alternative for women who are (or planning to become) pregnant
Simplicity	Twice- to thrice-daily dosing May require 2–4 tablets per dose

GI = gastrointestinal; STEPS = Safety, Tolerability, Efficacy, Preference (Pearls), Simplicity.

4. Other considerations: Routine monitoring of CBC, hepatic transaminases, and creatinine concentration when starting or adjusting DMARD therapy (methotrexate, leflunomide, sulfasalazine)
    a. Every 2–4 weeks for the first 3 months
    b. Every 8–12 weeks until month 6
    c. Every 12 weeks thereafter
5. Additional agents to consider
    a. Low disease activity and no poor prognostic factors
        i.   Hydroxychloroquine
        ii. Minocycline (diagnosis less than 6 months)
    b. Not recommended by the ACR
        i.   Azathioprine
        ii. Cyclophosphamide
        iii. Cyclosporine
        iv. D-penicillamine
        v.   Gold salts

Patient Case

7. T.D. is a 28-year-old, uninsured graduate student meeting with a rheumatologist regarding worsening RA symptoms. She currently takes methotrexate 20 mg by mouth weekly, folic acid 1 mg by mouth daily, and naproxen 500 mg by mouth twice daily as needed for pain. Her symptoms have been increasingly worse during the past 3 months, and she has been using naproxen around the clock for the past 30 days. Which is the best strategy to help T.D. control her symptoms?

    A. Recommend that she change to subcutaneous, injectable methotrexate.
    B. Increase methotrexate to 30 mg weekly.
    C. Replace methotrexate with adalimumab 40 mg subcutaneously every other week.
    D. Replace methotrexate with infliximab 3 mg/kg intravenously every 8 weeks.

---

infliximab – always with MTX

I. Biologic DMARDs
    1. TNF inhibitors
        a. Adalimumab (Humira)
        b. Certolizumab pegol (Cimzia)
        c. Etanercept (Enbrel)
        d. Golimumab (Simponi)
        e. Infliximab (Remicade)

Table 28. TNF Inhibitors STEPS

Safety	Increased risk of serious bacterial and/or fungal infections
	Associated with reactivation of tuberculosis
	May increase risk of malignancy, including melanoma, leukemia, and lymphoma
	Linked with new or worsening heart failure and possibly death in patients with heart failure
Tolerability	Headache
	Abdominal pain
	Injection site reactions
	Upper respiratory tract infection
	Infusion reactions (infliximab)

Table 28. TNF Inhibitors STEPS *(continued)*

Efficacy	First-line choice for biologic DMARDs on the basis of their ability to improve physical function and delay radiographic changes Superior to synthetic DMARDs with respect to radiographic outcomes Combination with methotrexate yields better outcomes than using TNF inhibitors as monotherapy
Preference (Pearls)	The ACR generally recommends biologic DMARDs after insufficient response to nonbiologic DMARDs or for patients with high disease activity and features of poor prognosis The EULAR recommends biologic DMARDs after insufficient response to methotrexate or other nonbiologic DMARDs All patients receiving biologic DMARDs should be tested for (and treated for) TB before starting RA therapy (see Figure 7 for TB screening recommendations) Treatment is expensive for patients without insurance or suboptimal coverage Infliximab should only be used in combination with methotrexate
Simplicity	Doses may be given subcutaneously weekly (etanercept), every other week (adalimumab), or every 4 weeks (golimumab) Certolizumab is dosed subcutaneously every other week when initiating therapy and may be extended to every 4 weeks for maintenance therapy Infliximab is dosed intravenously every 8 weeks after completing induction therapy at 0, 2, and 6 weeks; interval may be decreased to every 4 weeks if necessary

ACR = American College of Rheumatology; DMARD = disease-modifying antirheumatic drug; EULAR = European League Against Rheumatism; RA = rheumatoid arthritis; STEPS = Safety, Tolerability, Efficacy, Preference (Pearls), Simplicity; TB = tuberculosis; TNF = tumor necrosis factor.

2. Abatacept (Orencia)

Table 29. Abatacept STEPS

Safety	In patients with COPD, abatacept has been linked with more adverse pulmonary effects Increased risk of developing serious infections
Tolerability	Acute infusion reactions Upper respiratory tract infections
Efficacy	Should not be used in combination with other biologic DMARDs Effective for improving RA symptoms but should not be introduced until failure of at least one TNF inhibitor Combination with methotrexate results in higher rates of remission than methotrexate monotherapy
Preference (Pearls)	The ACR recommendations suggest abatacept as an option for patients with moderate to severe disease for >6 months or low disease activity with poor prognostic features who have not achieved response to methotrexate or another synthetic DMARD
Simplicity	IV regimen: After initial infusion, administer again at 2 weeks and then at 4 weeks; then begin administering every 4 weeks Subcutaneous regimen: Initial IV infusion; then subcutaneous injection within 24 hours; and then weekly thereafter

ACR = American College of Rheumatology; COPD = chronic obstructive pulmonary disease; DMARD = disease-modifying antirheumatic drug; IV = intravenous; RA = rheumatoid arthritis; STEPS = Safety, Tolerability, Efficacy, Preference (Pearls), Simplicity; TNF = tumor necrosis factor.

3.   Rituximab (Rituxan)

Table 30. Rituximab STEPS

Safety	Acute renal failure Cardiac arrhythmias Linked to fatal infusion-related adverse reactions Mucocutaneous reactions Progressive multifocal leukoencephalopathy Tumor lysis syndrome
Tolerability	Arthralgias Hematologic effects may include lymphopenia, neutropenia, leukopenia, thrombocytopenia, and anemia Hyperphosphatemia Hypertension Hyperuricemia
Efficacy	Has shown efficacy as monotherapy or as add-on therapy to methotrexate
Preference (Pearls)	Avoid use in patients who have not had an adequate trial with a TNF inhibitor Avoid administering live vaccines 3 months before or during treatment with rituximab
Simplicity	A two-dose therapeutic course (separated by 14 days) every 24 weeks (may be readministered every 16 weeks, if needed) Consider using acetaminophen and antihistamine before infusion

STEPS = Safety, Tolerability, Efficacy, Preference (Pearls), Simplicity; TNF = tumor necrosis factor.

4.   Tocilizumab (Actemra)

Table 31. Tocilizumab STEPS

Safety	Serious bacterial, fungal, and viral infections reported with use
	All patients should receive monitoring for tuberculosis before and after starting tocilizumab therapy
	GI perforation reported with concomitant use of tocilizumab and NSAIDs, corticosteroids, and/or methotrexate
	Avoid use in patients with the following:
	  Absolute neutrophil count < $2000/mm^3$
	  Platelet count < $100,000/mm^3$
	  Aminotransferase concentrations > 1.5 times the upper limit of normal

Tolerability	Dyslipidemias reported Hypersensitivity reactions starting with the second to fourth infusion Neutropenia or thrombocytopenia Transaminase elevations Upper respiratory tract infections
Efficacy	Effective treatment option for patients not achieving response, or with inadequate response, to methotrexate therapy Used in combination with methotrexate therapy
Preference (Pearls)	FDA approved for patients with an inadequate response to one or more TNF inhibitors
Simplicity	Intravenous infusion every 4 weeks

FDA = U.S. Food and Drug Administration; GI = gastrointestinal; NSAID = nonsteroidal anti-inflammatory drug; STEPS = Safety, Tolerability, Efficacy, Preference (Pearls), Simplicity; TNF = tumor necrosis factor.

5. Anakinra (Kineret)

Table 32. Anakinra STEPS

Safety	Increased risk of neutropenia when combined with TNF inhibitors High doses are associated with an increased risk of serious infection
Tolerability	Diarrhea Influenza-like reaction Injection site reactions
Efficacy	Effective for decreasing RA symptoms, but not as effective as TNF inhibitors
Preference (Pearls)	Do not administer live vaccines to patients receiving anakinra Not included in the ACR recommendations because of limited data available in the literature and not recommended in the EULAR guidelines because of lesser clinical efficacy in trials
Simplicity	Once-daily subcutaneous injection

ACR = American College of Rheumatology; EULAR = European League Against Rheumatism; RA = rheumatoid arthritis; STEPS = Safety, Tolerability, Efficacy, Preference (Pearls), Simplicity; TNF = tumor necrosis factor.

J. Janus-Associated Kinase Inhibitor – Tofacitinib (Xeljanz)

Table 33. Tofacitinib STEPS

Safety	Bone marrow suppression Gastrointestinal perforation in those with a history or at risk Hepatotoxicity Malignancy Tuberculosis	
Tolerability	Increased risk of infection Diarrhea	Headache Upper respiratory tract infections
Efficacy	Effective to reduce symptoms of RA Most studies evaluate efficacy by using ACR20 (20% improvement in RA symptoms), but others use ACR50 (50%) or ACR70 (70%) to assess symptom improvement	
Preference (Pearls)	The medication is too new (approved November 2012) to be included in ACR EULAR recommends using tofacitinib after other biologic treatments fail to control the disease	
Simplicity	Oral therapy, dosed twice daily Price (per month) is comparable to that of most biologic DMARDs	

ACR = American College of Rheumatology; DMARD = disease-modifying antirheumatic drug; EULAR = European League Against Rheumatism; RA = rheumatoid arthritis; STEPS = Safety, Tolerability, Efficacy, Preference (Pearls), Simplicity.

K. Other Considerations with Biologic DMARDs
   1. Tuberculosis

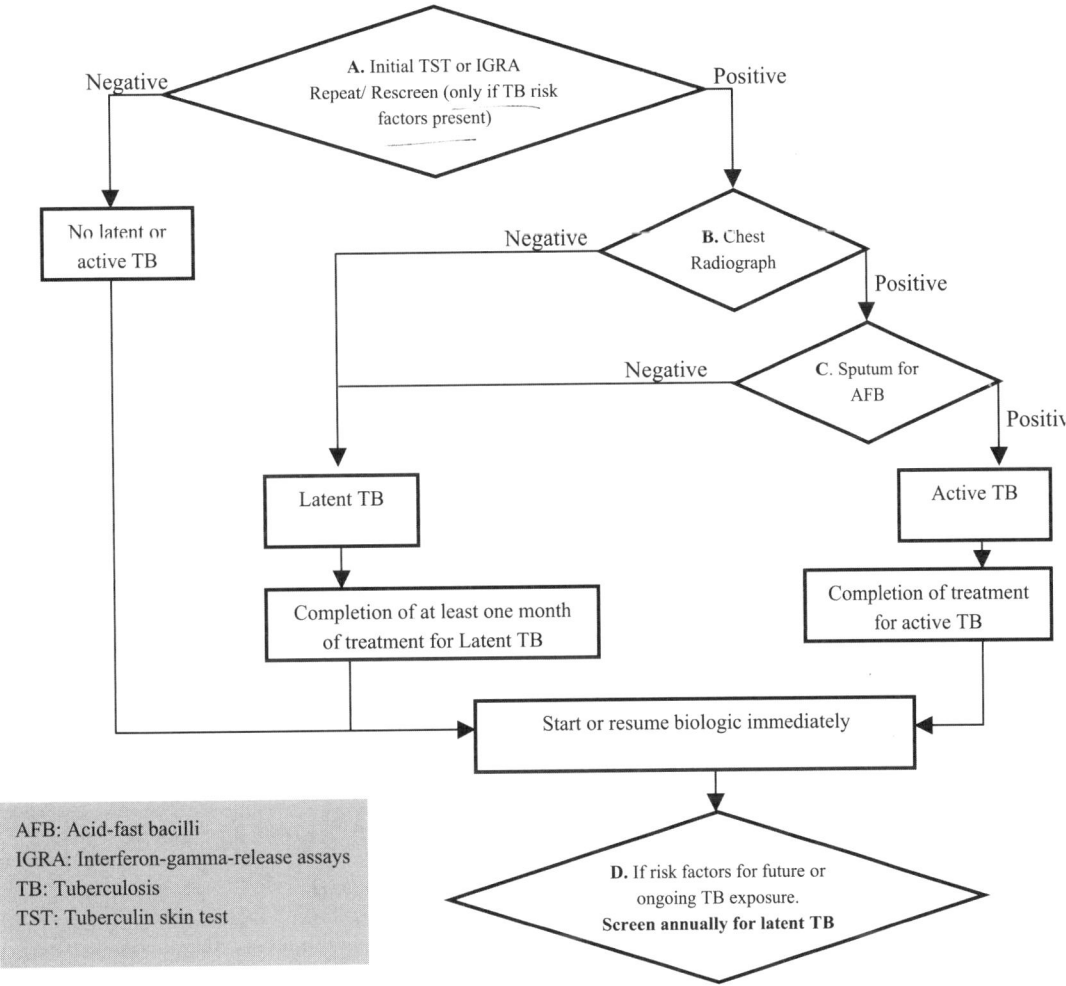

Figure 7. 2012 ACR recommendations for TB screening in patients using biologic DMARD therapy.

ACR = American College of Rheumatology; DMARD = disease-modifying antirheumatic drug; TB = tuberculosis

Reprinted with permission from: Singh JA, Furst DE, Bharat A, et al. 2012 update of the 2008 American College of Rheumatology recommendations for the use of disease-modifying antirheumatic drugs and biologic agents in the treatment of rheumatoid arthritis. Arthritis Care Res 2012;64:625-39.

   2. Medication assistance programs (www.needymeds.com) are available for those who qualify on the basis of financial need. *(Domain 2, Task 6, Knowledge 2)*
   3. Many pharmacy insurance providers require authorization paperwork before paying for biologic DMARD therapy. *(Domain 2, Task 6, Knowledge 3) (Domain 4, Task 6, Knowledge 6)*
      a. Step therapy: Documentation of unsuccessful treatment with one or several available conventional DMARDs
      b. Prior authorization: Documentation of symptom severity or contraindications requiring advancement of therapy beyond recommended first-line agents
      c. Authorization is usually temporary (12 months) and requires reevaluation to continue coverage.

4. Support groups are available, but patients who have used support groups have not shown significant improvements in disease or outcomes.
   a. Local group meetings
   b. Online chat or message boards
   c. Social networking groups

Patient Case

8. D.K. is a 37-year-old woman with RA for the past 8 years. She is currently treated with methotrexate and etanercept, but she returns to the rheumatology office today with worsening RA symptoms (classified as moderate to severe disease). Her concerns were the same 6 months ago, but she was given a course of oral corticosteroids in the hope that they would cause her symptoms to remit. However, her symptoms are still present and worsening. Which is the best next step to help control the patient's RA and symptoms?

   A. Start another course of prednisone, but increase the dose to 20 mg daily and continue indefinitely.
   B. Add another anti-TNF agent to the patient's regimen, such as adalimumab.
   C. Discontinue etanercept and initiate abatacept therapy for the patient.
   D. Continue etanercept and initiate abatacept therapy for the patient.

---

5. Patient resources *(Domain 5, Task 2, Knowledge 5)*
   a. Patient handouts from American Family Physician
   b. Online information from The Arthritis Foundation (www.arthritis.org)
   c. Online information from the ACR

L. Physician Quality Reporting System 2015 Quality Measures

Table 34. 2015 Physician Quality Reporting System Quality Measures *(Domain 5, Task 1, Knowledge 3)*

Number	Category	Criteria
108	RA: DMARD therapy	Percentage of patients ≥18 years who received a diagnosis of RA and were prescribed, dispensed, or administered at least one ambulatory prescription for a DMARD
176	RA: Tuberculosis screening	Percentage of patients ≥18 years with a diagnosis of RA who have documentation of a TB screening performed and results interpreted within 6 months before receiving a first course of therapy using a biologic DMARD
177	RA: Periodic assessment of disease activity	Percentage of patients ≥18 years with a diagnosis of RA who have an assessment and classification of disease activity within 12 months
178	RA: Functional status assessment	Percentage of patients ≥18 years with a diagnosis of RA for whom a functional status assessment was performed at least once within 12 months

Table 34. 2015 Physician Quality Reporting System Quality Measures (Domain 5, Task 1, Knowledge 3) *(continued)*

| 179 | RA: Assessment and classification of disease prognosis | Percentage of patients ≥18 years with a diagnosis of RA who have an assessment and classification of disease prognosis at least once within 12 months |
| 180 | RA: Glucocorticoid management | Percentage of patients ≥18 years with a diagnosis of RA who have been evaluated for glucocorticoid use and, for those taking prolonged doses of prednisone ≥10 mg daily (or equivalent) with improvement or no change in disease activity, documentation of glucocorticoid management plan within 12 months |

DMARD = disease-modifying antirheumatic drug; RA = rheumatoid arthritis; TB = tuberculosis.

Table 35. Drugs and Doses Reference Table

Medication Name	Brand Name	Dosing
Methotrexate		5–20 mg by mouth once weekly
Leflunomide	Arava	10–20 mg by mouth once daily
Sulfasalazine	Azulfidine	1–3 g by mouth once or twice daily
Tofacitinib	XELJANZ	5 mg by mouth twice daily
Hydroxychloroquine	Plaquenil	200–600 mg by mouth once daily
Minocycline		100 mg by mouth twice daily
Adalimumab	Humira	40 mg subcutaneously every other week
Certolizumab	Cimzia	200–400 mg subcutaneously every other week (or every 4 weeks)
Golimumab	Simponi	2 mg/kg intravenously at weeks 0 and 4; then every 8 weeks thereafter 50 mg subcutaneously once monthly
Etanercept	Enbrel	50 mg subcutaneously once weekly or 25 mg twice weekly
Infliximab	Remicade	3 mg/kg intravenously at weeks 0, 2, and 6 and then every 8 weeks thereafter
Abatacept	Orencia	Initial weight-based infusion and then: Intravenously at weeks 2 and 4 and then every 4 weeks thereafter 125 mg subcutaneously within 24 hours of infusion and then 125 mg subcutaneously every week thereafter
Rituximab	Rituxan	1000 mg intravenously at days 1 and 15 and then repeated every 24 weeks
Tocilizumab	Actemra	4–8 mg/kg intravenously every 4 weeks
Anakinra	Kineret	100 mg subcutaneously once daily

IV. PSORIATIC ARTHRITIS

A. Clinical Guidelines *(Domain 1; Tasks 3, 6, 7; Knowledge 2/1/2)*
   1. 2009 Group for Research and Assessment of Psoriasis and Psoriatic Arthritis (GRAPPA)
   2. 2008 American Academy of Dermatology guidelines on management of psoriasis and psoriatic arthritis

B. Clinical Presentation
   1. Subtypes
      a. Arthritis mutilans – Progressive disease with "telescoping digits"
      b. Distal interphalangeal disease (DIP arthritis) – Classic symptoms presentation
      c. Oligoarticular – Asymmetric arthritis, typically with dactylitis (sausage digits)
      d. Polyarticular – Symmetric arthritis
      e. Spondyloarthropathy – Symptoms predominantly in vertebrae, hip, and shoulder
   2. History and physical findings
      a. Articular pain, discomfort, and/or malformation
      b. Ocular inflammation
      c. Psoriatic lesions on body
      d. Skin and fingernail symptoms (e.g., fingernail begins to separate from nail bed)

C. Risk Factors
   1. Presence of psoriasis, specifically at sites such as the scalp, nails, and/or gluteus and perineum
   2. Environmental exposures – Trauma (Koebner effect) or infectious origin
   3. Genetic predisposition – First-degree relative with disease increases risk.

D. Disease Complications
   1. Rarely as severe as RA and not usually as debilitating (still painful and debilitating)
   2. May result in premature cardiovascular damage or pulmonary fibrosis

---

Patient Case

9. E.M. is a 35-year-old woman presenting to her primary care physician for a routine follow-up. She has no significant findings in her medical history and is usually without any health concern. However, today, she reports to her physician a 2- to-3 month history of worsening pain in her fingers, hands, hips, and knees. On physical examination, she has "thick" swollen fingers; brittle, pitted nails; and several small scaly lesions on her arms and lower back. The physician performs several blood tests and finds that she has a negative antinuclear antibody (ANA) and RF finding, but a slightly elevated high-sensitivity (hs)–CRP concentration (6.4 mg/dL). From the patient's presentation, physical examination, and laboratory tests, which evidence is the most useful for the physician to use to diagnose psoriatic arthritis in this patient?

   A. Dermatologic findings and hs-CRP concentration greater than 5 mg/dL.
   B. Dactylitis, nail dystrophy, psoriatic-like lesions, and negative RF finding.
   C. Swollen fingers, psoriatic-like lesions, and hs-CRP concentration greater than 5 mg/dL.
   D. Nail dystrophy, negative ANA finding, and negative RF finding.

E. Diagnostic Evaluation *(Domain 1, Task 2, Knowledge 1)*

    1. CASPAR (ClASsification criteria for Psoriatic ARthritis) criteria are both highly sensitive and specific for the diagnosis of psoriatic arthritis.

    2. Requires a score of at least 3 (of possible 6) points plus established articular inflammation

        a. Current (2 points) or history of (1 point) psoriasis

        b. Dactylitis (1 point)

        c. Juxta-articular new bone formation (1 point)

        d. Negative RF finding (1 point)

        e. Nail dystrophy (1 point)

    3. Negative prognostic indicators

        a. More than five actively inflamed joints

        b. Increased acute phase reactants

        c. Evidence of progressive radiographic changes

        d. Previous treatment with glucocorticoids

        e. Functional decline (or loss thereof)

        f. Deteriorated quality of life

F. Treatment Recommendations

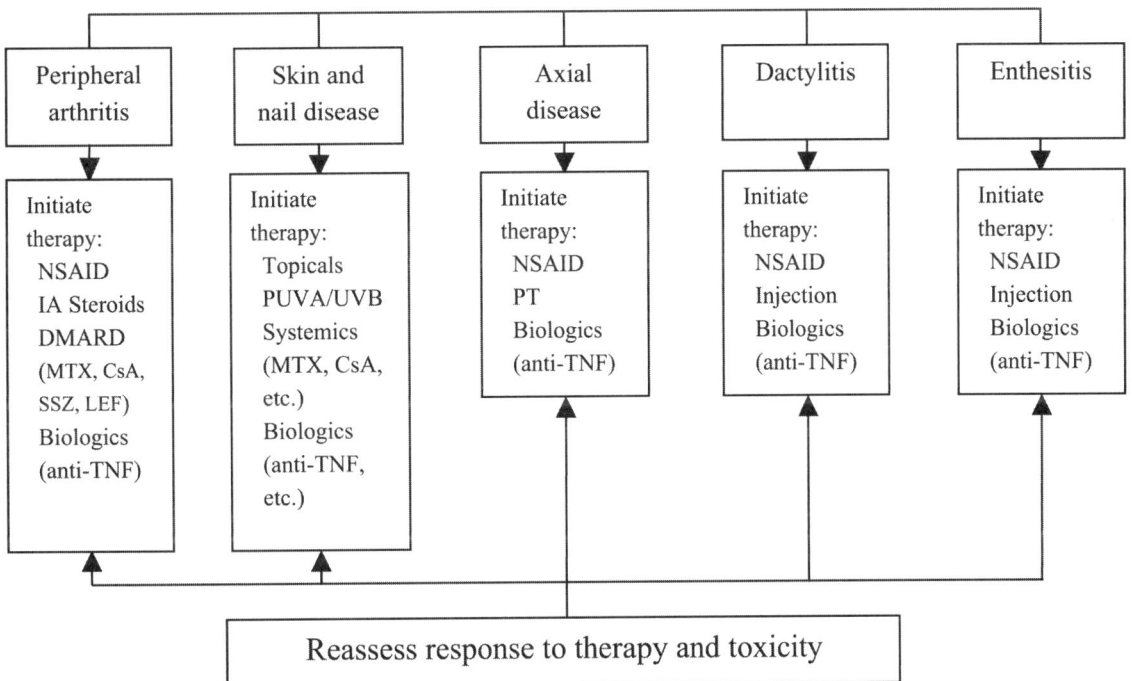

Figure 8. GRAPPA treatment guidelines for psoriatic arthritis.

Anti-TNF = anti–tumor necrosis factor; CsA = cyclosporine A; DMARD = disease-modifying antirheumatic drug; GRAPPA = Group for Research and Assessment of Psoriasis and Psoriatic Arthritis; IA = intra-articular; LEF = leflunomide, MTX = methotrexate; NSAID = nonsteroidal anti-inflammatory drug; PT = physical therapy; PUVA = psoralen ultraviolet A; SSZ = sulfasalazine; UVB = ultraviolet B.

Reprinted with permission from: Ritchlin CT, Kavanaugh A, Gladman DD, et al. Treatment recommendations for psoriatic arthritis. Ann Rheum Dis 2009;68:1387-94.

1. Treatment is based on agents for psoriasis and type of arthritis.
2. Initial therapy is determined by level of severity (mild, moderate, or severe).

Table 36. ACR Recommendations for Classification and Treatment of Psoriatic Arthritis[a]

Classification	Impact on Quality of Life	Therapy Choice(s)
Mild	Minimal	NSAID
Moderate	Affects daily tasks of living and physical/mental functions Lack of response to NSAID	DMARD Anti-TNF

Severe	Cannot perform major daily tasks without pain
	  or dysfunction
	Large impact on physical/mental functions
	Lack of response to either DMARD or TNF blockers
	  as monotherapy
		DMARD plus anti-TNF or
		  other biologic therapy

[a]See Rheumatoid Arthritis section for information about the safety, tolerability, and simplicity of the medications listed below to treat psoriatic arthritis.

ACR = American College of Rheumatology; DMARD = disease-modifying antirheumatic drug; NSAID = nonsteroidal anti-inflammatory drug; TNF = tumor necrosis factor.

Patient Case

10. T.M. is a 42-year-old man with a medical history significant for psoriasis and psoriatic arthritis. His current medications include topical betamethasone/calcipotriene and diclofenac extended release 150 mg daily. His psoriatic arthritis symptoms have been progressively worsening during the past 12 months, and he has been reluctant to use anything more than an NSAID. He has extreme debilitation more days than not and has some periods when he requires assistance with tasks such as dressing and simple cleaning. If he chooses to intensify his therapy, which would be the best approach to his treatment?

   A. Prednisone 10 mg once daily for 6 weeks.
   B. Methotrexate 10 mg once weekly.
   C. Golimumab 50 mg once monthly.
   D. Methotrexate 10 mg once weekly plus golimumab 50 mg once monthly.

---

3. Nonsteroidal anti-inflammatory drugs

Table 37. Efficacy and Preference/Pearls for NSAIDs in Psoriatic Arthritis

Efficacy	Monotherapy with NSAID is as effective as combination therapy with dual-NSAID or non-NSAID analgesic plus NSAID for pain associated with psoriatic arthritis
Preference (Pearls)	NSAIDs may worsen dermatologic symptoms/skin lesions in some patients

NSAID = nonsteroidal anti-inflammatory drug.

4. Nonbiologic DMARDs

Table 38. Efficacy and Preference/Pearls for Nonbiologic DMARDs in Psoriatic Arthritis

Efficacy	Methotrexate, leflunomide, and sulfasalazine all appear effective for reducing dermatologic and peripheral arthritic symptoms
Preference (Pearls)	May be used as first-line therapy in patients with moderate to severe psoriatic arthritis and/or an insufficient response to NSAID therapy

DMARD = disease-modifying antirheumatic drug; NSAID = nonsteroidal anti-inflammatory drug.

5. Biologic DMARDs

Table 39. Efficacy and Preference/Pearls for Biologic DMARDs in Psoriatic Arthritis

Efficacy	All agents (TNF inhibitors, T-cell inhibitor, and IL-12/IL-23 inhibitor) are effective for reducing the symptoms of psoriatic arthritis
Preference (Pearls)	Consider for first-line therapy in patients with moderate to severe symptoms and functional limitations with psoriatic arthritis May consider use in combination with a nonbiologic DMARD for severe or refractory cases of psoriatic arthritis

DMARD = disease-modifying antirheumatic drugs; IL = interleukin; TNF = tumor necrosis factor.

6. Alefacept (Amevive)

Table 40. Alefacept STEPS

Safety	HIV-infected patients should avoid because this medication actively reduces CD4$^+$ counts
	Increased risk of malignancy
	Liver failure
	Lymphopenia and infectious complications including the following:
	  Abscesses
	  Cellulitis
	  Pneumonia
	  Toxic shock syndrome
	  Herpes infection

Tolerability	Injection site reaction Shivering Myalgias
Efficacy	Effective as an add-on for patients with psoriatic arthritis with continued symptoms while treated with methotrexate
Preference (Pearls)	In clinical trials, alefacept was superior to placebo, when added to methotrexate, only in the ACR20 criteria and not the ACR50 or ACR70 criteria Predominantly indicated for psoriatic skin disease as opposed to peripheral arthritis symptoms
Simplicity	Once weekly intramuscular injection

ACR = American College of Rheumatology; HIV = human immunodeficiency virus; STEPS = Safety, Tolerability, Efficacy, Preference (Pearls), Simplicity.

7. Apremilast (Otezla)

Table 41. Apremilast STEPS

Safety	Depression and suicidal ideations
Tolerability	Unintentional weight loss Nausea Diarrhea
Efficacy	As monotherapy, demonstrated improvements in patients' arthritic symptoms and quality of life
Preference (Pearls)	Dose reduction required in patients with CrCl less than 30 mL/minute Dose titration required to help patients with gastrointestinal tolerance In clinical research, improvements over placebo were noted when using both the ACR20 and ACR50 response criteria
Simplicity	Oral medicine dosed once (renally impaired) to twice daily

ACR = American College of Rheumatology; CrCl = creatinine clearance; STEPS = Safety, Tolerability, Efficacy, Preference (Pearls), Simplicity.

8. Ustekinumab (Stelara)

Table 42. Ustekinumab STEPS

Safety	Infections reported in ≥27% of patients Severe infections (2%–3%) such as sepsis, tuberculosis, or opportunistic infections Hypersensitivity reactions Malignancy (Rare) neurotoxicity Many (potentially) significant drug-drug interactions	
Tolerability	Headache Fatigue Arthralgia	
Efficacy	Has demonstrated efficacy in patients with psoriatic arthritis	
Preference (Pearls)	Provide all necessary immunizations before starting therapy If necessary, may administer inactivated vaccines during therapy, but avoid all live vaccines May be used together or in combination with methotrexate In clinical research, improvements vs. placebo are noted in the ACR20 and ACR50 response criteria	
Simplicity	Intravenous administration every 12 weeks First two doses are administered 4 weeks apart	

ACR = American College of Rheumatology; STEPS = Safety, Tolerability, Efficacy, Preference (Pearls), Simplicity.

9. Several agents in the pipeline including brodaulmab
10. Surgery may be necessary for patients whose condition does not respond sufficiently to pharmacotherapy or who have progressive loss of joint function.
11. Psoralen ultraviolet A/ultraviolet B therapy may be helpful for patients with both (extensive) skin and articular disease.

G. Patient Information – Only a few resources are dedicated specifically to psoriatic arthritis because most originate from "arthritis" advocacy and information groups. *(Domain 5, Task 2, Knowledge 5)*
    1. The Arthritis Foundation (www.arthritistoday.org)
    2. The American College of Rheumatology (www.rheumatology.org)
    3. The Mayo Clinic (www.mayoclinic.com)

Table 43. Drugs and Doses Reference Table

Medication Name	Brand Name	Dosing
Methotrexate		5–20 mg by mouth once weekly
Leflunomide	Arava	10–20 mg by mouth once daily
Sulfasalazine	Azulfidine	2–3 g by mouth once or twice daily
Adalimumab	Humira	40 mg subcutaneously every other week
Golimumab	Simponi	50 mg subcutaneously once monthly
Etanercept	Enbrel	50 mg subcutaneously twice weekly for 3 months; then 25 mg twice weekly
Infliximab	Remicade	5 mg/kg IV at weeks 0, 2, and 6; then every 8 weeks thereafter
Abatacept	Orencia	Initial weight-based infusion and then: IV at weeks 2 and 4; then every 4 weeks thereafter 125 mg subcutaneously within 24 hours of infusion; then 125 mg subcutaneously every week thereafter
Alefacept	Amevive	15 mg intramuscular injection each week
Apremilast	Otezla	10 mg once daily on DAY 1 10 mg twice daily on DAY 2 10 mg in the morning and 20 mg in the evening on DAY 3 20 mg in the morning and 20 mg in the evening on DAY 4 20 mg in the morning and 30 mg in the evening on DAY 5 30 mg twice daily thereafter
Ustekinumab	Stelara	45 mg subcutaneously at weeks 0 and 4; then every 12 weeks thereafter

IV = intravenously.

V. OSTEOARTHRITIS

A. Treatment Guidelines
   1. Michigan Quality Improvement Consortium 2007 (updated 2011)
   2. National Institute for Health and Clinical Excellence
   3. American College of Rheumatology 2012

B. Common Sites
   1. Knees
   2. Hips
   3. Small joints of the hand
   4. Low back
   5. Ankle
   6. Elbow

C. Risk Factors
   1. Many risk factors are reversible and/or avoidable.
   2. Risk factors for developing disease are not always risk factors for clinical progression (e.g., a high bone density may be a risk factor for developing osteoarthritis, but a low bone density increases the chance of clinical progression).

Table 44. Factors Associated with Developing Osteoarthritis

Biomechanical	Joint injury Occupational/recreational use Joint laxity	Reduced muscle strength Joint malignancy
Constitutional	Ageing Obesity	Female sex High bone density
Genetic	40%–60% of hand, knee, and hip osteoarthritis is inherited through unknown genes	

Table 45. Clinical Findings in Osteoarthritis by Joint

	Back (chronic low back pain)	Knee	Hand (metacarpophalangeal)
Patient concerns	Low back pain for >3 months	Activity related Instability or buckling Morning stiffness <30 minutes Recurrent pain	Thumb or radial hand pain Difficulty with manual dexterity Gelling with inactivity <10 minutes Morning stiffness <30 minutes
Physical findings	Pain with straight leg raise examination (30–70 degrees)	Bony enlargement Crepitus Limited range of motion	Localized tenderness Limited range of motion
Imaging	Radiography is not routinely recommended for nonspecific back pain Consider MRI or CT for patients only if they are candidates for surgery	Radiography findings may be normal and are only adjunct to diagnosis CT or MRI is not indicated	Radiography (for staging)
Laboratory evaluation	Only in the presence of "red flags"[a]	Erythrocyte sedimentation rate (<40 mm/hour) Rheumatoid factor < 1:40 Synovial fluid aspiration unremarkable	Aspirate evaluation if suspected infection

[a]Red flags: Age at onset > 50 years, pain unrelenting at night or unrelated to activity, widespread symptoms, progressive motor or sensory deficit, unexplained weight loss, fevers/chills/infection, significant trauma, indications of nerve root problem, history of cancer, human immunodeficiency virus, steroids, osteoporosis, or substance abuse.

CT = computed tomography; MRI = magnetic resonance imaging.

D. Nonpharmacologic Interventions
   1. Education about expectations for therapy, importance of nonpharmacologic management strategies, and cognitive behavioral therapy (chronic low back pain)
   2. Weight loss (at least 5%)
   3. Low-impact exercise
   4. Physical therapy (mixed results as beneficial in the short term, but may lessen as patients provide self-care at home after stopping therapy)
   5. Support braces, orthotics, and assistive devices also have mixed results and are not strongly recommended by the American Academy of Orthopedic Surgeons (AAOS).

Patient Case

11. T.W. is a 67-year-old man with severe degenerative joint disease of his right knee. His medical history is significant for coronary artery disease (myocardial infarction 6 years earlier), heart failure (ejection fraction 32%), hypertension, erectile dysfunction, and gastroesophageal reflux disease. He takes lovastatin 40 mg daily, fosinopril 20 mg daily, carvedilol 12.5 mg twice daily, aspirin 81 mg daily, calcium carbonate chewable tablets as needed (around three times weekly), and sildenafil 25 mg as needed. His knee pain causes significant physical limitations, and he is embarrassed to use an electronic cart when he shops at grocery and department stores. He would like to be more active but has difficulty even with the activities of daily living. Given this information, which is the best initial choice for this patient's knee osteoarthritis?

A. Take acetaminophen 650 mg two tablets every 6 hours as needed for pain.

B. Take ibuprofen 400 mg one tablet every 6 hours as needed for pain.

C. Take naproxen 500 mg one tablet every 12 hours as needed for pain.

D. Apply diclofenac 1% gel to affected knee up to four times daily.

Table 46. Pharmacologic Interventions

Class/Agent	Comments
Topical applications	Capsaicin, NSAIDs Topical NSAIDs have proved short-term efficacy, but there is insufficient information to comment on long-term use (>12 weeks), and they are markedly more expensive than oral NSAIDs Topical NSAIDs are recommended over oral NSAIDs for patients >75 years Topical capsaicin should reduce pain in about 2 weeks
Acetaminophen	Recommended as the first-line pharmacologic agent for pain associated with (mild) OA (Exception: Acetaminophen is not recommended by the ACR for hand OA) Maximal dose of 4 g daily is still acceptable, though much more likely to see transaminase elevations with higher doses Most research finds acetaminophen more effective than placebo for OA pain, but only minimally effective overall and less effective than NSAIDs
NSAIDs	Naproxen, ibuprofen NSAIDs are more effective than acetaminophen at reducing pain, but their adverse event profile is less favorable No single NSAID is preferred to another, though the ACR does not recommend ibuprofen for patients using aspirin for cardiovascular disease prevention because of FDA documentation that ibuprofen interferes with aspirin activity The selective COX-2 inhibitor agent celecoxib may also be considered an alternative to nonselective NSAIDs; efficacy profile is the same as that for traditional NSAIDs, but with fewer reports of adverse GI events, and COX-2 agents do not affect platelet function For patients with a history of GI ulceration, a COX-2 inhibitor or an NSAID with a proton pump inhibitor is recommended as primary therapy For patients with a GI bleed in the past 12 months, the ACR recommends using a COX-2 inhibitor with a proton pump inhibitor

Table 46. Pharmacologic Interventions *(continued)*

Class/Agent	Comments
Controlled opioid analgesics	Opioid analgesics may be useful, but they should not be used routinely to treat pain associated with OA Patients may achieve response to therapy, but limit use to patients with severe pain that is inadequately controlled with previously mentioned therapies Likelihood of adverse event similar to that of NSAIDs NOT routinely recommended for OA because risk and severity of adverse events outweigh benefit potential
Glucosamine and chondroitin	Delayed onset of effects, cannot be used for immediate pain relief Glucosamine (with or without chondroitin) has questionable benefits from clinical trials Research is usually small and of variable quality, resulting in highly heterogeneous conclusions in meta-analyses and systematic reviews Chondroitin has demonstrated some benefit for knee OA in studies with high heterogeneity, but it appears to lose efficacy when paired with glucosamine NOT routinely recommended by the ACR
Low-dose corticosteroids	May help with short-term pain reduction and increased mobility for patients with moderate to severe OA of the knee

ACR = American College of Rheumatology; COX-2 = cyclooxygenase-2; FDA = U.S. Food and Drug Administration; GI = gastrointestinal; NSAID = nonsteroidal anti-inflammatory drug; OA = osteoarthritis.

E.   Tramadol (Con Zip, Rybix, Ryzolt, Ultram, Ultram ER [extended release])

Table 47. Tramadol STEPS

Safety	Avoid use (Rybix, Ultram, Ultram ER) in any situation where opioids are not indicated, including acute intoxication with alcohol, hypnotics, opioids, or psychotropic drugs Avoid use (Con Zip, Ryzolt) in patients with severe/acute asthma, hypercapnia, or severe respiratory depression in the absence of resuscitative equipment Contraindicated within 14 days of monoamine oxidase inhibitor therapy Seizures: As monotherapy or with greater risk when combined with other agents that lower the seizure threshold Limit immediate-release dose to 50 mg every 12 hours in patients with cirrhosis Avoid extended-release formulations in severe hepatic impairment (Child-Pugh class C) Cautious use in patients with mild to moderate renal impairment and avoid extended-release formulations in severe renal impairment (CrCl < 30 mL/minute) Risk of serotonin syndrome in patients concurrently using agents that act on the serotonin system	
Tolerability	CNS depression Constipation Dizziness Dyspepsia Flushing	Headache Nausea Postural hypotension Pruritus Somnolence
Efficacy	Provides small degree of pain relief	
Preference (Pearls)	Consider as an alternative in patients who do not receive adequate pain relief from acetaminophen and cannot tolerate it or for whom NSAID therapy is contraindicated	
Simplicity	May administer dose as needed up to four times daily (maximum 100 mg per dose) Classified by the DEA as Schedule IV in August 2014	

CNS = central nervous system; CrCl = creatinine clearance; DEA = Drug Enforcement Agency; ER = extended release; NSAID = nonsteroidal anti-inflammatory drug; STEPS = Safety, Tolerability, Efficacy, Preference (Pearls), Simplicity.

F.   Invasive Interventions
1.   Intra-articular corticosteroids may be effective for short-term pain relief (less than 4 weeks), but there is usually diminishing benefit beyond that time.
a.   Joint injections should not be performed more often than every 3 months.
b.   Osteoarthritis symptoms requiring regular use of corticosteroid injections (three or four a year) should be considered for surgical intervention.
2.   Intra-articular hyaluronic acid may be as effective as intra-articular corticosteroids for some patients, but with benefits observed up to 6 months.
a.   Benefits over corticosteroids not observed until 4 weeks after injections
b.   Much more costly alternative to intra-articular corticosteroids
c.   More frequent injections because many regimens require weekly injections for 3–5 consecutive weeks

G.   Surgery
1.   Total arthroplasty (joint replacement)
2.   Arthroscopic debridement
3.   Arthroscopic lavage

H.   Alternative Treatments *(Domain 1, Task 3, Knowledge 3)*
1.   S-adenosylmethionine may decrease pain and improve functional limitations in patients with osteoarthritis.
2.   Avocado/soybean unsaponifiables appear to help reduce pain in patients with osteoarthritis, but few trials with questionable supportive bias
3.   Devil's claw (*Harpagophytum procumbens*) has been associated with pain reduction in osteoarthritis in several low-quality clinical trials.

I.   Patient Resources
1.   Patient handouts from American Family Physician
2.   Online information from The Arthritis Foundation

Table 48. 2015 Physician Quality Reporting System Quality Measures

No.	Category	Criteria
109	OA: Function and pain assessment	Percentage of patient visits for patients ≥21 years with a diagnosis of OA with assessment for function and pain

OA = osteoarthritis.

VI. FIBROMYALGIA

A. Clinical Guidelines
   1. 2004 American Pain Society (APS) guideline on the management of fibromyalgia syndrome
   2. 2008 EULAR evidence-based recommendations for the management of fibromyalgia syndrome
   3. 2010 ACR preliminary diagnostic criteria for fibromyalgia and measurement of symptom severity

B. Patient Presentation and Symptoms
   1. Patients will experience the following:
      a. Physical symptoms (weakness, fatigue, decrements in physical function, morning stiffness, heat or cold disturbances, swelling in extremities)
      b. Psychological symptoms (mood disturbances)
      c. Cognitive problems (difficulty concentrating, diminished mental clarity, memory problems)
      d. Photophobia, phonophobia, and/or osmophobia

Patient Case

12. M.F. is a 32-year-old woman presenting to her primary care physician's office with fatigue, "pain all over," and headaches for the past 4 weeks. She has a history of major depression, but she has been successfully treated with regular counseling. She reports having a dull, aching pain most days in her shoulders and upper arms (bilateral), hips (bilateral), neck, and lower back. She says that she has fatigue daily (cannot play with children), difficulty sleeping 2 or 3 nights per week, and chronic headaches. She heard from a friend that she has all the symptoms of fibromyalgia and would like to be treated. Which is the best response for the physician to provide to the patient?

   A. Her symptoms do not meet the fibromyalgia diagnosis criteria.
   B. Her fibromyalgia would benefit most from tai chi.
   C. Her fibromyalgia requires drug therapy.
   D. Her fibromyalgia will require treatment with a two-drug regimen.

3 months.

---

   2. Diagnostic tools
      a. Widespread pain index (WPI): Award 1 point for each location a patient has experienced pain in the past 7 days.

Shoulder girdle, left	Shoulder girdle, right	Upper arm, left	Upper arm, right	Lower arm, left
Upper leg, left	Upper leg, right	Hip (buttock, trochanter), left	Hip (buttock, trochanter), right	Lower arm, right
Lower leg, left	Lower left, right	Jaw, left	Jaw, right	Chest
Abdomen	Upper back	Lower back	Neck	

    b. Symptom severity scale (SSS): Award 0–3 points for each level of severity of fatigue, waking unrefreshed, cognitive symptoms, and somatic symptoms.

        i.   0 = No problem/symptoms

        ii.   1 = Slight or mild problems/few symptoms

        iii. 2 = Moderate or considerable problems/moderate number of symptoms

        iv. 3 = Severe, pervasive, life-disturbing problems/great deal of symptoms

    c. ACR updated the diagnosis in 2010 to include the following:

        i.   Symptoms for more than 3 months PLUS

           (a) WPI of 7 or higher and an SSS of 5 or higher -OR-

           (b) WPI of 3–6 and an SSS of 9 or higher

        ii.   Absence of other disorders that could cause the same symptoms

C. Professional Treatment Recommendations (APS and EULAR)

    1. Educate patients about pain management and self-management.

    2. Cognitive behavioral therapy will help reduce pain, improve function, and enhance self-efficacy.

    3. Exercise programs should be of "moderate" intensity.

        a. High-intensity exercise will make symptoms of fibromyalgia worse.

        b. Exercise recommendations state the patient should exercise two to three times per week to a target of 60%–75% of his or her age-adjusted maximum heart rate (210 minus patient age).

        c. Patients should stretch before exercise to the point of mild resistance to reduce exercise-induced pain and injury.

    4. Other nonpharmacologic treatments

        a. Acupuncture

        b. Biofeedback

        c. Chiropractic manipulation

        d. Heated pool treatments (with or without exercise)

        e. Hypnosis

        f. Osteopathic manipulation

        g. Therapeutic massage

    5. Pharmacologic treatment strategy

        a. Tricyclic antidepressants, particularly amitriptyline, are the first-line treatment for reducing pain and symptoms associated with fibromyalgia.

        b. If patient has a contraindication to, cannot tolerate, or does not achieve response to therapy with a tricyclic antidepressant (at target does), consider therapy with an alternative agent.

        c. Additional classes with efficacy (vs. placebo) include the following:

           i. $\alpha2\delta$ Ligands (gabapentin, pregabalin)

           ii.   Dopamine D_3 receptor agonists (pramipexole)

           iii. Selective serotonin reuptake inhibitors (fluoxetine, paroxetine)

           iv. Serotonin and norepinephrine dual reuptake inhibitors (duloxetine, milnacipran)

           v.   Nonopioid μ-receptor antagonist (tramadol)

    6. Tricyclic antidepressants

        a. Amitriptyline

        b. Cyclobenzaprine

        c. Nortriptyline

Table 49. Tricyclic Antidepressant STEPS

Safety	FDA warns that antidepressants increase the risk of suicidal thinking and behavior in children, adolescents, and young adults with major depressive disorder Orthostatic hypotension Use with caution in patients with a history of cardiovascular disease, diabetes, hepatic impairment, mania/hypomania, renal impairment, seizure disorders, or thyroid dysfunction Patients should discontinue tricyclic antidepressants before general elective surgery that requires anesthesia

Tolerability	Anticholinergic effects Anorexia Dizziness Hypertension/hypotension Insomnia Numbness	Paresthesia Syncope Tachycardia Urticaria Weight gain

Efficacy	Tricyclic antidepressants, particularly amitriptyline, are the best medication intervention for improving the symptoms of fibromyalgia Have been proved to decrease symptoms of pain, fatigue, sleep, and depressed mood
Preference (Pearls)	Target dose of amitriptyline or cyclobenzaprine is 10–30 mg in the evening before sleep Likelihood of experiencing pain relief is about the same as the likelihood of experiencing an adverse event
Simplicity	Once-daily dosing in the evening, before sleep, to decrease adverse event severity

FDA = U.S. Food and Drug Administration; STEPS = Safety, Tolerability, Efficacy, Preference (Pearls), Simplicity.

Patient Case

13. S.E. is a 39-year-old woman with a medical history significant for minor depressive disorder. She is presenting to a medication management clinic after having initiated amitriptyline therapy for fibromyalgia. She raised the dose to 50 mg during the past 4 weeks and reports that she has not experienced a significant change in her symptoms. However, she does report that her negative feelings have lessened and that her sleep is much improved, but the pain and discomfort associated with her fibromyalgia remain. She is requesting a new medication to help control her symptoms. Which medication would be best to replace amitriptyline?

    A. Gabapentin titrated to 800 mg three times daily.
    B. Pregabalin 75 mg twice daily.
    C. Duloxetine 60 mg once daily.
    D. Tramadol 50 mg every 6 hours as needed for pain.

7. Selective serotonin reuptake inhibitors
   a. Fluoxetine
   b. Paroxetine

Table 50. Selective Serotonin Reuptake Inhibitor STEPS

Safety	See above for FDA warning about suicidal ideations with anitdepressants Allergic skin reactions May increase bleeding risk when used in conjunction with antiplatelet or anticoagulation therapy Use with caution in patients with a history of cardiovascular disease, diabetes, mania/hypomania, hepatic effects, renal impairment, and/or seizure disorders	
Tolerability	Anticholinergic effects Diarrhea Dizziness Dyspepsia	Headaches Insomnia Nausea Sexual dysfunction
Efficacy	Evidence is available to support use in fibromyalgia, but strength of recommendation is not as strong as with tricyclic antidepressants The combination of a selective serotonin reuptake inhibitor and a tricyclic antidepressant is better than either class alone	
Preference (Pearls)	Fluoxetine and paroxetine are the most often studied agents to have an effect in patients with fibromyalgia symptoms Small clinical trial with citalopram vs. placebo did not show significantly reduced symptoms	
Simplicity	Once-daily dosing	

FDA = U.S. Food and Drug Administration; STEPS = Safety, Tolerability, Efficacy, Preference (Pearls), Simplicity.

8. Serotonin and norepinephrine dual reuptake inhibitors
    a. Duloxetine
    b. Milnacipran

Table 51. Serotonin and Norepinephrine Dual Reuptake Inhibitor STEPS

Safety	See above for FDA warning about suicidal ideations with antidepressants Increased risk of bleeding when used with antiplatelet or anticoagulation therapy Severe skin reactions have been reported with duloxetine Blood pressure and heart rate may be increased with milnacipran	
Tolerability	Anticholinergic effects Dizziness Headache Hyperhidrosis Insomnia	Nausea Hot flashes (milnacipran) Sexual dysfunction

Efficacy	Agents equally improve pain, sleep, depressed mood, and quality of life in patients
	  with fibromyalgia
	Duloxetine 60 mg or 120 mg daily is effective for treating fibromyalgia syndrome
	Milnacipran's target dose is 50 mg twice daily (start with 12.5 mg twice daily and titrate
	  every 7 days to target dose)
	Class efficacy is equal to that of pregabalin, but assumed from indirect comparisons of all three agents	

Preference (Pearls)	Both duloxetine and milnacipran are FDA approved for treating fibromyalgia syndrome Duloxetine requires dose adjustments when creatinine clearance is <30 mL/minute	
Simplicity	Agents are dosed once or twice daily and have a relatively quick onset of effect	

FDA = U.S. Food and Drug Administration; STEPS = Safety, Tolerability, Efficacy, Preference (Pearls), Simplicity.

9. α2δ Ligand
    a. Gabapentin
    b. Pregabalin

Table 52. α2δ Ligand STEPS

Safety	Safety concerns are relatively rare, but still present:
	  Angioedema
	  Visual field disturbances have been reported
	Use with caution in patients with cardiac disease, particularly heart failure,
	  because of the risk of edema	

Tolerability	Dizziness Edema (peripheral)	Somnolence Weight gain
Efficacy	Both gabapentin and pregabalin are effective for improving pain, sleep, fatigue, and quality of life Poor tolerability reported in clinical trials	

Table 52. α2δ Ligand STEPS *(continued)*

Preference (Pearls)	Target dose: Gabapentin 2400 mg daily Pregabalin 300–450 mg daily Dosage adjustments are required in patients with renal impairment Pregabalin is registered as a schedule V substance (euphoria)
Simplicity	Pregabalin is dosed twice daily Titration schedule for gabapentin is relatively difficult and requires thrice-daily dosing

STEPS = Safety, Tolerability, Efficacy, Preference (Pearls), Simplicity.

10. Nonopioid μ-receptor antagonist (tramadol)
    a. See STEPS analysis and Osteoarthritis section.
    b. The APS recommends using tramadol when all other pain relief therapies have been exhausted.
11. Dopamine D_3 receptor agonists (pramipexole): One small clinical trial (60 patients) reported at least a 50% improvement in symptoms in significantly more patients using pramipexole titrated to 4.5 mg daily than with placebo.

D. Patient Information
1. Medications are effective for symptom relief, but all professional organizations advocate for education and cognitive behavioral therapy as the root of all treatments.
2. Most clinical trials evaluate and report symptom improvement and not complete symptom resolution.
3. Patient information resources available online
    a. Arthritis Foundation offers a variety of resources, including a self-help course, books, and educational videos (www.arthritis.org/conditions-treatments/disease-center/fibromyalgia-fms/).
    b. Exercise videos are available for purchase ($30 per video) through the Fibromyalgia Information Foundation (www.myalgia.com).

Table 53. Drugs and Doses Reference Table

Medication Name	Brand Name	Dosing
Amitriptyline	Elavil	25–100 mg once daily at bedtime
Nortriptyline	Pamelor	25–100 mg once daily at bedtime
Cyclobenzaprine	Flexeril	5–10 mg by mouth three times daily
Fluoxetine	Prozac	20–80 mg by mouth once daily
Paroxetine	Paxil	20–60 mg by mouth once daily
Duloxetine	Cymbalta	60 mg by mouth once daily
Milnacipran	Savella	50 mg by mouth twice daily
Gabapentin	Neurontin	300–1200 mg by mouth three times daily
Pregabalin	Lyrica	75–150 mg twice daily

VII. SYSTEMIC LUPUS ERYTHEMATOSUS

A. Clinical Guidelines
    1. 2008 EULAR recommendations on management of SLE
    2. 2008 EULAR recommendation on monitoring patients with SLE in clinical practice and in observational studies

Table 54. Definitions/Stages of SLE

Active SLE	The patient has signs/symptoms and tests that are attributed to inflammation and are reversible (target organ damage) with therapy
Mild SLE	The patient's condition is clinically stable without progressing organ damage or toxicity
Uncontrolled SLE	The patient's signs/symptoms of SLE continue despite pharmacologic treatment
Remission	The patient does not have signs/symptoms of SLE and is not receiving treatment
Complete response	Clinical remission with pharmacologic treatment

SLE = systemic lupus erythematosus.

Table 55. Organ Systems Involved and Potential Complications

Organ System	Potential Complications
Cardiovascular	Hypertension, dyslipidemia, endocarditis, pericardial effusion, valvular disease
Central nervous system	Cognitive disorders, neuropsychiatric disorders, depression, seizures
Gastrointestinal tract	Mesenteric vasculitis, pancreatitis
Hematologic/oncologic	Hemolytic anemia, neutropenia, thrombosis, thrombocytopenia, thrombotic thrombocytopenic purpura, non-Hodgkin lymphoma
Joints	Arthritis
Kidneys	Renal disease (lupus nephropathy or lupus nephritis)
Lungs	Pulmonary hypertension, pneumonitis, pulmonary embolus, interstitial fibrosis

B. Risk Factors for Disease
    1. Family history of SLE or other autoimmune disorders
    2. Exposure to silica, mercury, and/or pesticides
    3. Drug-induced disease
        a. Captopril
        b. Chlorpromazine
        c. Hydralazine
        d. Isoniazid
        e. Methyldopa
        f. Procainamide
        g. Quinidine
        h. Sulfasalazine
        i. Estrogens and oral contraceptives (not causative, but may provoke and worsen flares in patients with lupus)

C. Clinical Presentation: There are several clinical findings during a patient's history and physical examination, but some are more common than others.

Table 56. Frequency of Presenting Symptoms

Symptoms	Frequency, %
Arthritis	48.1
Malar rash	31.1
Active nephropathy	27.9
Neurologic changes	19.4
Fever	16.6
Raynaud phenomenon	16.3
Serositis	16
Thrombocytopenia	13.4
Thrombosis	9.2

D. Diagnosis
1. ACR criteria for classification require four positive (of possible 11) findings.
2. Findings may be present sequentially or at the same time.

Table 57. Eleven Criteria to Evaluate for the Diagnosis of Systemic Lupus Erythematosus

Malar (butterfly) rash	Discoid lupus	Photosensitivity
Oral or nasopharyngeal ulcers	Serositis	Nonerosive arthritis
Persistent proteinuria or casts	Immunologic abnormalities	Hematologic changes
Nonorganic seizures or psychosis	Positive ANA test result without drug-induced causes	

ANA = antinuclear antibody.

Table 58. Diagnostic Testing for Systemic Lupus Erythematosus

Antinuclear antibody	Anti–double-stranded DNA antibody	Anti-Ro antibody
Anti-La antibody	Anti-RNP antibody	Anti-Sm antibody
Anti-phospholipid	C3, C4	

RNP = ribonucleic protein.

Table 59. Other Pretreatment and "Routine" Testing for Systemic Lupus Erythematosus

Baseline		
Validated symptoms survey	Quality-of-life assessment	Ophthalmologic examination[a]
Routine every 6–12 months		
Complete blood cell count	Erythrocyte sedimentation rate	C-reactive protein
Albumin, serum	Creatinine, serum	Urinalysis
Creatinine/microalbumin ratio		

[a]See antimalarial drugs for more specific recommendations.

E.   Drug Treatment Strategies (EULAR recommendations)
1.   Antimalarial drugs are first-line therapy for all patients with newly diagnosed SLE and/or without major organ involvement, unless otherwise contraindicated.
2.   Systemic corticosteroids may be used to prevent flares and clinical relapse.
3.   Steroids can be used in addition to antimalarial agents to control symptoms and prevent seromarker elevation.
4.   NSAIDs may be used for a brief period, but patients need to be aware of gastrointestinal, cardiovascular, and/or renal complications.
5.   Immunosuppressive agents (methotrexate, azathioprine, and/or mycophenolate) are reserved for patients who cannot achieve disease control with antimalarial drugs and corticosteroids.

Patient Case

14.   D.B. is a 29-year-old woman with a medical history significant for SLE and lupus nephritis. Her current treatment is hydroxychloroquine 200 mg once daily, but she continues to have complications because of the disease, including persistent proteinuria and serositis. To control her symptoms, which intervention would be best?

A.   Increase the hydroxychloroquine dose to achieve a serum concentration greater than 1000 ng/mL.
B.   Add prednisone 40 mg daily for the next 6 months.
C.   Add omega-3 fatty acids (eicosapentaenoic acid [EPA] 1.8 g and docosahexaenoic acid [DHA] 1.2 g) per day.
D.   Add azathioprine 2 mg/kg/day.

6. Antimalarial agents
   a. Chloroquine
   b. Hydroxychloroquine

Table 60. Antimalarial Agents STEPS

Safety	Cardiomyopathy with long-term hydroxychloroquine use (rare)
	May cause the following:
	  Agranulocytosis, aplastic anemia, and/or thrombocytopenia
	  Exfoliative dermatitis, Stevens-Johnson syndrome
	  Myopathy and muscle weakness
	  Exacerbation of porphyria and/or psoriasis
	Loss of visual acuity and macular pigment changes (risk is highest with hydroxychloroquine doses > 6.5 mg/kg of lean body weight)
	Use with caution in patients with hepatic disease or receiving concurrent hepatotoxic agents

Tolerability	Abdominal cramping Nightmares Alopecia Psychosis Diarrhea Tinnitus Emotional changes Urticaria
Efficacy	Reduces disease activity in most patients and reduces the average dose of corticosteroids needed to control symptoms Associated with a reduction in mortality, irreversible organ damage, and progression to active disease
Preference (Pearls)	Recommended as first-line treatment by both EULAR (SLE without major organ involvement) and ACR (mild SLE) Dosing to achieve serum hydroxychloroquine concentration > 1000 ng/mL does not reduce the likelihood of disease flare American Academy of Ophthalmology recommends that patients have funduscopic and visual field examination within the first year of starting hydroxychloroquine; ophthalmologic screening recommendations are based on risk of drug-related disease (see Table 61)
Simplicity	Initially dosed once or twice daily until sufficient patient response Once-daily maintenance dosing

ACR = American College of Rheumatology; EULAR = European League Against Rheumatism; SLE = systemic lupus erythematosus; STEPS = Safety, Tolerability, Efficacy, Preference (Pearls), Simplicity.

Table 61. Ophthalmologic Screening Recommendations for Patients Treated with Antimalarial Agents

Risk Category	Recommendations	Criteria
Low	Screen as part of regular examination during the first 5 years Reevaluate if drug dose is increased or if there are changes in patient weight or renal/hepatic function	Dose < 6.5 mg/kg for hydroxychloroquine or 3 mg/kg for chloroquine Treatment for <5 years Lean or average fat level No renal or hepatic disease <60 years old

High	Annual screening
	May require additional testing for:
	    Extended therapy duration
	    Doses > 10 mg/day
		Dose > 6.5 mg/kg for hydroxychloroquine or 3 mg/kg for chloroquine
		Treatment for >5 years
		High fat level (unless dose adjusted for obesity)
		Renal or hepatic disease
		Current retinal disease
		>60 years old

7. Corticosteroids (see Rheumatoid Arthritis section for full STEPS analysis)
   a. Corticosteroids will delay the onset and prevent relapse or flares of SLE.
   b. May be dosed daily or on opposite days for patients with stable disease
   c. Doses of 20 mg or higher (prednisone equivalent) may be necessary for patients with progressive end-organ damage caused by lupus.
8. Immunosuppressive therapy (azathioprine, cyclosporine, methotrexate, mycophenolate mofetil)
   a. Agent of choice for patients when unable to prevent disease progression or induce remission with antimalarial drugs
   b. Recommended for patients with organ involvement (neuropsychiatric lupus, lupus nephritis, cutaneous lupus)
   c. Consider for use in patients who are unable to reduce their corticosteroid dose (to less than 10 mg of prednisone equivalent) per day
   d. Appears that azathioprine and cyclosporine are equal with respect to efficacy and safety in patients with SLE
   e. Both methotrexate and mycophenolate mofetil will decrease steroid requirements for patients treated with higher-than-acceptable corticosteroid doses.
   f. Rituximab, belimumab, or epratuzumab (investigational), added to standard therapy, has demonstrated benefits in patients with treatment refractory disease.

F. Nonpharmacologic Interventions
   1. Lifestyle modifications include smoking cessation, weight control, and exercise (where applicable).
      a. Omega-3 fatty acid intake (1.2 g of DHA and 1.8 g of EPA each day) reduced scores on validated SLE symptom surveys.
      b. Cardiovascular training programs may improve SLE symptom score surveys.
      c. Cognitive behavioral therapy and counseling may reduce fatigue and improve patient-reported mental health.
   2. Recommend that patients regularly use sunscreen in all outdoor exposure
   3. Do not use live vaccines in patients taking greater than 20 mg of corticosteroids (prednisone equivalents) each day.

G. Patient Information – Several online resources and professional groups provide patient information.
1. American College of Rheumatology (www.rheumatology.org)
2. Lupus Foundation of America (www.lupus.org)
3. National Institute of Arthritis and Musculoskeletal and Skin Disease (www.naims.nih.gov)

Table 62. Drugs and Doses Reference Table

Medication Name	Brand Name	Dosing
Hydroxychloroquine	Plaquenil	400–600 mg by mouth each day

VIII.   GOUT AND HYPERURICEMIA

A. Professional Treatment Recommendations and Guidelines
1. 2012 ACR guidelines for the management of gout
2. 2006 EULAR evidence-based recommendations for the diagnosis and management of gout
3. 2007 British Society for Rheumatology guideline for the management of gout

B. Gout and Hyperuricemia
1. Peak onset is between 40 and 60 years of age.
2. Men are 3–4 times more likely to develop gout and hyperuricemia, but the gender gap is less compared with postmenopausal women (estrogen stimulates renal elimination of uric acid).

Table 63. Characteristics of Gout

Type	Characteristics
Acute gout (gouty arthritis)	Severe pain and swelling with erythema First event is usually monoarticular (first metatarsophalangeal joint) and presents to patient overnight or in the early morning Subsequent attacks may involve more joints such as the ankle, finger(s), foot, knee, and/or wrist May resemble cellulitis
Chronic tophaceous gout	Persistent pain and swelling, accompanied by joint stiffness Polyarticular involvement Soft tissue mass composed of monosodium urate crystals and forming in areas of lowest body temperature (fingers, hands, ears) Frequent recurrent attacks Persistently elevated serum uric acid concentrations

Table 64. Risk Factors for Developing Gout and Hyperuricemia (uric acid, serum concentration greater than 6.8 mg/dL)

Conditions	Lifestyle	Medications
Alcoholism Cardiovascular disease Diabetes mellitus Dyslipidemia Hypothyroidism Lead exposure Metabolic syndrome Organ transplant Renal disease Myeloproliferative disorders Genetic disorders	Obesity Increased animal purine intake Consuming high-fructose foods and drinks Alcohol (beers, liquors more than wines)	Thiazide diuretics Low- to moderate-dose aspirin Ethambutol Nicotinic acid Vitamin B_{12} Cyclosporine Levodopa Pyrazinamide Cytotoxic agents Ethanol

Table 65. Factors Associated with the Underexcretion or Overproduction of Uric Acid

Underexcretion of urate	Primary	Dehydration Hypertension Hyperparathyroidism Hypothyroidism Lactic acidosis Renal insufficiency Lead exposure ("saturnine gout")
	Secondary	Ketosis Drug induced Aspirin ($\leq$325 mg daily) Cyclosporine Diuretics Ethambutol Ethanol Levodopa Niacin Pyrazinamide
Overproduction of urate	Primary	Hypoxanthine-guanine phosphoribosyltransferase deficiency, phosphoribosyl pyrophosphate enzyme synthase activity, type I glycogen storage disease (von Gierke disease)
	Secondary	Excessive purine intake Exfoliative psoriasis Hypertriglyceridemia Rapidly dividing tumors Tumor lysis syndrome Myeloproliferative/lymphoproliferative disorders Cytotoxic agents Vitamin B_{12} Alcohol/ethanol

C. Gout Complications
1. Uric acid nephrolithiasis
2. Acute uric acid nephropathy
3. Chronic kidney disease secondary to urate crystal deposition

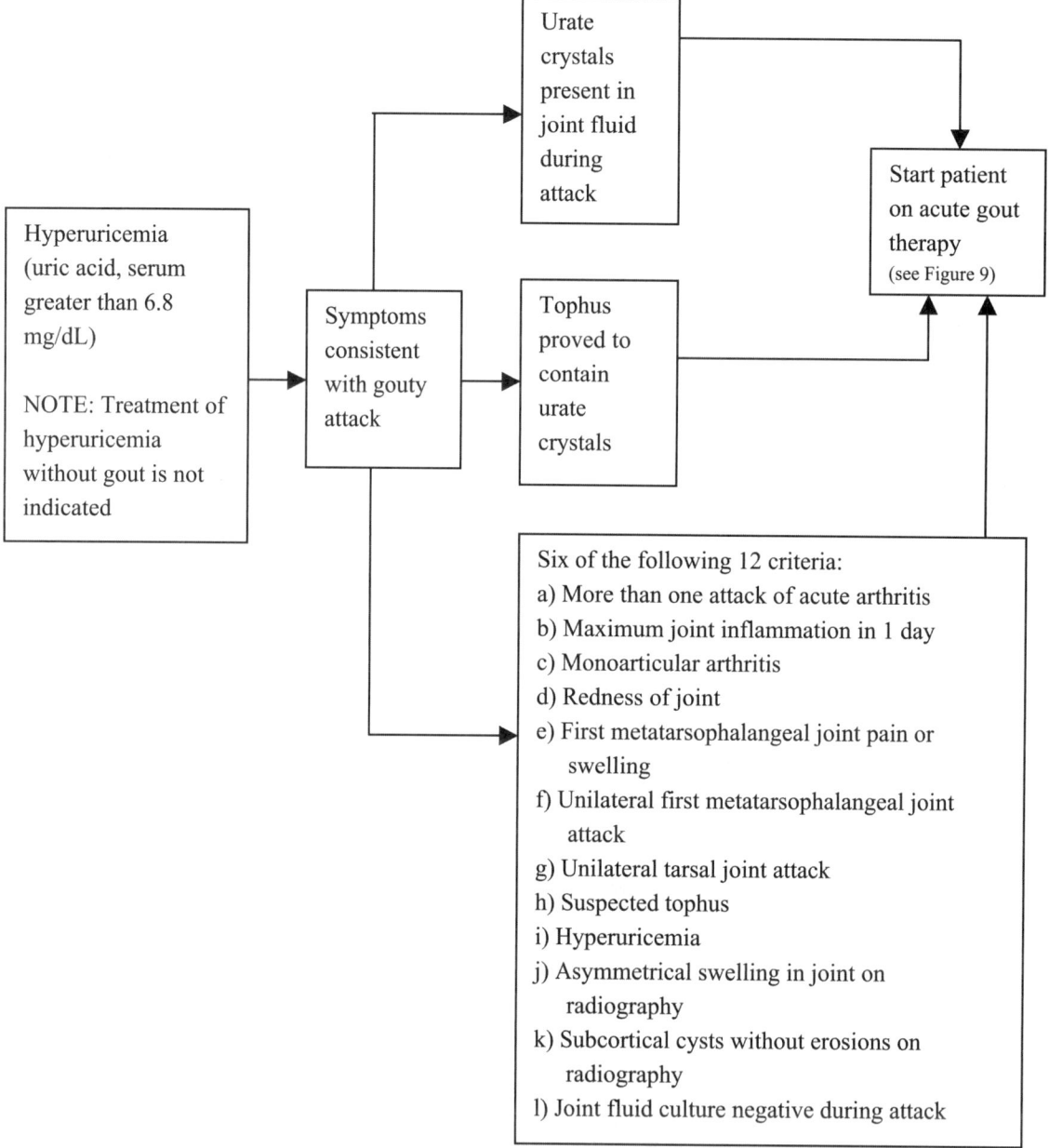

Figure 9. Decision to treat acute gout symptoms.

Based on the American College of Rheumatology preliminary criteria for the classification of the acute arthritis of primary gout (1977), as derived from: Wallace SL, Robinson H, Masi AT, et al. Preliminary criteria for the classification of the acute arthritis of primary gout. Arthritis Rheum 1977;20:895-900.

D. Treatment Options for Acute Attacks
    1. Nonpharmacologic
        a. Rest and elevate the affected joint(s).
        b. Ice packs

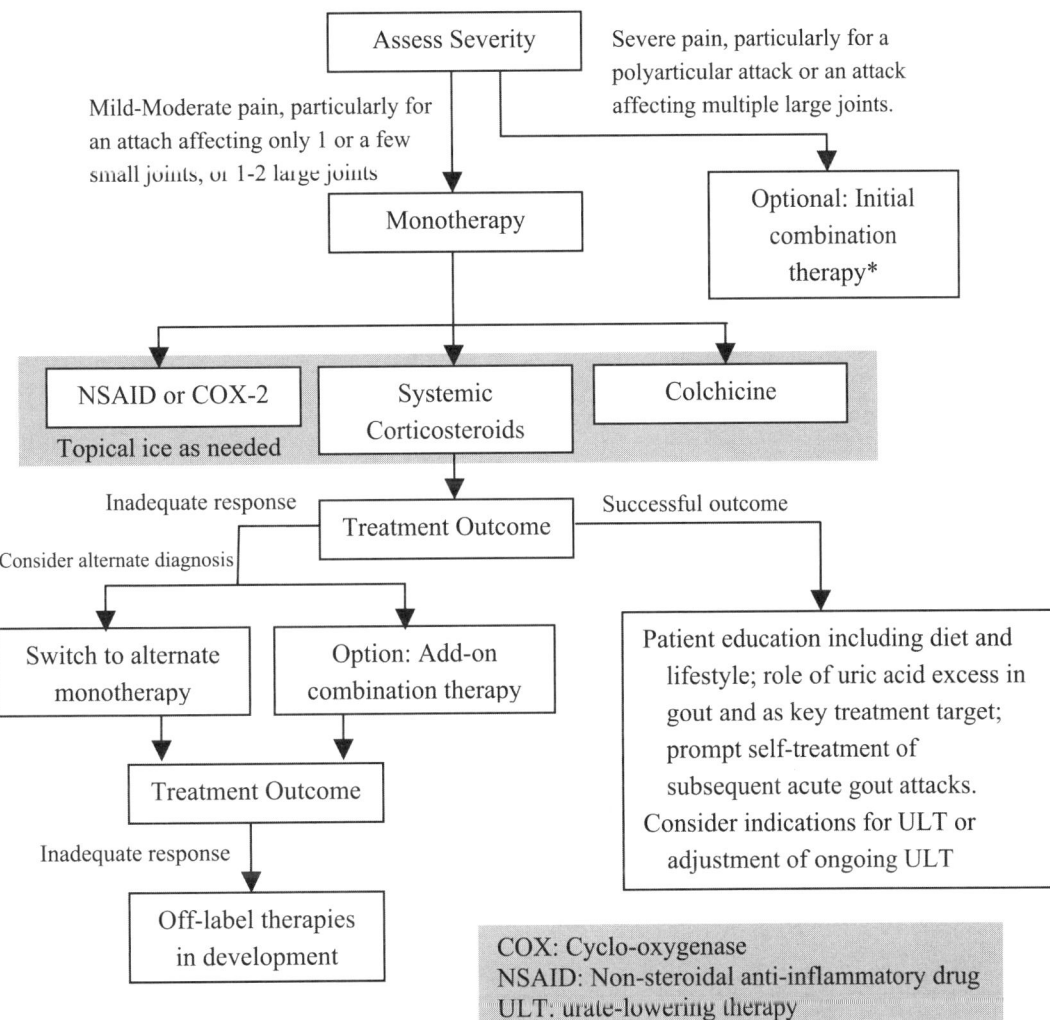

Figure 10. Management of acute gouty attack.

Reprinted with permission from: Khanna D, Khanna PP, Fitzgerald J, et al. 2012 American College of Rheumatology guidelines for the management of gout, part 2: therapy and anti-inflammatory prophylaxis of acute gouty arthritis. Arthritis Care Res 2012;64:1447-61.

    2. Pharmacologic
        a. Nonsteroidal anti-inflammatory drugs
            i. Safety and tolerability discussed above in the Rheumatoid Arthritis section
            ii. All NSAIDs appear equally effective.
            iii. Treatment should continue until symptoms subside (1–2 weeks).

Patient Case

15. M.K. is a 46-year-old man with a medical history significant for chest pain with exertion, dyslipidemia, impaired fasting glucose, hypertension, obesity, and gout (one episode, 5 months ago). His current medications include simvastatin 40 mg daily, nicotinic acid (extended release) 1000 mg at bedtime, lisinopril 40 mg daily, amlodipine 5 mg daily, and aspirin 81 mg daily. He presents to his primary care practitioner's office with symptoms consistent with gout in his left first metatarsophalangeal joint and left ankle, starting this morning. The metatarsophalangeal joint is swollen, inflamed, erythematous, and sensitive to light touch. Which is the best approach to therapy for M.K.?

   A. Colchicine 1.2 mg for first dose and then 0.6 mg 1 hour after.
   B. Colchicine 1.2 mg for first dose and then 0.6 mg 1 hour after; also, start allopurinol 300 mg once daily.
   C. Colchicine 1.2 mg for first dose and then 0.6 mg every hour thereafter as tolerated.
   D. Colchicine 1.2 mg for first dose and then 0.6 mg every hour thereafter as tolerated; also, start allopurinol 300 mg once daily.

    b.   Colchicine

Table 66. Colchicine STEPS

Safety	Doses > 4 mg may cause multiple organ failure and death
	Dose adjustment not necessary when CrCl > 30 mL/minute
	When CrCl < 30 mL/minute:
	  Do not use more than one acute treatment course every 2 weeks
	  Do not use >0.3 mg daily for prophylaxis initially
	Metabolized by the cytochrome P450 3A4 enzyme (elevated plasma colchicine concentrations can lead to fatal toxicity)
	Risk of adverse hematologic events includes myelosuppression, leukopenia, thrombocytopenia, and/or pancytopenia

Tolerability	GI discomfort Diarrhea
Efficacy	New(er) dosing strategy decreases the likelihood of adverse events without affecting efficacy
Preference (Pearls)	Slower to work than NSAIDs for pain relief, but still at least a 50% reduction in pain at 24 hours
Simplicity	Two tablets (0.6 mg each x 2 = 1.2 mg) within 12 hours of onset and one (0.6 mg) tablet 60 minutes later 2012 ACR recommendations suggest using 0.6 mg every 12 hours until acute symptoms resolve, starting immediately after the second 0.6-mg treatment dose

ACR = American College of Rheumatology; CrCl = creatinine clearance; GI = gastrointestinal; NSAID = nonsteroidal anti-inflammatory drug; STEPS = Safety, Tolerability, Efficacy, Preference (Pearls), Simplicity.

    c.   Corticosteroids
        i.   Safety and tolerability discussed above in the Rheumatoid Arthritis section
        ii.   Excellent option for patients with acute gout and renal insufficiency
        iii.   Prednisone is equal in efficacy to NSAIDs for reducing pain and discomfort.
        iv.   Intra-articular corticosteroids are especially effective with large joint involvement.
        v.   Intra-articular formulations show benefits superior to oral NSAIDs at 72 hours, but equal at 1 week.

E. Prevention Options for Recurrent Attacks
1. Nonpharmacologic
   a. Adequate hydration (2 L or more of water daily)
   b. Discontinue diuretic therapy whenever possible.
   c. Moderate, low-impact exercise
   d. Restrict dietary animal and yeast purine intake and alcohol (especially beer).
   e. Avoid highly refined carbohydrates and sugars.
   f. Weight reduction
2. Consideration and expectations of prevention
   a. Consider preventive therapy in individuals experiencing more than one acute gouty arthritis attack per year.
   b. Therapy goal is serum uric acid concentrations less than 5 mg/dL (with tophi) or 6 mg/dL (without tophi).
   c. 2012 guidelines suggest that prophylactic therapy can be initiated during an acute gouty attack, provided anti-inflammatory management has been started.
   d. Evaluate serum uric acid concentrations every 3 months for the first year after an attack and then annually thereafter.
   e. May try to discontinue agents at any time, but most will have at least one gouty attack (90%) during the next 10 years

3. Xanthine oxidase inhibitors
   a. Allopurinol (Zyloprim)
   b. Febuxostat (Uloric)

Table 67. Allopurinol STEPS

Safety	Exfoliative dermatitis Stevens-Johnson syndrome Hepatotoxicity	Mucositis Renal insufficiency Thiazides decrease excretion of allopurinol
Tolerability	Elevated transaminases or alkaline phosphatase values Transient rash	
Efficacy	Shown to prevent recurrent gouty arthritis attacks and reduce uric acid concentrations Useful to reduce tophi in patients with tophaceous gout	
Preference (Pearls)	First-line agent for prevention of recurrent gout and hyperuricemia Evaluate renal function for possible dose adjustments NOT for use in patients with asymptomatic hyperuricemia Do not stop therapy during an acute attack if the patient's condition is already managed with allopurinol Start at 100 mg daily and titrate by 100 mg daily every 2–4 weeks (maximum 800 mg daily) to achieve a uric acid concentration < 5–6 mg/dL Maximal dose should be 200 mg/day with CrCl < 20 mL/minute and <100 mg/day with CrCl < 10 mL/minute 2012 ACR guidelines suggest HALB*5801 testing for at-risk populations (patients of Korean descent with CKD stage 3 or worse, Han Chinese descent, or Thai descent)	
Simplicity	Daily dosing Relatively inexpensive (<$20 a month)	

ACR = American College of Rheumatology; CKD = chronic kidney disease; CrCl = creatinine clearance; STEPS = Safety, Tolerability, Efficacy, Preference (Pearls), Simplicity.

Table 68. Febuxostat STEPS

Safety	Contraindicated in patients using azathioprine, mercaptopurine, or theophylline (Canada only) Higher incidence of cardiovascular events observed compared with incidence in patients using allopurinol, though no causal relationship has been proved Hepatotoxicity
Tolerability	Arthralgias Nausea Rash
Efficacy	Approved to treat hyperuricemia in patients with gout
Preference (Pearls)	Greater efficacy for reducing uric acid concentration, but no more efficacious for preventing gout flares than allopurinol Used to reduce tophi in patients with tophaceous gout NOT for use in patients with asymptomatic hyperuricemia
Simplicity	Daily dosing Considerably more expensive than allopurinol (about $150–$200 per month)

STEPS = Safety, Tolerability, Efficacy, Preference (Pearls), Simplicity.

4. Uricosuric agent – Probenecid

Table 69. Probenecid STEPS

Safety	Avoid use in patients with uric acid kidney stones May worsen existing blood dyscrasias Many drug interactions and may increase the serum concentration of target agents
Tolerability	Dyspepsia Reflux esophagitis
Efficacy	Increases urate excretion and decreases serum uric acid concentrations Efficacy may be diminished when coadministered with salicylates
Preference (Pearls)	Ineffective in patients with even mild renal insufficiency Start with low doses to reduce the likelihood of precipitating another gouty attack
Simplicity	Coformulated with colchicine May cost $35–$100 per month (depending on daily dose and frequency)

STEPS = Safety, Tolerability, Efficacy, Preference (Pearls), Simplicity.

5. Other medications
   a. Colchicine
      i. For prophylaxis of gout induced by urate-lowering therapy
      ii. Not for use as monotherapy to prevent gouty attacks
      iii. Give during the first 6 months of urate-lowering therapy.

Patient Case

16. Y.W. is a 58-year-old man with a medical history significant for hypertension, type 2 diabetes mellitus, dyslipidemia, and obesity. His medications include glimepiride 2 mg daily, hydrochlorothiazide 12.5 mg daily, bisoprolol 5 mg daily, and simvastatin/ezetimibe 20/10 mg at night. During routine laboratory evaluation, his primary care provider finds his serum uric acid concentration to be 7.3 mg/dL. Which is the most appropriate strategy to decrease the patient's serum uric acid concentration?

A. Therapy is not indicated because the patient has not yet experienced a gouty attack.
B. Initiate allopurinol 100 mg daily and titrate to achieve a serum uric acid concentration less than 6 mg/dL.
C. Initiate febuxostat 40 mg daily and titrate to achieve a serum uric acid concentration less than 6 mg/dL.
D. Initiate probenecid 500 mg twice daily and titrate to achieve a serum uric acid concentration less than 6 mg/dL.

    b. Pegloticase

Table 70. Pegloticase STEPS

Safety	Contraindicated in patients with G6PD deficiency FDA black box warning regarding anaphylaxis and infusion reactions; patients should be closely monitored for at least 2 hours after infusion, though delayed reactions have been reported Risk of infusion reaction is increased when the patient's uric acid concentration is >6 mg/dL; consider discontinuing therapy if uric acid concentration is >6 mg/dL, especially if it is above this limit on two consecutive occasions Acute gout flare within the first 3 months of therapy Heart failure exacerbations have been reported in clinical trials Increased risk of anaphylaxis in patients who are restarting therapy after discontinuing it for >4 weeks	
Tolerability	Bruising Chest pain Constipation Dyspnea	Erythema Nausea Pruritus Urticaria
Efficacy	Showed decreased uric acid concentrations and number of gout flares in clinical trials	
Preference (Pearls)	Administer by intravenous infusion for 120 minutes Vials must be refrigerated and stored in a carton to protect them from light Elimination half-life is about 14 days Recommended to begin gout flare prophylaxis (NSAIDs or colchicine) 1 week before infusion and continue for at least 6 months	
Simplicity	120-minute infusion (8 mg) every 2 weeks	

FDA = U.S. Food and Drug Administration; G6PD = glucose-6-phosphate dehydrogenase; NSAID = nonsteroidal anti-inflammatory drug; STEPS = Safety, Tolerability, Efficacy, Preference (Pearls), Simplicity.

    c. Rasburicase
        i. Uricolytic agent, FDA approved only for tumor lysis syndrome
        ii. Seldom used for this indication
        iii. Some research shows rasburicase decreases tophi and uric acid concentrations in patients with gout.

d. Rilonacept
  i. Interleukin-1 inhibitor labeled for use in cryopyrin-associated periodic syndromes
  ii. When added to allopurinol therapy, it decreased the number of acute gout attacks.
  iii. Administered as a subcutaneous injection

6. Patient information
  a. Information from National Institute of Arthritis and Musculoskeletal and Skin Diseases (www.niams.nih.gov/Health_Info/Gout/default.asp)
  b. Gout and Uric Acid Education Society
    i. Web site for information and social networking
    ii. http://gouteducation.org/

Table 71. Drugs and Doses Reference Table

Medication Name	Brand Name	Dosing
Colchicine	Colcrys	0.6 mg twice daily (for prophylaxis)
Allopurinol	Zyloprim	200–300 mg by mouth each day
Febuxostat	Uloric	40–80 mg by mouth each day
Probenecid		250–500 mg by mouth twice daily
Pegloticase	Krystexxa	8 mg intravenously every 2 weeks

REFERENCES

Osteoporosis

1. Adachi JD, Adami S, Miller PD, et al. Tolerability of risedronate in postmenopausal women intolerant of alendronate. Aging (Milano) 2001;13:347-54.

2. Bischoff-Ferrari HA, Dawson-Hughes B, Willett WC, et al. Effect of vitamin D on falls: a meta-analysis. JAMA 2004;291:1999-2006.

3. Black DM, Greenspan SL, Ensrud KE, et al. The effects of parathyroid hormone and alendronate alone or in combination in postmenopausal osteoporosis. N Engl J Med 2003;349:1207-15.

4. Bolland MJ, Avenell A, Baron JA, et al. Effect of calcium supplements on risk of myocardial infarction and cardiovascular events: meta-analysis. BMJ 2010;341:c3691.

5 Calcitonin Salmon for the Treatment of Postmenopausal Osteoporosis: Joint Meeting of the Advisory Committee for Reproductive Health Drugs and the Drug Safety and Risk Management Advisory Committee. Washington, DC: Division of Reproductive and Urologic Products, U.S. Food and Drug Administration (FDA), 2013. Available at http://www.fda.gov/downloads/AdvisoryCommittees/Committees%C3%A5MeetingMaterials/Drugs/ReproductiveHealthDrugsAdvisoryCommittee/UCM343748.pdf. Accessed September 19, 2015.

6. Cartsos VM, Zhu S, Zavras AI. Bisphosphonate use and the risk of adverse jaw outcomes: a medical claims study of 714,217 people. J Am Dent Assoc 2008;139:23-30.

7. Clinician's Guide to Prevention and Treatment of Osteoporosis. Washington, DC: National Osteoporosis Foundation (NOF), 2014. Available at http://nof.org/files/nof/public/content/file/2791/upload/919.pdf. Accessed September 19, 2015.

8. Combs BP1, Rappaport M, Caverly TJ, et al. "Due" for a scan: examining the utility of monitoring densitometry. JAMA Intern Med. 2013;173:2007-9.

9. Cosman F, de Beur SJ, LeBoff MS, et al. Clinician's guide to preventions and treatment of osteoporosis. Osteoporosis Int 2014;25:2359-81.

10. Diagnosis and Treatment of Osteoporosis. Bloomington, MN: Institute for Clinical Systems Improvement (ICSI), 2013. Available at https://www.icsi.org/guidelines__more/catalog_guidelines_and_more/catalog_guidelines/catalog_musculoskeletal_guidelines/osteoporosis/. Accessed September 19, 2015.

11. DynaMed [Internet database]. Ipswich, MA: EBSCO Publishing. Available at www.ebscohost.com./dynamed. Accessed September 19, 2015.

12. Fosnight SM, Zafirau WJ, Hazelett SE. Vitamin D supplementation to prevent falls in the elderly: evidence and practical considerations. Pharmacotherapy 2008;28:225-34.

13. Grossman JM, Gordon R, Ranganath VK, et al. American College of Rheumatology 2010 recommendations for the prevention and treatment of glucocorticoid-induced osteoporosis. Arthritis Care Res (Hoboken) 2010;62:1515-26.

14. Howe TE, Shea B, Dawson J, et al. Exercise for preventing and treating osteoporosis in postmenopausal women. Cochrane Database Syst Rev 2011;7:CD000333.

15. Lewiecki EM. In the clinic. Osteoporosis. Ann Intern Med 2011;155:ITC1-15.

16. Oral Bisphosphonates: Ongoing Safety Review of Atypical Subtrochanteric Femur Fractures. In: MedWatch. Washington, DC: U.S. Food and Drug Administration. Available at www.fda.gov/Safety/MedWatch/SafetyInformation/SafetyAlertsforHumanMedicalProducts/ucm204127.htm. Accessed September 19, 2015.

17. Osteoporosis: Assessing the Risk of Fragility Fracture. London, England: National Institute for Health and Care Excellence (NICE), 2012. Available at www.nice.org.uk/guidance/cg146/resources/cg146-ostcoporosis-fragility-fracture-full-guideline3. Accessed September 19, 2015.

18. Raisz LG. Clinical practice: screening for osteoporosis. N Engl J Med 2005;353:164-71.

19. Screening for osteoporosis: U.S. Preventive Services Task Force recommendation statement. Ann Intern Med 2011;154:356-64.

20. Stenson WF, Newberry R, Lorenz R, et al. Increased prevalence of celiac disease and need for routine screening among patients with osteoporosis. Arch Intern Med 2005;165:393-9.

21. Torgerson DJ, Bell-Syer SE. Hormone replacement therapy and prevention of nonvertebral fractures: a meta-analysis of randomized trials. JAMA 2001;285:2891-7.

22. Watts NB, Bilezikian JP, Camacho PM, et al. American Association of Clinical Endocrinologists Medical Guidelines for Clinical Practice for the diagnosis and treatment of postmenopausal osteoporosis. Endocr Pract 2010;16(suppl 3):1-37.

Rheumatoid Arthritis

1. Abatacept (Orencia) for rheumatoid arthritis. Med Lett Drugs Ther 2006;48:17-8.

2. Aletaha D, Funovits J, Keystone EC, et al. Disease activity early in the course of treatment predicts response to therapy after one year in rheumatoid arthritis patients. Arthritis Rheum 2007;56:3226-35.

3. Aletaha D, Neogi T, Silman AJ, et al. 2010 rheumatoid arthritis classification criteria: an American College of Rheumatology/European League Against Rheumatism collaborative initiative. Ann Rheum Dis 2010;69:1580-8.

4. Combe B, Landewe R, Lukas C, et al. EULAR recommendations for the management of early arthritis: report of a task force of the European Standing Committee for International Clinical Studies Including Therapeutics (ESCISIT). Ann Rheum Dis 2007;66:34-45.

5. Donahue KE, Gartlehner G, Jonas DE, et al. Systematic review: comparative effectiveness and harms of disease-modifying medications for rheumatoid arthritis. Ann Intern Med 2008;148:124-34.

6. DynaMed [Internet database]. Ipswich, MA: EBSCO Publishing. Available at www.ebscohost.com./dynamed. Accessed September 21, 2015.

7. Huizinga TWJ, Pincus T. Rheumatoid arthritis. Ann Intern Med 2010;153:ITC1.

8. Hurkmans E, van der Giesen FJ, Vliet Vlieland TP, et al. Dynamic exercise programs (aerobic capacity and/or muscle strength training) in patients with rheumatoid arthritis. Cochrane Database Syst Rev 2009;4:CD006853.

9. Karlson EW, Chibnik LB, Tworoger SS, et al. Biomarkers of inflammation and development of rheumatoid arthritis in women from two prospective cohort studies. Arthritis Rheum 2009;60:641-52.

10. Osiri M, Shea B, Robinson V, et al. Leflunomide for treating rheumatoid arthritis. Cochrane Database Syst Rev 2003;1:CD002047.

11. Rheumatoid Arthritis: The Management of Rheumatoid Arthritis in Adults. National Institute for Health and Clinical Excellence (NICE), 2009. Available at http://guidance.nice.org.uk/CG79/NICEGuidance/pdf/English. Accessed September 21, 2015.

12. Singh JA, Saag KG, Bridges SL, et al. 2015 American College of Rheumatology Guideline for the Treatment of Rheumatoid Arthritis. Available online at: http://www.rheumatology.org/Portals/0/Files/ACR%202015%20RA%20Guideline.pdf. Accessed February 1, 2016.

13. Smolen JS, Aletaha D, Bijlsma JWJ, et al. Treating rheumatoid arthritis to target: recommendations of an international task force. Ann Rheum Dis 2010;69:631-7.

14. Smolen JS, Landewé R, Breedveld FC, et al. EULAR recommendations for the management of rheumatoid arthritis with synthetic and biological disease-modifying antirheumatic drugs: 2013 update. Ann Rheum Dis 2013;0:1-18.

15. Tocilizumab (Actemra) for rheumatoid arthritis. Med Lett Drugs Ther 2010;52:47-8.

16. van der Helm-van Mil AH, Detert J, Cessie SL, et al. Validation of a prediction rule for disease outcome in patients with recent-onset undifferentiated arthritis: moving toward individualized treatment decision-making. Arthritis Rheum 2008;58:2241-7.

17. Verstappen SM, Jacobs JW, van der Veen MJ, et al. Intensive treatment with methotrexate in early rheumatoid arthritis: aiming for remission: Computer Assisted Management in Early Rheumatoid Arthritis (CAMERA, an open-label strategy trial). Ann Rheum Dis 2007;66:1443-9.

18. Verstappen SM, McCoy MJ, Roberts C, et al. Beneficial effects of a 3-week course of intramuscular glucocorticoid injections in patients with very early inflammatory polyarthritis: results of the STIVEA trial. Ann Rheum Dis 2010;69:503-9.

19. Warrington TP, Bostwick JM. Psychiatric adverse effects of corticosteroids. Mayo Clin Proc 2006;81:1361-7.

Psoriatic Arthritis

1. DynaMed [Internet database]. Ipswich, MA: EBSCO Publishing. Available at www.ebscohost.com./dynamed. Accessed September 21, 2015.

2. Gottlieb A, Korman NJ, Gordon KB, et al. Guidelines of care for the management of psoriasis and psoriatic arthritis, section 2: psoriatic arthritis: overview and guidelines of care for treatment with an emphasis on the biologics. J Am Acad Dermatol 2008;58:851-64.

3. Jones G, Crotty M, Brooks P. Interventions for psoriatic arthritis. Cochrane Database Syst Rev 2000;3:CD000212.

4. Mease P, Goffe BS. Diagnosis and treatment of psoriatic arthritis. J Am Acad Dermatol 2005;52:1-19.

5. Mease PJ, Gladman DD, Keystone EC. Alefacept in combination with methotrexate for the treatment of psoriatic arthritis: results of a randomized, double-blind, placebo-controlled study. Arthritis Rheum 2006;54:1638-45.

6. Nijsten T, Wakkee M. Complexity of the association between psoriasis and comorbidities. J Invest Dermatol 2009;129:1601-3.

7. Ramiro S, Radner H, van der Heijde D, et al. Combination therapy for pain management in inflammatory arthritis (rheumatoid arthritis, ankylosing spondylitis, psoriatic arthritis, other spondyloarthritis). Cochrane Database Syst Rev 2011;10:CD008886.

8. Ravindran V, Scott DL, Choy EH. A systematic review and meta-analysis of efficacy and toxicity of disease modifying anti-rheumatic drugs and biological agents for psoriatic arthritis. Ann Rheum Dis 2008;67:855-9.

9. Ritchlin CT, Kavanaugh A, Gladman DD, et al. Treatment recommendations for psoriatic arthritis. Ann Rheum Dis 2009;68:1387-94.

10. Soriano ER, McHugh NJ. Therapies for peripheral joint disease in psoriatic arthritis: a systematic review. J Rheumatol 2006;33:1422-30.

11. Taylor W, Gladman D, Helliwell P, et al. Classification criteria for psoriatic arthritis: development of new criteria from a large international study. Arthritis Rheum 2006;54:2665-73.

Osteoarthritis

1. Agency for Heathcare Research and Quality, U.S. Department of Health and Human Services. Choosing nonopioid analgesics for osteoarthritis: clinician summary guide. J Pain Palliat Care Pharmacother 2009;23:433-57.

2. American Academy of Orthopaedic Surgeons Appropriate Use Criteria for Non-Arthroplasty Treatment of Osteoarthritis of the Knee. In: National Guidelines Clearinghouse (NGC). Rockville, MD: NGC, 2013. Available at http://www.guideline.gov/content.aspx?id=47819. Accessed September 22. 2015.

3. Bannuru RR, Natov NS, Obadan IE, et al. Therapeutic trajectory of hyaluronic acid versus corticosteroids in the treatment of knee osteoarthritis: a systematic review and meta-analysis. Arthritis Rheum 2009;61:1704-11.

4. The Care and Management of Osteoarthritis in Adults. National Institute for Health and Clinical Excellence (NICE) 2008. Available at http://www.nice.org.uk/guidance/cg59. Accessed September 22, 2015.

5. DynaMed [database online]. Ipswich, MA: EBSCO Publishing. Available at www.ebscohost.com./dynamed. Accessed September 22, 2015.

6. Fransen M, McConnell S, Bell M. Exercise for osteoarthritis of the hip or knee. Cochrane Database Syst Rev 2003;3:CD004286.

7. Heyneman CA, Lawless-Liday C, Wall GC. Oral versus topical NSAIDs in rheumatic diseases: a comparison. Drugs 2000;60:555-74.

8. Hochberg MC, Altman RD, April KT, et al. American College of Rheumatology 2012 recommendations for the use of nonpharmacologic and pharmacologic therapies in osteoarthritis of the hand, hip, and knee. Arthritis Care Res 2012;64:465-74.

9. Medical Management of Adults with Osteoarthritis. In: National Guideline Clearinghouse (NGC). Rockville, MD: NGC, 2007 (revised 2013). Available at http://www.guideline.gov/content.aspx?id=47806. Accessed September 22, 2015.

10. Nuesch E, Rutjes AW, Husni E, et al. Oral or transdermal opioids for osteoarthritis of the knee or hip. Cochrane Database Syst Rev 2009;4:CD003115.

11. Towheed TE, Maxwell L, Anastassiades TP, et al. Glucosamine therapy for treating osteoarthritis. Cochrane Database Syst Rev 2005;2:CD002946.

Fibromyalgia Syndrome

1. Carville SF, Arendt-Nielsen S, Bliddal H, et al. EU-LAR evidence-based recommendations for the management of fibromyalgia syndrome. Ann Rheum Dis 2008;67:536-41.

2. Chakrabarty S, Zoorob R. Fibromyalgia. Am Fam Physician 2007;76:247-54.

3. DynaMed [Internet database]. Ipswich, MA: EBSCO Publishing. Available at www.ebscohost.com./dynamed. Accessed September 23, 2015.

4. Goldberg DL, Burckhardt C, Crofford L. Management of fibromyalgia syndrome. JAMA 2004;292:2388-95.

5. Hauser W, Bernardy K, Uceyler N, et al. Treatment of fibromyalgia syndrome with antidepressants: a meta-analysis. JAMA 2009;301:198-209.

6. Hauser W, Bernardy K, Uceyler N, et al. Treatment of fibromyalgia syndrome with gabapentin and pregabalin--a meta-analysis of randomized controlled trials. Pain 2009;145:69-81.

7. Hauser W, Urrutia G, Tort S, et al. Serotonin and noradrenaline reuptake inhibitors (SNRIs) for fibromyalgia syndrome. Cochrane Database Syst Rev 2013;1:CD010292.

8. Holman AJ, Myers RR. A randomized, double-blind, placebo-controlled trial of pramipexole, a dopamine agonist, in patients with fibromyalgia receiving concomitant medications. Arthritis Rheum 2005;52:2495-505.

9. Li YH, Wang FY, Feng CQ, et al. Massage therapy for fibromyalgia: a systematic review and meta-analysis of randomized controlled trials. PLoS One 2014;9:e89304.

10. Lump MP, Hughes RA, Wiffen PJ. Duloxetine for treating painful neuropathy or chronic pain. Cochrane Database Syst Rev 2009;4:CD007115.

11. Lunn MP, Hughes RA, Wiffen PJ. Duloxetine for treating painful neuropathy, chronic pain and fibromyalgia. Cochrane Database Syst Rev 2014;1:CD007115.

12. Meyer BB, Lemley KJ. Utilizing exercise to affect the symptomatology of fibromyalgia: a pilot study. Med Sci Sports Exerc 2000;32:1691-7.

13. Moore RA, Derry S, Aldington D, et al. Amitriptyline for neuropathic pain and fibromyalgia in adults. Cochrane Database Syst Rev 2012;12:CD008242.

14. Moore RA, Wiffen PJ, Derry S. Gabapentin for chronic neuropathic pain and fibromyalgia is adults. Cochrane Database Syst Rev 2014;4:CD007938.

15. Wolfe F, Clauw DJ, Fitzcharles MA, et al. The American College of Rheumatology preliminary diagnostic criteria for fibromyalgia and measurement of symptom severity. Arthritis Care Res (Hoboken) 2010;62:600-10.

16. Wolfe F, Smythe HA, Yunus MB, et al. The American College of Rheumatology 1990 criteria for the classification of fibromyalgia: report of the Multicenter Criteria Committee. Arthritis Rheum 1990;33:160-72.

Systemic Lupus Erythematosus

1. [No authors listed]. Guidelines for referral and management of systemic lupus erythematosus in adults: American College of Rheumatology Ad Hoc Committee on Systemic Lupus Erythematosus Guidelines. Arthritis Rheum 1999;42:1785-96.

2. Bertsias G, Ioannidis JP, Boletis J, et al. EULAR recommendations for the management of systemic lupus erythematosus: report of a Task Force of the EULAR Standing Committee for International Clinical Studies Including Therapeutics. Ann Rheum Dis 2008;67:195-205.

3. Cervera R, Khamashta MA, Font J, et al. Morbidity and mortality in systemic lupus erythematosus during a 10-year period: a comparison of early and late manifestations in a cohort of 1,000 patients. Medicine (Baltimore) 2003;82:299-308.

4. Costedoat-Chalumeau N, Galicier L, Aumaître O, et al. Hydroxychloroquine in systemic lupus erythematosus: results of a French multicentre controlled trial (PLUS Study). Ann Rheum Dis 2013;72:1786-92.

5. DynaMed [Internet database]. Ipswich, MA: EBSCO Publishing. Available at www.ebscohost.com./dynamed. Accessed September 25, 2015.

6. Griffiths B, Emery P, Ryan V, et al. The BILAG multicentre open randomized controlled trial comparing ciclosporin vs azathioprine in patients with severe SLE. Rheumatology (Oxford) 2010;49:723-32.

7. Haq I, Isenberg DA. How does one assess and monitor patients with systemic lupus erythematosus in daily clinical practice? Best Pract Res Clin Rheumatol 2002;16:181-94.

8. Madhok R, Wu O. Systemic lupus erythematosus. Am Fam Physician 2007;76:1351-3.

9. Marmor MF, Carr RE, Easterbrook M, et al. Recommendations on screening for chloroquine and hydroxychloroquine retinopathy: a report by the American Academy of Ophthalmology. Ophthalmology 2002;109:1377-82.

10. Mosca M, Tani C, Aringer M, et al. European League Against Rheumatism recommendations for monitoring patients with systemic lupus erythematosus in clinical practice and in observational studies. Ann Rheum Dis 2010;69:1269-74.

11. Rahman A, Isenberg DA. Systemic lupus erythematosus. N Engl J Med 2008;358:929-39.

12. Ruiz-Irastorza G, Ramos-Casals M, Brito-Zeron P, et al. Clinical efficacy and side effects of antimalarials in systemic lupus erythematosus: a systematic review. Ann Rheum Dis 2010;69:20-8.

13. Wallace DJ, Kalunian K, Petri MA, et al. Efficacy and safety of epratuzumab in patients with moderate/severe active systemic lupus erythematosus: results from EMBLEM, a phase IIb, randomised, double-blind, placebo-controlled, multicentre study. Ann Rheum Dis 2014;73:183-90.

14. Wright SA, O'Prey FM, McHenry MT, et al. A randomised interventional trial of omega-3-polyunsaturated fatty acids on endothelial function and disease activity in systemic lupus erythematosus. Ann Rheum Dis 2008;67:841-8.

Gout

1. DynaMed [Internet database]. Ipswich, MA: EBSCO Publishing. Available at www.ebscohost.com./dynamed. Accessed September 25, 2015.

3. Harris MD, Siegel LB, Alloway JA. Gout and hyperuricemia. Am Fam Physician 1999;59:925-34.

4. Jordan KM, Cameron JS, Snaith M, et al. British Society for Rheumatology and British Health Professionals in Rheumatology guideline for the management of gout. Rheumatology (Oxford) 2007;46:1372-4.

5. Khanna D, Fitzgerald J, Khanna PP, et al. 2012 American College of Rheumatology guidelines for the management of gout, part 1: systematic nonpharmacologic and pharmacologic therapeutic approaches to hyperuricemia. Arthritis Care Res 2012;64:1431-46.

6. Khanna D, Khanna PP, Fitzgerald J, et al. 2012 American College of Rheumatology guidelines for the management of gout, part 2: therapy and anti-inflammatory prophylaxis of acute gouty arthritis. Arthritis Care Res 2012;64:1447-61.

7. Sivera F, Andrés M, Carmona L, et al. Multinational evidence-based recommendations for the diagnosis and management of gout: integrating systematic literature review and expert opinion of a broad panel of rheumatologists in the 3e initiative. Ann Rheum Dis 2014:328-35.

8. Terkeltaub RA, Furst DE, Bennett K, et al. High versus low dosing of oral colchicine for early acute gout flare: twenty-four-hour outcome of the first multicenter, randomized, double-blind, placebo-controlled, parallel-group, dose-comparison colchicine study. Arthritis Rheum 2010;62:1060-8.

9. University of Texas at Austin School of Nursing, Family Nurse Practitioner Program. Management of Chronic Gout in Adults. Austin, TX: University of Texas at Austin, School of Nursing, 2012. Available at www.guideline.gov/content.aspx?id=37278. Accessed September 25, 2015.

10. Wallace SL, Robinson H, Masi AT, et al. Preliminary criteria for the classification of the acute arthritis of primary gout. Arthritis Rheum 1977;20:895-900.

11. Wilson JF. Gout. Ann Intern Med 2010;152:ITC2-1.

12. Zhang W, Doherty M, Bardin T, et al. EULAR evidence based recommendations for gout, part II: management: report of a task force of the EULAR Standing Committee for International Clinical Studies Including Therapeutics (ESCISIT). Ann Rheum Dis 2006;65:1312-24.

ANSWERS AND EXPLANATIONS TO PATIENT CASES

1. Answer: C

Many medications contribute to BMD loss by either accelerating bone resorption or inhibiting osteogenesis. For this patient, levothyroxine most significantly affected her BMD by speeding up the bone resorption process. Excessive thyroid hormone supplementation or drug-induced hyperthyroidism puts patients at risk of osteoporosis and fracture. Practitioners should be cognizant of TSH and free thyroid hormone concentrations, treating patients to a euthyroid state and a TSH concentration of around 2.0–3.0 mIU/L. This suggestion does not apply for patients who require maximal thyroid hormone suppression (i.e., history of thyroid cancer).

2. Answer: B

The patient in question has not yet undergone a DEXA scan and received a T-score for her lumbar spine or femoral neck. Therefore, antiresorptive therapy is not warranted until the results are available. However, according to the USPSTF, the patient is a candidate for undergoing DEXA scan before age 65 years, given that her FRAX score for major osteoporotic fracture is greater than 9.3%. She should also begin treatment with calcium and vitamin D to preserve BMD. If the DEXA findings show osteopenia (T-score between −1.0 and −2.5), bisphosphonate therapy will be initiated because the patient's risk of hip fracture in the next 10 years is greater than 3%.

3. Answer: D

Because the patient has an extensive history of GI disease and receives chronic therapy with a proton pump inhibitor, she will most likely benefit from treatment with a calcium citrate supplement. Calcium carbonate salts, when administered with an acid-suppressing agent, yield less calcium availability than a calcium citrate formulation. However, when converting from a calcium carbonate tablet to a calcium citrate tablet, the "serving size" is usually doubled, and the patient requires two tablets of calcium citrate to equal the elemental calcium in one calcium carbonate tablet.

4. Answer: A

This patient's inability to be mobile (and possibly upright) drastically limits the medication choices for the primary prevention of an osteoporotic fracture. Zoledronic acid seems to be the most appropriate agent because there are data to support its ability to maintain vertebral bone density, and patients do not have to adhere to strict postdosing restrictions when using it. Risedronate is appropriate if the patient can remain upright for 30–60 minutes, but this may be too physically demanding for the patient. The calcitonin nasal spray is less effective than the bisphosphonate options and would be a poor choice for the patient. Raloxifene has a high incidence of venous thromboembolism and, in conjunction with the patient's limited mobility, might increase her risk of a venous thromboembolism.

5. Answer: C

Rheumatoid factor is one of four clinically relevant markers when predicting disease prognosis. The other indicators include functional limitations, positive anti–citrullinated protein antibody (or positive RF finding) finding, radiographic evidence of bony erosions, and extra-articular disease. These prognostic factors are then used when determining initial therapy using the ACR algorithms. Joint involvement, ESR, and CRP are important when classifying RA, but they are not good indicators of prognosis.

6. Answer: C

To assess the most appropriate therapy for the patient, the provider must identify that she has high disease activity, poor prognostic factors, and disease duration of less than 6 months. Monotherapy with a nonbiologic DMARD would be inappropriate, given her level of disease activity and poor prognosis. The use of anakinra is not supported by the ACR 2012 recommendations because of the lack of sufficient efficacy data since the 2008 publication. For this patient, the use of a TNF inhibitor plus methotrexate is appropriate and meets the recommendations from the ACR for a person with high disease activity for less than 6 months and poor prognostic factors.

7. Answer: C

Although the maximal studied dose of methotrexate for patients with RA can be up to 30 mg weekly, the maximal recommended dose is 20 mg weekly. If a patient reaches the 20-mg dose by mouth without sufficient clinical effect, a prescriber should begin to reconsider the effectiveness of the current therapeutic approach. Although it is possible to switch to injectable methotrexate, this approach is not preferred and should be reserved for patients who cannot afford a TNF inhibitor. Both adalimumab and infliximab are TNF inhibitors, but only adalimumab may be used as monotherapy (between the two agents). Infliximab should always be given in combination with methotrexate.

8. Answer: C

The patient should discontinue etanercept and begin therapy with abatacept. The ACR recommends using abatacept for patients without an adequate rheumatologic response to methotrexate and an anti-TNF agent. Increasing and continuing prednisone may help alleviate some pain, but long-term treatment with corticosteroids is not warranted for everyone, and efforts should focus on the best way to maximally suppress bone deformation. Adding another anti-TNF agent or combining abatacept with an anti-TNF agent is also not recommended.

9. Answer: B

The CASPAR criteria are used to assist in the diagnosis of psoriatic arthritis. These criteria are based on five questions that have a total cumulative score of up to 6 points. Patients are given 2 points if they have active psoriasis (1 point for a history of psoriasis) and 1 point for each of the following: dactylitis ("sausage digits"), negative RF findings, juxta-articular new bone formation, and/or nail dystrophy. If the score is greater than 3 points, the patient is considered to have psoriatic arthritis. In this particular case, the patient scored 5 of 6 points: active psoriasis, dactylitis, negative RF findings, and nail dystrophy.

10. Answer: D

The patient presents with severe psoriatic arthritis and requires treatment with a combination biologic and nonbiologic DMARD, in this case golimumab and methotrexate. Although using either agent alone may help alleviate the symptoms, the extreme severity of the patient's symptoms requires an aggressive treatment approach that could eventually be decreased, once his symptoms are lessened with combination therapy. The use of systemic corticosteroids is not recommended in patients with psoriatic arthritis. This is an insufficient dose of burst therapy, and systemic corticosteroids should not be used as chronic maintenance therapy for controlling the symptoms of psoriatic arthritis.

11. Answer: D

The man in this case has moderate to severe osteoarthritis of the knee that causes considerable limitations in the activities of daily living. Given his history of a myocardial infarction, ibuprofen is discouraged by the ACR for pain control because of its potential interaction to decrease the cardioprotective efficacy of aspirin. Although naproxen is recommended over ibuprofen, the patient's heart failure may be made worse with scheduled use. The acetaminophen dose exceeds 4 g daily. The topical NSAID is appropriate for this person because of its low likelihood of adverse events and interactions with other medications and disease states.

12. Answer: A

Although the patient's physical symptoms meet the criteria for diagnosing fibromyalgia (WPI score 8 and SSS estimated to be greater than 5), she has experienced these symptoms for only the past 4 weeks. According to the ACR, the patient must have symptoms for at least 3 months and elevated WPI and SSS scores. If these symptoms continue, the patient will qualify for a diagnosis of fibromyalgia, and she should be treated with a tricyclic antidepressant such as amitriptyline to start. If she is unable to achieve sufficient pain relief or if she has adverse events, she may try one of the alternative agents such as duloxetine, fluoxetine, or gabapentin.

13. Answer: C

This patient may benefit most from a trial of duloxetine 60 mg once daily. She has minor depressive disorder and states that some of her symptoms (sad feelings and sleep issues) have improved with the tricyclic antidepressant, but the main reason for the medication (her pain) was unaffected. When patients do not achieve response to the first-line treatment, alternative agents should be used. The α2δ ligands (gabapentin and pregabalin) are acceptable agents, but her beneficial response for non-pain symptoms with the antidepressant would warrant a trial of another agent with antidepressant properties. In addition, tramadol is recommended only for patients with fibromyalgia when all other alternative agents have been tried and have failed.

14. Answer: D

In this patient's situation, adding azathioprine will offer more benefit to the patient than the other listed options. In patients with SLE and evidence of lupus-related organ damage, adding an immunologic agent is warranted when the patient lacks a sufficient response to an antimalarial agent such as hydroxychloroquine. The practice of treating patients to a serum hydroxychloroquine concentration of greater than 1000 mg/mL has not proved beneficial. In addition, using systemic corticosteroid doses greater than 10 mg daily for extended periods is not recommended. The purpose of introducing an immunologic agent is to control symptoms and limit the amount of systemic corticosteroid use in the patient.

15. Answer: A

Because this patient is experiencing an acute gouty attack, the use of allopurinol is inappropriate. Allopurinol should be initiated at a starting dose (100 mg), but the time separating acute attack and prophylaxis remains unanswered (immediate vs. 1 to 2 weeks later). With respect to the colchicine dose, recent information indicates that both of the doses listed are equally effective, but the lower cumulative dose causes considerably fewer GI adverse events. The "as-tolerated" instructions for Option C and Option D put the patient at risk of overdosing and could cause the patient to experience GI adverse effects and even life-threatening hematologic effects.

16. Answer: A

The patient should not receive treatment for his hyperuricemia. Patients should not receive therapy until they have experienced their first gouty attack. One to 2 weeks after the first attack, patients may begin uric acid–lowering therapy, and they should be treated until a serum uric acid concentration of less than 6 mg/dL is attained. Until their first attack, treatment with a xanthine oxidase inhibitor or uricosuric agent is not indicated.

ANSWERS AND EXPLANATIONS TO SELF-ASSESSMENT QUESTIONS

1. Answer: D

According to her DEXA scan results, the patient would traditionally be classified as having osteopenia in her lumbar spine. In many cases, this would require her to be treated only with calcium and vitamin D supplementation. However, because her 10-year risk of a hip fracture is greater than 3% with the FRAX tool, the NOF would consider this patient as having osteoporosis and recommend she receive antiresorptive therapy. Of the choices, alendronate is the only agent to have antiresorptive properties, and of the two doses, 70 mg once weekly is the recommended treatment dose. Alendronate 35 mg once weekly is considered a prevention dose for bisphosphonates.

2. Answer: C

The patient should restart therapy but change to a different bisphosphonate. The use of a bisphosphonate for this patient is important because of her history of a fragility fracture. Reinitiating alendronate at 70 mg may be appropriate, but the likelihood of the same adverse event is high. Reducing the dose would not be appropriate for secondary fracture prevention. Although raloxifene is efficacious for secondary fracture prevention, its usefulness is limited to vertebral fractures, not hip fractures. Changing bisphosphonates may decrease the chances of the adverse drug event recurring, and the dose and dosing interval for risedronate are appropriate for this patient and her medical condition. The patient should be counseled on the proper way to take bisphosphonate.

3. Answer: C

According to the latest edition of the ACR's guidelines for managing glucocorticoid-induced osteoporosis, bisphosphonates should be used for postmenopausal women with moderate fracture risk (based on age and T-score) if they are using 7.5 mg or more of prednisone daily for more than 1 month. Because the patient meets these criteria, risedronate 150 mg monthly plus calcium and vitamin D supplementation are warranted.

4. Answer: D

The use of raloxifene may increase a woman's risk of a venous thromboembolism. Because the patient had an idiopathic (unprovoked) deep venous thromboembolism 18 months earlier, SERM use is not warranted. The use of raloxifene, which has been beneficial for patients with invasive breast cancer, has not been linked to lower extremity edema. In addition, despite the possible recurrence of hot flashes and spotting, raloxifene has not been associated with significant uterine abnormalities.

5. Answer: D

Patients with RA receiving biologic DMARDs should not be administered live vaccines such as varicella zoster. Nor should live vaccines be administered for 3 months after discontinuing biologic DMARDs. The trivalent seasonal influenza vaccine and 23-valent pneumococcal vaccine are acceptable to give to all patients, according to the schedule recommended by the Centers for Disease Control and Prevention (CDC) and Advisory Committee on Immunization Practices (ACIP). The Tdap vaccine may also be safely administered to patients who are considered (non-HIV) immune compromised or receiving immune system–compromising agents.

6. Answer: D

According to the ACR recommendations, patients with newly diagnosed RA should begin DMARDs within the first 3 months of diagnosis to achieve the best prognosis. The EULAR does not recommend a time frame for treatment initiation but states that patients should begin therapy with a DMARD immediately.

7. Answer: C

For a patient who wants to have a baby in the next 24 months, it is appropriate to rule out the use of all agents with a high potential of being teratogenic. Methotrexate, leflunomide, and minocycline all may cause abnormal or fatal fetal outcomes and should be avoided in pregnancy. Although sulfasalazine is not considered a first-line agent for treating RA, it is effective and likely the safest (though not without risk) in pregnancy. For patients receiving sulfasalazine during pregnancy, there have been reports of an increased risk of kernicterus, jaundice, and hemolytic anemia when used near term. Although the benefits appear to outweigh the risks in this situation, patient education and understanding of risk are essential.

8. Answer: B

This patient has risk factors for a poor prognosis with RA and has not achieved a sufficient response with methotrexate alone. The best choice for this patient is to change to an injectable form of methotrexate to possibly increase drug delivery and efficacy. Ideally, the patient's medication would be transitioned to TNF inhibitor, but the significant cost of these agents is prohibitive for patients without adequate prescription insurance coverage. Rituximab should not be recommended until the patient has an adequate trial with and subsequent failure with TNF-inhibitor therapy.

9. Answer: A

According to the ACR and GRAPPA, patients with minimal to no functional limitations from the psoriatic arthritis should be treated only with NSAIDs or other analgesics. When the symptoms progress to moderate severity and affect the patient's activities of daily living, or when the symptoms do not respond to simple analgesics, providers should consider adding either a DMARD (e.g., sulfasalazine) or a biologic agent (e.g., etanercept). Combination DMARD and biologic agent should be reserved for patients with severe disease or for those whose condition does not respond to either agent alone.

10. Answer: B

For this patient, the next best choice for pain relief is topical diclofenac 1% gel. The ACR 2012 guidelines do not recommend the routine use of glucosamine and chondroitin or opiate analgesia for osteoarthritis pain. In addition, treatment recommendations prefer topical NSAID therapy to systemic NSAIDs for patients older than 75 years.

11. Answer: C

Patients who are treated with hydroxychloroquine require ophthalmologic evaluations regularly, but the initial evaluation and follow-up depends on the weight-based dose, duration of therapy, and several other factors. Patients who are younger than 60 years, nonobese, without renal or hepatic disease, treated for less than 5 years, and with treatment of less than 6.5 mg/kg will need an initial screening within the first 5 years of therapy and then annually after 5 years. Annual evaluations are not required before year 5 unless one of the above criteria is not met.

12. Answer: C

It would be best for the patient to begin treatment with pregabalin 75 mg twice daily. Although all the medications listed are appropriate for treating fibromyalgia syndrome, several issues need to be considered. Nortriptyline and duloxetine would create a significant drug-drug interaction with selegiline, most likely resulting in hypertensive crisis and/or serotonin syndrome. The gabapentin dose is too low for the patient and would most likely not produce a clinically significant change in her symptoms. The target dose for gabapentin for fibromyalgia is 1800–2400 mg daily (divided three times).

13. Answer: B

The patient has chronic kidney disease, thereby limiting the choice of medications and doses that may be used to prevent recurrent gouty attacks. The patient is a candidate for gout prevention and treatment of hyperuricemia. The number of attacks per year does not factor into initiating therapy. Probenecid should be avoided in patients with a CrCl of less than 50 mL/minute. Colchicine has no effect on tophi formation. Xanthine oxidase inhibitors are the drug of choice for patients with tophi. Because the patient has a CrCl between 21 and 40 mL/minute, the suggested maximal dose of allopurinol is 150 mg daily. Some recommendations do not start limiting allopurinol's dose until the CrCl is less than 20 mL/minute, but the general therapeutic rule for allopurinol is to start at 100 mg daily and titrate to a serum uric acid concentration of less than 6 mg/dL.

Health Maintenance and Public Health

Julie M. Sease, Pharm.D., FCCP, BCPS, BCACP, CDE

Presbyterian College School of Pharmacy
Clinton, South Carolina

Health Maintenance and Public Health

Julie M. Sease, Pharm.D., FCCP, BCPS, BCACP, CDE

Presbyterian College School of Pharmacy

Clinton, South Carolina

Learning Objectives

1. Recommend appropriate first-aid therapy for common scenarios, including initial patient positioning, bleeding, asthma, anaphylaxis, seizures, musculoskeletal injuries, chest pain, burns, thermal and heat injuries, and ocular injuries. *(Domain 1; Tasks 3, 6, 7)*

2. Develop and execute a plan to deliver appropriate cardiopulmonary resuscitation according to guideline recommendations. *(Domain 1; Tasks 3, 6, 7)*

3. Use knowledge of the patterns of drug poisoning, including implicated drugs and patient characteristics, in order to recommend strategies to prevent and treat opioid overdose. *(Domain 5, Task 2)*

4. Recommend drugs to prevent infection from exposures to category A bioterrorism threats. *(Domain 5, Task 3)*

5. Using knowledge of vaccines that are routinely administered, including their route of administration, number of doses, indication, contraindications, and common adverse effects, assess a patient's vaccine history and recommend the necessary vaccines. *(Domain 1, Task 5) (Domain 4, Task 5) (Domain 5, Task 2)*

6. Develop a process to design and implement interventions for addressing nonadherence, and integrate these interventions into pharmacy practice. *(Domain 2; Tasks 3, 4)*

7. Integrate knowledge of complementary and alternative medicines to educate patients and make appropriate recommendations for their use. *(Domain 1; Tasks 2, 3, 4, 6) (Domain 3, Task 1)*

Self-Assessment Questions

Answers and explanations to these questions can be found at the end of the chapter.

1. What age group is at highest risk of death from foreign-body airway obstruction?

    A. Younger than 5 years.
    B. Five to 10 years.
    C. Eleven to 16 years.
    D. Seventeen years and older.

2. Based on national trends, what drug class is most likely to cause overdose drug deaths in the next year?

    A. Anticoagulants.
    B. Tricyclic antidepressants.
    C. Benzodiazepines.
    D. Opioids.

3. What element of disaster preparedness is most likely to lead to an effective disaster response?

    A. Flexible plan based on type of disaster.
    B. Availability of on-call pharmacists.
    C. Collaborative practice agreement for vaccine administration by pharmacists.
    D. Surge supply of doxycycline and ciprofloxacin.

4. Which of the following vaccines should not be given to a pregnant woman because of a theoretical risk of infection in the fetus?

    A. Inactivated influenza vaccine (IIV).
    B. Meningococcal conjugate vaccine (MenACWY-D).
    C. Measles, mumps, and rubella (MMR).
    D. Diphtheria and reduced tetanus toxoids and acellular pertussis (Tdap).

5. Which of the following statements best represents the medication possession ratio (MPR) measure?

    A. The duration of time from initiation to discontinuation of therapy.
    B. Sum of days' supply of a medication over a defined period.
    C. The value is increased proportionately to a patient's failure to fill a medication.
    D. The degree of a patient's ability to demonstrate understanding of health information in order to make a health decision.

6. Which of the following statements is correct regarding The Dietary Supplement Health and Education Act (DSHEA) of 1994?

    A. Supplements are categorized as drugs and must go through the new-drug approval process before being sold in the market place.
    B. Dietary supplements must be proven safe and effective and submitted for U.S. Food and Drug Administration (FDA) approval.
    C. Dietary supplement manufacturers may claim that the product may affect body structure or function.
    D. Labeling must contain a seal of approval to demonstrate safety testing has occurred for the product.

I. FIRST AID

A. Evidence and Recommendations
1. Where available, the size of treatment effect and level of evidence (LOE) are included according to the American Heart Association methodology (Circulation 2010;122:S657-64).
   a. Class I: Benefit >>> risk (should be done)
   b. Class IIa: Benefit >> risk (reasonable to do)
   c. Class IIb: Benefit ≥ risk (may be considered)
   d. Class III: Risk ≥ benefit (may be harmful)
   e. Level of evidence
      i. A: Several randomized trials or meta-analyses
      ii. B: Single randomized trial or nonrandomized studies
      iii. C: Limited evaluations available (case reports, standard of care, expert opinion)
2. Recommendations for first aid are based on the First Aid: 2010 American Heart Association and American Red Cross Guidelines for First Aid.
3. Recommendations for cardiopulmonary resuscitation (CPR) are based on the Adult and Pediatric Basic Life Support Guidelines.

B. General First-Aid Principles
1. Obtain help by contacting emergency medical services (EMS) (i.e., call 911) when indicated.
2. In cases of poisoning, the poison center should also be contacted by dialing 1 (800) 222-1222 (see Section II for more details).
3. Positioning: In general, individuals should not be moved. Situations in which a specific position is recommended are listed below.
   a. Potential spinal injury—In general, a person should not be moved if there is any suspicion of a spinal injury.
      i. Secondary injury from moving or manipulating a patient can occur because the spinal cord is unprotected.
      ii. Most spinal injuries are caused by motor vehicle collisions and falls.
      iii. Spinal injury should be suspected if any of the following risk factors are present after a traumatic injury:
         (a) The person is 65 years or older.
         (b) Involved in a motor vehicle or bicycle crash
         (c) Fall greater than standing height
         (d) Pain or tenderness in the neck or back
         (e) Paresthesia symptoms in the extremities
         (f) Upper extremity or torso weakness
         (g) Altered level of consciousness
         (h) Sustained other injuries causing pain in the head or neck
         (i) Children 2 years or older with trauma involving the head or neck
      iv. The head should be stabilized to restrict motion and prevent secondary injury by manually restricting head and neck movement (Class IIb, LOE C).
   b. If there is evidence of shock, the legs should be raised 6–12 inches while the person is supine (Class IIb, LOE C).
      i. Raising the legs may increase blood pressure by shifting volume.

      ii.   Evidence of shock may include altered level of consciousness, decreased urine output, cool or mottled skin, weak/rapid pulse, nausea/vomiting, and hypotension. Not all of the preceding signs will be present, and some may be difficult to assess (e.g., decreased urine output) in first-aid situations.

      iii.   If there is pain when the legs are raised, there could be internal trauma, and no further efforts to raise the legs should be made.

   c. The individual should be put in the High Arm IN Endangered Spine (HAINES) position (one arm is extended, and the person's head is rested on the arm) (Class IIb, LOE C). The person's legs are bent, and the person is placed on his or her side, when any of the following conditions are present:

      i.   Difficulty breathing because of vomiting or secretions

      ii.   The individual is unresponsive and should be left alone while help is hailed.

   d. The individual is found in a prone position (face down) and is unconscious and should be placed in the supine position (face up).

C. Specific Emergencies and First-Aid Recommendations

  1. Asthma

   a. Clinical features of a severe asthma attack that can be assessed by a bystander

      i.   The person is only able to speak in words or phrases

      ii.   Prefers to sit forward (tenting)

      iii.   Agitation

      iv.   Increased respiratory rate

      v.   Peak flow less than 40% of predicted (may be difficult to obtain in some situations)

   b. Help patients administer their rescue inhalers according to physician prescription (Class IIa, LOE C).

   c. Management of asthma exacerbations at home (Expert Panel 3 recommendations)

      i.   May decrease length and severity of exacerbation

      ii.   Initial treatment is a short-acting β-agonist (e.g., albuterol), using a metered-dose inhaler MDI (2–6 puffs) or nebulizer.

      iii.   Up to two treatments are recommended separated by 20 minutes.

      iv.   Physician follow-up is recommended in all cases, based on severity (contact physician to emergency department [ED] transport).

      v.   All patients should have a written action plan.

  2. Anaphylaxis

   a. Clinical features

      i.   Rapid onset: Symptoms start in less than 1 minute to several hours after exposure to an allergen.

      ii.   Life-threatening respiratory or cardiovascular collapse

      iii.   Systemic symptoms

        (a) Skin involvement is reported in up to 90% of cases. Urticaria (i.e., hives), rash, swelling, pruritus (lips, tongue, uvula, ears, genitals, palms of the hands, soles of the feet, periorbital)

        (b) Respiratory involvement in up to 70% of cases. Signs of upper airway involvement may include swelling, pruritus, hoarseness, dysphonia, dysphagia, or stridor. Lower-respiratory signs and symptoms may include shortness of breath, chest tightness, or wheezing.

        (c) Nasal symptoms may be the earliest signs and include rhinorrhea and sneezing.

        (d) The gastrointestinal tract is involved in up to 45% of cases. Symptoms include nausea, vomiting, diarrhea, and abdominal pain.

        (e) The cardiovascular system is involved in up to 45% of cases. Symptoms may include chest pain, tachycardia, bradycardia, hypotension, and shock. A fluid shift of up to 50% from the intravascular compartment can occur in 10 minutes.

b. Treatment

    i. Treatment recommendations for the first-aid provider include administering an epinephrine autoinjector or helping patients self-administer their own epinephrine autoinjector (Class IIb, LOE B).

    ii. Administration and dosing of self-injectable autoinjectors

      (a) Inject into the anterolateral aspect of the thigh and hold for 10 seconds; autoinjector can be administered through clothing.

      (b) Use caution to avoid inadvertent administration into digits and hands.

      (c) Dosing is weight based in children. A child weighing less than 30 kg will be prescribed the 0.15-mg product, and others weighing 30 kg or more will be prescribed the 0.3-mg product

3. Seizures

  a. The primary treatment for patients experiencing a seizure is to prevent potential injuries.

  b. Avoid restraining patients because this may contribute to muscle or soft tissue injury. Ease patients to the ground, and clear the area around them.

  c. Do not try to place items in the patient's mouth because this can cause damage to the patient's teeth or to the bystander (Class IIa, LOE C).

  d. A postictal state (confusion, decreased level of consciousness, or unresponsiveness) is a common and expected finding after seizures.

4. Chest pain or pressure

  a. Presumed to be cardiac until proved otherwise so the EMS should be activated. Patients should not be transported by private vehicle.

  b. The chest discomfort may radiate down the left jaw or arm; it may be described as pain or pressure, and it can be accompanied by symptoms such as diaphoresis and shortness of breath.

  c. Aspirin 162–325 mg is recommended if there are no allergies or other contraindications (e.g., active bleeding, acute stroke) and aspirin is readily available (Class IIa, LOE A).

    i. Early aspirin administration (within 24 hours) decreases mortality.

    ii. The patient should chew and swallow the dose (use chewable aspirin if available).

    iii. Enteric-coated products should be avoided.

  d. Nitroglycerin sublingual can be administered to patients for whom it is prescribed.

    i. Do not use someone else's nitroglycerin.

    ii. It can be administered every 3–5 minutes up to three doses.

5. Bleeding

  a. The best treatment is direct and manual pressure over the area that is bleeding. To be effective, the manual pressure must be firm and held for a significant amount of time. Gauze should be placed over the affected area and more added, if necessary. No attempt should be made to remove old gauze.

  b. An alternative to manual pressure is using elastic bandages over gauze, but this may not be as effective.

  c. Tourniquets are not generally recommended unless control of bleeding cannot be achieved or is not possible with manual pressure.

    i. Improperly placed tourniquets can lead to secondary injury of muscles and nerves, and to limb ischemia. Limb ischemia can contribute to electrolyte aberrations, leading to cardiac arrhythmias, metabolic acidosis, shock, and death.

    ii. If they are used, the time they were applied should be conspicuously noted and communicated to health care professionals taking over care.

  d. Using pressure points (indirect pressure at a distal location) is less effective than other techniques and should not be used routinely.

6. Wounds and abrasions
    a. Wash with warm soap and water while removing foreign matter from the wound (Class I, LOE A). Although cold and warm water are equally effective, warm water is more comfortable.
    b. Superficial injuries should be covered with a topical antibiotic cream or ointment and a dressing to keep the wound moist (Class IIa, LOE A).
        i. Consider potential allergies to antibiotics before application.
        ii. Wounds have less infection risk when covered.
7. Thermal burns
    a. Thermal burns should be cooled with cool to room-temperature (not cold) tap water as soon as possible after the injury (Class I, LOE B).
        i. Treat burns within 30 minutes to help reduce pain, edema, depth of injury, and need for grafting procedures.
        ii. Ice or ice water should not be used because it can cause secondary injuries, including tissue ischemia.
    b. Blisters caused by burns should be left intact, and no attempt should be made to remove or drain them. Place a sterile dressing over the blister to help speed healing and decrease pain (Class IIa, LOE B).
8. Electrical injuries
    a. Electric current traveling through the body can cause a variety of injuries of differing severities, including a tingling sensation, burns, respiratory arrest, and life-threatening cardiac arrhythmias. Prolonged exposure can occur when sufficient current travels through the individual and causes tetany and an inability to let go of the electrical source.
    b. The first step for treating the injured person is to ensure the power is turned off at the source (e.g., breaker box). Failure to do this may contribute to the bystander's injury. Use of other materials (e.g., wooden board) is not recommended to move electric wires from the injured person or to move the person from the electrical source because there is still a risk of electrical conduction through the board.
    c. Do not touch the injured person while the power is on (Class III, LOE C).
    d. After the power has been turned off, the individual has to be assessed and CPR efforts initiated, if indicated. Do not move the injured person unless there is immediate danger.
    e. People who have received an electrical shock should be assessed for non-apparent injuries in a health care setting such as an ED.
9. Ocular injuries
    a. If the eye is exposed to chemicals
        i. Remove contact lenses.
        ii. Irrigate for 10–15 minutes with copious amounts of water with an eyewash station (Class I, LOE C).
        iii. If an eyewash station is not immediately available, the eyelid can be retracted and water poured onto the eye by using a drinking cup.
    b. Mechanical injuries to the globe or foreign objects embedded in the eye are treated initially by covering the affected eye, if possible, and the patient is then referred to an ophthalmologist. No attempt to remove foreign objects should be made.
10. Temperature-related emergencies
    a. Hypothermia caused by exposure to cold is treated by rewarming the affected individual.
        i. The initial treatment is to remove all wet clothing and wrap exposed body parts with blankets or other articles of clothing.
        ii. If there is a delay in medical care
            (a) The person with hypothermia should be actively rewarmed (warm environment, immersion in warm water) (Class IIa, LOE B).
            (b) Frozen parts of the body can be rewarmed by placing them in warm water (e.g., body temperature) for 20–30 minutes (Class IIb, LOE C).

        (c)   Do not use chemical warmers directly on frostbite because they can cause burns (Class III, LOE C).

        (d)   If there is a chance of refreezing, rewarming should not be attempted (Class III, LOE C). Any potential benefit is replaced by potential harm if refreezing occurs.

     iii.   Benefits of rewarming include return of venous circulation and decreased tissue loss.

  b.   Heat-related injuries include cramps, heat exhaustion, and heat stroke.

     i.   Heat cramps are muscle spasms affecting the legs, arms, abdominal muscles, and muscles of the back. Treatment recommendations are to have the affected person rest, cool off, and drink an electrolyte- and carbohydrate-based drink, if available. Massage and stretching are other strategies that can be used in combination with rehydration and cooling.

     ii.   Heat exhaustion is characterized by nausea, muscle cramps, dizziness, headache, diaphoresis, and fatigue. The affected person should be moved to a cool, shaded place with clothing removed. External cooling using cool water sprays can also be used. Similar to a person who has had heat cramps, the person who has had heat exhaustion should be encouraged to drink electrolyte- and carbohydrate-based solutions.

     iii.   Heat stroke includes exhaustion-related effects in addition to more severe central nervous system involvement, including syncope, altered mental status, and seizures. Because of the severity of the injury, people with heat stroke should be placed in cold water up to their chin, with EMS transport to an ED.

11. Musculoskeletal trauma

  a.   Sprains and strains should be treated with external cooling because it decreases pain, swelling, and healing time. The best method to use is a plastic bag filled with ice water covered with a thin towel (Class IIb, LOE C). Refreezable ice packs are less effective. To prevent secondary injury, no more than 20 minutes per application should be used. Heat is inferior to cold and is not recommended.

  b.   Bone fractures should be suspected when there is injury to any extremity. No attempt should be made to reduce or straighten bone fractures (Class III, LOE C). There is no evidence of better outcomes such as decreased pain or deformity. Splinting the injured extremity may decrease pain and prevent secondary injury until definitive therapy (Class IIa, LOE C). The injured person should avoid bearing weight on the extremity.

  c.   If the extremity is blue or pale, the EMS should be activated because it may indicate a more severe injury requiring prompt medical attention.

Patient Cases

1. A scouting troop is hiking on a trail along a mountainside. One of the adolescent boys slips and falls about 6 ft onto a rocky ledge. He has pain in his left leg. There is obvious injury, including several abrasions, and a likely fracture to both the tibia and the fibula. Which is the most appropriate first-aid therapy for his apparent fracture?

   A. Try to set his leg manually to decrease pain.
   B. Splint his leg with available materials.
   C. Encourage ambulation to maintain circulation.
   D. Apply ice to the fracture to decrease pain.

2. At the ambulatory care clinic, an adult patient known to have a seizure disorder falls to the floor from a seated position. The patient appears to be having tonic-clonic muscle contractions consistent with a generalized seizure. Which action is best to take?

   A. Try to place a wallet or other object in the patient's mouth to help the patient avoid biting his or her tongue.
   B. Ensure the area is clear of obstacles that could cause secondary injury.
   C. Try to hold the patient still, and speak words of reassurance.
   D. Try to administer the patient's antiseizure medication.

D. Cardiopulmonary Resuscitation
   1. In out-of-hospital arrests, CPR should be initiated unless the following occurs:
      a. There are signs of obvious irreversible death (e.g., rigor mortis, decomposition).
      b. The person performing CPR would be in physical danger.
      c. The patient has an advanced directive indicating that he or she does not wish to receive resuscitative efforts.
   2. Sequence for rescuers: Verify that the patient is unresponsive and not breathing normally.
      a. Patient is not moving or does not respond after tapping on the shoulder and shouting at the patient.
      b. A patient with gasping breaths or absent breathing is assumed to be in cardiac arrest (Class I, LOE C).
   3. If one person is present at an arrest
      a. Adults: Activate the emergency response system (ERS) and obtain an automated external defibrillator (AED), if easily accessible.
      b. Infants and children: Perform 2 minutes of CPR; then activate the ERS.
   4. If more than one person is present at an arrest
      a. One person should activate the ERS and obtain an AED.
      b. One person should initiate CPR (see Table 1).
   5. After activating the ERS
      a. Compressions; then airway; then breathing (CAB) is the preferred sequence (see Table 1).
      b. If a rescuer is untrained or unwilling to provide ventilations, compression-only CPR is recommended.

Table 1. Initial Sequence of Actions After a Person Collapses

	Lay Rescuer	**Health Care Provider**
Unresponsive adult	1. Activate ERS and obtain an AED, if immediately available 2. Provide 30 chest compressions at a rate of at least 100/minute OR continuously at a rate of at least 100/minute if rescuer is untrained in giving rescue breaths 3. Open the airway and give two breaths if rescuer is trained in giving rescue breaths 4. Repeat steps 2 and 3 5. Use the AED, when available	1. Activate ERS and obtain an AED 2. Check pulse (no more than 10 seconds) 3. Provide 30 chest compressions at a rate of at least 100/minute 4. Open the airway and give two breaths 5. Repeat steps 3 and 4 6. Use the AED, when available Note: If the cause of the collapse is respiratory (e.g., drowning), the health care provider should perform CPR with an emphasis on rescue breathing
Unresponsive infant or child	1. Provide 30 chest compressions 2. Open the airway and give two breaths (omit if rescuer untrained or unwilling) 3. Repeat steps 1 and 2 for a total of five cycles (~2 minutes) 4. Activate ERS and obtain an AED, if available	1. Check pulse (brachial for infants and carotid or femoral in a child; no more than 10 seconds) 2. Provide 30 chest compressions 3. Open the airway and give two breaths 4. Repeat steps 2 and 3 for a total of five cycles (~2 minutes) 5. Activate ERS and obtain an AED, if available

AED = automated external defibrillator; CPR = cardiopulmonary resuscitation; ERS = emergency response system.

6. Compression-only CPR
   a. Compression-only CPR is superior to no CPR.
   b. The recommended chest compression rate is at least 100/minute.
   c. Instructions can be given by telephone by emergency medical dispatchers, even for people untrained in giving CPR (Class I, LOE B).
   d. Survival rates with conventional CPR compared with compression-only CPR are similar.
   e. Indicated for lay rescuers responding to a person in presumed adult cardiac arrest. Asphyxial (e.g., drowning) causes for arrest and pediatric arrests should include rescue breaths (Class I, LOE B).
7. Effective chest compressions
   a. Ensure the patient is lying on his or her back (supine) on a hard surface.
   b. Correct rate is *at least* 100 compressions per minute for all patients—Push fast (Class IIa, LOE B).
   c. Minimize interruptions (Class IIa, LOE B). Time performing chest compressions should be at least 80%.
   d. Allow complete chest recoil after each compression (adults: Class IIa, LOE B; pediatric: Class IIb, LOE B).
      i. Incomplete chest recoil is associated with increased intrathoracic pressure.
      ii. Decreased cerebral and coronary perfusion occurs with higher intrathoracic pressures.
      iii. As rescuers become fatigued, incomplete chest recoil is more common because rescuers lean over the patient.
   e. Infants (younger than 1 year)
      i. Lay rescuers and lone health care providers: Two fingers on the sternum just below the nipple line (Class IIb, LOE C)
      ii. Compression/ventilation ratio 30:2

      iii.   Two health care providers should use the two-thumb encircling technique; compression/ventilation ratio 15:2

      iv.   Depth should be about 1½ inches (one-third the depth of the chest); push hard.

   f.   Children (1 year of age until puberty)

      i.   Puberty: Hair under the arms for male individuals and breast development in female individuals

      ii.   Lay rescuers and lone health care providers: One or two hands over the sternum between the nipples

      iii.   Compression/ventilation ratio 30:2

      iv.   Two health care providers: One or two hands over the sternum between the nipples; compression/ventilation ratio 15:2

      v.   Depth should be about 2 inches (one-third of the depth of the chest); push hard.

   g.   Adults (at and beyond puberty)

      i.   Lay rescuers and health care providers should use two hands over the sternum between the nipples (Class IIa, LOE B).

      ii.   Compression/ventilation ratio 30:2

      iii.   Depth should be at least 2 inches; push hard (Class IIa, LOE B).

      iv.   Compression and relaxation times should be equal (Class IIb, LOE C).

Table 2. Chest Compression Techniques

	Chest Compression Technique	**Landmarks**	**Depth of Compressions, inches**
Infant (<1 year)	Two fingers over sternum Two-thumb encircling if two health care rescuers	Just below nipple line	~1½
Child (1 year to prepubescent)	Heel of one hand or heel of one hand with the other hand on top, as for adults	Over sternum at nipple line	~2
Adult (postpubescent)	Heel of one hand with the other hand on top	Over sternum at nipple line	At least 2

   8.   Rescuer role change

     a.   Fatigue can cause deterioration in the quality of CPR in both ventilations and chest compressions.

     b.   Change ventilator and chest compression roles every 2 minutes to prevent fatigue (Class IIa, LOE B).

     c.   Role changes should take no more than 5 seconds.

   9.   Airway and breathing

     a.   Open the airway (for lay rescuers): Head tilt–chin lift for the injured and uninjured individuals (Class IIa, LOE B).

     b.   Open the airway (for health care providers).

       i.   Head tilt–chin lift for individuals without suspected head or neck trauma (Class IIa, LOE B)

       ii.   Jaw thrust for patients with suspected head or neck trauma (Class IIb, LOE C). If the jaw thrust maneuver fails, the head tilt–chin lift should be used (Class I, LOE C).

    c.   Evaluate effective ventilations by ensuring a visible chest rise with each breath (Class IIa, LOE C). Ineffective breaths may require repositioning the airway and reattempting ventilations.

    d.   Ventilatory techniques

       i.   Mouth-to-mouth for child and adult

       ii.   Mouth-to-mouth-and-nose for infant. If unable to ventilate, then use mouth-to-mouth or mouth-to-nose (Class IIb, LOE C).

       iii.   Face shield (i.e., plastic film that acts as a barrier)

       iv.   Face mask: Contains a one-way valve to allow air to flow from the rescuer to the person in cardiopulmonary distress and diverts the person's exhaled air from the rescuer

       v.   Bag-mask

          (a)   Contains a reservoir and a mask designed to cover the mouth and nose

          (b)   Adult and pediatric sizes are available.

          (c)   If oxygen is available, provide 100% at a rate of 10–12 L/minute.

          (d)   Most effective with two rescuers

       vi.   Each breath should be delivered during 1 second to avoid excessive ventilation leading to complications (Class IIa, LOE C).

          (a)   Increased intrathoracic pressure, which leads to decreased venous return and decreased perfusion

          (b)   Increased risk of aspiration and regurgitation of gastric contents

          (c)   Barotrauma

    e.   If gasps of breath are present, the patient should be treated in the same way as if he or she were not breathing.

    f.   Even if a patient has a pulse, rescue breaths may be required.

       i.   Infant or child—Twelve to 20 breaths/minute (one breath every 3–5 seconds)

       ii.   Adult—Ten to 12 breaths/minute (one breath every 5–6 seconds) (Class IIb, LOE C)

    g.   Complications of improper ventilation: Gastric inflation that can cause regurgitation and aspiration and restrict lung compliance

10. An AED is the most likely source of externally applied electricity outside a hospital environment.

    a.   The efficacy of a single shock is greater than 90%.

    b.   Use as soon as it is available (Class IIa, LOE C). The time from discontinuing CPR for a shock should be minimized. The shorter the time between the shock and CPR, the more likely the shock is to be successful.

    c.   CPR should be started immediately with chest compressions after a shock.

    d.   AEDs: Available in public areas (e.g., casinos, airports, sports facilities, shopping malls)

    e.   AEDs provide voice and visual prompts to aid in the successful use of the AED.

    f.   Infants

       i.   A manual defibrillator is preferred (initial dose 2 J/kg; second dose 4 J/kg).

       ii.   A pediatric attenuator or an AED can be used if a manual defibrillator is unavailable.

       iii.   If neither a manual defibrillator nor a pediatric attenuator system on an AED is available, a standard AED can be used (Class IIb, LOE C).

    g.   Children 1–8 years of age

       i.   Use a pediatric attenuator system, if available.

       ii.   Use adult systems if pediatric attenuator system is unavailable.

    h.   Children older than 8 years and adults: Use an adult pad system.

    i.   The first step to using an AED is to turn it on, then follow the audio and visual prompts.

    j.   Pad placement: Pads should be placed on the right upper chest (sternolateral position) and the left lateral chest. If medication patches are present, they should be removed and the medication wiped from the skin to maximize the electricity delivered to the heart. If an implanted device is felt or visualized beneath the skin (e.g., an internal cardiac defibrillator), the pad should be placed no closer than 1 inch to the device.

11. Foreign-body airway obstruction

    a.   Children younger than 5 years are at highest risk of death caused by foreign-body airway obstruction.

       i.   This age group accounts for 90% of deaths from foreign-body airway obstruction.

      ii.   Common causes include balloons, small objects, food (e.g., hot dogs, grapes, nuts, candy).

    b.   Mild airway obstruction – Audible sounds are noted.

    c.   Severe airway obstruction – No sounds are heard, and no cough is evident.

    d.   The person choking may show the universal choking sign (two hands encircling the neck).

    e.   Verbally ask the patient whether he or she is choking.

    f.   Intervention should be done only for severe choking.

       i.   An audible cough that becomes silent

      ii.   Respiratory difficulty

     iii.   The person choking becomes unconscious.

    g.   Activate the ERS for severe choking.

    h.   Perform abdominal thrusts (i.e., Heimlich maneuver) until the foreign body is expelled or the person becomes unresponsive.

    i.   Abdominal thrusts should not be used in the following groups:

       i.   Infants (younger than 1 year)

      ii.   A woman in the late stages of pregnancy

     iii.   The rescuer is unable to encircle his or her arms around the patient (e.g., in obesity).

     iv.   Apply rapid abdominal thrusts until the foreign body is relieved or the patient becomes unconscious.

      v.   Chest thrusts can be considered if abdominal thrusts are ineffective.

     vi.   Abdominal thrusts can cause internal injury, and survivors may need to be assessed by a physician to determine any extent of injuries.

    j.   Chest thrusts

       i.   Use for patients for whom abdominal thrusts are contraindicated (infants, women in the late stages of pregnancy, people who are too obese for the rescuer to encircle his or her arms around the person's abdomen).

      ii.   Infants: Five back blows are alternated with five chest thrusts.

     iii.   Consider using if abdominal thrusts fail

    k.   If the patient becomes unconscious

       i.   Ensure the ERS has been activated.

      ii.   Begin CPR.

     iii.   Examine the mouth for evidence of foreign bodies that can be removed before each series of rescue breaths.

12. Rescuers

    a.   The person delivering a shock must ensure all personnel stay clear of the patient while a shock is being delivered.

    b.   Careful coordination is necessary to minimize interruptions in good-quality CPR.

E. Pharmacist Roles
   1. Become trained and maintain certification in providing CPR.
   2. Recognize and manage the pitfalls of CPR.
      a. Chest compressions that are too slow, that are too shallow, or that do not allow complete recoil
      b. Too much time without CPR being performed (e.g., when the defibrillator pads are being applied or the defibrillator is being charged)
      c. CPR that does not start immediately after a shock
      d. Chest compressor fatigue
      e. Excessive or ineffective ventilation

F. Guidelines: Available at www.circulationaha.org

Patient Cases

3. A 71-year-old man well known to the hypertension clinic presents for his follow-up appointment. While in the lobby, he tells the clerk about the pressure he feels in his chest and appears pale and somewhat diaphoretic. Just before coming to the clinic, he took all of his morning medications, including aspirin 162 mg, metoprolol 100 mg, lisinopril 20 mg, atorvastatin 20 mg, and glipizide 5 mg orally. The clerk goes to get help from the pharmacist, and when they arrive in the lobby, they see the patient become unresponsive. The pharmacist instructs the clerk to call 911 and obtain the AED. Which is the most appropriate action for the pharmacist to take next?

   A. Wait for the AED to arrive.
   B. Cycle 30 chest compressions with two rescue breaths.
   C. Cycle one rescue breath with 15 chest compressions.
   D. Start chest-compression-only CPR.

Patient Cases (continued)

4. At the scene of a car crash, an adult man is unresponsive and not breathing. There is concern about a cervical spine injury. Emergency medical response is already en route, and another bystander (a nurse, trained in CPR) offers to help with the airway. After initiating chest compressions, the nurse is unable to open the airway with a jaw thrust. Which is the best action to take?

   A. Try opening the airway with the jaw thrust until successful.
   B. Continue with chest-compression-only CPR.
   C. Try to open the airway with the head tilt–chin lift maneuver.
   D. Increase ventilation efforts by blowing more forcefully.

II. TOXICOLOGY

A. Poison Control Centers
   1. More than 50 poison control centers exist, covering all 50 states, as well as American Samoa, Micronesia, Guam, Puerto Rico, and the U.S. Virgin Islands.
   2. Single telephone number routes to the poison control center serving that area: (800) 222-1222

3. All information from calls is logged and ultimately captured in the National Poison Data System.
    a. Real-time database that can help disseminate public health concerns as they unfold (e.g., contaminated food)
    b. An annual report is published that summarizes data related to calls to poison centers.
4. Patients undergo initial management on the telephone, with appropriate triage for further evaluation and treatment at a medical facility, if necessary.
    a. Poison control centers are staffed 24 hours per day.
        i. Board-certified medical toxicologist available
        ii. Nurses and pharmacists who are specialists in poison information must pass a national certification examination every 7 years.
    b. Serve as a resource for medical professionals

B. National Toxicology Statistics
    1. The top five drug classes most commonly implicated in overdoses are listed below.
        a. Opioids: 75.2%
        b. Benzodiazepines: 29.4%
        c. Antidepressants: 17.6%
        d. Antiepileptic and antiparkinson drugs: 7.8%
        e. Systemic and hematologic drugs: 7.2%
    2. Opioids were also commonly implicated in pharmaceutical-related deaths when combined with drugs from other classes. The data that follow describe the percentage of cases in which opioids were also involved. For example, 77.2% of deaths involving benzodiazepines also involved the use of opioids.
        a. Benzodiazepines: 77.2%
        b. Antiepileptic and antiparkinson drugs: 65.5%
        c. Antipsychotic and neuroleptic drugs: 58%
        d. Antidepressants: 57.6%
        e. Other analgesics, antipyretics, and antirheumatics: 56.5%
    3. Most (50%–80%) people who die of prescription opioid overdoses have a history of chronic pain.
    4. Opioids
        a. Detection of opioids is commonly done with the use of immunoassays that detect the class of drugs.
        b. Morphine, codeine, and related drugs such as hydrocodone are detected. However, sensitivity differs between them such that detection of hydrocodone requires higher concentrations to produce a positive result.
        c. Oxycodone is also poorly detected.
        d. Some opioids are not detected by the assay because they do not contain a phenanthrene ring (e.g., fentanyl and methadone).
        e. For these reasons, specific rules as to how long an opioid is detectable will vary by drug, dose, and timing. If additional information is necessary about urine detection of a particular opioid, specific assays (qualitative or quantitative) can be obtained.
    5. Substance Abuse and Mental Health Services Administration (SAMHSA) recommended strategies to combat opioid-related deaths (http://store.samhsa.gov/shin/content//SMA13-4742/Overdose_Toolkit_2014_Jan.pdf).
        a. Education for providers, patients, family members, and other individuals at high risk of opioid overdose
            i. Providers should be educated by using evidence-based practices to prevent and manage overdose.
            ii. Others should be educated about potential drug interactions (e.g., alcohol, benzodiazepines), safe storage, signs of overdose, and proper disposal.
        b. Treatment access for those with substance abuse disorders
        c. Access to naloxone

d. Bystanders of suspected opioid overdose should be encouraged to call 911.

e. Use prescription drug monitoring programs.

6. Naloxone

    a. Several laws have been enacted that allow laypersons access to this drug and address liability issues for prescribers and bystanders. The most up-to-date information on laws by jurisdiction is available through www.lawatlas.org.

    b. Pharmacology: Pure opioid antagonist that displaces opioids from binding sites (e.g., μ receptors)

    c. Overdose is classically characterized by respiratory depression, altered mental status, miosis (pinpoint pupils), and decreased bowel motility.

    d. Traditionally, given by intravenous or intramuscular routes in emergency departments

    e. Kits containing injectable naloxone and mucosal atomization devices have been used for intranasal drug administration.

        i. Advantages include decreased risk of needlestick injuries and ease of administration.

        ii. Using 2-mg doses, intranasal and intramuscular administration produce similar response rates within 10 minutes; however, duration may be shorter for the intranasal route, requiring more supplemental naloxone doses.

    f. Commercially available naloxone intramuscular autoinjector was approved by U.S. Food and Drug Administration (FDA) in April 2014, and commercially available nasal spray was approved by FDA in November 2015 and is expected to be marketed in early 2016.

        i. Tradename: Evzio

        ii. Each carton for dispensing contains two autoinjectors and one training device.

        iii. Each autoinjector contains 0.4-mg naloxone. Similar to other autoinjectors, it can be administered through clothing. After actuation, the device should be held in place for 5 seconds.

        iv. Autoinjectors have electronic voice instructions when activated.

7. Public health implications

    a. Providers need to be aware of the effect of pharmaceuticals on health care utilization because of misuse, abuse, and deaths from overdose.

    b. Health care professionals should be aware of and use prescription drug monitoring databases in their state to detect potential abuse.

    c. Pharmacists should play an active role in the care of patients to ensure they are receiving safe and optimal care, especially with opioids. Organizations such as the American Pain Society have issued recommendations for the long-term use of opioids in noncancer pain. Recommendations include proper patient selection and risk stratification, management plans, and monitoring for intended and adverse effects.

    d. Opioid overdose prevention strategies are multipronged and naloxone is an emerging strategy. With the expansion of naloxone use, providers should be aware of naloxone intranasal kits and naloxone autoinjectors.

C. Pediatric Toxicology (Am J Prev Med 2009;37:181-7)

  1. 1. Pediatric patients (18 years and younger) presenting to the ED with poisoning (medication overdose or overexposure to a nonpharmaceutical consumer product) predominate in the young (5 years or younger).

    a. The most common medications, listed in descending order, causing ED visits because of unsupervised ingestion are listed below.

        i. Acetaminophen

        ii. Opioids and benzodiazepines

        iii. Cough and cold preparations

        iv. Nonsteroidal anti-inflammatory drugs

        v. Antidepressants

  b. The results of this investigation highlight the need for pharmacists to educate patients who are around children on the importance of poison prevention strategies and the need for close supervision of children.

 2. Flow restrictors may be another layer of safety for pediatric medications (J Pediatr 2013;1134:39).

 D. Poison Prevention Strategies: May reduce unintentional poisonings from drugs and household products

  1. Child-resistant packaging (e.g., caps on medication containers and poisons)

  2. Identify all poisons around the house and maintain them in a locked cabinet.

  3. Keep all potential poisons in their original containers.

  4. Never store food with poisons.

  5. Keep plants away from animals and children.

  6. Have poison control number easily accessible.

  7. Use carbon monoxide detectors.

III. BIOTERRORISM/NATURAL DISASTERS

 A. Emergency Response Starts Locally: The most effective response is through advanced preparation and through disaster drills.

  1. Pharmacists are essential and highly accessible health care providers.

  2. Incidents are first managed locally.

   a. Additional government support is used as required by the effects of the disaster.

   b. Facilities should prepare disaster plans, including contact lists, calling trees, backup communication, medication storage (if applicable), recordkeeping, and emergency supplies.

   c. Disaster plans are facility-specific, but many have common themes, including the ability to flex according to the situation. Examples of plans:

    i. Community pharmacy: J Am Pharm Assoc 2013;53:432-7

    ii. Hospital pharmacy: CJHP 2007;September/October:6-15

   d. Personal disaster plans should be made as well. A useful resource for guiding individuals in this process is available at www.ready.gov.

  3. The pharmacist will be faced with critical issues during a disaster, including the following:

   a. Limited formulary

   b. Increased need for therapeutic substitution

   c. Management of adverse effects caused by medication changes

   d. Disruption in continuity of care

   e. Patient's ability to store medications properly is diminished.

   f. How to keep records if there is disruption in electronic and Internet connectivity

   g. Communication disruptions

  4. Role of the pharmacist

   a. American Society of Health-System Pharmacists (ASHP) statement on the role of health-system pharmacists in emergency preparedness includes the following recommendations:

    i. Pharmaceutical control and distribution, including planning efforts

    ii. Management of drug therapy for patients during disasters

    iii. Assist with developing guidelines for the diagnosis and treatment of affected individuals.

    iv. Help select pharmaceuticals and supplies for local, regional, and national stockpiles.

    v. Ensure proper storage, packaging, labeling, and handling of pharmaceuticals.

    vi. Ensure pharmaceutical deployment.

    vii. Educate individuals who receive pharmaceuticals.

        viii. Advise public health officials about appropriate messages related to pharmaceuticals to be shared with the public.

        ix. Collaborate with prescribers in the management of patients.

  b. Other roles identified through experience (Public Health Rep 2009;124:217-23)

        i. Prevention of ED overcrowding by caring for patients with nonemergency needs through collaborative protocols that allow pharmacists to refill limited supplies of medications for chronic therapy

        ii. Assess patients for appropriate level of care through triage activities.

        iii. Provide care for minor injuries and other health needs with over-the-counter medications and appropriate use of vaccinations.

        iv. Partner with a doctor of pharmacy educational program as a source of additional personnel.

  c. Pharmacists with clinical responsibilities can be broadly classified into one of three general categories.

        i. Ambulatory readiness pharmacists: Practice in the community setting; the patients they serve include those with low-acuity conditions and chronic diseases

        ii. Pharmacotherapy readiness pharmacists: Practice in the hospital setting and help care for patients with moderate acute conditions and chronic diseases

        iii. Critical care readiness pharmacists: Practice in the hospital setting, delivering intensive care to patients with high-acuity medical conditions

5. Locations where pharmacists may serve during a disaster

  a. Usual place of work is most likely, but may also include shelters, clinics, hospitals, other outreach sites, or temporary medical centers

  b. Points of distribution

        i. Mass distribution of prophylactic medications or vaccines

        ii. Locations include schools, shopping malls, schools, community centers, and stadiums.

        iii. To be effective, patient flow, triage, staffing, recordkeeping, and medication dispensing or immunization administration must be considered.

6. National coordination

  a. The National Incident Management System was established under the Homeland Security Presidential Directive (HSPD)–5: Management of Domestic Incidents

        i. Nationwide template to coordinate efforts, including preparation, response, and recovery

        ii. Provides the basis for the National Response Framework (NRF)

  b. National Response Framework

        i. Part of the National Preparedness System, which was mandated by Presidential Policy Directive (PPD)–8: National Preparedness

        ii. The NRF is a document that addresses response to a disaster, which is one of the five mission areas—prevention, protection, mitigation, response, and recovery—defined by PPD-8.

        iii. Fourteen core capabilities are defined that must be addressed to respond to any incident.

           (a) Planning

           (b) Public information and warning

           (c) Operational coordination

           (d) Critical transportation

           (e) Environmental response/health and safety

           (f) Fatality management services

           (g) Infrastructure systems

           (h) Mass care services

           (i) Mass search and rescue

           (j) On-scene security and protection

(k) Operational communications

(l) Public and private resources

(m) Public health and medical services

(n) Situational assessment

iv. The NRF uses emergency support functions (ESFs) to manage resources and deliver core capabilities. Each ESF may address several core capabilities.

(a) Fifteen ESFs: Transportation; Communications; Public Works and Engineering; Firefighting; Information and Planning; Mass Care; Emergency Assistance, Temporary Housing, and Human Services; Logistics; Public Health and Medical Services; Search and Rescue; Oil and Hazardous Materials Response; Agriculture and Natural Resources; Energy; Public Safety and Security; External Affairs

(b) Pharmacists are most likely to be involved with the Public Health and Medical Services (ESF8) because one of the main core capabilities is public health and medical services.

(c) ESF8 is primarily coordinated by the Department of Health and Human Services (HHS), but local, state, and tribal officials retain primary responsibility for health and medical needs. Medical care is just one of the many functions of ESF8.

(d) There are several areas where pharmacists may serve on the federal level. Disaster medical assistance teams and national pharmacy response teams incorporate pharmacists into emergency response, including mass chemoprophylaxis or immunizations. In addition, the U.S. Public Health Service Ready Reserve Corps was established in 2010. In time of national need, those in the Reserve Corps may be deployed on short notice (www.usphs.gov). While deployed, pharmacists are considered federal employees and are paid a government salary, reimbursed for travel and other expenses, and provided liability coverage while practicing outside their state. During national emergencies when these teams are activated, licensure in one state is recognized by all states.

7. Strategic National Stockpile (SNS)

a. Local and regional supplies are used initially, but these may become exhausted, necessitating the utilization of the SNS.

b. Managed by HHS, with the Centers for Disease Control and Prevention (CDC) as the agency in charge of the SNS

c. Repository of medications, including antibiotics, antitoxins, antidotes, and other drugs to support an ill-defined threat

d. Deployment of SNS assets includes a 12-hour push pack and vendor-managed inventory. SNS assets are deployed in response to a request by the state governor's office to HHS or CDC.

e. Twelve-hour push package

i. First line of support

ii. Can be delivered anywhere in the United States within 12 hours of the decision to deploy

iii. Contains pharmaceuticals and medical supplies

iv. Personnel are also deployed to ensure efficient receipt and deployment of assets at the site.

v. Located at 12 strategic and secure locations within the United States

f. Vendor-managed inventory is a secondary source of supplies, including medications that are tailored according to continued needs.

B. Weapons of Mass Destruction
1. Bioterrorism
   a. The CDC classifies bioterrorism agents as category A, B, or C according to their threat to national security.
   b. Category A diseases: Category A agents are the highest priority because they can be easily disseminated or transmitted from person to person, are associated with high mortality rates with public health impacts, can cause public panic/social disruption, and require public health preparedness efforts.

      These include anthrax (*Bacillus anthracis*), botulism (*Clostridium botulinum*), plague (*Yersinia pestis*), smallpox (*Variola major*), tularemia (*Francisella tularensis*), and viral hemorrhagic fevers (Filoviruses and arenaviruses). Table 3 highlights the clinical characteristics of the diseases and postexposure prophylaxis for category A agents when many individuals are affected.
   c. Category B diseases are moderately easy to disseminate and have moderate morbidity but low mortality rates, requiring enhanced disease surveillance and diagnostics; they include diseases mediated by *Clostridium perfringens* toxin, brucellosis, food safety (e.g., *Salmonella, Shigella*), glanders, Q fever, ricin poisoning, melioidosis, typhus fever, equine viral encephalitis, and waterborne diseases (e.g., *Vibrio*).
   d. Category C diseases can be engineered for mass dissemination with the potential for high morbidity and mortality; they can cause a major health impact and include Nipah virus infection, hantavirus infection, tick-borne viral infections, yellow fever, and multidrug-resistant tuberculosis.

Table 3. Summary of High-Priority Bioterrorism Agents with Recommendations for Postexposure Prophylaxis

Clinical Manifestations	Adult Postexposure Prophylaxis	Pediatric Postexposure Prophylaxis
Anthrax (*Bacillus anthracis*)		
Inhalational form: Starts with flulike symptoms; then respiratory symptoms progressively worsen; death ensues within 5–7 days, but can take up to 2 months	Postexposure prophylaxis for pneumonic (i.e., inhalational) anthrax is most effective when antimicrobials and vaccines are used in combination The vaccine uses a protein to induce immunity and does not contain any dead or live bacteria; it is in limited supply and is only available through CDC	
Cutaneous form: Typically occurs from a break in the skin; pruritic rash and edema at infection site that forms a black eschar; 1–7 days from exposure Gastrointestinal form: Rare, but may occur in conjunction with inhalational form, causing abdominal pain and ulcerations; can also occur from raw/ undercooked meats; 1–7 days after exposure No person-to-person transmission Spores may germinate for up to 60 days after exposure, so prophylaxis for many patients may be necessary for up to 60 days	Ciprofloxacin 500 mg PO q12h *Or* Doxycycline 100 mg PO q12h *Or* Amoxicillin 500 mg PO tid if the strain is sensitive to penicillin Duration: 60 days Because of the severity of the disease, pregnant women and those who are immunocompromised should receive the same therapy Anthrax vaccine adsorbed is recommended for all adults (18–65 years), including pregnant woman, as a three-dose subcutaneous series; the first dose is administered no later than 10 days after exposure, and the remaining doses are given 2 and 4 weeks after the initial dose	Ciprofloxacin 10–15 mg/kg PO q12h *Or* >8 years and >45 kg: Doxycycline 100 mg PO q12h ≤8 years or ≤45 kg: Doxycycline 2.2 mg/kg PO q12h (not to exceed 100 mg/dose) Duration: 60 days Although fluoroquinolones and tetracyclines are usually avoided in children, their use is indicated because of the severity of the disease Vaccine recommendations are made when the event occurs

Table 3. Summary of High-Priority Bioterrorism Agents with Recommendations for Postexposure Prophylaxis *(continued)*

Clinical Manifestations	Adult Postexposure Prophylaxis	Pediatric Postexposure Prophylaxis
Botulism *(Clostridium botulinum)*		
Portal of entry is through the ingestion of contaminated food, or it is inhalational, with the earliest onset of symptoms at 6 hours; however, it can be delayed by more than a week The toxin inhibits the release of acetylcholine; symptoms include visual difficulties and trouble with speech, swallowing, breathing, and muscle control No person-to-person transmission	An antitoxin is available through the CDC and may halt clinical progression and shorten disease duration; limited supply of the antitoxin may limit its use in postexposure prophylaxis when many patients may require therapy	
Plague *(Yersinia pestis)*		
Fleas are the vector to spread natural disease; they cause disease in small rodents and humans through bites; in cases of bioterrorism, aerosolization and resultant inhalation will cause disease Pneumonic form: Caused by primary inhalation or hematogenous spread; the clinical course includes a severe pneumonia with high fevers, chills, malaise, cough that progresses to respiratory failure and death; even with treatment, mortality is around 60% Pneumonic plague can be transmitted from person to person; droplet precautions should be used for infected individuals Bubonic form: High fevers, malaise, buboes (painful and swollen lymph nodes), may progress to bacteremia, sepsis, or pneumonia; with treatment, mortality is around 5%	Preferred Doxycycline 100 mg PO q12h Ciprofloxacin 500 mg PO q12h *Or* Alternative Chloramphenicol 25 mg/kg PO qid Duration: 7 days Indicated only for pneumonic form	Preferred >45 kg: Doxycycline 100 mg PO q12h ≤45 kg: Doxycycline 2.2 mg/kg PO q12h (not to exceed 100 mg/dose) Ciprofloxacin 20 mg/kg PO bid (up to 1 g/day) *Or* Alternative Chloramphenicol 25 mg/kg PO qid Duration: 7 days Indicated only for pneumonic form

Table 3. Summary of High-Priority Bioterrorism Agents with Recommendations for Postexposure Prophylaxis *(continued)*

Clinical Manifestations	Adult Postexposure Prophylaxis	Pediatric Postexposure Prophylaxis
Smallpox *(Variola DNA virus)*		
Prodrome of illness includes headache, malaise, myalgia, and a temperature of >102°F; lesions first appear in the mouth, and then spread to the skin; the rash (macules, papules, and vesicles) progressively spreads from the hands, face, and forearms to the trunk and lower extremities; lesions have a more dense appearance on the extremities and face; lesions eventually crust over and leave pitted scars; unlike chickenpox, smallpox lesions are commonly found on the palmar aspect of hands and the soles of the feet High person-to-person transmission through close contact and possible airborne spread Early vaccination can prevent or decrease the severity of disease if given within 4 days of exposure	Vaccine indications • Exposure to the virus • Close contact (<2 m) with a person with confirmed or suspected smallpox, including those with medical or public health responsibilities • Laboratory personnel who may come in contact with clinical specimens from patients with known or suspected smallpox Vaccine administration • Bifurcated needles are inserted into the vial • A droplet is suspended between the prongs and is the required dose • The needle is used to puncture the skin 15 times over the deltoid muscle • Patients are evaluated 6–8 days after vaccine administration to ensure an immune response with a lesion at the injection site • The CDC Web site contains detailed administration instructions (http://emergency.cdc.gov/agent/smallpox/vaccination/vaccination-method.asp) In cases of high exposure to smallpox, including acts of bioterrorism, the benefits of the vaccine outweigh risks and therefore no absolute contraindications exist in this setting	
Tularemia *(Francisella tularensis)*		
The mode of delivery for bioterrorism is likely to be aerosolization Symptoms include fever, chills, rigors, headache, myalgia, sore throat, with progression to pneumonia; other organs can also be affected including spleen, liver, and kidney Untreated, mortality is 30%–60% No person-to-person transmission	Ciprofloxacin 500 mg PO q12h *Or* Doxycycline 100 mg PO q12h Duration: 14 days	Ciprofloxacin 15 mg/kg PO q12h *Or* >45 kg: Doxycycline 100 mg PO q12h ≤45 kg: Doxycycline 2.2 mg/kg PO q12h (not to exceed 100 mg/dose) Duration: 14 days

bid = twice daily; CDC = Centers for Disease Control and Prevention; PO = orally; qid = four times daily; q12h = every 12 hours; tid = three times daily.

Patient Cases

5. Aerosolization of an unknown bioterrorism category A agent occurred in a large metropolitan area. Initial symptoms of individuals exposed to this agent have been primarily respiratory and pneumonia-like after several days. The only people who seem to be affected are those who were in the original area. Family members who were not primarily exposed did not seem to contract illness after contact with their loved ones who were exposed. This category A agent is most likely to cause which of the following diseases?

   A. Botulism.
   B. Plague.
   C. Smallpox.
   D. Tularemia.

6. A man presents to the chemoprophylaxis point-of-dispensing tent after confirmed inhalational exposure to anthrax. He has no known allergies to medications. Which postexposure prophylaxis regimen is best?

   A. Single vaccine dose in addition to oral ciprofloxacin for 60 days.
   B. Vaccination today and then in 2 and 4 weeks.
   C. Oral doxycycline for 60 days.
   D. Oral ciprofloxacin for 60 days plus vaccination today, with two additional doses at 2 and 4 weeks.

  2. Chemical agents

    a. The CDC categorizes chemical agents into various categories, mostly according to the primary signs/symptoms humans would experience. Below are the main categories and representative examples.

      i. Biotoxins: Ricin, digitalis, strychnine, nicotine, tetrodotoxin

      ii. Blister agents/vesicants: Nitrogen and sulfur mustards, lewisite, phosgene oxime

      iii. Blood agents: Arsine, carbon monoxide, cyanide

      iv. Caustics: Hydrogen fluoride, hydrogen chloride

      v. Pulmonary agents: Ammonia, chlorine, bromine, phosphorus

      vi. Incapacitating agents: 3-Quinuclidinyl benzilate, opioids

      vii. Long-acting warfarins: "Super warfarin"

      viii. Metals: Arsenic, mercury, barium

      ix. Nerve agents: Sarin, soman, tabun, VX

      x. Organic solvents: Benzene

      xi. Riot control: Bromobenzylcyanide, chloroacetophenone

      xii. Toxic alcohols

    b. Patient presentation and treatment depend on the causative agent. Specific information regarding recognition, testing, and treatment can be found at www.bt.cdc.gov.

C. Useful Resources

  1. Rx Response (www.rxresponse.org): An online tool that can be used to locate the closest open pharmacy during an emergency, find information about supply-chain issues, and print wallet cards for patients that contain basic medical information, including medications

  2. Emergency preparedness and response (emergency.cdc.gov): An extensive CDC resource that reviews issues related to planning and response to disasters

  3. Federal Emergency Management Agency (FEMA) (www.fema.gov): Content important for planning and responding to disasters. The approach is very broad and includes all aspects of disasters. The NRF and details of each emergency support function can be found at this Web site.

4. Emergency preparedness (www.fda.gov/Drugs/EmergencyPreparedness/default.htm): A resource for consumers and health professionals that details important issues related to the preparation and response to natural and man-made threats

IV. IMMUNIZATIONS

Guidelines

Kim DK, Bridges CB, Harriman KH. Advisory Committee on Immunization Practices recommended immunization schedule for adults aged 19 years or older: United States, 2015. Ann Intern Med 2015;162:214–23.

Centers for Disease Control and Prevention. Advisory Committee for Immunization Practices (ACIP). Recommended Adult Immunization Schedule—United States, 2015. Available at www.cdc.gov/vaccines/schedules/hcp/adult.html.

Centers for Disease Control and Prevention. Advisory Committee for Immunization Practices (ACIP). Recommended Immunization Schedules for Persons Aged 0 Through 18 Years—United States, 2015. Available at www.cdc.gov/vaccines/schedules/hcp/child-adolescent.html.

A. Definitions
 1. Immunity: The ability of the body to detect material endogenous to itself and to eliminate foreign materials
 2. Antigen: A live or inactivated substance capable of producing an immune response
 3. Antibody: Protein molecules produced by B lymphocytes to help eliminate an antigen
 4. Two basic mechanisms for acquiring immunity
    a. Passive: The transfer of antibody produced by animal or human and transferred to another human (e.g., injection or from mother to infant through the placenta or breast milk)
    b. Active: The stimulation of the immune system to produce an antigen-specific antibody
    c. Methods
       i. Survive infection: Memory B cells remember the antigen and, when exposed to it again, replicate and produce antibodies.
       ii. Vaccination: The injection of a small amount of antigen to produce an immune response

B. General Recommendations
 1. Live, attenuated: Contains modified and weakened live virus
    a. Produces an immune response similar to a natural infection by replicating in a vaccinated person
    b. Immune response is produced after the first dose for most people; however, some patients may need more than one dose to provide a high level of immunity.
    c. Can cause adverse effects (e.g., fever, malaise, myalgias), such as the disease being vaccinated against but typically not as severe
    d. Contraindicated in immunosuppressed patients because of the risk of causing uncontrolled replication
    e. Contraindicated in pregnancy because of concern about infecting the fetus
    f. Children younger than 1 year cannot develop an immune response to live vaccines.
    g. Live, attenuated vaccines
       i. Virus
          (a) Measles, mumps, and rubella (MMR)
          (b) Varicella
          (c) Zoster
          (d) Yellow fever

           (e) Rotavirus

           (f) Intranasal influenza

           (g) Oral polio – Not available in the United States

      ii. Bacteria—Oral typhoid

2. Inactivated: Contains virus that has been inactivated by heat and/or chemicals

    a. Not alive; therefore, cannot replicate in the body

    b. Usually requires several doses to prime the immune system and then to produce response

    c. Examples of inactivated vaccines

      i. Polio (injection only)

      ii. Hepatitis A/B

      iii. Influenza (injection only)

      iv. Human papillomavirus (HPV)

      v. Rabies

      vi. Pneumococcal conjugate or polysaccharide

      vii. Meningococcal conjugate or polysaccharide

3. Polysaccharide vaccines: Inactivated vaccines that contain long chains of sugar molecules that make up the surface capsule protein of the bacteria

    a. Pure polysaccharide

      i. Immune response does not require T-helper cells; is mediated through B cells

      ii. Children younger than 2 years are unable to form an immune response by this method because of immaturity of the immune system.

      iii. Types of pure polysaccharide vaccines

           (a) Pneumococcal (PPSV23)

           (b) Meningococcal (MPSV4)

    b. Conjugate polysaccharide

      i. A polysaccharide vaccine combined with protein that changes the response to a T cell–mediated response

      ii. Allows children younger than 2 years to form an immune response

      iii. Types of conjugate polysaccharide vaccines

           (a) *Haemophilus influenzae* type B (Hib)

           (b) Pneumococcal (PCV13)

           (c) Meningococcal vaccine (MenACWY)

4. Recombinant vaccines

    a. Produced by inserting part of the gene of the antigen into the gene of another cell (e.g., a yeast cell)

    b. Types of recombinant vaccines available

      i. Human papillomavirus

      ii. Hepatitis B

      iii. Live typhoid vaccine (attenuated *Salmonella typhi*)

      iv. Egg-free influenza

5. Timing and spacing

    a. Antibody-vaccine interactions

      i. Live, attenuated vaccines may be affected by circulating antibodies.

           (a) Vaccine given first: Wait 2 weeks before administering antibody.

           (b) Antibody given first: Wait 3 months before administering vaccine. (Exception: Zoster vaccine is not known to be affected by circulating antibody at any time before or after receipt of antibody-containing blood product.)

      ii. Does not apply to inactivated vaccines

    b. Simultaneous administration

        i. There is no limit to the number of vaccines that can be administered in one visit.

        ii. Live, attenuated injectable vaccines not given during the same visit must be separated by at least 4 weeks.

           (a) If administered too closely together, the first vaccine given could interfere with the immune response of the second.

           (b) Does not apply to oral live, attenuated vaccines (i.e., rotavirus)

           (c) Does not apply to inactivated vaccines

    c. Interval between multidose vaccines

        i. Increasing the interval between multidose vaccines will not diminish the effect of the vaccine.

        ii. Decreasing the interval between multidose vaccines may interfere with the immune response.

        iii. Exception: Vaccines may be given up to 4 days before the next scheduled dose.

    d. Age requirements: Vaccines should not be given earlier than the minimum age requirement for the vaccine.

        i. Exception: During a measles outbreak, the MMR vaccine may be given before 12 months of age; however, this dose will not count toward the series.

        ii. Exception: Vaccines may be given up to 4 days before the minimum age because doing so is unlikely to result in a decreased immune response.

6. Number of doses

    a. Live, attenuated vaccine

        i. Provides an immune response after one dose

        ii. A second dose, if recommended, is usually given to ensure 100% immunity.

    b. Inactivated vaccines

        i. Usually require two or three doses before an immune response is complete

        ii. Immune response may wane over time, thus requiring a booster dose.

7. Certain vaccines are recommended for people traveling outside the United States: The CDC's Yellow Book is the definitive reference for recommended vaccines (http://wwwnc.cdc.gov/travel/yellowbook/2016/table-of-contents).

8. Adverse reactions

    a. Local injection site reactions: Most common and least severe

        i. Pain, redness, and swelling at the injection site

        ii. Occur within 4 hours of injection

        iii. More common with inactivated vaccines

    b. Systemic

        i. Generalized symptoms of fever, rash, headache, malaise, myalgias, and/or loss of appetite

        ii. More common with live, attenuated vaccines because the immune response takes on a mild form of the disease vaccinated against

        iii. Manifests within 7–21 days

    c. Allergic: Least common and most severe

        i. Life-threatening; seek medical assistance immediately

        ii. May be caused by vaccine itself or one of its components (i.e., eggs, neomycin, latex)

        iii. Rate: Less than 1 in 500,000

        iv. Symptoms may occur within seconds of exposure or may be delayed an hour or more after exposure.

    d. Reporting adverse reactions

        i. Vaccine Adverse Event Reporting System (VAERS), a subunit of the CDC

        ii. Report any clinically significant adverse event

        iii. Access Web site online at http://vaers.hhs.gov/esub/index.

9. Precautions
   a. Definition—Condition in a recipient that might increase the chance or severity of a serious adverse reaction, or might compromise the ability of the vaccine to produce immunity
   b. Risk-benefit assessment before administration
      i. Pertussis-containing vaccines—Diphtheria and tetanus toxoids and acellular pertussis (DTaP) vaccine only
         (a) Temperature greater than 105°F within 48 hours of a dose and no other identifiable cause
         (b) Collapse or shock-like state within 48 hours of a dose
         (c) Persistent, inconsolable crying lasting more than 3 hours within 48 hours of a dose
         (d) Seizure without fever within 3 days of a dose
      ii. Guillain-Barré syndrome within 6 weeks of a vaccine
         (a) DTaP, diphtheria and reduced tetanus toxoids and acellular pertussis (Tdap), tetanus and diphtheria (Td) vaccines: Should receive if benefits outweigh risks
         (b) Influenza vaccine: Benefits of receiving likely outweigh risks
         (c) Meningococcal conjugate vaccine – Avoid, except in individuals with high risk of contracting meningitis.
   c. Temporary—Those who may receive a vaccine when conditions improve or change
      i. Moderate to severe acute illness
      ii. Recent receipt of antibody-containing blood products (applies only to MMR, rotavirus, and varicella-containing vaccines)
10. Contraindications
   a. Permanent—Those who should avoid vaccination with a specific vaccine
      i. Severe allergic reaction after a previous dose (e.g., anaphylaxis)
      ii. Encephalopathy not attributable to another cause occurring 7 days after a pertussis vaccine
   b. Temporary contraindications to live, attenuated vaccines—Those who may receive a vaccine once conditions improve or change
      i. Pregnancy
         (a) Live, attenuated vaccines should not be given because of the theoretical risk of infection to the fetus (documented only with vaccinia).
         (b) Inactivated vaccines cannot replicate; therefore, they cannot cause fetal infection and are safe to give (exception: HPV because its safety has not been studied).
      ii. Immunosuppression
         (a) Live, attenuated vaccines should not be administered because of the risk of uncontrolled replication.
         (b) Inactivated vaccines may be given; however, the immune response may be diminished, and revaccination when immune competence is regained is recommended.
         (c) Chronic therapy with high-dose oral steroids: Defined as prednisone 20 mg/day (or ≥2 mg/kg/day) for more than 14 days; is contraindicated with live, attenuated vaccines (may vaccinate once discontinued for more than 1 month)
         (d) Aerosolized, topical steroids or short-term steroid bursts are not a contraindication to live, attenuated vaccines.
         (e) Live, attenuated vaccines can be given 3 months after the cessation of chemotherapy or at least 2 weeks before the initiation of immunosuppressive therapy.
   c. Household contacts of individuals with altered immunocompetence may be given live vaccines, if indicated. An exception to this: Contacts of severely immunocompromised patients requiring care in a protective environment
11. Invalid contraindications
   a. Mild illness
   b. Antimicrobial therapy

    c. Disease exposure
    d. Household contact with pregnant or immunosuppressed person
    e. Breastfeeding
    f. Preterm birth
    g. Family history of adverse events
    h. Many simultaneous vaccines
    i. Current administration of tuberculin skin test

Patient Case

7. H.H. is a 4-year-old boy who presents with a runny nose. He does not have a fever today. Medical history is significant for asthma exacerbation 3 months ago. Which combination of vaccines will most likely be given to H.H. at this visit?

    A. Live, attenuated influenza vaccine (LAIV), MMR vaccine.
    B. Inactivated influenza vaccine (IIV), varicella vaccine.
    C. LAIV and HPV vaccine.
    D. IIV and MenACWY.

    C. Influenza Vaccine
        1. Influenza infection
            a. Usually results in a respiratory illness
            b. Incubation: 1–4 days
        2. Virus types
            a. Type A: Moderate to severe illness that affects all age groups (human and animal virus origins)
            b. Type B: Typically, milder illness that affects children only (human-only virus)
            c. Type C: Rarely seen, never attributed to epidemics
        3. Common clinical features include fever, chills, body aches, malaise, and sore throat.
        4. Vaccine composition
            a. Contains different influenza viruses, based on surveillance forecasts by the World Health Organization (WHO) of the virus likely to be prevalent in the coming year
                i. LAIV is available as a quadrivalent vaccine.
                    (a) Two influenza type A strains
                    (b) Two influenza type B strains
                ii. Inclusion of two influenza type B lineages should increase the likelihood of providing antibodies against a higher number of circulating types.
                iii. IIV is available in the quadrivalent or trivalent inactivated influenza vaccine composition.
            b. Vaccine development takes about 6 months; therefore, decisions must be made in January to have a vaccine available by October.
        5. Types of influenza vaccine
            a. Inactivated influenza vaccine
                i. Administered intramuscularly
                    (a) 0.25 mL for children 6–35 months of age
                    (b) 0.5 mL for children 3 years and older
                ii. Grown in chicken embryos
                iii. Available in multidose vials or in preservative-free, single-dose vials
                iv. Immunity after administration is generally less than 1 year

   v. Adverse reactions

    (a) Local injection site reactions (15%–20%)

    (b) Systemic reactions are uncommon.

    (c) Immediate hypersensitivity is usually associated with a component of the vaccine.

  b. Live, attenuated influenza vaccine

   i. Administered as 0.1-mL spray per each nostril

   ii. Grown in chicken embryos

   iii. Available in a single-dose, preservative-free sprayer unit

   iv. Indicated only for individuals 2–49 years of age

   v. Contraindications and precautions

    (a) Pregnant women

    (b) Patients receiving immunosuppressive therapy

    (c) Patients with chronic medical conditions

    (d) People with history of egg allergy

    (e) Children 2–4 years of age with asthma or wheezing episode documented in past 12 months

    (f) People who take antiviral medication within past 48 hours

    (g) People who care for severely immunocompromised individuals who require a protective environment

   vi. Adverse reactions are localized and/or may present as mild influenza-type symptoms.

  c. High-dose IIV

   i. Administered intramuscularly

   ii. Grown in chicken embryos

   iii. Available in multidose vials or in preservative-free, single-dose vials and syringes

   iv. Contains 4 times the amount of antigen compared with IIV

   v. Approved for use in individuals older than 65 years

   vi. Developed to increase immunogenicity in older populations because the ability to form an immune response wanes with age

   vii. The CDC does not give this vaccine preference over IIV because of the lack of clinical efficacy data.

  d. Intradermal influenza vaccine

   i. Administered by intradermal route

   ii. Grown in chicken embryos

   iii. Available in a single-dose, prefilled microinjection system

   iv. Approved for use in individuals 18–64 years of age

   v. Preservative-free

  e. Recombinant influenza vaccine (RIV3) (egg-free)

   i. Trivalent vaccine administered intramuscularly

   ii. Flu shot produced without using chicken eggs was approved by the FDA in 2013.

   iii. May be administered to patients with true severe hypersensitivity reactions to eggs

   iv. Preservative-free, approved for individuals 18 years of age and older

6. Recommendations

  a. Influenza vaccine administration should begin before onset of influenza activity (by October if possible).

  b. All individuals 6 months or older should get a yearly influenza vaccine.

  c. Individuals at high risk of complications should be certain to get the vaccine.

   i. Pregnant women (IIV only)

   ii. Children younger than 5 years, especially children younger than 2 years

   iii. Adults 50 years and older (IIV only)

        iv.   Individuals of any age with certain medical conditions (IIV only)

(a) Diabetes

(b) Asthma

(c) Chronic obstructive pulmonary disease

(d) Neurologic and neurodevelopmental conditions

(e) Cystic fibrosis

(f) Heart disease (congenital heart disease, congestive heart failure, coronary artery disease)

(g) Kidney and liver disorders

(h) Weakened immune system

(i) Morbid obesity

(j) Individuals younger than 19 years receiving chronic aspirin therapy

        v.   Individuals in close contact with those at high risk of complications

(a) Health care workers

(b) Household contacts of high-risk individuals

(c) Household contacts and caregivers of children younger than 6 months (i.e., those who cannot receive the vaccine)

    d.   With the advent of RIV3, all patients with severe egg allergies can receive the influenza vaccine with RIV3. Those with a hives-only reaction may receive IIV or RIV3.

    e.   All children 6 months to 8 years of age who are receiving their first influenza vaccine should receive a total of two doses, at least 4 weeks apart.

D. Pneumococcal Vaccine

    1.   Pneumococcal infection

        a.   Usually results in pneumococcal pneumonia (less commonly, otitis media or meningitis)

        b.   Incubation period is 1–3 days for pneumonia.

    2.   Caused by the bacterium *Streptococcus pneumoniae*

        a.   Ninety known serotypes, but only a few account for severe disease

        b.   Encapsulated bacteria

    3.   Clinical features of pneumonia commonly include fever, chills, productive cough, dyspnea, and tachypnea.

    4.   Pneumococcal vaccine

        a.   Inactivated vaccine

        b.   Administration route

           i.   Pneumococcal polysaccharide may be administered intramuscularly or subcutaneously.

          ii.   Pneumococcal conjugate may be administered intramuscularly.

        c.   Types of vaccine

           i.   Pneumococcal conjugate vaccine (PCV13)

(a) Contains polysaccharide, conjugated antigen for 13 serotypes of pneumococcal bacteria

(b) Available only in single-dose, preservative-free syringes

(c) Previously contained seven serotypes (PCV7); however, changed to PCV13 because of an increased incidence of infections with serotypes outside those contained in PCV7

(d) FDA approved for use in patients aged 6 weeks to 5 years (four-dose series), 6–17 years (single dose), and 50 years and older (single dose)

          ii.   Pneumococcal polysaccharide vaccine (PPSV23)

(a) Contains purified capsular polysaccharide antigen from 23 serotypes of pneumococcal bacteria

(b) Available in single prefilled syringes and single-dose and multidose vials

(c) Accounts for about 88% of pneumococcal disease

    (d) Around 80% of patients will develop antibodies after one dose.

    (e) FDA approved for individuals 2 years of age and older and adults 50 years of age or older

  d. No information regarding safety in pregnancy—It is best to give the vaccination to women of childbearing age at high risk of pneumococcal disease before conception.

  e. Adverse reactions are usually localized injection site reactions. Systemic reactions are rare.

 5. Recommendations

  a. Pneumococcal conjugate vaccine (PCV13)

   i. All children younger than 2 years

    (a) Series of four doses

    (b) Given at 2, 4, 6, and 12–15 months

   ii. Children 2–5 years of age should receive one dose of PCV13 if three or four doses of PCV7 were received and two doses of PCV13 at least 8 weeks apart, if less than three doses of PCV7 were received, if they have chronic heart disease, diabetes mellitus, chronic lung disease, sickle cell disease, asplenia, human immunodeficiency virus (HIV) infection, chronic renal failure, or diseases treated with immunosuppressive therapy or radiation.

   iii. Children and adolescents 6–18 years of age who are PCV13 naive and asplenic with cochlear implants, chronic renal failure, HIV infection, diseases treated with immunosuppressive therapy or radiation, cerebrospinal fluid (CSF) leaks, or who are immunocompromised receive one dose.

   iv. Adults 65 years of age and older

    (a) Receive one dose of PCV13 followed by one dose of PPSV23, 6–12 months later

    (b) Adults who have not previously received PCV13 and who have previously received one or more doses of PPSV23 should receive one dose of PCV13 at least 1 year after receipt of the most recent PPSV23.

  b. Pneumococcal polysaccharide vaccine (PPSV23)

   i. When PCV is also indicated, PCV13 should be given first

   ii. All patients 65 years and older

   iii. Patients between 2 and 64 years of age with the following conditions should receive one dose:

    (a) Chronic lung disease

     (1) Asthma—Children and adolescents 2–18 years of age who are using high-dose oral corticosteroids or adults 19 years and older

     (2) Chronic obstructive pulmonary disease

     (3) Emphysema

    (b) Chronic heart disease

    (c) Diabetes mellitus

    (d) Chronic renal failure or nephrotic syndrome

    (e) Anatomic or functional asplenia

    (f) Cochlear implants

    (g) CSF leak

    (h) Immunocompromising conditions

    (i) HIV infection

   iv. All patients 19–64 years of age (in addition to those included above),

    (a) Smoke cigarettes

    (b) Reside in nursing homes or long-term care facilities

    (c) Chronic liver disease

    (d) Alcoholism

     v.   Revaccination

        (a)   Individuals receiving one or two PPSV23 doses before age 65 years should receive another dose at age 65 years or in 5 years, whichever is longer.

        (b)   Individuals with chronic renal failure, functional/anatomic asplenia, immunocompromising conditions, sickle cell disease, HIV infection, or nephrotic syndrome should receive a one-time revaccination 5 years after the initial dose.

        (c)   No further doses are needed if patients were vaccinated at or after age 65 years.

  c.   Recommendations for adults 19 years and older with immunocompromising conditions, functional or anatomic asplenia, CSF leaks, or cochlear implants

     i.   Pneumococcal vaccine–naive individuals

        (a)   PCV13 first

        (b)   PPSV23 at least 8 weeks later with revaccination as outlined above

     ii.   Previous vaccination with PPSV23

        (a)   PCV13 at least 1 year after PPSV23

        (b)   Revaccination with PPSV23 should occur 5 years after original vaccination with PPSV23 and at least 8 weeks after vaccination with PCV13.

Patient Case

8. L.D. is a 40-year-old man with HIV infection. He received one dose of PPSV23 5 years ago. Which pneumococcal vaccine would be best to give him currently?

  A. Give one dose of PCV13.

  B. Give one dose of PPSV23.

  C. Either vaccine is appropriate.

  D. Neither vaccine is recommended.

  E. Meningococcal Vaccine

    1. Meningococcal infection

      a. Typically presents as meningococcal meningitis

      b. Incubation period is 2–10 days.

    2. Caused by the bacterium *Neisseria meningitidis*—Encapsulated bacteria

    3. Common clinical features include fever, headache, and neck stiffness (may progress to sepsis)

    4. Meningococcal vaccine

      a. Inactivated vaccine

      b. Two-dose series; minimal interval between doses is 8 weeks

      c. Types of meningococcal vaccine

        i.   Meningococcal polysaccharide vaccine (MPSV4 [Menomune])

           (a)   Quadrivalent vaccine that contains serogroups A, C, Y, W

           (b)   Administered subcutaneously

        ii.   Meningococcal conjugate vaccine (MenACWY-D [Menactra] and MenACWY-CRM [Menveo])

           (a)   Contains four *N. meningitidis* serogroups conjugated to either a diphtheria toxoid (MenACWY-D) or a CRM197 (MenACWY-CRM)

           (b)   Administered intramuscularly

           (c)   Available in single-dose, preservative-free vials

           (d)   Is the preferred formulation of the vaccine because it provides a better immune response than MPSV4

           (e)   MenACWY-D is approved for individuals 9 months–55 years of age, whereas MenACWY-CRM is used in children as young as 2 months and through age 55 years.

      iii.   Combination vaccine also available—Meningococcal groups C and Y and *Haemophilus* b tetanus toxoid conjugate vaccine Hib-MenCY-TT (MenHibrix)

    d. Adverse reactions

      i.   Local injection site reactions

      ii.   Systemic reactions: Fever (less than 3%), headache, and malaise

      iii.   There have been some case reports of Guillain-Barré syndrome occurring after the administration of meningococcal conjugate vaccine, but the association with the vaccine is unclear.

5.   Recommendations

    a. Meningococcal conjugate vaccine

      i.   High-risk children with functional/anatomic asplenia (including sickle cell)

        (a)   For children younger than 19 months administer four-dose series of Menveo or MenHibrix at 2, 4, 6, and 12–15 months of age.

        (b)   For children 19–23 months of age with incomplete series of MenHibrix or Menveo, ensure completion of series with two doses at least 3 months apart.

        (c)   For children 24 months or older with incomplete series, administer two-dose series at least 2 months apart. If MenACWY-D is given, wait until 2 years of age and at least 4 weeks after completion of PCV13.

      ii.   High-risk children with persistent complement component deficiency

        (a)   For children younger than 19 months, administer four-dose series of Menveo or MenHibrix at 2, 4, 6, and 12–15 months of age.

        (b)   For children 7–23 months with complement component deficiency and no vaccination

           (1)   If MenACWY-CRM is given, a two-dose series should be given with the second dose after 12 months of age and at least 3 months after the first dose.

           (2)   If MenACWY-D is given at 9–23 months of age, a two-dose series should be given with the second dose at least 3 months after the first dose.

        (c)   For children 24 months or older with complement component deficiency with incomplete vaccination, give two doses of either MenACWY-D or MenACWY-CRM at least 2 months apart.

      iii.   For children who travel to high endemic areas, administer the age-appropriate formulation and series.

      iv.   Administer one dose of MenACWY-D or MenACWY-CRM to all children 11–12 years of age and one booster dose at 16 years.

      v.   Administer one dose of MenACWY-D or MenACWY-CRM at age 13–18 years if not previously vaccinated.

        (a)   If first dose is given at 13–15 years of age, a booster dose should be given at 16–18 years.

        (b)   If first dose is given when older than 16 years, a booster dose is not necessary.

      vi.   Unvaccinated college freshmen living in a dormitory through age 21 years

      vii.   Individuals 2–55 years of age at increased risk of meningococcal disease

        (a)   Microbiologists routinely using *N. meningitidis* isolates (single dose)

        (b)   Military recruits (single dose)

        (c)   Patients traveling to countries with *N. meningitidis* epidemics (single dose)

        (d)   Patients with terminal complement component deficiency (two doses administered at least 2 months apart)

        (e)   Patients with anatomic or functional asplenia or complement component deficiencies (two doses administered at least 2 months apart)

        (f)   Patients at risk during an outbreak because of a vaccine serogroup

       viii. For adults 56 years and older

         (a) MenACWY (either option) is preferred if previously vaccinated with MenACWY and have indication for revaccination.

         (b) Multiple doses are anticipated.

       ix. Infection with HIV is not an indication for a routine MenACWY vaccination, but if a vaccination is given, two doses of MenACWY should be administered 2 months apart.

    b. Meningococcal polysaccharide vaccine (MPSV4)

      i. Acceptable alternative for patients 2–55 years of age if the conjugate vaccine is unavailable

      ii. Preferred vaccine in patients 56 years and older who have not received MenACWY previously and require a single dose

    c. Revaccination every 5 years is recommended for patients who remain at high risk.

Patient Case

9. A.J. is a 17-year-old female adolescent who is planning to attend college next fall. Her admission process requires documentation of completed vaccination history. A.J. received her most recent vaccine when she was 13 years of age. Which vaccine option would be best to give to A.J. today?

    A. Give one dose of MenACWY-D.

    B. Give one dose of Hib-MenCY-TT.

    C. A.J. is not a candidate for the vaccine because she already received the necessary vaccines.

    D. A.J. is not a candidate for the vaccine because she does not meet the age requirements.

  F. Varicella Vaccine

    1. Varicella infection

      a. Caused by the varicella zoster virus—Has the ability to lie dormant in the nervous system

        i. Primary infection: Chickenpox with incubation period of 14–16 days

        ii. Secondary infection: Herpes zoster (shingles)

      b. Clinical features include rash, fever, and pruritus.

    2. Varicella vaccine

      a. Live, attenuated vaccine

      b. Administered subcutaneously as a series of two doses

      c. Approved for use in patients 12 months and older

      d. Contains a small amount of neomycin

      e. Among patients 12 months to 12 years of age, 97% develop an immune response; however, in those 13 years and older, two doses are necessary to achieve a similar response.

      f. Adverse reactions

        i. Local injection site reactions

        ii. Varicella-like rash at injection site

      g. Contraindications/precautions

        i. Avoid in those who are severely immunocompromised or pregnant.

        ii. Avoid use in those receiving an antiviral (e.g., acyclovir, famciclovir) 24 hours before vaccination.

        iii. Avoid use of antiviral agents for 14 days after vaccine administration.

    3. Recommendations

      a. Children younger than 13 years

        i. First dose should be given to all children 12–15 months of age.

      ii.   Second dose should be given to all children 4–6 years of age. Second dose may be administered before age 4 years if 3 months have elapsed since first dose. If second dose is administered at least 4 weeks after the first dose, it may be accepted as valid.

  b. Adolescents and adults 13 years and older

      i.   Should be given if there is no history of varicella immunity, defined as follows:

        (a) U.S. citizens born before 1980 are considered immune (exceptions: Health care personnel and pregnant women).

        (b) Documentation of two varicella vaccinations, at least 4 weeks apart

        (c) History of diagnosis confirmed by a health care provider

        (d) History of herpes zoster diagnosis confirmed by a health care provider

        (e) Laboratory diagnosis

      ii. Should give special consideration to those who have close contact with individuals at high risk of severe disease or of exposure or transmission

  c. Pregnant women should be assessed for varicella immunity and, if not immune, they should receive the first dose after completion of pregnancy and the second dose 4–8 weeks later.

  d. Postexposure prophylaxis—Can be 70%–100% effective in preventing disease if given within 3 days of exposure to varicella virus; especially useful in controlling outbreaks in hospitals, schools, and day care centers

G. Herpes Zoster Vaccine

  1. Herpes zoster infection

    a. Caused by reactivation of a latent varicella zoster virus associated with aging and immunosuppression

    b. Clinical features include unilateral lesions on trunk or trigeminal nerve, pain, and paresthesia.

  2. Herpes zoster vaccine

    a. Live, attenuated vaccine

    b. Administered subcutaneously

    c. Contains the same antigen as the varicella vaccine, but is at least 14-times more potent

    d. Available in a preservative-free powder for reconstitution

    e. Contains neomycin

    f. Use of the vaccine can decrease the incidence of herpes zoster infection by 50%—Efficacy is best in those 50–59 years of age and decreases with increasing age.

    g. The duration of protection from herpes zoster infection is currently unknown.

    h. Adverse reactions—Local injection site reactions

      i. Contraindications

        (a) Avoid use in pregnancy.

        (b) Severe hypersensitivity to neomycin or other vaccine component

        (c) Avoid in severely immunocompromised individuals, including those taking high-dose prednisone (or equivalent) of 20 mg or more for more than 14 days.

      ii. Precautions

        (a) Avoid use in those receiving an antiviral (e.g., acyclovir, famciclovir) 24 hours before vaccination.

        (b) Avoid use of antiviral agents for 14 days after vaccine administration.

  3. Recommendations

    a. All individuals 60 years and older regardless of their history of chickenpox or herpes zoster infection

    b. The herpes zoster vaccine was approved for use in patients 50 years and older by the FDA. The CDC has not changed its recommendations to date.

H. Tetanus, Diphtheria, and Pertussis Vaccines
1. Tetanus
   a. Caused by the neurotoxic exotoxin tetanospasmin, which is produced by *Clostridium tetani,* gram-negative anaerobe in soil
   b. Enters the body through open wounds, with an incubation period of 3–21 days
   c. Common clinical features include lockjaw (trismus), neck stiffness, difficulty swallowing, abdominal muscle rigidity, fever, and sweating.
2. Diphtheria
   a. Caused by a toxin produced by *Corynebacterium diphtheriae* that commonly presents as pharyngeal/tonsillar diphtheria
   b. Incubation period is 2–5 days.
   c. Common clinical features in pharyngeal diphtheria include malaise, sore throat, fever, exudative pharyngitis, and anorexia.
3. Pertussis (whooping cough)
   a. Caused by *Bordetella pertussis*
   b. Incubation period is 7–10 days.
   c. Clinical features present in progressive stages of respiratory infection, starting with runny nose, fever, and mild cough and progressing to rapid, prolonged coughing spells, often causing cyanotic episodes and vomiting.
   d. Immunity after disease is not always permanent.
4. Types of vaccine
   a. Inactivated vaccine
   b. Available in combination vaccines (composition and age indicated are shown in Table 4)
   c. Uppercase letters signify a full-strength dose; lowercase letters signify a partial dose.
   d. Pertussis is found in its acellular form within the vaccine because the whole-cell vaccine was previously associated with severe adverse reactions.
   e. Adverse effects
      i. DTaP/diphtheria-tetanus (DT)
         (a) Local injection site reaction (increase in severity with each dose)
         (b) Temperature as high as 101°F
         (c) Swelling of the entire leg/arm where the vaccine was administered; seen after fourth or fifth dose
      ii. Tdap/Td vaccine
         (a) Local injection site reactions
         (b) Mild fever
         (c) Headache
         (d) Tiredness
         (e) Swelling of the entire leg/arm where the vaccine was administered

Table 4. Formulations of Vaccines Containing Diphtheria, Tetanus, and Pertussis

Vaccine	Diphtheria	Tetanus	Pertussis	Age
DTaP	7–8 Lf-units	5–12.5 Lf-units	2–25 mcg	Birth to 7 years
DT	7–8 Lf-units	5–12.5 Lf-units	–	Birth to 7 years
Td	2–2.5 Lf-units	5 Lf-units	–	7 years and older
Tdap	2–2.5 Lf-units	5 Lf-units	2.5–8 mcg	7 years and older

DT = diphtheria-tetanus; DTaP = diphtheria and tetanus toxoids and acellular pertussis vaccine; Lf = limit of flocculation unit; Td = tetanus and diphtheria vaccine; Tdap = diphtheria and reduced tetanus toxoids and acellular pertussis.

5. Recommendations
   a. Children, birth to 6 years—Total of five doses of DTaP
      i. Given at 2, 4, 6, and 15–18 months and at 4–6 years
      ii. Fourth dose may be given at 12 months as long as 6 months have elapsed between doses 3 and 4.
      iii. DT may be substituted if child does not tolerate pertussis portion of the vaccine (including inconsolable crying, temperature greater than 105°F, or seizures).
   b. Adolescents, 11–12 years of age
      i. One dose of Tdap
      ii. Then, one dose of Td every 10 years as a booster vaccine
   c. Adults, 18 years and older
      i. One dose of Tdap if not already received
      ii. Then, one dose of Td every 10 years as a booster vaccine
   d. Pregnant women
      i. One dose of Tdap with each pregnancy, regardless of Tdap/Td history
      ii. Preferably between 27 and 36 weeks of gestation
      iii. Recommended to protect the infant because the first dose of DTaP is not given until 2 months of age, and the full series is not completed until 5–6 years
   e. Adults 65 years and older
      i. One dose of Tdap if not already received
      ii. Then, one dose of Td every 10 years as a booster vaccine

---

Patient Case

10. K.T. is a 45-year-old man who presented with a laceration to his arm after a car accident. He is unsure of the date of his most recent tetanus booster, but believes it was more than 10 years ago. Which form of vaccine would be best to give this patient today?
    A. DTaP.
    B. DT.
    C. Td.
    D. Tdap.

I. HPV Vaccine
   1. Human papillomavirus
      a. Most common sexually transmitted infection in the United States, with 20 million reported infections
         i. Current estimates show that 80% of women will be infected by age 50 years.
         ii. Up to 20% prevalence in heterosexual men
      b. More than 100 types of HPV have been isolated.
         i. Types 6 and 11 have been associated with benign cervical cell abnormalities, genital warts, and laryngeal papillomas.
         ii. Types 16 and 18 together account for 70% of cases of cervical cancer.
      c. Clinical features are generally asymptomatic, but patients may have anogenital warts and cervical cancer precursors.
      d. High-risk sexual behavior is the only verifiable risk factor for HPV disease.
   2. HPV vaccines
      a. Recombinant, inactive vaccine
      b. Intramuscular injection in single-dose, preservative-free syringes and vials

    c.   Dosing schedule of three doses with second dose administered 4 to 8 weeks after first dose and third dose administered at least 12 weeks after second dose and at least 24 weeks (6 months) after first dose

    d.   Infection with a specific type of HPV before vaccination will not decrease the effectiveness of the vaccine to the other types contained within the vaccine.

    e.   Vaccine will not help treat previous HPV infection.

    f.   Not studied in pregnancy and therefore not recommended

    g.   Three vaccine types available

        i.   Quadrivalent vaccine (Gardasil, HPV4)

           (a) Contains proteins of HPV types 6, 11, 16, and 18

           (b) Approved for use in male and female individuals 9–26 years of age

        ii.   9-Valent vaccine (Gardasil 9)

           (a) Contains proteins of HPV types 6, 11, 16, 18, 31, 33, 45, 52, and 58

           (b) Approved for use in male individuals 9–15 years of age and female individuals 9–26 years of age

        iii. Bivalent vaccine (Cervarix, HPV2)

           (a) Contains proteins of HPV types 16 and 18

           (b) Approved for use in female individuals 9–25 years of age

    h.   Adverse reactions

        i.   Local injection site reactions

        ii.   Systemic reactions: Nausea, dizziness, myalgia, and malaise

        iii. To avoid syncope, it is recommended that patients be observed in the clinic for 15–20 minutes after vaccination.

3. Recommendations

    a.   Female recipients

        i.   All girls should receive vaccine (quadrivalent, bivalent, or 9-valent) at 11 or 12 years of age.

        ii.   All female individuals 13–26 years of age if not previously vaccinated

    b.   Male recipients

        i.   All should receive the quadrivalent vaccine at 11 or 12 years.

        ii.   All male individuals 13–21 years of age if previously unvaccinated or whose three-dose series was incomplete

        iii. All men 22–26 years of age may also receive the vaccine.

Patient Case

11. Which of the following individuals is a candidate for the HPV vaccine?

    A. 32-year-old health care worker.

    B. 27-year-old pharmacy school student.

    C. 40-year-old woman not in a monogamous relationship.

    D. 13-year-old male adolescent.

J. MMR Vaccine

    1. Measles

        a.   Caused by a paramyxovirus

        b.   Incubation period is 14–18 days.

        c.   Clinical features are the progression of a prodrome of high-grade fever and cough to blue-white Koplik spots on mucous membranes, hairline rash spreading downward/outward, and diarrhea.

2. Mumps
   a. Caused by a paramyxovirus acquired through the nasopharynx by respiratory droplets
   b. Incubation is 14–18 days.
   c. Clinical features are the progression of a prodrome of low-grade fever, headache, and malaise to unilateral or bilateral parotitis.
3. Rubella (German measles)
   a. Caused by a togavirus
   b. Incubation period is 14 days.
   c. Clinical features are the progression of a prodrome (not seen in children) of a low-grade fever, malaise, and upper respiratory symptoms to a rash starting on the face and spreading to the rest of the body (symptoms are more faint than those of measles).
4. MMR vaccine
   a. Live, attenuated vaccine
   b. Administered subcutaneously
   c. About 2%–5% may not respond (especially to measles and mumps viruses) to full immunity after the first dose; therefore, two doses are recommended.
   d. Grown in chick embryo fibroblast culture but has been given to egg-allergic patients without incident
   e. Adverse events
      i. Local injection site reactions
      ii. Systemic reactions: Fever, rash, joint pain
5. Rubella vaccine
   a. RA 27/3 (Meruvax II)
   b. Live, attenuated vaccine
   c. Only one dose is necessary to confer immunity.
   d. Use of the single agent is not recommended.
6. Recommendations
   a. All children should receive the MMR vaccine (two-dose series).
      i. First dose is given at 12 months or older.
      ii. Second dose is usually given at 4–6 years but can be given as soon as 28 days after first dose.
      iii. Administer one dose at age 6–11 months before departure from the United States for international travel. Revaccinate with two doses with first dose starting at 12 months or older and second dose at least 4 weeks later.
   b. Adults not receiving MMR as a child should be given at least one dose of the vaccine unless they were born before 1957 (considered immune).

K. Hepatitis A Vaccine
   1. Hepatitis A infection
      a. Caused by the hepatitis A virus
      b. Acquired through fecal-oral transmission
      c. Replicates in the liver and is detected in the blood and excreted in the feces by the biliary system within 10–12 days; however, symptoms do not present until about 28 days after infection and resolve in about 2 months
      d. Clinical features include fever, malaise, jaundice, dark urine, abdominal pain, and nausea.
   2. Types of vaccine
      a. Inactivated whole-cell virus vaccine
      b. Havrix and Vaqta are available with no preference given to one vaccine over the other.
         i. Havrix is a two-dose series given at 0 and 6–12 months.
         ii. Vaqta is a preservative-free vaccine given at 0 and 6–18 months.
         iii. Twinrix is a three-dose, combination hepatitis A and hepatitis B vaccine given at 0, 1, and 6 months.

      c.   Pediatric versions approved for individuals 12 months to 18 years of age

      d.   Adult versions approved for individuals 19 years and older

      e.   Seroconversion is 100% after two doses.

      f.   Adverse reactions

          i.   Local injection site reactions

          ii.   Systemic symptoms include malaise, fever, and fatigue.

3.   Recommendations

      a.   Since 2005, it has been recommended that all children 12–23 months of age receive this vaccine.

      b.   All patients at high risk of the disease

          i.   Travelers to countries with a high rate of the disease or close contact with international adoptee

          ii.   Men who have sex with men

          iii.   Illicit drug use

          iv.   Patients with chronic liver disease

          v.   Patients who are treated with clotting factor concentrates

          vi.   Patients who work with hepatitis A–infected animals or in a hepatitis A research laboratory

      c.   Given as a two-dose series, at least 6 months apart

L.   Hepatitis B Vaccine

   1.   Hepatitis B infection

      a.   Caused by the hepatitis B virus (HBV)

      b.   Clinical feature is a progression from a prodrome of malaise, nausea/vomiting, fever, right upper quadrant pain, rash, dark urine to the ictal phase of jaundice, and hepatomegaly to potentially chronic hepatitis.

      c.   Most HBV infections result in complete elimination of the hepatitis B surface antigen (HBsAg) from the body and replacement with HBV antibodies.

   2.   Types of vaccine

      a.   Two available vaccines

          i.   Recombivax HB

              (a)   Pediatric formulation: Can be used for any age group

             (b)   Adult formulation: Can be used for any age group

             (c)   Single-dose vials (preservative-free)

          ii.   Engerix-B

              (a)   Pediatric formulation: Approved for use in patients 20 years and younger

             (b)   Adult formulation: Approved for use in patients 11 years and older

             (c)   Does not contain thimerosal as a preservative, but does contain it as a residual from the manufacturing process

      b.   Recombinant, inactive vaccine administered as a three-dose injection series

      c.   After three doses, up to 95% of patients 19 years and younger develop an immune response, and up to 90% of adults develop an immune response. This effect wanes over time, with a significant drop-off in patients older than 60 years.

      d.   Adverse reactions

          i.   Local injection site reactions

          ii.   Systemic: Fatigue, headache, irritability, and fever

3. Recommendations
   a. All children at birth, 1–2 months, and 6–18 months. Unlike most vaccines, the recommended period between doses 2 and 3 is at least 8 weeks for optimization of anti–hepatitis B antigen titers.
   b. All children at 11–12 years (and up to 18 years as catch-up), if not vaccinated as an infant
      i. Given at baseline, 1 month, and 6 months
      ii. Alternative (only with Recombivax vaccine): Baseline and 4 months later only in patients 11–15 years of age
   c. Adults at high risk of HBV if not previously vaccinated
      i. High-risk patients
         (a) Individuals with diabetes as soon as diabetes is diagnosed, up to age 60 years; after age 60 years, they may be vaccinated at the discretion of the primary care provider
         (b) Sexual partners of HBsAg-positive individuals
         (c) Sexually active people not in a mutually monogamous relationship
         (d) Men who have sex with men
         (e) Current or recent illicit intravenous drug users
         (f) Household contacts of HBsAg-positive individuals
         (g) Health care workers
         (h) Individuals with end-stage renal disease
         (i) Travelers to places where hepatitis B infection is prevalent
         (j) Those infected with HIV
      ii. Usually given at baseline, 1 month, and 6 months

Patient Case

12. C.C. is a 33-year-old woman who will be traveling to Beijing to manage a start-up manufacturing company. Which of the following recommendations would you offer C.C. regarding vaccination against hepatitis A?

   A. C.C. is not a candidate for this vaccine because of her age.
   B. C.C. should receive a three-dose series of hepatitis A vaccine because she will be moving to a country with high rate of the disease.
   C. C.C. should receive a two-dose series of hepatitis A vaccine because she will be moving to a country with high rate of the disease.
   D. C.C. will not be at high risk of hepatitis A, and her risks in receiving the vaccine outweigh the benefit.

M. Hib Vaccine
   1. Hib infection
      a. Caused by the encapsulated bacterium *H. influenzae* by entering the body through the nasopharynx, where it can be dormant for several months before causing disease
      b. Disease is not very common in children older than 5 years.
      c. Common clinical feature of meningitis (common manifestation) include fever, decreased mental status, and stiff neck.
      d. Risk factors for disease
         i. Household crowding
         ii. Large household size
         iii. Day care attendance
         iv. Low socioeconomic status
         v. Low parental education
         vi. School-aged siblings

2. Hib vaccine
   a. Polysaccharide vaccine was removed from the market in 1988 because a more useable conjugate vaccine was developed.
   b. Polysaccharide-protein conjugate vaccines
      i. Approved for use in children 6 weeks and older
      ii. Clinical efficacy is 95%–100% after two or three doses.
      iii. Types
         (a) Polyribosylribitol phosphate chemically conjugated to tetanus toxoid (PRP-T)
         (b) *Haemophilus* B conjugate (PRP-OMP), conjugated to meningococcal group B outer membrane protein
   c. Adverse reactions—Local injection site reactions
3. Recommendations
   a. All children should start the vaccine series at 2 months.
      i. PRP-T: Intramuscular
         (a) Ideally, should be used only as the final (booster) dose in children 12 months to 4 years of age with one dose of Hib vaccine
         (b) Otherwise, series of three doses at 2, 4, and 6 months with one booster dose at 12–15 months
      ii. PRP-OMP: Intramuscular
         (a) Series of two doses at 2 and 4 months
         (b) One booster dose at 12–15 months
   b. The two vaccines are interchangeable because they are equally efficacious. If using a combination of both vaccines, a total of three doses should be given.
   c. If the vaccination series is started late, not all doses may be necessary; the number of doses can be determined by using Table 5.
   d. Patients with asplenia or sickle cell disease and those undergoing splenectomy should receive one dose.
   e. Patients who receive a hematopoietic stem cell transplant should receive three doses 6 months after transplantation with at least 4 weeks between doses.
   f. Hib vaccination is not recommended for adults with HIV infection because the risk of infection is low.

Table 5. Dosing Schedule for *Haemophilus influenzae* Type B Vaccines

Vaccine	Age at First Dose, months	Primary Series	Booster
PRP-T	2–6	Three doses, 2 months apart	12–15 months
	7–11	Two doses, 2 months apart	12–15 months
	12–14	One dose	2 months later
	15–59	One dose	Unnecessary
PRP-OMP	2–6	Two doses, 2 months apart	12–15 months
	7–11	Two doses, 2 months apart	12–15 months
	12–14	One dose	2 months later
	15–59	One dose	Unnecessary

PRP-OMP = *Haemophilus* B conjugate; PRP-T = polyribosylribitol phosphate chemically conjugated to tetanus toxoid.

N. Polio Vaccine
   1. Poliomyelitis
      a. Caused by the polio virus that enters by mouth and attaches to the throat; within 1 week, it invades the lymph nodes and, eventually, the bloodstream

    b. It may then infect the central nervous system, causing replication in motor neurons, resulting in cell destruction and clinical symptoms of the disease.

    c. Clinical features of infection are usually asymptomatic but, in rare cases, may result in symptoms of meningitis (1%–2%) or paralytic symptoms (less than 1%).

2. Types of vaccine

    a. Oral poliovirus vaccine

       i. Live, attenuated vaccine that contains all three serotypes of poliovirus

       ii. No longer used in the United States because of limited cases of vaccine-associated paralytic poliomyelitis

    b. Inactivated poliovirus vaccine

       i. Contains all three serotypes of poliovirus

       ii. Administered subcutaneously or intramuscularly

       iii. Available in a multidose vial, containing 2-phenoxyethanol as a preservative

       iv. Contains trace amounts of neomycin, streptomycin, and polymyxin B

       v. Considered 99% effective after three doses

       vi. Adverse reactions—Localized injection reactions

3. Recommendations for inactivated poliovirus vaccine

    a. Vaccinate all children starting at age 2 months.

    b. Series of four doses given at 2 months, 4 months, 6–18 months, and 4–6 years

O. Rotavirus Vaccine

1. Rotavirus infection

    a. Enters the body through the mouth and replicates directly in the small intestine, resulting in severe gastroenteritis caused by rotavirus (usually more severe in infants)

    b. Incubation period of around 2 days

    c. Clinical features typically include watery diarrhea with or without fever/vomiting.

    d. Infection with rotavirus seldom leads to immunity from the disease, but subsequent infections are less severe.

2. Rotavirus vaccine

    a. Live oral vaccine

    b. Types

       i. RV5 (RotaTeq)

         (a) Contains five strains of rotavirus suspended in a buffer solution

         (b) Administered as three doses at 2, 4, and 6 months (completed by 32 weeks)

         (c) Contains trace amounts of bovine fetal serum but is preservative-free

         (d) In studies, has been up to 74% effective in decreasing any gastroenteritis symptoms and 98% effective in decreasing severe gastroenteritis symptoms

       ii. RV1 (Rotarix)

         (a) Contains one strain of rotavirus

         (b) Two doses at 2 and 4 months (completed by 24 weeks)

         (c) Available as a lyophilized powder for reconstitution that must be used within 24 hours of reconstitution

         (d) Latex rubber in packaging

3. Virus can shed in the feces up to 15 days after administration.

4. Immunity duration is unknown; has been studied for 2 consecutive years, with waning protection in the second year

5. Adverse reactions

    a. Intussusception, which occurred in previously marketed rotavirus vaccine; however, this has occurred as often as with placebo in the current vaccines

   b. Vomiting

   c. Diarrhea

   d. Irritability

   e. Fever

  6. Recommendations

   a. The Advisory Committee on Immunization Practices, the American Academy of Pediatrics, and the American Academy of Family Practice have no preference for the use of one vaccine over the other.

   b. The vaccines should be administered routinely at 2 months but can be initiated as early as 6 weeks, with at least 4 weeks between doses.

   c. Infants receiving a diagnosis of rotavirus before or during vaccine administration should still complete the full treatment recommendations.

   d. It is not recommended to re-dose if part of dose, or the entire dose, is spit out.

 P. Summary of Vaccine Recommendations

Table 6. Childhood Immunization Schedule, Birth to 6 Years

Vaccine	Birth	1 mo	2 mo	4 mo	6 mo	12 mo	15 mo	18 mo	19–23 mo	2–3 yr	4–6 yr
Hepatitis B	1st dose	2nd dose			3rd dose						
Rotavirus			1st dose	2nd dose	3rd dose[a]						
DTaP/DT			1st dose	2nd dose	3rd dose	4th dose					5th dose
Hib			1st dose	2nd dose	3rd dose[b]	3rd or 4th dose[b]					
PCV/PPSV			1st PCV	2nd PCV	3rd PCV	4th PCV				PPSV[c]	
IPV			1st dose	2nd dose	3rd dose						4th dose
Influenza						Annually (IIV only)				Annually (IIV or LAIV)	
MMR					[d]	1st dose					2nd dose
Varicella						1st dose					2nd dose
Hepatitis A						2-dose series[e]				[f]	
Meningococcal			Give only if high risk								

☐ Recommended for all individuals in this category who meet the age requirements and who lack documentation of vaccination or have no evidence of previous infection.

▨ Recommended if some other risk factor is present.

[a]If RV5 or unknown, give third dose.

[b]If PRP-OMP is given at 2 and 4 months, a dose at 6 months is not indicated. Only a booster at 12–15 months of age.

[c]Only if at high risk.

[d]Administer one dose to infants aged 6–11 months before departure from the United States for international travel.

[e]Give the second dose 6–18 months after the first dose.

[f]May give if immunity desired.

DTaP/DT = diphtheria and tetanus toxoids and acellular pertussis vaccine/diphtheria-tetanus; Hib = *Haemophilus influenzae* type B; IIV = inactivated influenza vaccine; IPV = inactivated poliovirus vaccine; LAIV = live, attenuated influenza vaccine; MMR = measles, mumps, and rubella; mo = month(s); PCV/PPSV = pneumococcal conjugate vaccine/pneumococcal polysaccharide vaccine; PRP-OMP = *Haemophilus* B conjugate, conjugated to meningococcal group B outer membrane protein; RV5 = rotavirus vaccine; yr = years.

Table 7. Childhood Immunization Schedule, 6–18 Years

Vaccine	7–10 Years	11–12 Years	13–18 Years
Tdap		Tdap	
Human papillomavirus		Three-dose series	
Meningococcal		First dose	Booster[a]
Influenza	One dose annually		
Pneumococcal	One or two doses[b]		
Hepatitis A	Two doses[b]		

[a]Booster dose at 16 years.

[b]If at high risk and not previously vaccinated.

Tdap = diphtheria and reduced tetanus toxoids and acellular pertussis.

Table 8. Adult Immunization Schedule

Vaccine	19–21 Years	22–26 Years	27–49 Years	50–59 Years	60–64 Years	≥65 Years
Influenza	1 dose annually					
Tdap/Td	Substitute 1-time dose of Tdap for Td booster; then boost with Td every 10 years					
Varicella	2 doses[a]					
HPV	3 doses					
Zoster					1 dose	
MMR	1 or 2 doses[a]					
PCV13	1 dose[b]					1 dose
PPSV23	1 or 2 doses[c]					1 dose
Meningococcal	1 or more doses[c]					
Hepatitis A	2 doses[c]					
Hepatitis B	3 doses[c]					
Hib	1 to 3 doses[d]					

☐ Recommended for all individuals in this category who meet the age requirements and who lack documentation of vaccination or have no evidence of previous infection.

▨ Recommended if some other risk factor is present.

[a]Without evidence of immunity.

[b]Only in immunocompromising conditions, functional or anatomic asplenia, CSF leaks, or cochlear implants.

[c]Only in at-risk individuals and those not previously vaccinated.

[d]Only in functional or anatomic asplenia, sickle cell disease, elective splenectomy, or hematopoietic stem cell transplant.

CSF = cerebrospinal fluid; Hib = *Haemophilus influenzae* type B; HPV = human papillomavirus; MMR = measles, mumps, and rubella; PCV = pneumococcal conjugate vaccine; PPSV = pneumococcal polysaccharide vaccine; Td = tetanus and diphtheria; Tdap = diphtheria and reduced tetanus toxoids and acellular pertussis.

Q. Vaccine Storage
   1. Most vaccines need to be stored at refrigerator temperatures (2°C–8°C) and not frozen. Exception: Varicella-containing vaccines should be kept frozen until reconstituted.
   2. Multidose vials may be used until the expiration date on the package unless otherwise stated in the manufacturer's product information.

R. Pharmacists as Immunizers
  1. Authority
     a. Pharmacists may administer the influenza vaccine in every state.
     b. The authority to administer other vaccines varies greatly by state.
     c. To administer a vaccine, a pharmacist must have an order from a physician or other provider to do so. This varies among states and is usually a standing order and/or a written prescription.
  2. Certificate programs
     a. Most states require pharmacists to have completed a certificate program to administer vaccines.
     b. Most state pharmacy boards allow immunization training in college of pharmacy curricula to be used in place of a formal certificate program.
     c. Several immunization delivery continuing education programs exist for pharmacists.
        i. Most notable is a program through the American Pharmacists Association
        ii. www.pharmacist.com/pharmacy-based-immunization-delivery

S. Safety
  1. Clinical Laboratory Improvements Amendment (CLIA) waiver
     a. All places that perform diagnostic tests are considered a laboratory.
     b. Laboratories that perform only tests with an insignificant risk of erroneous results may apply for a CLIA waiver.
     c. A CMS-116 form may be completed to obtain this waiver.
     d. An alphabetized list of waived laboratory tests is available at www.accessdata.fda.gov/scripts/cdrh/cfdocs/cfClia/analyteswaived.cfm.
  2. Bloodborne pathogen safety
     a. All bodily fluids should be considered hazardous—All employees with exposure to bodily fluids should be provided with, and use, personal protective equipment (PPE) appropriate to the task (e.g., gloves, gowns, laboratory coats, face shields or masks, eye protection, mouthpieces, resuscitation bags, pocket masks, or other ventilation devices).
     b. Gloves should always be worn when it can be reasonably anticipated that the employee will have hand contact with blood, other potentially infectious materials, mucous membranes, and nonintact skin (does not apply to administering vaccines). The employer should make running water accessible for employees to wash their hands immediately after removing PPE. If running water is not immediately available, an antiseptic cleaner is an appropriate alternative as long as employees can eventually get to running water.
     c. Sharps/needles should not be bent, recapped, or clipped after use.
     d. Sharps/needles should be disposed of in a container that is puncture-resistant, red, leakproof, and closeable for transport.
     e. Food and drink should not be kept in the same location (refrigerator, freezer, countertops) where potentially hazardous materials are kept.
     f. Employers shall make the hepatitis B vaccine available to all employees with potential exposure to bloodborne pathogens. This shall be provided at no cost to the employee. The employee has the right to decline this vaccine but must sign a statement attesting to his or her refusal.

V. ADHERENCE

Guidelines

World Health Organization. Adherence to Long-term Therapies: Evidence for Action. Available at www.who.int/chp/knowledge/publications/adherence_full_report.pdf.

The American College of Preventive Medicine. Medication Adherence: Improving Health Outcomes Time Tool: A Resource from the American College of Preventive Medicine. Available at www.acpm.org/?page=MedAdhereTTProviders.

A. Definitions
   1. Adherence: The extent to which a person's behavior (taking medication, following a diet, or making healthy lifestyle changes) coincides with recommendations from a health care provider
   2. Medication adherence: The patient's conformance with the provider's recommendation with respect to timing, dosage, and frequency of medication-taking during the prescribed length of time
      a. Primary nonadherence is when a prescription is written but the patient does not fill the prescription.
         i. Harder to quantify because of a lack of claims data
         ii. Now able to identify never-filled prescriptions because of electronic prescriptions
      b. Secondary nonadherence is when a prescription is filled but the patient does not continue to conform to the provider's recommendation.
   3. Compliance: Patient's passive following of provider's orders
   4. Persistence: Duration of time a patient takes medication, from therapy initiation to discontinuation
   5. Measuring adherence
      a. Medication possession ratio (MPR)
         i. Historically, the most common way for measuring adherence using claims data
         ii. Defined as the summation of a medication days' supply across a defined interval
         iii. Does not account for actual patient discontinuation of medication
         iv. Varying definitions of the numerator and denominator
         v. May overestimate adherence, depending on defined intervals
         vi. In general, a patient is considered adherent if the MPR is greater than 80%.
      b. Proportion of days covered (PDC)
         i. Method of assessing adherence using claims data
         ii. Defined as the number of days with drug on hand divided by the number of days in a specified time interval. It may be multiplied by 100 to yield a percentage.
         iii. The denominator does not use a simple summation of days' supply as MPR, which ensures that the calculation is both more conservative and more consistent (e.g., if the measurement period is 365 days, and if the patient's first fill of the medication is on day 20 of the year, then the denominator period is 345 days (365 − 20 = 345).
         iv. In general, a patient is still considered adherent if the PDC is greater than 80%.
      c. Comparison of MPR and PDC
         i. PDC and MPR result in similar results when examining adherence to a single drug.
         ii. PDC will be a more conservative estimate to adherence when examining adherence to a class of drugs that is prone to frequent switching and concomitant therapy with several drugs within a class.

B. Burden of Nonadherence
   1. Nonadherence rate
      a. 2003 report by the WHO estimates adherence rates to be about 50%.
         i. Adherence rates tend to significantly decline after 6 months.
         ii. After 1–2 years, nonadherence rates may reach up to 75% with some medications.
      b. Primary nonadherence has been estimated to be up to 24% across medication classes.

    c. Adherence rates among various medication classes
- i. Primary nonadherence
  - (a) Antihyperlipidemic medications between 13% and 34%
  - (b) Antidiabetic medications between 11% and 32%
  - (c) Antihypertensive medications between 7% and 28%
- ii. Secondary nonadherence
  - (a) Antihyperlipidemic medications up to 39%
  - (b) Antidiabetic medications up to 28%
  - (c) Antihypertensive medications up to 34%
  - (d) Rates with medications continue to decline over time and may reach up to 50%.

2. Outcomes related to nonadherence
- a. Estimated costs to the health care system are thought to be $290 billion annually.
- b. Associated with as many as 40% nursing home admissions
- c. 5.4 times increase of hospitalizations, rehospitalizations, or premature death in patients with high blood pressure
- d. 2.5 times increased risk of hospitalization for patients with diabetes

C. Reasons for Nonadherence

1. Sources contributing to nonadherence
- a. Provider and health care system factors
  - i. Ineffective communication
  - ii. Failure to recognize health literacy issues and/or cultural beliefs
  - iii. Lack of positive reinforcement
  - iv. Continuity or access to care
- b. Medication- and condition-related factors
  - i. Complexity of administration
  - ii. Number of medications
  - iii. Therapy duration or frequent changes in therapy
  - iv. Fear of or experienced adverse effects
  - v. Lack of immediate benefits
  - vi. Asymptomatic disease
  - vii. Social stigma with certain medications
  - viii. Cost of medications
- c. Patient-related factors
  - i. Lack of knowledge about the disease state, medications, and outcomes
  - ii. Cost of medication, copayment or both
  - iii. Social support
  - iv. Health literacy
  - v. Physical
    - (a) Blind, deaf, cognitive impairment
    - (b) Dysphagia
  - vi. Cultural

2. Characteristics related to nonadherence with cardiovascular medication
- a. Cost
- b. Concerns about medication adverse effects
- c. Lack of belief in benefits of medications
- d. Lack of knowledge about the severity of a cardiovascular-related disease
- e. Sex—Male individuals tend to have a higher occurrence.

  f. Ethnicity—Nonwhite race

  g. Age—Younger

 3. The National Community Pharmacists Association identified six predictors of adherence in a recent analysis.

  a. Personal connection with pharmacist or staff

  b. Cost

  c. Continuity of care

  d. Patients' beliefs about the importance of the medication

  e. Patients' knowledge about their disease state(s)

  f. The risk of adverse effects

D. Strategies and Interventions to Improve Adherence

 1. Strategies should be multifactorial and address characteristics of nonadherence.

  a. Patient interventions

   i. Pillboxes

   ii. Visual aids

   iii. Electronic reminder systems

   iv. Education about medication and disease state(s)

   v. Financial assistance programs

  b. Provider or health care systems intervention

   i. Introduce team-based care with pharmacists or nurses.

   ii. Improve communication.

   iii. Improve access to care (i.e., telemedicine).

   iv. Use of technology to improve monitoring of adherence

   v. Use of generic or preferred formulary medications

  c. Policy-based interventions (i.e., cost coverage for certain disease states)

 2. Interventions have been difficult to design for broad-spectrum approaches to address adherence and improve clinical outcomes.

 3. Population-based interventions for improving adherence to cardiovascular medications

  a. Collaboration, education, decision aids all have low or insufficient methods for assessing adherence and outcomes.

  b. Pharmacist-led hypertension clinics

   i. Improved blood pressure control

   ii. Improved adherence to hypertension medications

   iii. Long-term outcomes lacking

  c. Improving the cost of cardiovascular medications

  d. Blister packaging

   i. Improvement in adherence and persistence

   ii. Widespread applicability difficult to judge because limited trials exist

  e. Use of interactive voice response system

   i. Improved first fill compared with usual care

   ii. Outcomes too early to predict, as is long-term persistence with medications

E. Integrating Adherence into Pharmacy Practice

 1. Use of mnemonics to help aid with assessing and addressing nonadherence

  a. SIMPLE technique by the American College of Preventive Medicine

   i. S – Simplify the regimen.

   ii. I – Impart knowledge.

   iii. M – Modify patient beliefs and behavior.

    iv.   P – Provide communication and trust.
    v.   L – Leave the bias.
    vi.   E – Evaluate adherence.
  b. B-SMART
    i.   B – Barriers
    ii.   S – Solutions
    iii.   M – Motivation (necessary only if not ready for change)
    iv.   A – Adherence tools
    v.   R – Relationship
    vi.   T – Triage

Table 9. Examples of Addressing Adherence Issues Through SIMPLE and B-SMART

SIMPLE	B-SMART
Simplifying Regimen -Adjusting medication frequency, dosage, and timing with patient activities -Customized packaging -Use of adherence aids	**Barriers** (questions to identify barriers) -During the past week, how many days have you missed taking any of your medications? -Have you stopped or started taking any of your medications on your own? -Have you experienced any problems or had any adverse effects while taking your medication?
Impart Knowledge -Involving the patient's family or caregiver -Helping to cope with medication costs -Providing instructions in writing and verbally	**Solutions** -Use of devices to address individual concerns -Education on the benefits and risks of not taking medication -Tips to reduce adverse effects -Referral to financial services -Use of interpreter lines -Simplify regimen
Modify Patient Beliefs and Behavior -Self-management -Shared decision-making -Addressing fears and concerns -Ensuring comprehension of risks with nonadherence -Asking patients to restate the positives and negatives	**Motivation** (necessary only if the patient is unwilling to change) -Assessing the patient's willingness to change (determined in barrier identification) -Ask additional questions to confirm adherence -Discern if related to not taking the medication at all -Guide the discussion -Validate self-efficacy and self-management -Convey hopefulness
Provide Communication and Trust -Listen -Interview patients -Use plain language -Work with the patient	**Adherence Tools** -Using solutions identified and offering individualized solutions -Collaborate with the patient, provider and family -Ensure understanding -Ask the patient to restate (active participation)

Table 9. Examples of Addressing Adherence Issues Through SIMPLE and B-SMART *(continued)*

SIMPLE	B-SMART
Leave the Bias -Understand health literacy -Communicate in a patient-centered manner	**Establishing Relationships** -Eye contact -Active listening and being nonjudgmental -Communicate in an open adult-to-adult style -Seek to understand -Be on time and follow up
Evaluate Adherence -Ask patients at each encounter -Periodically review patient's refill history -Use medication adherence scales	**Triage** -Refer for case management -Behavior and social medicine/social services -Health education classes -Community programs -Physician follow-up

---

Patient Case

13. W.M. is a 57-year old man with a diagnosis of hypertension who was given a prescription for lisinopril. After 1 week, he stopped taking the medication because he was too dizzy to function at work. He presents today asking for a blood pressure check. His blood pressure reading is 175/95 mm Hg. After discussing goals, W.M. demonstrates understanding and has been implementing other lifestyle behaviors to improve blood pressure. Which barrier to adherence have you identified?

    A. Financial.
    B. Concerns about medication adverse effects.
    C. Social support.
    D. Health literacy.

---

    2. Tools available for patients and providers
        a. Addressing forgetfulness or complex medication regimens
            i. Calendars
                (a) MyMedSchedule (www.mymedschedule.com [free—Need to register])
                (b) Use of Microsoft Office programs
                (c) Wallet cards
            ii. Pillboxes
                (a) Inexpensive to moderately priced
                (b) Readily available
                (c) E-Pill—Calendar and pillbox (www.epill.com/chart.html)
            iii. Alarms
        b. Addressing physical concerns
            i. Talking Rx (www.talkingrx.com)
                (a) Attaches to the bottom of a pill vial
                (b) Allows a pharmacist or caregiver to leave a 60-second recorded message
            ii. Prodigy diabetes devices that are fully audible (www.prodigymeter.com)

    c. Financial Support
        i. Online resource: www.needymeds.org, www.rxassist.org, www.pparx.org, www.benefitscheckup.org
        ii. Medicare plan resource: www.medicare.gov
    d. Organizational tools and support
        i. American Heart Association (http://scriptyourfuture.org/file/4dc82ede7ea0a.pdf)
           (a) Medicine management tool
           (b) Worksheet to keep track of patient's daily medicines, glucose readings, and blood pressure
        ii. American College of Cardiology (https://www.cardiosmart.org/Tools/Med-Reminder)
           (a) CardioSmart Med Reminder (mobile application)
           (b) The CardioSmart Med Reminder is to be used for educational purposes only.
        iii. American Society of Consultant Pharmacists Foundation (www.adultmeducation.com)
           (a) Focus on improving medication adherence in older adults
           (b) Tools for assessing medication knowledge and readiness for change
           (c) Consumer information (i.e., Questions You Should Ask About Your Medicines)
    e. Improving health literacy
        i. Agency for Healthcare Research and Quality's (AHRQ's) Health Literacy Universal Precautions Toolkit (http://www.ahrq.gov/literacy)
        ii. National Council on Patient Information and Education (www.talkaboutrx.org)

VI. COMPLEMENTARY AND ALTERNATIVE MEDICINE

  A. Definitions
    1. Complementary and alternative medicine (CAM)—Diverse group of medical and health care systems, practices, and products not considered part of conventional medicine
    2. Complementary—Used together with conventional medicine
    3. Alternative—Used in place of conventional medicine
    4. Dietary supplement—Intended to supplement the diet
        a. Contains vitamin, mineral, herb/botanical, amino acids, enzymes, metabolite as replacements, and other ingredients intended to supplement the diet
        b. Does not meet definition of food

  B. Types of CAM
    1. Natural products
        a. Botanicals
        b. Animal-derived extracts
        c. Vitamins, minerals, fatty acids, amino acids, and proteins
        d. Prebiotics and probiotics
    2. Mind and body practices (i.e., tai chi, medication, hypnosis)
    3. Manipulative/body based (i.e., chiropractic manipulation, massage therapy)
    4. Energy medicine (i.e., acupuncture, cupping)

  C. Dietary Supplement Regulations
    1. Before 1994, dietary supplements were subject to same regulatory requirements as other foods under the FDA.
    2. The Dietary Supplement Health and Education Act of 1994 (DSHEA)
        a. Dietary supplements can be marketed without FDA approval.
        b. Manufacturer responsible for safety and efficacy, but not required to submit to the FDA

      c. The FDA monitors for adverse events once on the market, but no regulations are designated before postmarketing surveillance period.

      d. Must follow good manufacturing practices for foods

      e. May make three types of claims

          i. Health claims—The FDA authorizes scientific-based literature.

          ii. Structure/function claims—Not subject to FDA review or authorization

          iii. Nutrient content claims—Describes the level of substance in the product

   3. Label requirements

      a. Must contain supplement facts

      b. Legislation requires supplement manufacturers to have substantiation of label claims carry a disclaimer: "This statement has not been evaluated by the FDA. This product is not intended to diagnose, treat, cure, or prevent any disease."

      c. Supplement seal of approval to ensure additional testing and safety by manufacturer

          i. Not required, but ideal because it ensures additional testing

          ii. United States Pharmacopeia (USP) Convention

          iii. NSF International (formerly known as National Sanitation Foundation)

          iv. Consumer laboratories

D. Concerns with CAM

   1. Estimated that only 33%–45% of patients report CAM use to a health care professional

   2. Those more likely to use CAM

      a. Women

      b. Higher income

      c. Self-assessed good health

      d. Higher education levels

      e. Former smokers

      f. Hospitalized in the past year

      g. Access to health care (insured)

   3. Few studies have critically evaluated some of the most common CAM agents.

      a. Most CAM agent interactions remain largely unknown.

      b. The most common supplements studied for interactions include the following:

          i. Garlic

          ii. Gingko

          iii. Ginseng

          iv. St. John's wort

   4. It is estimated that up to 60% of patients do not report adverse events associated with CAM, and many do not recognize that the adverse events they experience are associated with the CAM product.

E. Examples of Dietary Supplements

   1. The National Health Interview Survey in 2007 surveyed more than 20,000 U.S. citizens on supplement use.

      a. The top five supplements used were the following:

          i. Glucosamine/chondroitin—For joint pain

          ii. Fish oil/omega-3 fatty acid supplements—For cholesterol and cardiovascular health

          iii. Echinacea—For immunity

          iv. Flaxseed oil—For cholesterol

          v. Garlic—For cholesterol

      b. In the 2002 survey, both ginseng and gingko biloba were in the top 5 in place of flaxseed and fish oil.

2. Management of dyslipidemia with herbal supplements
   a. Fish oil/omega-3 fatty acid supplements
      i. Indication: Hypertriglyceridemia, cardiovascular protection
      ii. Mechanism
         (a) Lower triglycerides (TGs) by decreasing hepatic secretion of very-low-density lipoprotein (VLDL), increasing VLDL clearance, and reducing TG transport
         (b) Anti-inflammatory and antithrombotic effects because they compete with arachidonic acid in the cyclooxygenase and lipoxygenase pathways
      iii. Dose
         (a) Average dose required is between 2 and 4 g/day of docosahexaenoic acid (DHA) and eicosapentaenoic acid (EPA).
         (b) Typical fish oil capsule contains 120 mg of DHA and 180 mg of EPA.
      iv. Adverse effects
         (a) Fishy aftertaste, stomach upset, belching, heartburn, halitosis
         (b) Doses greater than 3 g/day may increase bleeding risk in some individuals.
         (c) Some reports exist that fish oil may worsen glycemic control in diabetes.
      v. Interactions
         (a) Antiplatelets—Increased bleeding risk
         (b) Antihypertensives—May lower blood pressure
      vi. Effectiveness
         (a) Hypertriglyceridemia
            (1) Decreased TG values by 20%–50% in a dose-dependent manner
            (2) Doses of 4 g/day do not seem to be as effective as gemfibrozil 1200 mg/day.
         (b) Cardiovascular protection
            (1) A recent 2012 meta-analysis showed no benefit of fish oil for secondary prevention in patients with existing cardiovascular disease.
            (2) Likely because of the widespread use of statins now as compared with when fish oil was first studied
            (3) This new study conflicts with previous information regarding the overall cardioprotective benefits of fish oil.
   b. Flaxseed oil
      i. Indication—Cardiovascular disease, hypercholesterolemia
      ii. Mechanism
         (a) Hypercholesterolemia
            (1) Contains high content of α-linolenic acid, which is a precursor to omega-3 fatty acids
            (2) Possibly affects the synthesis of bile acids from cholesterol
            (3) Overall, not well understood
         (b) Cardiovascular disease: May increase systemic arterial elasticity, which may improve circulatory function
      iii. Dose
         (a) Ground flaxseed up to 50 g/day (for hypercholesterolemia)
         (b) Flaxseed oil 1.2–3.6 g/day (for hypercholesterolemia and cardiovascular disease)
      iv. Adverse effects—Diarrhea, allergic reactions, questionable increased risk of prostate cancer
      v. Interactions—Antiplatelets with increased risk of bleeding

vi. Effectiveness

    (a) Hypercholesterolemia—Some research shows that flaxseed oil significantly reduces cholesterol or TG values in patients with or without baseline elevations. Other research does not.

    (b) Cardiovascular disease—Some evidence suggests benefit in combination with a low-fat diet. However, it has not been well studied, and overall studies assessing outcomes are lacking.

c. Garlic

  i. Mechanism: Inhibits hepatic cholesterol synthesis through the active ingredient allicin

  ii. Dose: 0.4–1.2 g/day of dried garlic powder; 2–5 mg of garlic oil; 300–1000 mg of garlic extract

  iii. Adverse effects: Stomach upset, garlic breath, reports of bleeding, and body odor

  iv. Interactions

    (a) Increased international normalized ratios (INRs) with warfarin

    (b) Mixed evidence on the impact of the cytochrome P450 (CYP) isoenzyme system

  v. Effectiveness

    (a) Meta-analysis of 13 randomized, double-blind, placebo-controlled studies with a statistically significant reduction of 5.8% in total cholesterol (TC) in favor of garlic

    (b) Systematic review of studies for at least 4 weeks with a decrease in TC by 17.1 mg/dL and a decrease in low-density lipoprotein cholesterol (LDL-C) by 6.2 mg/dL

d. Other supplements for high cholesterol

  i. Plant sterols/stanols

    (a) Indication: Hypercholesterolemia

    (b) Mechanism: Inhibits the absorption of dietary and biliary cholesterol

    (c) Dose: From 800 mg to 6 g per day

    (d) Adverse effects: Nausea, indigestion, diarrhea, constipation

    (e) Interactions: Ezetimibe may reduce stanols/sterols values up to 41%.

    (f) Effectiveness

      (1) Significantly reduces TC and LDL-C values

      (2) Recommended as part of lifestyle modification in American Diabetes Association's (ADA's) Standards of Medical Care in Diabetes—2015

  ii. Red yeast rice (several products contain lovastatin)

    (a) Indication: Hypercholesterolemia

    (b) Mechanism: Inhibits endogenous cholesterol synthesis (like statins)

    (c) Dose—600 mg twice daily to 2400 mg once or twice daily

    (d) Adverse effects

      (1) Stomach discomfort, heartburn, flatulence, headache, and dizziness

      (2) Concerns about myopathy and liver toxicity exist because it contains lovastatin.

    (e) Interactions

      (1) Statins—Duplicate therapy

      (2) CYP 3A4 inhibitors (e.g., clarithromycin, ketoconazole, protease inhibitors)

      (3) Gemfibrozil—Increased risk of myopathies

    (f) Effectiveness

      (1) Some research has shown decreases in TC of up to 20% and in LDL-C of up to 26%.

      (2) However, these products provided up to about 10 mg daily of statins.

      (3) The FDA has tried to remove red yeast rice products from the market, yet they remain available, despite containing variable amounts of prescription medications.

  iii. Soy, fiber, policosanol, and krill oil may also be widely used by patients for potential cholesterol-lowering effects with varying levels of evidence and impact on hypercholesterolemia.

Patient Case

14. R.T. is a 58-year-old man with coronary artery disease, hypertension, obesity, and impaired fasting glucose. Current medications include aspirin, metoprolol, lisinopril, and pravastatin. The lipid panel is as follows: TC 152 mg/dL, LDL 59 mg/dL, TG 349 mg/dL. R.T.'s primary care provider has recommended that R.T. start taking fish oil. Which of the following counseling points will you offer R.T.?

A. Omega-3 fatty acids increase intestinal cholesterol absorption.

B. Recommend ginseng instead of fish oil to improve triglycerides.

C. Avoid over-the-counter fish oil products because of the risk of hepatotoxicity.

D. Improved triglyceride benefits are associated with a fish oil product containing EPA and DHA at 2–4 g/day.

---

3. Glucosamine/chondroitin
   a. Indication: Osteoarthritis
   b. Mechanism
      i. Glucosamine sulfate—Stimulates the metabolism of chondrocytes in cartilage and of synovial cells in the synovium
      ii. Chondroitin sulfate—Protects cartilage from degradation by inhibiting leukocyte elastase, decreasing migration of polymorphonuclear leukocytes, and increasing synthesis of proteoglycans and hyaluronic acid
   c. Dose
      i. Glucosamine: 1500 mg once daily or divided three times daily
      ii. Chondroitin: 1000–1200 mg once daily or divided two or three times daily
   d. Adverse effects
      i. Glucosamine: Mild stomach concerns
      ii. Chondroitin: Mild stomach concerns
   e. Interactions
      i. Glucosamine
         (a) May induce resistance to etoposide, teniposide, and doxorubicin
         (b) Doses greater 3000 mg/day may enhance the effects of warfarin.
      ii. Chondroitin: Doses greater than 2400 mg/day may enhance the effects of warfarin.
   f. Effectiveness—A recent 2-year study showed that, during a 2-year period, glucosamine and chondroitin alone or in combination showed no clinically significant benefit on pain or function scales, compared with placebo.
4. Echinacea
   a. Indication—Treatment and prevention of the common cold and other upper respiratory infections
   b. Mechanism—Activates phagocytosis and increases the number of circulating lymphocytes
   c. Dose
      i. Capsules containing freeze-dried extract: 100 mg three times daily
      ii. Herbal compound tea: 5–6 cups of tea the first day; then 1 cup daily for 5 days
      iii. Liquid: Use 20 drops every 2 hours for the first day; then three times daily for up to 10 days
   d. Adverse effects—Allergic reactions, fever, stomach disturbances, dry mouth, sore throat, tingling and numb tongue, mouth ulcers
   e. Interactions
      i. Possible CYP3A4 inhibitor
      ii. May interfere with immunosuppressants
   f. Effectiveness—Several randomized placebo-controlled trials showed no difference in symptoms.

5. Other significant supplements
    a. Ginseng
        i. Indication—Mental performance/memory, immunity
        ii. Mechanism
            (a) May work against stress by affecting the hypothalamic-pituitary-adrenal axis
            (b) Seems to increase serum cortisol concentrations and stimulate adrenal function
        iii. Dose—100–200 mg once or twice daily
        iv. Adverse effects—Insomnia, tachycardia, mania, Stevens-Johnson syndrome
        v. Interactions
            (a) May lower blood glucose values and may enhance hypoglycemic effects of some antidiabetes medications
            (b) May enhance effectiveness of anticoagulants, causing reduction of blood coagulation
        vi. Effectiveness
            (a) Mental performance/memory
                (1) Several studies report improvement in reaction time, concentration, learning, math, and logic.
                (2) Most studies are small and not well designed.
                (3) In addition, a small amount of negative evidence
            (b) Immunity
                (1) A few studies suggest ginseng stimulates T lymphocytes and neutrophils.
                (2) Improves the effectiveness of antibiotics in acute bronchitis and enhances the body's response to influenza vaccine
            (c) If patients use it, recommend short-term use (less than 3 months).
    b. Gingko biloba
        i. Indication: Claudication, dementia, tinnitus
        ii. Mechanism: Protects tissues from oxidative damage
        iii. Dose: 40–80 mg three times daily
        iv. Adverse effects—Stomach disturbances, headache, dizziness, palpitations, vertigo, allergic skin reactions, spontaneous bleeding
        v. Interactions
            (a) Anticonvulsants—May lower seizure threshold
            (b) Antiplatelets—Increased bleeding risk
            (c) Aminoglycosides—Increased ototoxicity
            (d) Thiazide—Increased blood pressure
        vi. Effectiveness
            (a) For dementia
                (1) Studies lasting 3 months to 1 year show stabilization or improvement in some cognitive and social functioning measures in many types of dementia.
                (2) Improvement appears to be less than that found with prescription drugs.
            (b) For claudication
                (1) May increase pain-free walking distance
                (2) Most studies used ginkgo 120 mg/day divided in two or three doses for 6 months, which may increase the risk of adverse effects.
                (3) Additional studies are needed to compare the use of gingko with exercise therapy and prescription medications.
    c. St. John's wort
        i. Indication—Depression, anxiety
        ii. Mechanism—Serotonin receptor antagonist (serotonin-3 and serotonin-4)

     iii.   Dose—300 mg three times daily

     iv.   Adverse effects—Photosensitivity, insomnia, vivid dreams, restlessness, anxiety, diarrhea, fatigue, dry mouth

     v.   Interactions

       (a) Induces CYP3A4, CYP2C9, CYP1A2, and P-glycoprotein

       (b) Marginal effect on CYP2D6

       (c) Antidepressants—As it works on similar neurochemicals

     vi.   Contraindications— Should be avoided during pregnancy or lactation

     vii.   Effectiveness

       (a) St. John's wort extract is likely as effective as the selective serotonin reuptake inhibitors.

       (b) Short-term response rates appear to be between 65% and 100%, but long-term rates appear to be closer to 60%–69%.

       (c) Although beneficial outcomes exist, drug interactions likely preclude the use of this supplement; moreover, there is a need for provider management of depression and mood disorders.

  d.   Black cohosh

     i.   Indications—Hot flashes, premenstrual syndrome, painful menstruation

     ii.   Mechanism—Estrogen-like effects by an unknown mechanism, possibly some serotoninergic-type effects

     iii.   Dose—20–40 mg twice daily (according to manufacturer, 20 mg provides results similar to 40 mg)

     iv.   The use of black cohosh should not exceed 6 months' period because of the lack of safety data.

     v.   Adverse effects—Stomach upset, rash, headache, dizziness, weight gain, cramping, hepatotoxicity

     vi.   Interactions

       (a) Mixed evidence that black cohosh inhibits CYP2D6

       (b) Hepatotoxic drugs—Because of case reports of liver toxicity, caution is needed when using black cohosh with other agents with potential hepatotoxicity (e.g., isoniazid, methotrexate, acetaminophen), and liver function test monitoring is recommended.

       (c) Avoid use in patients with breast cancer—Although relatively unknown, best to avoid in patients with breast cancer because of unknown risks of possible estrogen-like effects.

     vii.   Effectiveness

       (a) Studies funded by the German manufacturer of Remifemin, a branded form of an alcohol extract of black cohosh, found this specific product helpful in reducing the frequency of hot flashes and in alleviating mood disorders with no difference in liver function test findings.

       (b) Several meta-analyses since then have failed to provide consistent evidence that black cohosh provides symptomatic improvement in the management of menopausal symptoms.

       (c) Liver function test monitoring is recommended because of increased case reports of hepatotoxicity.

  e.   Saw palmetto

     i.   Indication—Benign prostatic hypertrophy (BPH)

     ii.   Mechanism—Noncompetitively inhibits 5-α-reductase types 1 and 2 and prevents conversion of testosterone to dihydrotestosterone

     iii.   Dose—160 mg twice daily or 320 mg once daily

     iv.   Adverse effects

       (a) Mild and comparable with placebo

       (b) Impotence rate similar to placebo and less than with finasteride

       (c) High doses may cause stomach upset and diarrhea.

     v.   Interactions—None specifically proved

      vi.   Effectiveness

          (a) Research on saw palmetto is inconsistent for treating BPH, with some positive results and others showing no difference compared with placebo.

          (b) Positive studies suggest a 25% improvement in nocturia.

          (c) Other studies show effects of saw palmetto comparable with those of finasteride in improving peak and mean urine flow and residual volume.

          (d) α-Adrenergic blockers appear more effective in head-to-head trials.

          (e) May take up to 1–2 months to show effectiveness

  f.   Melatonin

      i.   Indication—Sleep disorders (e.g., circadian rhythm, insomnia, jet lag)

      ii.   Mechanism—Shifts circadian rhythm by increasing the binding of GABA (γ-aminobenzoic acid) to its receptors

      iii.   Dose

          (a) For jet lag: 0.5–5 mg at bedtime on arrival of the destination day and continuing for 2–5 days

          (b) For insomnia: 0.3–5 mg at bedtime in either immediate-release or extended-release form

      iv.   Adverse effects—Daytime sleepiness, dizziness, and headache, but no different from placebo

      v.   Interactions

          (a) Anticoagulants—Some case reports of minor bleeding with melatonin and warfarin

          (b) Fluvoxamine—May increase bioavailability of exogenous melatonin by up to 20 times; may be beneficial in difficult-to-treat insomnia

          (c) Immunosuppressants (e.g., cyclosporine, tacrolimus, azathioprine)—Melatonin stimulates immune function and may interfere with therapy; avoid using in combination.

      vi.   Effectiveness

          (a) Insomnia

             (1) Research on melatonin is inconsistent for treating insomnia.

             (2) Some studies report decreased sleep latency onset time by 4–7½ minutes, with clinical significance being a reduction of 5–10 minutes.

             (3) On average, melatonin significantly increases total sleep duration by about 13 minutes.

             (4) Other studies fail to show changes in objective measurements.

          (b) Jet lag

             (1) Most evidence shows melatonin can positively improve alertness and psychomotor performance.

             (2) Traveling westward: May take melatonin 0.5 mg on the night of arrival during the second half of the night until adapted (shifts body clock to later time)

             (3) Traveling eastward: May take melatonin 0.5–3 mg on the night of arrival at local bedtime until adapted (shifts body clock to earlier time)

             (4) The American Academy of Sleep Medicine recommends the use of melatonin in conjunction with other methods as a viable treatment option.

Patient Case

15. C.B. is a 56-year-old woman who presents to the pharmacy after watching a daytime talk show. She is excited to learn about the menopausal management options available over the counter to help alleviate hot flashes. She asks about black cohosh and whether there is any information she should know about before taking this product. What is the best recommendation that you will give to C.B.?

    A. It is as effective as a selective serotonin reuptake inhibitor.
    B. This product should not be used by patients with a history of asthma.
    C. Recommend to discontinue use after 6 months.
    D. This product may be safely recommended for patients with a history of breast cancer.

F. Counseling Tips for CAM
   1. Encourage open communication between patient and health care providers.
   2. Target one medical problem.
   3. Assess regularly.
   4. Avoid in pregnancy and lactation.
   5. Avoid combination or proprietary blend products.
   6. Stop dietary supplements 2–3 weeks before elective surgery.
   7. Same potential as prescription drugs for adverse effects and drug interactions

G. Tools for Evaluating CAM

Table 10. Overview of Tools for Evaluating CAM

	Monograph Components	**Rating Scales**	**Additional Pearls**
Natural Medicines Database[a]	-Safety -Effectiveness -Adverse reactions -Dosage/administration -Interactions with drugs, herbs, food, laboratory tests, and diseases -Interactions with herbs -Mechanism of action -Editor's comments -Patient handout	**Safety** -Likely safe -Possibly safe -Possibly unsafe -Likely unsafe -Unsafe **Efficacy** -Effective -Likely effective -Possibly effective -Possibly ineffective -Likely ineffective -Ineffective	-Evidence based, links provided to references within monograph—Clinical Management Series (CE presentations) -Links to Pharmacist Letter -USP-verified products -Subscription necessary http://naturaldatabase.therapeuticresearch.com/

Table 10. Overview of Tools for Evaluating CAM *(continued)*

	Monograph Components	Rating Scales	Additional Pearls
AltMedDex	-Overview -Dosing information -Dosage forms, drug storage + stability, adult and pediatric doses -Pharmacokinetics -Cautions/contraindications -Adverse reaction -Pregnancy and lactation -Drug interactions -Clinical applications -Monitoring guidelines -Place in therapy -Mechanism of action -Comparative -References	**Not categorized by effectiveness or safety** **Variables not defined**	-Evidence based, but WITHOUT links to references within monograph—More detailed efficacy information provided in monograph without having to look up the article -AltMedDex protocols -Part of the Micromedex resources (www.micromedex.com/ products/) -Subscription necessary

Natural Standard[a]	-Historical/theoretical uses
	-Dosing/toxicology
	-Precautions
	-Contraindications
	-Adverse effects
	-Interactions
	-Mechanism of action
	-History
	-Evidence table
	-Evidence discussion
	-Products studied
		-Safety
		-Similar to natural medicines
		-Efficacy
		  A: Strong scientific evidence
		  B: Good scientific evidence
		  C: Unclear/conflicting scientific evidence
		  D: Fair negative scientific evidence
		  F: Strong negative scientific evidence
		-Lack of evidence
			-Three available monographs
			-Professional monograph – Bottom Line Monograph (available in Spanish)
			-Flashcard (specifically for patients)
			-News items
			-Interactive tools
			-www.naturalstandard.com
			-Subscription required

Quackwatch.com *(founded 1996)*	-Rather than individual product monographs, topics are presented in the format of articles	-No standardized categories for evaluating effectiveness or safety of individual alternative therapies	-Lists of Quackwatch-recommended and sources of health advice are available on this Web site (www.quackwatch.com/) -Free weekly e-mail newsletter -A health fraud discussion list is available -Quackwatch Web pages are also available in German, French, and Portuguese

CAM = complementary and alternative medicine; CE = continuing education; USP = United States Pharmacopeia.

[a]Natural Medicines Database and Natural Standard were recently merged into a product called Natural Medicines.

REFERENCES

First Aid

1. Berg MD, Schexnayder SM, Chameides L, et al. Part 13: pediatric basic life support: 2010 American Heart Association guidelines for cardiopulmonary resuscitation and emergency cardiovascular care. Circulation 2010;122:S862-75.

2. Berg RA, Hemphill R, Abella BS, et al. Part 5: adult basic life support: 2010 American Heart Association guidelines for cardiopulmonary resuscitation and emergency cardiovascular care. Circulation 2010;122:S685-705.

3. Markenson D, Ferguson JD, Chameides L, et al. Part 13: first aid: 2010 American Heart Association and American Red Cross international consensus on first aid science with treatment recommendations. Circulation 2010;122:S585-605.

4. Markenson D, Ferguson JD, Chameides L, et al. Part 17: first aid: 2010 American Heart Association and American Red Cross guidelines for first aid. Circulation 2010;122:S934-46.

5. Sampson HA, Munoz-Furlong A, Campbell RL, et al. Second symposium on the definition and management of anaphylaxis: summary report—Second National Institute of Allergy and Infectious Disease/Food Allergy and Anaphylaxis Network Symposium. Ann Emerg Med 2006;47:373-80.

6. U.S. Department of Health and Human Services, National Institutes of Health, National Heart, Lung, and Blood Institute. Expert Panel Report 3: Guidelines for the Diagnosis and Management of Asthma [monograph on the Internet]. Bethesda, MD: National Heart, Lung, and Blood Institute, 2007. Available at www.nhlbi.nih.gov/health-pro/guidelines/current/asthma-guidelines/full-report/. Accessed September 28, 2015.

Toxicology

1. Cobaugh DJ, Gainor C, Gaston CL, et al. The opioid abuse and misuse epidemic: implications for pharmacists in hospitals and health-systems. Am J Health Syst Pharm 2014;71:e82-97.

2. Jones CM, Mack KA, Paulozzi LJ. Pharmaceutical overdose deaths, United States, 2010. JAMA 2013;309:657-9.

3. Lovegrove MC, Hon S, Geller RJ, et al. Efficacy of flow restrictors in limiting access of liquid medications by young children. J Pediatr 2013;163:1134-9.

4. Schillie SF, Shehab N, Thomas KE, et al. Medication overdoses leading to emergency department visits among children. Am J Prev Med 2009;37:181-7.

Bioterrorism/Natural Disasters

1. American Society of Health-System Pharmacists. ASHP statement on the role of health-system pharmacists in emergency preparedness. Am J Health Syst Pharm 2003;60:1993-5.

2. Bardas SL, Cooper E, Vongspanich A. Emergency preparedness in health-system pharmacies. CJHP 2007;September/October:6-15.

3. Hogue MD, Hogue HB, Lander RD, et al. The nontraditional role of pharmacists after hurricane Katrina: process description and lessons learned. Public Health Rep 2009;124:217-23.

4. Noe B, Smith A. Development of a community pharmacy disaster preparedness manual. J Am Pharm Assoc 2013;53:432-7.

5. Pincick LL, Montello MJ, Tarosky MJ, et al. Pharmacist readiness roles for emergency preparedness. Am J Health Syst Pharm 2001;68:620-3.

6. Setlak P. Bioterrorism preparedness and response: emerging role for health-system pharmacists. Am J Health Syst Pharm 2004;61:1167-75.

7. Terriff CM, Schwartz MD, Lomaestro BM. Bioterrorism: pivotal clinical issues: consensus review of the Society of Infectious Diseases Pharmacists. Pharmacotherapy 2003;23:274-90.

8. Wright JG, Quinn CP, Shadomy S, et al. Use of anthrax vaccine in the United States: recommendations of the Advisory Committee on Immunization Practices (ACIP), 2009. MMWR 2010;59:1-30.

Immunizations

1. Centers for Disease Control and Prevention. Advisory Committee for Immunization Practices (ACIP). Recommended Immunization Schedules for Persons Aged 0 Through 18 Years and Adults Aged 19 Years and Older—United States, 2015. Available at www.cdc.gov/vaccines/schedules/. Accessed September 29, 2015.

2. Centers for Disease Control and Prevention. Atkinson W, Hamborsky J, Wolfe S, eds. Epidemiology and Prevention of Vaccine-Preventable Diseases, 12th ed. Washington, DC: Public Health Foundation, 2012.

3. Centers for Disease Control and Prevention. General recommendations for immunization: recommendations by the Advisory Committee for Immunization Practices (ACIP). MMWR 2011;60:1-64.

4. Centers for Disease Control and Prevention. Immunization Tables. Available at www.cdc.gov/vaccines/schedules/hcp/index.html. Accessed September 29, 2015.

5. Centers for Disease Control and Prevention Prevention and control of influenza with vaccines: recommendations of the Advisory Committee on Immunization Practices—(ACIP)—United States. MMWR 2015;64:818-25.

6. Centers for Disease Control and Prevention. Prevention and control of meningococcal disease: recommendations of the Advisory Committee on Immunization Practices (ACIP). MMWR 2013;62(RR02):1-22.

7. Centers for Disease Control and Prevention. Summary recommendations: preventing tetanus, diphtheria, and pertussis among adolescents: use of tetanus toxoid, reduce diphtheria toxoid and acellular pertussis vaccines: recommendations of the Advisory Committee on Immunization Practices—(ACIP)—United States. MMWR 2006;55(RR3):1-50.

8. Centers for Disease Control and Prevention. Summary recommendations: updated recommendations for use of tetanus toxoid, reduced diphtheria toxoid, and acellular pertussis vaccine (Tdap) in pregnant women—Advisory Committee on Immunization Practices—(ACIP)—United States. MMWR 2012;61:468-70.

9. Centers for Disease Control and Prevention. Updated recommendations for prevention of invasive pneumococcal disease among adults using the 23-valent pneumococcal polysaccharide vaccine (PPSV23): recommendations of the Advisory Committee on Immunization Practices—(ACIP)—United States. MMWR 2010;59:1102-6.

10. Centers for Disease Control and Prevention. Updated recommendations for use of tetanus toxoid, reduced diphtheria toxoid, and acellular pertussis (Tdap) vaccine in adults aged 65 years and older—Advisory Committee on Immunization Practices (ACIP), 2012. MMWR 2012;61:468-70.

11. Centers for Disease Control and Prevention. Updated recommendations for use of tetanus toxoid, reduced diphtheria toxoid, and acellular pertussis (Tdap) vaccine in adults—Advisory Committee on Immunization Practices (ACIP), 2012. MMWR 2006;55(RR17):1-33.

12. Centers for Disease Control and Prevention. Use of 13-valent pneumococcal conjugate vaccine and 23-valent pneumococcal polysaccharide vaccine among adults aged 65 years: recommendation of the Advisory Committee on Immunization Practices. MMWR 2014;63:822-5.

13. Centers for Disease Control and Prevention. Use of 13-valent pneumococcal conjugate vaccine and 23-valent pneumococcal polysaccharide vaccine for adults with immunocompromising conditions: recommendations of the Advisory Committee on Immunization Practices. MMWR 2012;61:816-9.

14. Centers for Medicare and Medicaid Services. Brochure 6 – How to Obtain a CLIA Certificate of Waiver. Available at www.cms.gov/Regulations-and-Guidance/Legislation/CLIA/. Accessed December 10, 2014.

15. Kim DK, Bridges CB, Harriman KH. Advisory Committee on Immunization Practices recommended immunization schedule for adults aged 19 years or older: United States, 2015. Ann Intern Med 2015;162:214–23.

16. U.S. Department of Labor, Occupational Safety and Health Administration. Bloodborne Pathogens. Available at www.osha.gov/pls/oshaweb/owadisp.show_document?p_table=STANDARDS&p_id=10051. Accessed December 15, 2014.

17. U.S. Food and Drug Administration. A Guide to Informed Consent – Information Sheet. Available at www.fda.gov/RegulatoryInformation/Guidances/ucm126431.htm. Accessed December 15, 2014.

Adherence

1. Agency for Healthcare Research and Quality. Medication Adherence Interventions: Comparative Effectiveness. Closing the Quality Gap: Revisiting the State of Science. Available at www.effectivehealthcare.ahrq.gov/reports/final.cfm. Accessed December 15, 2014.

2. American College of Preventive Medicine. 2011. Medication Adherence: Improving Health Outcomes Time Tool: A Resource from the American College of Preventive Medicine [excerpted with permission from the ACPM]. Available at www.acpm.org/?MedAdhereTTProviders. Accessed December 14, 2014.

3. Brown MT, Bussell JK. Medication adherence: who cares? Mayo Clin Proc 2011;86:304-14.

4. Cheetham TC, Niu F, Green K, et al. Primary non-adherence to statin medications in a managed care organization. J Manag Care Pharm 2013;19:367-73.

5. Derose SF, Green K, Marrett E, et al. Automated outreach to increase primary adherence to cholesterol lowering medications. JAMA Intern Med 2013;173:38-43.

6. Fischer MA, Choudhry NK, Brill G, et al. Trouble getting started: predictors of primary medication nonadherence. Am J Med 2011;124:1081.e9-e22.

7. Fischer MA, Stedman MR, Lii J, et al. Primary medication nonadherence: analysis of 195,930 electronic prescriptions. J Gen Intern Med 2010;25:284-90.

8. Gwadry-Sridhar FH, Manias E, Zhang Y, et al. A framework for planning and critiquing medication compliance and persistence using prospective study designs. Clin Ther 2009;31:421-35.

9. Ho PM, Bryson CL, Rumsfeld JS. Medication adherence. Circulation 2009;119:3028-35.

10. Lau DT, Nau DP. Oral antihyperglycemic medication nonadherence and subsequent hospitalization among individuals with type 2 diabetes. Diabetes Care 2004;27:2149-53.

11. Levine DA, Morgenstern LB, Langa KM, et al. Recent trends in cost-related medication nonadherence among stroke survivors in the United States. Ann Neurol 2013;73:180-8.

12. Martin MY, Kim Y, Kratt P, et al. Medication adherence among rural, low-income hypertensive adults: a randomized trial of a multimedia community-based intervention. Am J Health Promot 2011;25:372-8.

13. National Community Pharmacists Association. 2013. Medication Adherence in America. A National Report Card. Available at www.ncpanet.org/membership/benefits/preview-of-simplify-my-meds-/medication-adherence-in-america-a-national-report-card. Accessed December 14, 2014.

14. Nau DP. Proportion of Days Covered (PDC) as a Preferred Method of Measuring Medication Adherence. Available at http://pqaalliance.org/resources/adherence.asp. Accessed December 10, 2014.

15. Osterberg L, Blaschke T. Adherence to medication. New Engl J Med 2005;353:487-97.

16. Oyekan E, Nimalasuriya A, Martin J, et al. The B-SMART appropriate medication-use process: a guide for clinicians to help patients, part 1: barriers, solutions, and motivation. Perm J 2009;13:60-9.

17. Oyekan E, Nimalasuriya A, Martin J, et al. The B-SMART appropriate medication-use process: a guide for clinicians to help patients, part 2: adherence, relationships, and triage. Perm J 2009;13:50-4.

18. Peterson AM, Nau DP, Cramer JA, et al. A checklist for medication compliance and persistence and studies using retrospective databases. Value Health 2007;10:3-12.

19. Raebel MA, Ellis JL, Carroll NM, et al. Characteristics of patients with primary nonadherence to medications for hypertension, diabetes, and lipid disorders. J Gen Intern Med 2012;27:57-64.

20. Viswanathan M, Golin CE, Jones CD, et al. Interventions to improve adherence to self-administered medications for chronic diseases in the United States. Ann Intern Med 2012;157:785-95.

21. World Health Organization. 2003. Adherence to Long-term Therapies: Evidence for Action. Available at www.who.int/chp/knowledge/publications/adherence_full_report.pdf. Accessed October 4, 2014.

22. Yeaw J, Benner J, Wait J, et al. Comparing adherence and persistence across 6 chronic medication classes. J Manag Care Pharm 2009;15:728-40.

Complementary and Alternative Medicine

1. Bailey RL, Gahche JJ, Letino CV, et al. Dietary supplement use in the United States, 2003-2006. J Nutr 2011;141:261-6.

2. Bent S, Ko R. Commonly used herbal medicines in the United States: a review. Am J Med 2004;116:478-8.

3. Borrelli F, Ernst E. Black cohosh (Cimicifuga racemosa) for menopausal symptoms: a systematic review of its efficacy. Pharmacol Res 2008;58:8-14.

4. Boyle P, Robertson C, Lowe F, et al. Meta-analysis of clinical trials of Permixon in the treatment of symptomatic benign prostatic hyperplasia. Urology 2000;55:533-9.

5. Brouwer IA, Katan MB, Zock PL. Dietary alpha-linolenic acid is associated with reduced risk of fatal coronary heart disease, but increased prostate cancer risk: a meta-analysis. J Nutr 2004;134:919-22.

6. Brzezinski A, Vangel M, Wurtman RJ, et al. Effects of exogenous melatonin on sleep: a meta-analysis. Sleep Med Rev 2005;9:41-50.

7. Buscemi N, Vandermeer B, Hooton N, et al. The efficacy and safety of exogenous melatonin for primary sleep disorders: a meta-analysis. J Gen Intern Med 2005;20:1151-8.

8. Buscemi N, Vandermeer B, Pandya R, et al. Melatonin for Treatment of Sleep Disorders. Summary, Evidence Report/Technology Assessment No. 108. (Prepared by the University of Alberta Evidence-Based Practice Center, under Contract No. 290-02-0023.) AHRQ Publication No. 05-E002-2. Rockville, MD: Agency for Healthcare Research and Quality, November 2004.

9. Carraro JC, Raynaud JP, Koch G, et al. Comparison of phytotherapy (Permixon) with finasteride in the treatment of benign prostate hyperplasia: a randomized international study of 1,098 patients. Prostate 1996;29:231-40.

10. Chow ECY, Teo M, Ring J, et al. Liver failure associated with the use of black cohosh for menopausal symptoms. MJA 2008;188:420-2.

11. Cohen M. Complementary and integrative medical therapies, the FDA, and the NIH: definitions and regulation. Dermatol Ther 2003;16.77-84.

12. Colato C. Herbal interactions on absorption of drugs: mechanisms of action and clinical risk assessment. Pharm Res 2010;62:207-27.

13. Foster S. Black cohosh: *Cimicifuga racemosa*; a literature review. HerbalGram 1999;45:35-49.

14. Gardiner P, Phillips R, Shaughnessy AF. Herbal and dietary supplement-drug interaction in patients with chronic illnesses. Am Fam Physician 2008;77:73-8.

15. Harper CR, Edwards MC, Jacobson TA. Flaxseed oil supplementation does not affect plasma lipoprotein concentration or particle size in human subjects. J Nutr 2006;136:2844-8.

16. Hartter S, Grozinger M, Weigmann H, et al. Increased bioavailability of oral melatonin after fluvoxamine coadministration. Clin Pharmacol Ther 2000;67:1-6.

17. Hernandez MG, Pluchino S. *Cimicifuga racemosa* for the treatment of hot flashes in women surviving breast cancer. Maturitas 2003;44(suppl 1):S59-65.

18. Herxheimer A, Petrie KJ. Melatonin for preventing and treating jet lag. Cochrane Database Syst Rev 2002;2:CD001520.

19. Hooper L, Thompson RL, Harrison RA, et al. Omega 3 fatty acids for prevention and treatment of cardiovascular disease. Cochrane Database Syst Rev 2004;4:CD003177.

20. Hu FB, Manson JE. Omega-3 fatty acids and secondary prevention of cardiovascular disease – is it just a fish tale? Arch Intern Med 2012;172:694-6.

21. Izzo AA, Ernst E. Interactions between herbal medicines and prescribed drugs: a systemic review. Drugs 2001;61:2163-75.

22. Jacobson JS, Troxel AB, Evans J, et al. Randomized trial of black cohosh for the treatment of hot flashes among women with a history of breast cancer. J Clin Oncol 2001;19:2739-45.

23. Kris-Ehterton PM, Harris WS, Appel LJ, et al. Fish consumption, fish oil, omega-3 fatty acids, and cardiovascular disease. Circulation 2002;106:2747-57.

24. Kwak SM, Myung SK, Lee YJ, et al. Efficacy of omega-3 fatty acid supplements (eicosapentaenoic acid and docosahexaenoic acid) in the secondary prevention of cardiovascular disease: a meta-analysis of randomized, double-blind, placebo-controlled trials. Arch Intern Med 2012;172:686-94.

25. Levitsky I, Alli TA, Wisecarver J, et al. Fulminant liver failure associated with the use of black cohosh. Dig Dis Sci 2005;50:538-9.

26. Lissoni P, Barni S, Mandala M, et al. Decreased toxicity and increased efficacy of cancer chemotherapy using the pineal hormone melatonin in metastatic solid tumor patients with poor clinical status. Eur J Cancer 1999;35:1688-92.

27. Marinac JS, Buchinger CL, Godfry LA, et al. Herbal products and dietary supplements: a survey of use, attitudes, and knowledge among older adults. J Am Osteopath Assoc 2007;107:13-20.

28. Mehta DH, Gardiner PM, Phillips RS, et al. Herbal and dietary supplement disclosure to healthcare providers by individuals with chronic conditions. J Altern Complement Med 2008;14:1263-9.

29. Messina BAM. Herbal supplements: facts and myths – talking to your patients about herbal supplements. J Perianesth Nurs 2006;21:268-78.

30. Nappi RE, Malavasi B, Brundu B, et al. Efficacy of *Cimicifuga racemosa* on climacteric complaints: a randomized study versus low-dose transdermal estradiol. Gynecol Endocrinol 2005;20:30-5.

31. National Center for Complementary and Alternative Medicine (NCCAM). U.S. Department of Health and Human Services. National Institute of Health. Available at www.nccam.nih.gov/health/whatiscam. Accessed December 15, 2014.

32. Nies LK, Cymbala AA, Kasten SL, et al. Complementary and alternative therapies for the management of dyslipidemia. Ann Pharmacother 2006;40:1094-992.

33. Osmers R, Friede M, Liske E, et al. Efficacy and safety of isopropanolic black cohosh extract for climacteric symptoms. Obstet Gynecol 2005;105:1074-83.

34. Palacio C, Masri G, Mooradian A. Black cohosh for the management of menopausal symptoms: a systematic review of clinical trials. Drugs Aging 2009;26:23-6.

35. Roche HM, Gibney MJ. Effect of long-chain n-3 polyunsaturated fatty acids on fasting and postprandial triacylglycerol metabolism. Am J Clin Nutr 2000;71:232S-7S.

36. Sack R. Jet lag. N Engl J Med 2010;362:440-7.

37. Sawitzke AD, Shi H, Finco MF, et al. Clinical efficacy and safety of glucosamine, chondroitin sulfate, their combination, celecoxib or placebo taken to treat osteoarthritis of the knee: 2-year results from GAIT. Ann Rheum Dis 2010;69:1459-64.

38. Schachter SC. Complementary and alternative medical therapies. Curr Opin Neurol 2008;21:184-9.

39. Su D, Li L. Trends in the use of complementary and alternative medicine in the United States: 2002-2007. J Health Care Poor Underserved 2011;22:296-310.

40. U.S. Food and Drug Administration. Dietary Supplements. Available at www.fda.gov/Food/DietarySupplements/. Accessed December 10, 2014.

41. van Dam M, Stalenhoef AFH, Wittekoek J. Efficacy of concentrated n-3 fatty acids in hypertriglyceridaemia: a comparison with gemfibrozil. Clin Drug Invest 2001;21:175-81.

42. Warshafsky S, Kamer Rs, Sivak SL. Effect of garlic on total serum cholesterol: a meta-analysis. Ann Intern Med. 1993;119(7 pt 1):599-605.

43. Wilt TJ, Ishani A, Stark G, et al. Saw palmetto extracts for treatment of benign prostatic hyperplasia: a systematic review. JAMA 1998;280:1604-9.

44. Wu CH, Wang CC, Kennedy J. Changes in herb and dietary supplement use in the U.S. adult population: a comparison of the 2002 and 2007 National Health Interview Surveys. Clin Ther 2011;33:1749-58.

45. Yilmaz MB, Yontar OC, Turgut OO, et al. Herbals in cardiovascular practice: are physicians neglecting anything? Int J Cardiol 2007;122:48-51

46. Zhdanova IV, Wurtman RJ, Regan MM, et al. Melatonin treatment for age-related insomnia. J Clin Endocrinol Metab 2001;86:4727-30.

ANSWERS AND EXPLANATIONS TO PATIENT CASES

1. Answer: B

The American Heart Association and American Red Cross guidelines for first aid recommend splinting potential fractures (Answer B). Option A is incorrect because setting bone fractures may induce more pain, and there is no evidence that it will decrease pain or deformity. Ambulation is not recommended; in fact, any weight bearing should be avoided until further evaluation and treatment (Option C). Ice is recommended when there is a sprain or strain (Option D), but the priority is to immobilize the leg with splints.

2. Answer: B

According to first-aid guidelines, the initial management of a patient with a seizure is to prevent injury, which includes keeping the area clear (Answer B). Although the lay public might think of placing an object such as a wallet into the patient's mouth to prevent tongue biting, the risk of being bitten and of causing harm to the patient outweighs any potential benefit (Option A). Holding the patient still is not recommended, and in fact, the patient should not be restrained because of potential secondary injuries (Option C). Although this patient probably requires adjustment in his or her seizure medications, administering a dose acutely is not recommended because it would probably be an oral medication, and the patient is unlikely to be able to swallow (Option D).

3. Answer: B

When an AED is immediately available, it should be used as rapidly as possible, but the clerk will be slightly delayed as he or she calls 911 and grabs the AED; waiting for it to arrive will decrease the chances for survival (Option A). This situation involves a man with a witnessed arrest, when an AED and immediate CPR are most likely to be effective. While the pharmacist waits for the AED to be obtained and set up, CPR can be initiated with chest compressions and ventilations in the correct ratio (Answer B). Option C is not the correct ratio for any CPR effort, according to the most recent guidelines. Chest-compression-only CPR (Option D) would be appropriate for a non–health care rescuer to provide if an AED was unavailable.

4. Answer: C

In this case, two rescuers are providing health care, allowing the nurse to focus on the airway. The best choice to open the airway if the jaw thrust is not effective is to open the airway with the head tilt–chin lift maneuver (Answer C). Continuing with the jaw thrust might prevent secondary injury by limiting neck movement, but guidelines recommend rescue breaths with the head tilt–chin lift procedure if the jaw thrust is unsuccessful (Option A). Chest-compression-only CPR can be used for witnessed arrests when a bystander is not trained in rescue breaths; however, two health care providers are responding, so this is not the best choice (Option B). Increased pressure would lead to gastric distention and a risk of aspiration and vomiting (Option D).

5. Answer: D

Many of the category A agents, when aerosolized, can cause pneumonia-like illnesses. Botulism (Option A) is less likely because there was no mention of associated symptoms affecting the muscles. Smallpox would also cause skin lesions and is highly contagious (Option C). Pneumonic plague can be transmitted from person to person by droplets; however, because none of the family members developed the illness after exposure to the affected individuals, the likelihood of plague is diminished (Option B). The most likely disease is tularemia (Answer D).

6. Answer: D

The best choice for postexposure prophylaxis against inhalational anthrax is a combination of antibiotics and the vaccine. The recommended vaccine schedule is a three-dose series (Answer D). The regimen in Option A is not optimal because it does not constitute a full vaccine schedule and is limited to a single dose. Option C and Option D are not optimal because these regimens are inferior to using the combination of antibiotic and vaccine in this setting.

7. Answer: B

Patients 2–4 years of age with a documented wheezing episode in the past 12 months should not receive LAIV. This patient should not receive the meningococcal vaccine until his 11-year checkup. In addition, the IIV is more appropriate for this patient. He should receive all vaccines as recommended. He is eligible to receive both his MMR and varicella vaccines at this visit. Option A is not the correct choice because although H.H. is a candidate for MMR vaccine, he is not a candidate for LAIV. The HPV vaccine will not be offered until the patient is 11 years of age.

8. Answer: A

This patient has a diagnosis of HIV and is considered an immunocompromised person. This makes him a candidate for both PPSV23 and PCV. Although this patient has already received the first dose of PPSV23, the patient should receive one dose of PCV13 now and then one dose of PPSV23 at least 8 weeks after receiving the dose of PCV13. The patient will be eligible for a third dose of PPSV23 at age 65 years.

9. Answer: A

A.J. should receive one booster dose when possible before college entry. One booster dose is recommended because her first dose was administered before her 16th birthday. Either type of meningococcal conjugate vaccine (MenACWY-D or MenACWY-CRM) would be appropriate for her to receive. Hib-MenCY is not indicated at her age.

10. Answer: D

Until 2005, guidelines stated that Td vaccine was necessary only when administering tetanus boosters after the 11- to 12-year checkup. Because of recent pertussis outbreaks, guidelines have changed to include a one-time revaccination with Tdap vaccine to booster pertussis immunity. It is likely that this patient received Td vaccine with his most recent booster dose; thus, he requires Tdap vaccine today. The DTaP and DT vaccines are not recommended because they are approved only for patients younger than 7 years.

11. Answer: D

The quadrivalent HPV vaccine may be administered to both male and female individuals aged 9–26 years. The bivalent vaccine is administered to female individuals 9–25 years of age. Although other vaccines may be appropriate, the 32-year-old health care worker and the 40-year old woman reporting a non-monogamous relationship are not candidates for this vaccine. The 27-year-old pharmacy school student would not be a candidate for this vaccine, if just starting the vaccine series. If the series was started before the student reached 27 years of age, the vaccine series may be completed; however, the best choice is Answer D. The HPV vaccine series should be initiated at the 11- or 12-year checkup before onset of sexual activity.

12. Answer: C

The Advisory Committee on Immunization Practices (ACIP) states that susceptible people traveling to or working in countries that have high or intermediate hepatitis A endemicity are at increased risk of hepatitis A

virus infection and should be vaccinated before departure. Hepatitis A vaccine is a two-dose series.

13. Answer B

W.M. discontinued his medication because of the adverse effects that he is experiencing. He does come with the request to check his blood pressure, understands goals, and has implemented lifestyle changes. These actions demonstrate his understanding of the importance to manage the hypertension. W.M. does not mention financial concerns and from the information provided, it seems that he has means to access the prescribed medication. The case does not identify any social concerns (e.g., unstable living conditions, low health literacy, inability to access pharmacy) and is not the best answer choice. The next step to assist W.M. is to contact his provider and discuss appropriate options and an action plan to resolve adverse reactions.

14. Answer: D

Omega-3 fatty acids improve hyperlipidemia by decreasing intestinal cholesterol absorption. Ginseng is a herbal product that may be used for mental performance or memory. Fish oil is typically not associated with hepatotoxicity, unlike red yeast rice. The recommended dose for triglyceride lowering is 2–4 g/day in divided doses. Fish oil is a source of omega-3 fatty acids, primarily EPA and DHA, that is used to lower triglycerides and improve cardiac health.

15. Answer: C

The North American Menopause Society recommends that if black cohosh is selected for management of mild vasomotor symptoms, the product should be used on a short-term trial. Adverse effects of black cohosh include gastrointestinal disturbances, headache, rash, and weight gain. Because of the number of case reports of acute hepatitis with black cohosh, the Dietary Supplement Information Expert Committee recommended that a cautionary statement be included on products, alerting consumers to the potential for hepatotoxicity. The use of black cohosh is not recommended beyond a 6 months' period because of the lack of safety data. Option A is not correct because there is no current evidence to support that black cohosh is as effective as select serotonin reuptake inhibitors (SSRIs) in the management of hot flashes. A few studies have shown SSRI therapy to be effective in reducing hot flash symptoms (JAMA 2003;289:2827-34, J Clin Oncol 2002;20:1578-83, JAMA 2011;305:267-74); however, the efficacy of black cohosh has not been well established and has not been compared to the efficacy of SSRIs. Option B is not correct because there is no warning to the use of black cohosh in patients with a history of asthma. It is unclear how black cohosh may interact with estrogen or progesterone therapy. The safety of black cohosh for patients with a medical history significant for breast cancer is controversial. To date, studies have been inconclusive to support efficacy and safety; therefore, Option D is not the best recommendation that can be offered to patients.

ANSWERS AND EXPLANATIONS TO SELF-ASSESSMENT QUESTIONS

1. Answer A
Although foreign-body airway obstruction can occur at any age (Options B–D), deaths occur most commonly in those younger than 5 years of age (Answer A).

2. Answer D
All of the listed drugs are commonly implicated in overdose. However, the overwhelming majority of overdose deaths are caused by opioids (Answer D). Anticoagulants fall under the systemic and hematologic drug category, which accounts for about 7% of drug deaths (Option A). Tricyclic antidepressants are a class within the antidepressant category that accounts for less than 20% of drug-related overdose deaths (Option B). Benzodiazepines are the second leading cause of overdose deaths caused by drugs (Option C).

3. Answer A
All of the elements listed are important for an effective disaster plan. Pharmacists will invariably be required as part of the plan, but they may not need to be "on-call" because a disaster may require use of calling trees and other mechanisms to engage important personnel (Option B). Each disaster will be specific. Although vaccinations and antibiotic supplies are important, they are only applicable to a subset of disasters (Options C and D). The most important element is flexibility of the plan to allow an effective local response (Answer A).

4. Answer C
Live, attenuated vaccines are not recommended in pregnant women because of the theoretical risk of infection to the fetus. Of the vaccines listed, the only live, attenuated vaccine is the MMR vaccine. Therefore, Options A, B, and D are incorrect and Answer C is the best answer. In fact, the Tdap (Option D) vaccine is now recommended for administration to women between weeks 27 and 36 of pregnancy in order to protect the infant, because the first dose of DTaP is not given until 2 months of age and the full series is not completed until 5–6 years of age. Whereas live, attenuated influenza vaccine should be avoided in pregnant women, IIV (Option A) does represent a vaccine that pregnant women should receive if pregnant during the usual period for annual influenza vaccination.

5. Answer: B
Medication possession ratio is defined as the sum of days' supply of a medication for a defined period. A patient is considered adherent if MPR is 0.8 (80%) or higher; therefore, a higher MPR value is an indication of a patient's adherence to prescribed therapy. Option C is not correct because the MPR value is increased proportionally to a patient's refills. If a patient fails to refill a medication, the MPR would decrease over time. The duration of time from start to end of a medication regimen is defined as persistence. Health literacy is defined by the patient's ability to interpret and understand health information in order to make an informed decision regarding his or her health.

6. Answer: C
The DSHEA of 1994 defines dietary supplements as food, not drugs. DSHEA does not require that the safety or efficacy of supplements be established before they are marketed, nor is this requirement mandated by the FDA. Three types of claims may be made: health claims, structure/function claims, and description of the contents in the product. A supplement may be certified for quality by a third party certifier, although this is not required under DSHEA rules. Products that undergo this additional testing will include a quality "seal" authorized by the certifier.

Dermatologic & Eyes, Ears, Nose, and Throat, and Immunologic Disorders

Jamie L. McConaha, Pharm.D., BCACP

Duquesne University
Pittsburgh, Pennsylvania

Dermatologic & Eyes, Ears, Nose, and Throat, and Immunologic Disorders

Jamie L. McConaha, Pharm.D., BCACP

Duquesne University
Pittsburgh, Pennsylvania

Learning Objectives

1. Evaluate antioxidant and multivitamin supplements for components and doses consistent with the AREDS (Age-Related Eye Disease Study) formulation for preventing the progression of macular degeneration.

2. Formulate an ophthalmologic drug therapy regimen for a patient that will decrease the patient's elevated intraocular pressures using agents that work synergistically (increased aqueous outflow and decreased production).

3. Create criteria to evaluate dry eye symptom treatment beyond traditional artificial tears.

4. Evaluate a medication profile to determine whether the signs and symptoms of vertigo are medication induced or a component of organic disease.

5. Construct an individualized pharmacy care plan for a patient with allergic rhinitis who has not received relief from intranasal corticosteroids.

6. Discuss the risks and benefits of agents used in addition to nonsedating histamine-1 blockers/antagonists for the treatment of urticaria.

7. Recommend immunizations for patients receiving injectable medications for the treatment and/or prevention of angioedema.

8. Determine how patients with acne should initiate, switch, or modify topical or oral therapeutic agents using a treatment algorithm.

9. Educate a patient using isotretinoin about therapy and the various monitoring variables that will take place to ensure drug safety and efficacy.

10. Recommend single or multiple topical agents for treating plaque psoriasis given a patient's disease presentation, severity, and (if applicable) prior therapies.

11. Effectively educate a patient on an infestation and the purpose, proper use, and potential adverse reactions of the first-line treatment options for scabies and/or lice.

12. Create a pain management strategy for a patient with first-degree or superficial second-degree burns.

13. Create a monitoring plan for a patient using becaplermin for the treatment and healing of a decubitus ulcer.

Self-Assessment Questions

Answers and explanations to these questions may be found at the end of the chapter.

1. J.R. is a 68-year-old man with a medical history significant for type 2 diabetes. He presents to his ophthalmologist for his annual eye examination and is told he has signs of moderate (intermediate) macular degeneration. His ophthalmologist wishes to prescribe supplements for the patient. Which combination best resembles the formulation proven to decrease the progression of macular degeneration?

   A. Vitamin C, vitamin E, beta-carotene, and zinc.
   B. Vitamin C, beta-carotene, and zinc.
   C. Vitamin C, vitamin E, and beta-carotene.
   D. Vitamin C, vitamin E, and zinc.

2. A.A. is a 54-year-old man with a medical history significant for open-angle glaucoma, diabetes, and obesity, all of which are appropriately treated. At his most recent visit to the ophthalmologist (6 months earlier), he was noted to have increased intraocular pressures (IOPs) without changes in visual field or acuity. He was initiated on latanoprost therapy at that visit; now, he is returning for a follow-up. Today, his IOP is significantly decreased, but it still is not within an acceptable range to prevent progressive vision changes. Which medication is most appropriate to add to his therapy?

   A. Travoprost; one drop in each eye in the evening.
   B. Betaxolol; one drop in each eye twice daily.
   C. Dorzolamide; one drop in each eye three times daily.
   D. Brimonidine; one drop in each eye three times daily.

3. F.T. is a 52-year-old woman who works in a retail shop. She presents to an ophthalmologist with "scratching" in her eyes, constant irritation, and difficulty making it through the workday, leaving early once per week because of eye irritation and headaches. She has tried to use artificial teardrops, but they soothe her symptoms only temporarily. The ophthalmologist considers that F.T. has mild to moderate dry eyes and wants to adjust her therapy to better address the symptoms. Which is the best next step to recommend for therapy?

   A. Artificial tear ointment.
   B. Topical cyclosporine 0.05%.
   C. Topical cyclosporine 0.1%.
   D. Systemic cholinergic agents.

4. P.W. is a 45-year-old man who presents to the pharmacy and states that he has been having episodes of "dizziness" for the past several months. His medical history is significant for hypertension, seizures, type 2 diabetes, and headaches. He has discussed the matter with his physician and has undergone many tests, only to find that there is no readily identifiable cause for his symptoms. All radiographic study results of his head are normal, all of his laboratory values are within normal limits, and his blood pressure readings are "at target." He believes his dizziness may be caused by one of the medications he takes. In the past several months, he has started using hydrochlorothiazide, naproxen, fluoxetine, and metformin. Which medication is most likely associated with his dizziness?

   A. Hydrochlorothiazide.
   B. Acetaminophen.
   C. Carbamazepine.
   D. Metformin.

5. A.T. is a 9-year-old girl presenting to her pediatrician's office with her mother. The mother believes that A.T. has allergies because she has had a "runny nose and puffy and watery eyes" for the past few weeks. The child's nose has continuous, clear, thin discharge, and she is constantly sniffling. Her mother reports "waves" of sneezes two or three times daily. During the interview, the pediatrician observes several instances of the patient sniffling, rubbing her eyes, and making the "allergic salute" and wishes to prescribe an intranasal corticosteroid.

The patient's mother refuses this medication because her daughter has frequent bloody noses, so instead, she requests an oral agent. Which would be the best oral agent for the child?

   A. Clemastine 1.34 mg once daily.
   B. Fexofenadine 30 mg twice daily.
   C. Montelukast 5 mg once daily.
   D. Pseudoephedrine 30 mg every 6 hours as needed.

6. Y.A. is a 26-year-old woman with a medical history significant only for dysmenorrhea, for which she takes naproxen 500 mg as needed, and low-dose oral contraceptive therapy. She is a schoolteacher at the local middle school and regularly contracts respiratory viral illnesses from her students. She is returning to work after being out with the influenza virus infection. She currently takes fexofenadine 60 mg twice daily for residual nasal symptoms and an urticarial rash she developed with the influenza virus. However, even though she may return to work, the rash has not completely resolved, and it is causing her moderate discomfort (noticeable, but not interfering with daily activities). She requests something to help further alleviate the symptoms of the urticaria. Which is the best agent for her (in addition to fexofenadine)?

   A. Montelukast 10 mg once daily.
   B. Diphenhydramine 25 mg every 6 hours as needed.
   C. Famotidine 20 mg once daily.
   D. Doxepin 25 mg once daily.

7. A.R. is a 24-year-old woman with a history of hereditary angioedema (HAE). She is treated with a plasma-derived C1 inhibitor (C1 INH) (Cinryze) every 3–4 days to prevent symptom onset. Given her medical condition and treatment regimen, which immunization is most important for her to receive?

   A. Influenza annually.
   B. Pneumonia (pneumococcal vaccine polyvalent) now and after age 55 years.
   C. Herpes zoster now.
   D. Hepatitis B series now.

8. F.D. is a 17-year-old female adolescent with a 5-year history of inflammatory acne conglobata on her face, neck, and upper torso. Since her initial diagnosis, she has been treated with a variety of topical and systemic agents such as benzoyl peroxide (with and without antibacterials), topical retinoids, and oral minocycline. Although these agents have partly controlled her symptoms, they have not offered sufficient relief. After much consideration, she and her family have agreed to try isotretinoin therapy. They have been counseled on the adverse events associated with its use and are ready to begin therapy. Which additional measure best represents the next step before the clinician prescribes therapy?

   A. Enroll the patient in the iPledge program to help avoid teratogenicity in the event of an unplanned or planned pregnancy.

   B. Have the patient obtain clearance from a mental health provider to begin using the agent because it has been associated with suicidal ideations.

   C. Remain diligent to testing hepatic transaminase concentrations every other week until therapy is discontinued; discontinue the medication if the patient does not adhere to testing.

   D. Have the patient agree to avoid driving after sunset for 6 months secondary to vision changes associated with the drug.

9. J.F. is a 22-year-old man with moderate psoriasis of his back and legs. He has received treatment with topical corticosteroids intermittently for the past 9 years. Each treatment course has been successful at alleviating his symptoms of itching and burning. His most recent symptom flare is the worst to date and is not responding to topical corticosteroids as it did previously. Which agent is best to add to his topical corticosteroid?

   A. Prednisone 20 mg daily for 14 days.
   B. Topical calcipotriene twice daily.
   C. Methotrexate 20 mg once weekly.
   D. Adalimumab 40 mg once every other week.

10. D.T. is a 46-year-old woman with severe and sometimes debilitating psoriasis with arthritis symptoms. She has been having painful psoriatic arthritis complications in her hands, wrists, hips, and knees for the past 6 months and has gained only limited relief from nonsteroidal anti-inflammatory drugs (NSAIDs) and oral corticosteroids. She underwent a hysterectomy with a bilateral salpingo-oophorectomy 4 years ago and has poorly controlled hypertension, despite being treated with fosinopril, hydrochlorothiazide, and amlodipine. She is employed and has medical and prescription insurance. Which is the first choice to help lessen this patient's symptoms?

   A. Methotrexate 20 mg once weekly.
   B. Cyclosporine (equaling 1.25 mg/kg) twice daily.
   C. Acitretin 50 mg once daily.
   D. Etanercept 50 mg twice weekly.

Questions 11 and 12 pertain to the following case.
L.L. is a 14-year-old male adolescent visiting his aunt and uncle for a few weeks in the summer. He is up to date with his immunizations and has had a relatively unremarkable childhood. He attends a sleep-away camp every summer for 2 weeks and then visits his cousins the following week. On the second day of his visit with his relatives, L.L. begins to experience itching between his fingers, under his arms, and on the underside of his buttocks. The itching is unrelieved with bathing, loratadine, or hydrocortisone cream. His aunt takes him to her children's pediatrician for evaluation and is surprised to hear that he has contracted scabies. He has not experienced an infestation such as this before; most likely, he contracted it during the first few days of camp.

11. Which is the best first choice to eradicate this infestation?

   A. Permethrin 1%.
   B. Permethrin 5%.
   C. Malathion 0.5%.
   D. Lindane 1%.

12. L.L.'s aunt is concerned that her family may have also contracted scabies and wants everyone in the house to be treated. Which is the most appropriate response to this request?

    A. All individuals in the house should be empirically treated, regardless of the presence of symptoms.

    B. Household prophylaxis is unnecessary in scabies infestations, and patients should seek treatment on an individual basis.

    C. Only those in the house who have had close contact with the patient's clothing or bedding need prophylactic therapy.

    D. The family should have an "on-call" prescription for a scabicide and use it at the first sign of itching and discomfort.

13. T.S. is a 38-year-old man with no significant medical history. After a long weekend of working outside and not wearing sunscreen, he has developed sunburn on his upper arms, neck, face, and back. He is relatively uncomfortable and cannot wear a shirt or sleep on his back without discomfort. The sunburned areas are not blistering or weeping. They are erythematous and warm to the touch, and they blanch with pressure. Which would be the best way to relieve his pain and make him more comfortable?

    A. Topical silver-based cream applied once or twice daily.

    B. Topical aloe vera and an occlusive dressing over the back, arms, and neck.

    C. Ibuprofen 400 mg every 6 hours as needed for pain.

    D. Hydrocolloid dressings (DuoDERM) for 5–10 days.

14. E.C. is a 73-year-old man with an extensive medical history. Most notably, the patient has poorly controlled type 2 diabetes, severe peripheral arterial disease, and a below-the-knee amputation on his left leg 6 months prior. Since the amputation, the patient has chosen to spend most of his time in bed and uses a wheelchair for activities outside the house. He has developed a 1 in. x 2 in. decubitus ulcer on his right hip that requires surgical debridement and medical management. He is prescribed becaplermin to promote wound healing. Ten weeks after starting the medication, he returns to the wound management group and is reported to have a 35% reduction in ulcer size. Which is the best way to continue with the patient's treatment?

    A. Continue the current regimen for another 10 weeks.

    B. Increase the becaplermin dose to 1.5 times his original dose (length of gel ribbon).

    C. Decrease his becaplermin dose to 0.75 times his original dose (length of gel ribbon).

    D. Discontinue this therapy because he has not experienced sufficient wound healing in the first 10 weeks.

I. MACULAR DEGENERATION

A. Professional Treatment Guidelines *(Domain 3)*
   1. 2008 American Academy of Ophthalmology (AAO) guideline on age-related macular degeneration (AMD)
   2. 2004 update of the American Optometric Association clinical practice guideline; care of the patient with AMD

B. Types *(Domain 1)*
   1. Dry (atrophic or non-neovascular); most common type
   2. Wet (exudative or neovascular); more damaging
   3. Best disease (rare genetic disease in children and/or adolescents)

C. Factors Associated with Developing Macular Degeneration *(Domains 1 and 2)*
   1. Age
   2. Family history of macular degeneration
   3. Women have a higher incidence and earlier onset than do men
   4. White race
   5. Cigarette smoking
   6. Cumulative light exposure
   7. Hypertension
   8. Higher summer sun exposure
   9. Excessive alcohol intake
   10. Genetic/familial predisposition
       a. Complement factor H (CFH) gene variant Y402H
       b. LOC387715 polymorphism
       c. Complement C3 variant (Arg80Gly)
       d. SERPING1 gene
   11. After diagnosis
       a. Obesity associated with an increased risk of disease progression
       b. Physical activity associated with a decreased risk of disease progression

Table 1. Presentation and Diagnosis

Patient Presentation	Funduscopic Changes	Diagnostic Tests
Loss of visual acuity Poor color vision Central scotoma (blind/blurry spot in field of view) Metamorphopsia (wavy lines)	Retinal atrophy Retinal pigment abnormalities Soft drusen Choroidal neovascularization Retinal detachment (wet) Subretinal hemorrhage (wet) Exudates (wet)	Color fundus photography Fluorescein angiographic imaging Optical coherence tomography

Patient Case

1. M.C. is a 76-year-old man with a medical history of hypertension, type 2 diabetes, cerebrovascular accident with residual left-sided hemiparesis, peripheral neuropathy, and renal insufficiency. He has smoked 1 pack/day for the past 50 years and is not ready or willing to quit. He is treated for neovascular (wet) AMD with intravitreal bevacizumab. His ophthalmologist recommends that he begin an antioxidant vitamin regimen, but the patient is unsure what he is supposed to take. Which combination of products is best to recommend for this patient?

    A. Vitamin C, vitamin E, beta-carotene, and zinc.
    B. Vitamin C, beta-carotene, and zinc.
    C. Vitamin C, vitamin E, and beta-carotene.
    D. Vitamin C, vitamin E, and zinc.

  D. Treatment *(Domains 1 and 3)*
    1. AREDS formula (vitamin C 500 mg, vitamin E 400 international units, beta-carotene 15 mg or 25,000 international units of vitamin A, and zinc 80 mg)

Table 2. Antioxidant STEPS

Safety	Increased risk of cardiovascular event in patients taking higher doses (> 400 international units) of vitamin E daily Increased risk of lung cancer in patients who smoke and use high doses of beta-carotene Potential increase in genitourinary disease with high-dose zinc supplementation
Tolerability	Excessive vitamin C will increase urinary oxalate (risk of nephrolithiasis) Carotenodermia reported in > 10% of patients using beta-carotene
Efficacy	No benefit for disease prevention or progression in patients with mild AMD Antioxidant plus zinc is effective for preventing patients with intermediate disease from progressing to advanced macular degeneration or visual acuity loss
Preference (Pearls)	Least invasive intervention for macular degeneration Antioxidants with or without zinc do not treat macular degeneration, but only prevent disease progression Patients who smoke should use the AREDS formulation without beta-carotene because of the increased risk of lung cancer, but this regimen lacks good evidence to fully support its use
Simplicity	OTC formulation (comparable to the AREDS formulation) is available for $10 a month

AMD = age-related macular degeneration; AREDS = Age-Related Eye Disease Study; OTC = over the counter.

    2. Intravitreal drug therapy
      a. Bevacizumab (Avastin)
      b. Pegaptanib (Macugen)
      c. Ranibizumab (Lucentis)
      d. Aflibercept (Eylea) – Recently U.S. Food and Drug Administration (FDA) approved

Table 3. Intravitreal Therapy STEPS

Safety	Increased IOP Stroke, MI, or thrombotic event Endophthalmitis and retinal detachment
Tolerability	Endophthalmitis (erythema, photophobia, vision changes) Conjunctival hemorrhage Corneal edema (pegaptanib) Vitreous floaters (pegaptanib)
Efficacy	Reduced visual acuity loss (< 15 letters on Snellen chart) Significantly more individuals gaining visual acuity ($\geq$ 15 letters on Snellen chart)
Preference (Pearls)	These agents should only be used for neovascular (wet) AMD First class of agents to improve visual acuity in patients with neovascular (wet) AMD Ranibizumab is the most extensively studied of the three options Bevacizumab is not FDA labeled for AMD; however, it is more widely used and is covered by third-party payers because of its major cost advantage over ranibizumab
Simplicity	Intravitreal injections (traumatic) performed once monthly to once every 3 months Ranibizumab costs $2100 per month Bevacizumab costs $30/dose Periodic eye examinations are needed

IOP = intraocular pressure; MI = myocardial infarction.

3. Other considerations
   a. Photodynamic therapy
      i. Verteporfin infusion followed by laser therapy
      ii. Reduces visual acuity loss (greater than 15 lines on Snellen chart) at 24 months
      iii. Questionable benefit of adding intravitreal triamcinolone to therapy
   b. Laser photocoagulation
   c. Surgery
   d. Over-the-counter (OTC) vitamin preparations also include lutein and zeaxanthin, but there is no evidence to support their supplementation (outside dietary intake) to prevent the progression of macular degeneration.
   e. Self-management and problem-solving treatment sessions may help patients adjust to life with macular degeneration.

II. GLAUCOMA

A. Professional Treatment Guidelines *(Domain 3)*
   1. AAO 2010 guidelines on primary open-angle glaucoma (POAG)
   2. National Institute for Health and Clinical Excellence (NICE) 2009 review on diagnosis and management of chronic open-angle glaucoma and ocular hypertension

B. Types of Glaucoma *(Domain 1)*
   1. POAG (most common)
   2. Acute angle-closure glaucoma
   3. Congenital glaucoma
   4. Secondary glaucoma

C. Factors Associated with Developing POAG – Prediction tool available through Ocular Hypertension Treatment Study for 5-year risk of conversion from ocular hypertension to glaucoma *(Domains 1, 2 and 3)*
1. Advanced age
2. African ancestry or Latino/Hispanic ethnicity
3. Family history and genetic predisposition
4. Elevated IOPs (ocular hypertension)
5. Thinner central cornea
6. Low ocular perfusion pressures
7. Various optic nerve characteristics (size and shape of optic cup, thickness of neuroretinal rim, and symmetry of optic cups)
8. Myopia
9. Type 2 diabetes (controversial)

D. Disease Prevention *(Domains 1 and 2)*
1. The AAO does not recommend community screenings because they are not a cost-effective intervention.
2. May be beneficial to target high-risk populations for screening instead of screening the general population.
   a. Older adults
   b. Diabetes
   c. Family history of glaucoma

E. Presentation and Diagnosis *(Domain 1)*
1. Patient findings
   a. Ocular hypertension (21 mm Hg or greater) often precedes the diagnosis of (chronic) open-angle glaucoma.
   b. POAG is usually asymptomatic in early stages, but it develops to noticeable tunnel vision and scotomas (visual field defect) over time.
   c. Patients with acute angle-closure glaucoma present with ocular pain, blurry vision, halos, and headache.
   d. Congenital glaucoma causes patients to have light sensitivity and excessive lacrimation.
2. Screening procedures for glaucoma may include, but are not limited to, the following:
   a. Goldmann applanation tonometry is the reference standard for diagnosis and should be performed before pupil dilation to assess IOP.
      i. Normal IOP is 13–18 mm Hg.
      ii. IOP and time of day should be recorded to assess for diurnal variations.
   b. Gonioscopy should be used to evaluate the anterior chamber angle as well as to identify/rule out secondary causes of glaucoma and IOP.
   c. Pachymetry measures central corneal thickness and is indicated in the evaluation of the patient with glaucoma or suggestion of glaucoma.
   d. Use of a biomicroscope with ancillary lens is the preferred method to assess the optic nerve (preferably through a dilated pupil).
3. Diagnosis is based on several factors.
   a. Physical examination will reveal an increased cupping diameter in the optic nerve.
   b. IOP is usually elevated, though some patients may have a normal value.
   4. Disease severity is usually related to disease duration. Follow-up examination of patients with a diagnosis of POAG should occur within the first 1–2 years.

Patient Case

2. E.K. is a 67-year-old woman with a medical history significant for type 2 diabetes, hypertension, osteoar-thritis, hypothyroidism, asthma, and osteopenia. At her most recent ophthalmologist appointment, she had increased IOPs and findings consistent with POAG. Her IOP is 35 mm Hg, and she has optic nerve changes. Her ophthalmologist recommends therapy to decrease her IOPs and prevent the progression of glaucoma. Which regimen is best for E.K. to start?

    A. Travoprost eyedrop; one drop in each eye at bedtime.
    B. Travoprost eyedrop; two drops in each eye at bedtime.
    C. Timolol eyedrop; one drop in each eye twice daily.
    D. Timolol eyedrop; two drops in each eye twice daily.

F. Treatment of POAG *(Domain 1)*
    1. IOP lowering is individually determined but typically targets a reduction of 25% or more from baseline IOP to delay visual field loss.
    2. Early, aggressive management of elevated IOP may delay progression.
    3. Topical ocular rules
        a. Only one drop is necessary per dosing.
        b. Wait about 5 minutes between agents if using several drops.
    4. At each patient contact, counsel patient regarding treatment adherence and proper administration of eyedrops (including nasolacrimal occlusion techniques).

Table 4. Therapeutic Considerations for Drug Classes

Reduce Aqueous Outflow Resistance	Decrease Aqueous Production
Prostaglandin analogs Adrenergic agents (epinephrine) Miotics (pilocarpine) Adrenergic agonists	β-Blockers Carbonic anhydrase inhibitors Adrenergic agonists (primary)

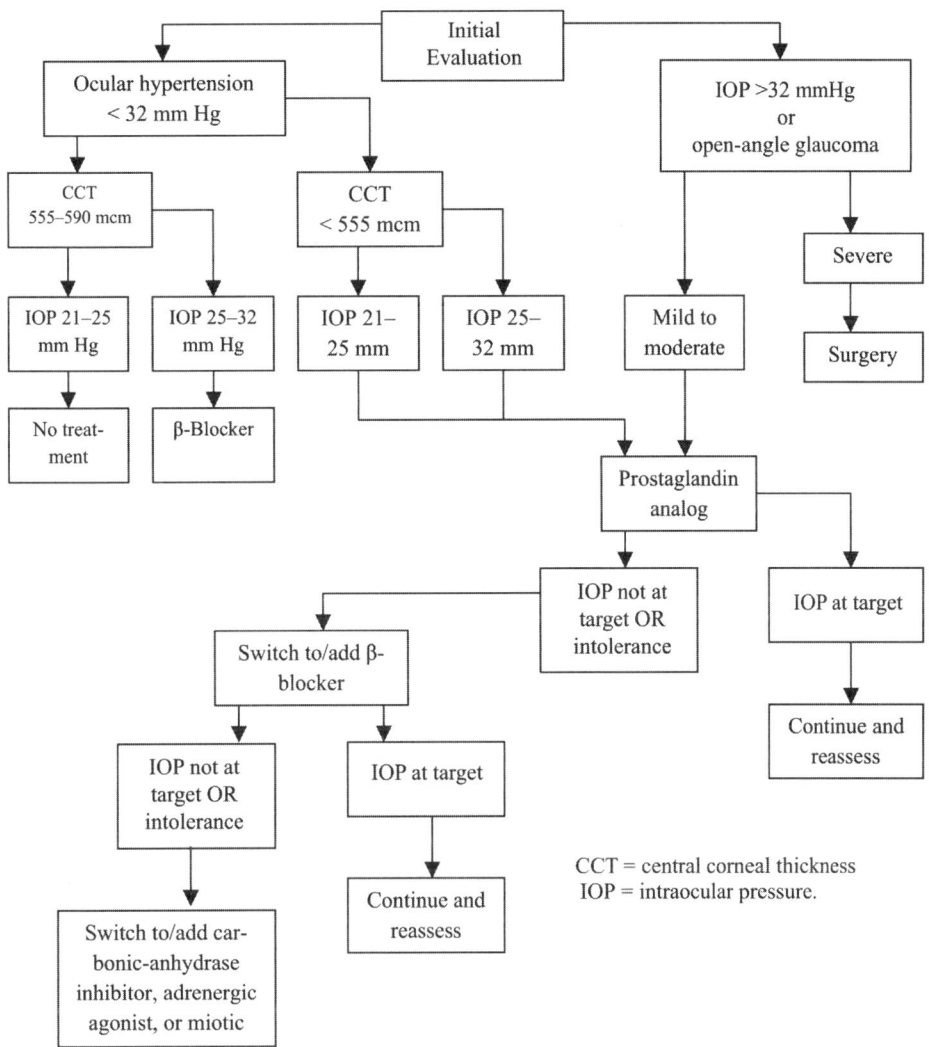

Figure 1. Ocular hypertension and primary open-angle glaucoma treatment algorithm.

CCT = central corneal thickness.

5. Prostaglandin analogs
   a. Bimatoprost (Lumigan)
   b. Latanoprost (Xalatan)
   c. Tafluprost (Zioptan)
   d. Travoprost (Travatan)
   e. Unoprostone (Rescula)

Table 5. Ocular Prostaglandin Analog STEPS

Safety	Contraindicated in macular edema or history of herpetic keratitis
Tolerability	Increased brown pigmentation of iris (especially blue or multicolored irises) Increased number, thickness, curvature, and pigmentation of eyelashes Ocular pruritus/dryness/blurring Eyelid erythema
Efficacy	Greatest IOP reduction potential of all available pharmacologic agents
Preference (Pearls)	In patients who do not achieve adequate IOPs with a single agent, add a second agent (from a different class) to further lower IOP Caution when using with ophthalmologic NSAIDs because they may decrease the therapeutic effect of the prostaglandin analog
Simplicity	Once-daily application in the evening Available as a combination with a topical β-antagonist for patients who require additional therapy Administer 15 minutes before inserting contact lenses secondary to benzalkonium chloride (will adsorb to contact lenses)

NSAID = nonsteroidal anti-inflammatory drug.

6. β-Antagonists (topical)
   a. Betaxolol (Betoptic S)
   b. Timolol (Timoptic)
   c. Levobunolol (Betagan)
   d. Metipranolol (OptiPranolol)
   e. Carteolol (Ocupress)

Table 6. Ocular β-Antagonists STEPS

Safety	Severe cardiovascular and respiratory events reported with topical β-antagonists Not to be used as monotherapy in patients with angle-closure glaucoma
Tolerability	Ocular burning and stinging with application Reported bradycardia, depression, and bronchospasm
Efficacy	Adding to a prostaglandin analog appears to decrease the variations in IOP throughout the day
Preference (Pearls)	May be used as monotherapy, but would be best used as add-on therapy for patients without adequate IOP lowering with a prostaglandin analog
Simplicity	Once- or twice-daily application Available as a combination with a prostaglandin analog for patients who require additional therapy Administer 15 minutes before inserting contact lenses secondary to benzalkonium chloride (will adsorb to contact lenses)

7. Selective α_2-agonists
   a. Apraclonidine (Iopidine)
   b. Brimonidine (Alphagan P)

Table 7. Selective α-Agonists STEPS

Safety	Caution with use around children < 5 years secondary to serious systemic adverse events with ingestion Use with caution in patients with cardiovascular disease, cerebrovascular disease, depression, orthostatic hypotension, or Raynaud phenomenon Ocular hypersensitivity reactions (hyperemia, swelling, pruritus)
Tolerability	Tearing Foreign body sensation Ocular inflammation Dry mouth Altered taste
Efficacy	Reported to have IOP-lowering properties similar to β-antagonists
Preference (Pearls)	Third-line agent for treating glaucoma (brimonidine preferred) May be efficacious for a limited time (less than 1 month; apraclonidine)
Simplicity	Application three times daily Administer 15 minutes before inserting contact lenses secondary to benzalkonium chloride (will adsorb to contact lenses)

8. Carbonic anhydrase inhibitors
   a. Topical brinzolamide (Azopt)
   b. Topical dorzolamide (Trusopt)
   c. Oral acetazolamide (Diamox)
   d. Oral methazolamide (Neptazane)

Table 8. Carbonic Anhydrase Inhibitor STEPS

Safety	Systemic agents may cause serious dermatologic adverse events; recommend to avoid or discontinue topical preparation if the patient has a history of Stevens-Johnson syndrome or toxic epidermal necrolysis with systemic agent Contraindications (mainly systemic use) include aplastic anemia, nephrolithiasis, sulfonamide allergy, thrombocytopenia
Tolerability	Stinging Blurry vision Corneal edema Altered taste sensation
Efficacy	Least potential for IOP lowering of all available classes to treat glaucoma Agents in this class are equally effective and may switch within class if the patient develops adverse reactions to one
Preference (Pearls)	Third-line agent for treating glaucoma Topical formulations are typically used before oral formulations Oral formulations are reserved for patients who have an inadequate response or cannot tolerate the topical formulations
Simplicity	Available as a combination with a β-antagonist for patients who require additional therapy Application two or three times daily

9. Marijuana – IOP-lowering effects last about 3 hours with each marijuana cigarette (3000 marijuana cigarettes per year).
10. Surgical intervention
    a. Trabeculectomy
        i. Consider when two or more agents fail to control rising IOPs.
        ii. Increased risk of developing cataracts
    b. Laser trabeculoplasty
    c. Implantable valves

III. DRY EYES (XEROPHTHALMIA)

A. Professional Treatment Guidelines: 2013 AAO Preferred Practice Pattern: Dry Eye Syndrome *(Domain 3)*

B. Factors Associated with Developing Dry Eye Syndrome *(Domain 1)*
1. Advanced age (older than 65 years)
2. Female sex
3. Concurrent use of medications that have anticholinergic effects
4. Postmenopausal estrogen therapy
5. LASIK (laser-assisted in situ keratomileusis) and refractive excimer laser surgery
6. Vitamin A deficiency
7. May be associated with the following medical conditions:
    a. Rheumatoid arthritis
    b. Sarcoidosis
    c. Sjögren syndrome
    d. Systemic lupus erythematosus

C. Presentation and Diagnosis *(Domain 1)*
1. Patient will have dry and irritated eyes, redness, excess watering, photophobia, gritty, scratchy, burning, or a foreign body sensation.
2. Physical examination will show an irritated (red) but otherwise normal-looking eye.
3. Diagnostic tests include the following:
    a. Tear break-up time test
    b. Ocular surface dye staining
    c. Aqueous tear production (Schirmer test)
    d. Fluorescein clearance test/tear function index
    e. Lacrimal gland function test
    f. Tear osmolarity test

D. Potential Complications *(Domains 1 and 2)*
1. Corneal ulceration
2. Functional vision loss
3. Infections
4. Neovascularization
5. Scarring

E. Treatment *(Domain 1)*
1. Nonpharmacologic interventions include the following:
    a. Avoiding medications with anticholinergic or diuretic properties
    b. Smoking cessation and avoidance of secondhand smoke
    c. Avoiding drafts or low-humidity environments
    d. Hot compresses
    e. Frequent breaks from reading/television/computer screen
    f. Eyelid scrub/massage

Table 9. Severity Classification for Dry Eye Syndrome

Dry Eye Severity	1	2	3	4
Discomfort, severity, and frequency	Mild and/or episodic; occurs under environmental stress	Moderate episodic or chronic; stress or no stress	Severe frequent or constant without stress	Severe and/ or disabling and constant
Visual symptoms	None or episodic mild fatigue	Annoying and/or activity limiting, episodic	Annoying, chronic, and/or constant, limiting activity	Constant and/or possibly disabling
Conjunctival injection	None to mild	None to mild	+/−	+/++
Conjunctival staining	None to mild	Variable	Moderate to marked	Marked
Corneal staining (severity/location)	None to mild	Variable	Marked central	Severe punctate erosions
Corneal/tear signs	None to mild	Mild debris, decrease meniscus	Filamentary keratitis, mucus clumping, increased tear debris	Filamentary keratitis, mucus clumping, increased tear debris, ulceration
Lid/meibomian glands	MGD variably present	MGD variably present	Frequent	Trichiasis, keratinization, symblepharon
TFBUT, seconds	Variable	≤ 10	≤ 5	Immediate
Schirmer score, mm/5 minutes	Variable	≤ 10	≤ 5	≤ 2

MGD = meibomian gland disease; TFBUT = fluorescein tear break-up time.

Reproduced with permission from: The definition and classification of dry eye disease: report of the Definition and Classification Subcommittee of the International Dry Eye Workshop (2007). Ocul Surf 2007;5:75-92.

Patient Case

3. When classifying patients with xerophthalmia in order to choose the best treatment, which patient would be best suited to receive ophthalmologic cyclosporine?

    A. A 63-year-old woman with bothersome dry eyes once weekly who receives adequate relief from artificial tear solution.

    B. A 54-year-old woman with daily dry eyes who receives adequate relief from artificial tear ointment.

    C. A 58-year-old woman with twice-weekly dry eyes unrelieved with artificial tears, leading to lost productivity.

    D. A 61-year-old woman with dry eyes, dry mouth, fatigue, and other dry mucous membranes.

Table 10. Treatment Recommendations Based on Dry Eye Syndrome Severity[a]

Mild	Education and environmental modifications
	Elimination of offending topical or systemic medications
	Aqueous enhancement using artificial tear substitutes, gels/ointments
	Eyelid therapy (warm compresses and eyelid hygiene)
	Treatment of contributing ocular factors such as blepharitis or meibomianitis
	Correction of eyelid abnormalities
Moderate[b]	Anti-inflammatory agents (topical cyclosporine and corticosteroids), systemic omega-3 fatty acid supplements
	Punctal plugs
	Spectacle side shields and moisture chambers
Severe[b]	Systemic cholinergic agents
	Systemic anti-inflammatory agents
	Mucolytic agents
	Autologous serum tears
	Contact lenses
	Permanent punctual occlusion
	Tarsorrhaphy

[a]Note: Tear replacement therapy is often unsuccessful when used as the sole treatment for dry eye syndrome if additional causative factors are not concomitantly addressed.

[b]In addition to the above treatments.

Reproduced with permission from: Management and therapy of dry eye disease: report of the Management and Therapy Subcommittee of the International Dry Eye Workshop (2007). Ocul Surf 2007;5:163-78.

2. Artificial tears usually consist of normal saline, methylcellulose, or hydroxypropyl methylcellulose.
    a. Available in liquid, gel, and ointment forms
    b. Preservative-free forms are often recommended; however, they may be more expensive.
3. Topical cyclosporine (0.1%, 0.05%)

Table 11. Topical Cyclosporine STEPS

Safety	Remove contact lenses before use and wait 15 minutes before reinserting them
Tolerability	Blurry vision Burning sensation Foreign body sensation	Hypersensitivity reaction Large, evident conjunctiva blood vessels

Efficacy	Effective for patients with moderate to severe disease that is refractory
	  to conventional therapy
	0.1% concentration may be more effective than 0.05% formulation for
	  patients with moderate to severe symptoms

Preference (Pearls)	0.05% formulation is FDA approved in the United States Higher-dose formulations may require special preparation and compounding
Simplicity	Dosed every 12 hours May use artificial tears concurrently, allowing a 15-minute interval between administration of the two products

4. Systemic cholinergic agonists – FDA approved to treat xerostomia in patients with Sjögren syndrome, but also appear to improve tear production
   a. Cevimeline
   b. Pilocarpine

Table 12. Systemic Cholinergic Agonist STEPS

Safety	Use with caution in patients with a history of: Cardiovascular disease Cholelithiasis Nephrolithiasis Respiratory disorders
Tolerability	Abdominal pain Diaphoresis Dyspepsia Edema Excessive salivation Flushing/headache	Nausea Sinusitis Upper respiratory tract infection symptoms Urinary tract infection Vomiting
Efficacy	Improves symptoms of dry eyes better than artificial tears
Preference (Pearls)	Most research for treating dry eye symptoms was with patients with Sjögren disease and other symptoms of hyper-anticholinergic activity (e.g., xerostomia, fatigue)
Simplicity	Dosed three or four times daily

5. Topical pilocarpine (2%) is also an option for patients who cannot tolerate or afford topical cyclosporine or systemic cholinergic agonists.
6. Oral omega-6 fatty acid (6 capsules per day of evening primrose oil) showed benefit in a small cohort of women who wore contact lenses.
7. Topical tamarind seed polysaccharide (0.5%, 1%) is effective for short-term symptoms.

IV. VERTIGO

A. Professional Treatment Guidelines *(Domain 3)*: 2008 American Academy of Otolaryngology–Head and Neck Surgery (AAO-HNS) clinical practice guideline on benign paroxysmal positional vertigo (BPPV)

B. Vertigo: A Symptom of Another Underlying Condition – Is not a lone treatable condition *(Domain 1)*

C. The Condition May Be Caused by the Following: *(Domain 1)*
   1. Centrally originating causes (cerebral ischemia such as stroke, carotid artery stenosis, migraine headaches, tumors, neurodegenerative disorders, epilepsy, intoxication, positional changes)
   2. Peripherally originating causes (BPPV, vestibular neuronitis, Ménière disease, otosclerosis, whiplash)
   3. Medications such as Mysoline, carbamazepine, and phenytoin; antihypertensives; and cardiovascular medications

D. Benign Paroxysmal Positional Vertigo *(Domain 1)*
   1. Most common disorder of the inner ear's vestibular system; benign condition
   2. Presents most often in men in their 50s; lasts an average of 3–4 years and then subsides
   3. Typically, there are no precipitating events or findings leading up to symptom presentation.
   4. Symptoms tend to present in episodes and last for less than 1 minute.
   5. Complications of the condition may include falls, nausea, vomiting, or dehydration.
   6. Treatment
      a. First-line therapy is repositioning and vestibular exercises and rehabilitation.
      b. Antihistamines and benzodiazepines should not be used routinely to treat BPPV.

E. Ménière Disease *(Domain 1)*
   1. First presentation generally occurs between age 20 and 50 years and affects both sexes equally.
   2. Patients will present with episodes of sustained vertigo, (progressive) hearing loss, and/or tinnitus.
   3. May be caused by genetic predisposition, trauma, viral infection, and/or vasculopathies
   4. Symptoms may be triggered by barometric changes, allergies, hormonal changes, or increased sodium intake.

Table 13. American Academy of Otolaryngology–Head and Neck Surgery Diagnostic Criteria for Ménière Disease

Diagnosis	Criteria	Staging
Possible	Other causes excluded and … episodic vertigo without documented hearing loss	N/A
Probable	Other causes excluded and … one definitive episode of vertigo one or more episode of hearing loss, tinnitus, or aural fullness	
Definite	Other causes excluded and … two or more definitive spontaneous episodes of vertigo lasting > 20 minutes one or more episodes of hearing loss, tinnitus, or aural fullness	Audiogram findings Stage 1: < 25 dB Stage 2: 26–40 dB Stage 3: 41–70 dB Stage 4: > 70 dB
Certain	All criteria for definite Ménière disease plus confirmation of endolymphatic hydrops (excess endolymph fluid in ears)	

N/A = not applicable.

5. Treatment options *(Domain 1)*
   a. Nonpharmacologic interventions include the following:
      i. Reduce or restrict sodium, alcohol, and caffeine intake.
      ii. Affects mainly women between their fifth and seventh decade
   b. Thiazides (hydrochlorothiazide), in addition to sodium restriction, may be of benefit in reducing symptoms of dizziness and hearing loss.
   c. Betahistine (not available in the United States) has shown effective reduction of vertigo, but no effect on hearing loss, in Ménière disease.
   d. Intratympanic injections include the following:
      i. Gentamicin: Will reduce vertigo, but may cause decreased auditory response
      ii. Dexamethasone: Will reduce vertigo less effectively than gentamicin, but may have only a small effect on patient hearing
      iii. Options such as latanoprost and lidocaine show positive results in small studies (of 10 and 40 patients).
   e. Surgery may be necessary for patients whose condition does not respond to dietary, activity, and pharmacologic interventions.
   f. Positive pressure devices (deliver air pulsations to inner ear periodically throughout the day) showed a significant reduction in vertigo symptoms and sick days.

F. Patient Resources: National Institute on Deafness and Other Communication Disorders (www.nidcd.nih.gov/)

V. ALLERGIC RHINITIS

A. Professional Guidelines and Published Reviews *(Domain 3)*
   1. Joint Task Force on Practice Parameters for Allergy and Immunology: The Diagnosis and Management of Rhinitis: An Updated Practice Parameter 2008
   2. British Society for Allergy and Clinical Immunology guidelines for the management of allergic and nonallergic rhinitis 2008

B. Types of Allergic Rhinitis *(Domain 1)*
   1. Seasonal
   2. Perennial
   3. Occupational

Table 14. Factors Associated with Developing Symptoms of Rhinitis

Allergic Irritants	Nonallergic Irritants
Dust mites (late fall and throughout winter)	Infection
Trees (oak or maple in late winter and spring)	Pollution
Grasses (spring and early summer)	Stress
Mold (summer)	Tobacco smoke
Ragweed (late summer and early fall)	Weather
Insect debris (throughout the year)	
Pet dander	

Table 15. Presentation and Diagnosis of Rhinitis

Age at onset	Onset of allergic rhinitis is common in childhood, adolescence, and early adult years, with a mean age onset of 8–11 years In childhood, it is more common in boys than in girls, but in adulthood, it is more common in women In 80% of cases, allergic rhinitis develops by age 20 years About 50% of patients with allergic rhinitis will be able to manage without medications within 10 years of their initial diagnosis

Symptoms	Nasal congestion/obstruction Sneezing Thin rhinorrhea Pruritus	Ocular discharge (lacrimation) Decreased or loss of smell and/or taste Postnasal drip with or without nausea

Physical findings	Mouth breathing at rest Swollen turbinates with evidence of clear secretions Conjunctival swelling

     a.   Presence of purulent discharge or fever probably indicates a nonallergic disease.

     b.   Diagnosis is best made using the skin prick test.

         i.   Current recommendation is to make the diagnosis on the basis of symptoms, examination, and response to therapy.

        ii.   Unreasonable to perform on everyone with concerns consistent with allergic rhinitis

     c.   May consider the following tests for individuals thought to have atypical disease:

         i.   Skin testing

        ii.   IgE (immunoglobulin E) (blood) evaluation

        iii.   Pulmonary function test (asthma)

        iv.   Sweat test (cystic fibrosis)

        v.   Computed tomography of sinuses

  C.   Nonpharmacologic Treatment *(Domains 1 and 2)*

     1.   Control for dust mites and other insect refuse

     2.   Control moisture to reduce likelihood of mold spores

     3.   Pet management

        a.   Removal of pet

        b.   Limiting pet areas (not in bedroom or on furniture)

     4.   Manage pollen exposure

Patient Case

4. T.B. is a 21-year-old college student presenting to his local urgent care clinic for allergic rhinitis. He has taken intranasal fluticasone (2 sprays in each nostril once daily) and oral loratadine as needed for the past 6 years with success. However, during the past 1–2 weeks, his symptoms have been unrelieved by scheduled intranasal fluticasone and daily loratadine. He knows his symptoms are out of control because his roommate is cat-sitting for his parents, but he cannot ask the roommate (and cat) to leave. He has to cat-sit for only 1 more week. Yet he cannot live with this degree of discomfort any more. In addition to household hygiene and dander management, which is the best short-term option to help T.B. control his symptoms?

    A. Double the intranasal corticosteroid dose until the feline is out of the house.
    B. Change loratadine to fexofenadine plus pseudoephedrine twice daily until the allergen is gone.
    C. Add prednisone 10 mg once daily to his current regimen and continue for the duration of the cat-sitting.
    D. Add montelukast 10 mg once daily to his regimen for the next 7 days.

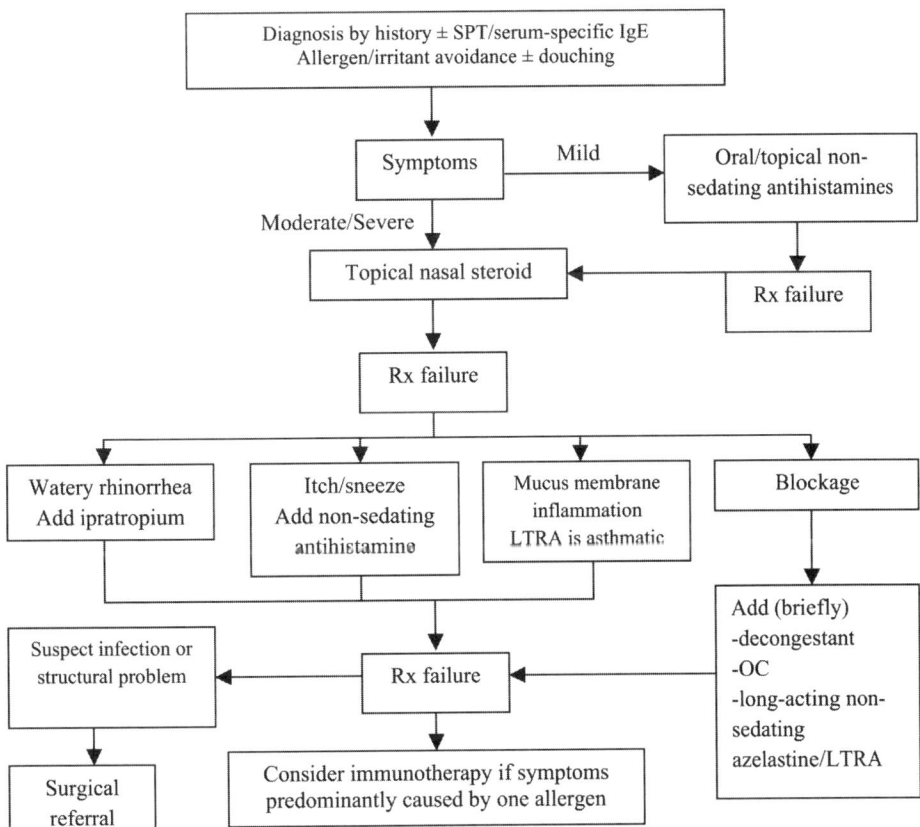

Figure 2. BSACI 2008 allergic rhinitis treatment algorithm.

BSACI = British Society for Allergy & Clinical Immunology; IgE = immunoglobulin E; LTRA = leukotriene receptor antagonist; OC = oral corticosteroid; Rx = prescription; SPT = skin prick test.

Reprinted with permission from: Scadding GK, Durham SR, Mirakian R, et al. BSACI guidelines for the management of allergic and non-allergic rhinitis. Clin Exp Allergy 2008;38:19-42.

D. Topical Pharmacologic Treatment *(Domain 1)*
1. Intranasal antihistamines
   a. Azelastine (Astepro)
   b. Olopatadine (Patanase)

Table 16. Intranasal Antihistamines STEPS

Safety	Although topical, associated with somnolence and drowsiness
Tolerability	Abnormal taste (bitter) Postnasal drainage Sneezing
Efficacy	Less effective than intranasal corticosteroids for nasal symptoms Possibly better than systemic antihistamines for symptoms of allergic rhinitis
Preference (Pearls)	Recommended as first-line therapy for patients with mild disease Reserve for patients with a preference for non-corticosteroid treatment options or for those with mucosal irritation or nosebleeds with intranasal corticosteroids
Simplicity	Once- or twice-daily dosing

2. Intranasal corticosteroids
   a. Beclomethasone (Beconase AQ; Qnasl)
   b. Budesonide (Rhinocort Aqua)
   c. Ciclesonide (Omnaris; Zetonna)
   d. Fluticasone (Flonase; Veramyst)
   e. Mometasone (Nasonex)
   f. Triamcinolone (Nasacort AQ-Rx; Nasacort Allergy 24 Hour-OTC)
   g. Flunisolide

Table 17. Intranasal Corticosteroids STEPS

Safety	Safe for use in pregnancy Intranasal corticosteroids are not associated with increased likelihood of fractures in postmenopausal women Conflicting evidence regarding growth deceleration in adolescents (mometasone, fluticasone, and triamcinolone approved < 6 years)
Tolerability	Epistaxis (appears to be directly related to agent potency) Headache Cough Pharyngitis
Efficacy	Most effective treatment for seasonal and perennial allergic rhinitis Treatment of choice for patients with moderate to severe allergic rhinitis Has shown efficacy over oral/intranasal antihistamines, oral leukotriene inhibitors, and a combination of these
Preference (Pearls)	Patients may receive benefit with as-needed use, but maximal efficacy when used on a schedule No intranasal steroid has been proved superior to another, so choice should be based on formulary, cost, and response to therapy
Simplicity	Once- or twice-daily dosing

E. Systemic Pharmacologic Options *(Domain 1)*
   1. Oral antihistamines, second generation
      a. Cetirizine (Zyrtec)
      b. Levocetirizine (Xyzal)
      c. Fexofenadine (Allegra)
      d. Loratadine (Claritin)
      e. Desloratadine (Clarinex)

Table 18. Oral Antihistamine, Second-Generation STEPS

Safety	Loratadine and cetirizine are FDA pregnancy category B
Tolerability	Dry mouth Headache Somnolence
Efficacy	Recommended as first-line agent, but most expert guidelines note they are ineffective for nasal congestion alone Most agents are effective for treating symptoms of seasonal or perennial allergic rhinitis Continuous use is most effective, but appropriate for PRN use
Preference (Pearls)	Second-generation agents are preferred to first-generation agents because they cause less sedation and fewer anticholinergic adverse effects All second-generation oral antihistamines are equally efficacious, except for desloratadine because it has not yet shown equal efficacy to other agents in the class Combining first-generation antihistamines (bedtime dosing) with second-generation antihistamines (daytime dosing) has not been well studied, and next-day sedation has been observed
Simplicity	Once- or twice-daily dosing Some in combination with decongestants

PRN = as needed

   2. Oral decongestants
      a. Phenylephrine (Sudafed PE)
      b. Pseudoephedrine (Sudafed)

Table 19. Oral Decongestants STEPS

Safety	Caution in use with patients with preexisting cardiovascular disease, diabetes, hyperthyroidism, closed-angle glaucoma, or bladder neck obstruction
Tolerability	Insomnia Palpitations Irritability
Efficacy	Effective in relieving nasal congestion symptoms
Preference (Pearls)	Pseudoephedrine is preferred to phenylephrine to relieve symptoms of nasal congestion
Simplicity	Extended-release formulations Available as combination Federal regulations limit the amount of pseudoephedrine a person may purchase with a valid photo ID: 3.6 g daily or 9 g monthly

3. Leukotriene receptor antagonists
   a. Montelukast (Singulair)
   b. Zafirlukast (Accolate) – FDA-approved asthma treatment
   c. Zileuton (Zyflo) – FDA-approved asthma treatment

Table 20. Leukotriene Receptor Antagonists for Allergic Rhinitis STEPS

Safety	Neuropsychiatric disorders have been reported in postmarketing reports, but they are considered rare events
Tolerability	Headache Abdominal pain/discomfort Nasal congestion/cold-like symptoms
Efficacy	Less effective than intranasal corticosteroids, but as effective as oral antihistamines
Preference (Pearls)	May be used in combination with an oral antihistamine, but the clinical significance of this improvement is not well evaluated In general, recommended for patients who lack adequate symptom control with an oral antihistamine, intranasal corticosteroid, or combination Montelukast is approved for both rhinitis and asthma, and therefore may be useful for patients with both conditions
Simplicity	Once-daily (montelukast) or twice-daily (zafirlukast, zileuton) administration Zileuton requires regular monitoring of hepatic transaminases

4. Systemic corticosteroids
   a. Oral steroids may be recommended for patients with an insufficient response to all other treatment options.
   b. Limit treatment to 5–7 days.
   c. Depot corticosteroid therapy is not recommended.
5. Allergen immunotherapy
   a. Consider for patients who have the following:
      i. Symptoms despite systemic corticosteroid therapy
      ii. An inadequate response to high-dose medication, several medications, or both
      iii. Coexisting conditions such as sinusitis, asthma, or both
   b. Provided as subcutaneous injection, sublingual tablet, or transcutaneous skin prick
      i. Effective for the treatment of allergic rhinitis
      ii. Treatment options for patients with identifiable and relevant allergens (consistent exposure) who require high doses of medications to avoid symptoms
      iii. Treatment for less than 5 years increases the chance of symptom relapse.
   c. Systemic adverse reactions have been reported in 5%–10% of individuals receiving allergen immunotherapy.
6. Other pharmacologic options
   a. Intranasal cromolyn (available only OTC as NasalCrom)
   b. Intranasal ipratropium (Atrovent)
7. Herbal medicines
   a. Butterbur (Petasites hybridus)
   b. Guduchi (Tinospora cordifolia)
   c. Green shiso (Perilla frutescens)
   d. Huáng qí (Astragalus propinquus)

VI. URTICARIA ("HIVES")

A. Professional Treatment Guidelines *(Domain 3)*
1. European Academy of Allergy and Clinical Immunology/Global Allergy and Asthma European Network/European Dermatology Forum/World Allergy Organization (EAACI/GA(2)LEN/EDF/WAO) guideline on management of urticaria 2009
2. British Association of Dermatologists guidelines for evaluation and management of urticaria in adults and children 2007

Table 21. Identifiable Causes of Urticaria *(Domains 1 and 3)*

Immunologic Causes	
Type 1 IgE mediated	Foods Tree nuts, legumes, shellfish, eggs, milk, soy, wheat
	Organic substances Preservatives, latex
	Medications Penicillins and penicillin-like agents, aspirin, NSAIDs
	Aeroallergens Dust mites, pollen, animal dander, molds
Type 2 cytotoxic-antibody mediated	Transfusion reaction
Type 3 antibody-antigen mediated	Serum sickness reaction
Type 4 delayed hypersensitivity	Medication, food handling, animal exposure
Autoimmune disease	Hashimoto disease, systemic lupus erythematosus, vasculitis, hepatitis
Infection	Viral, parasitic, bacterial, fungal
Nonimmunologic causes	
Physical stimuli	Exposure to sun, water, or extreme temperatures, delayed pressure, or vibration
Mast cell degranulation	Opiates, vancomycin, aspirin, radiocontrast media, dextran, muscle relaxants, bile salts, NSAIDs
Foods (histamine containing)	Strawberries, tomatoes, shellfish, cheese, spinach, eggplant

---

Patient Case

5. J.T. is a 13-year-old male adolescent presenting to his pediatrician with his father. It is spring, and the family has just opened the pool for the season. J.T. has been swimming daily for the past 4 days, but he has been getting out after 15 minutes because of excessive itching all over his body. His father describes J.T.'s symptoms as "giant welts" on his arms, legs, and stomach that are erythematous on the border. They cause J.T. significant discomfort, and the "welts" (wheals) last 4–6 hours. He has no significant medical history and no recent vaccinations, illness, or exposure to sick individuals. He takes no medications for chronic therapy; has not changed clothing materials, soaps, or detergents; and has no other symptoms. He once before developed these symptoms during the winter months when he was wet from playing in the melting snow. The pediatrician gives J.T. a diagnosis of acute cold urticaria and would like to prescribe a drug for him that he can take 60 minutes before swimming to decrease the chances or intensity of the symptoms. Which is the best choice of drug in this situation?

A. Diphenhydramine 25 mg.
B. Loratadine 10 mg.
C. Prednisone 50 mg.
D. Famotidine 10 mg.

B. Additional Causes May Include the Following: *(Domains 1 and 3)*
1. Alcohol
2. Connective tissue diseases
3. Menses
4. Stress

C. Physical Presentation and Evaluation *(Domain 1)*
1. Well-defined wheals on the skin
   a. Pruritic with or without burning sensation
   b. Central swelling with or without surrounding erythema
   c. Skin returns to "normal" within 24 hours
2. When collaborating with a diagnostician, be sure to rule out dermatologic reactions that are more serious.
3. Consider some testing if the cause is not readily identifiable (American College of Allergy, Asthma, and Immunology).
   a. Complete blood cell count
   b. Erythrocyte sedimentation rate
   c. Urinalysis
   d. Liver function testing

D. Nonpharmacologic Treatment *(Domains 1 and 2)*
1. Discontinue and/or avoid triggers to urticarial reactions.
2. When a trigger is unavoidable and the result is severe (e.g., exercise induced, cold induced), use pharmacologic treatment options to prevent symptoms and ensure that patient is not alone.

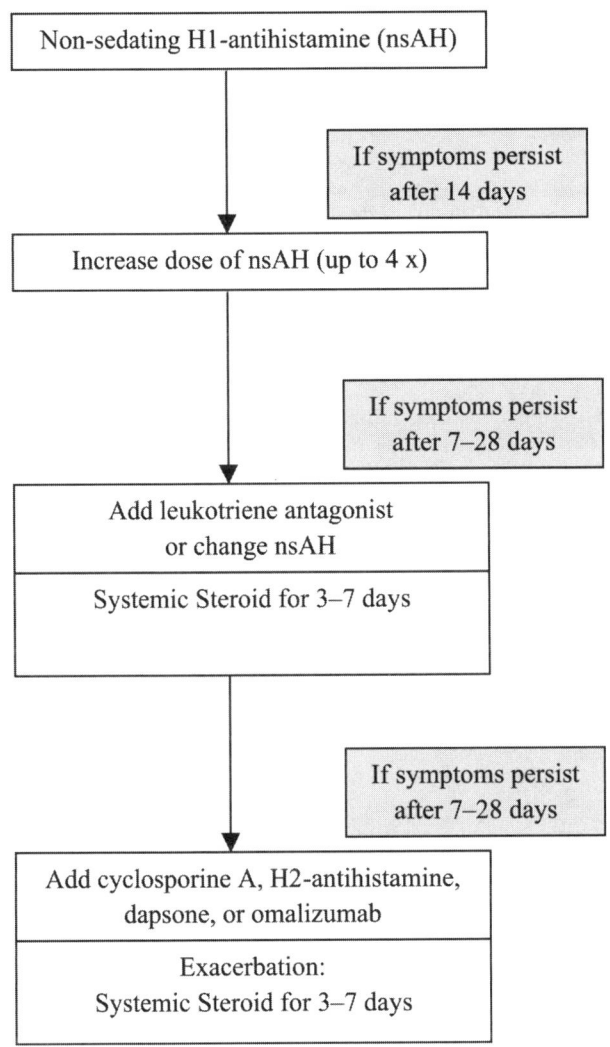

Figure 3. Urticaria treatment algorithm.

Source: The EAACI/GA2LEN/EDF/WAO guideline: management of urticaria (2009).

E. Pharmacologic Options *(Domain 1)*
1. All professional treatment guidelines recommend a nonsedating histamine-1 (H₁) antihistamine (nsAH) as first-line therapy.
2. In patients with an inadequate response to an nsAH, consider adding the following:
    a. First-generation (sedating) H₁ antihistamine
    b. Histamine-2 (H₂) receptor antagonist
    c. Corticosteroids
    d. Tricyclic antidepressants
    e. Leukotriene modifier
3. First-line options: nsAHs – Loratadine (Claritin), cetirizine (Zyrtec), fexofenadine (Allegra), levocetirizine (Xyzal), desloratadine (Clarinex)

Table 22. Nonsedating H_1 Antihistamine STEPS

Safety	In pregnancy, loratadine and cetirizine are FDA pregnancy category B
Tolerability	Dry mouth Headache Somnolence
Efficacy	Appears that most agents in this class are equally effective for treating urticaria, though few head-to-head comparisons exist
Preference (Pearls)	May need to increase dose to greater than recommended (up to 4 times) to achieve desired effect
Simplicity	Once-daily dosing with limited adverse drug reactions Available OTC

4. Second-line or additional options
   a. (First-generation) H_1 antihistamines – Diphenhydramine (Benadryl), chlorpheniramine (Chlor-Trimeton), clemastine (Tavist Allergy), hydroxyzine (Atarax), cyproheptadine

Table 23. (First-Generation) H_1 Antihistamine STEPS

Safety	Contraindications in pregnancy (hydroxyzine) or breastfeeding (diphenhydramine) Chlorpheniramine is FDA pregnancy category C
Tolerability	Excessive sedation Discoordination Dry mouth or secretions (anticholinergic adverse effects)
Efficacy	As effective as the nonsedating antihistamines for treating urticarial
Preference (Pearls)	N/A
Simplicity	Require many daily doses Most available OTC

b. H_2 antagonists – Ranitidine (Zantac), famotidine (Pepcid), nizatidine (Axid), cimetidine (Tagamet)

Table 24. H_2 Antagonists

Safety	Associated with an increased risk of developing community-acquired pneumonia
Tolerability	Constipation or diarrhea Dizziness Headache
Efficacy	Significant increase in resolution when added to histamine-1 (H_1) antagonist
Preference (Pearls)	Not justified to add to nsAH therapy initially Reserve for patients whose condition does not sufficiently respond to nsAH or (first-generation) H_1 antihistamine
Simplicity	Once- or twice-daily dosing Available OTC

nsAH = nonsedating H_1 antihistamine.

c. Corticosteroids (short-term or "burst" therapy)

Table 25. Corticosteroid (burst) STEPS

Safety	Gastrointestinal toxicity Prolonged use increases risk of osteoporotic fracture
Tolerability	Acute hyperglycemia Appetite changes Mood and sleep disturbance
Efficacy	May expedite time to remission (< 3 days) for patients with acute urticaria
Preference (Pearls)	Studied doses were 50 mg of prednisone daily for 3 days, but may be possible to use lower doses Follow with H_1 receptor antagonist
Simplicity	Once-daily dosing for 3–7 days, followed by step-up therapy

5. Other agents to consider
   a. Tricyclic antidepressants (doxepin, oral) – May use doses of up to 75 mg daily for patients with insufficient response to H_1 receptor antagonists
   b. Leukotriene modifier – Inconsistent evidence from small-scale studies to support use of montelukast and zafirlukast in urticaria

VII. ANGIOEDEMA

A. Professional Treatment Guidelines *(Domain 3)* – 2012 International Collaboration in Asthma, Allergy and Immunology consensus document on hereditary and acquired angioedema

B. Classification of Angioedema *(Domain 1)*
   1. Acquired component (C)1 inhibitor (C1 INH) deficiency
   2. Allergic
   3. Hereditary angioedema (HAE) Type 1 – Low C1 inhibitor values and function; type II – Normal C1 inhibitor values but low function
   4. Idiopathic
   5. Medication induced

C. Risk Factors and Patient Presentation *(Domains 1 and 2)*
   1. Typically caused by exposure to the following:
      a. Foods: Peanuts, tree nuts, wheat, eggs, milk, seafood
      b. Medications: Angiotensin-converting enzyme (ACE) inhibitors, fibrinolytics, NSAIDs, oral contraceptives, paroxetine, or risperidone
         i. NSAIDs may be most likely to cause angioedema.
         ii. Angioedema occurs in less than 1% of the population using ACE inhibitors (occurs more commonly in ACE inhibitor users who are female, smokers, or of African American descent).
   2. May not require instigation and may be strictly hereditary
      a. C1 inhibitor
      b. Estrogen-related HAE

3. Other risk factors include the following:
   a. African American race
   b. History of drug rash or seasonal allergies
   c. Patient older than 65 years
4. Patients will present with the following:
   a. Skin swelling that may occur on the body
      i. Mucus membranes are usually involved.
      ii. ACE inhibitor–induced angioedema will present only in the face, lips/mouth, and tongue.
   b. Urticaria
   c. Dyspnea and/or wheezing
   d. Others that occur less than 10% of the time: Nasal congestion, pain, loss of consciousness (or fainting), and/or abdominal pain

D. Diagnostic Evaluation *(Domain 1)*
   1. C1 INH deficiency screening
   2. C4 complement will help if C1 INH deficiency screening is unremarkable and angioedema continues.
   3. In patients with other suspected rheumatologic conditions, may consider checking the following:
      a. Antinuclear antibody
      b. Rheumatoid factor
      c. C3/C4 complement
      d. C1q antibodies

E. Treatment Strategies *(Domains 1 and 2)*
   1. Remove patient from instigating factor.
   2. Emergency care (if needed)
      a. Rapid fluid replacement (1–2 L of normal saline)
      b. Epinephrine (0.2–0.5 mg intramuscularly) every 5–10 minutes as needed
      c. Diphenhydramine (25–50 mg intravenously or intramuscularly)
      d. Ranitidine (50 mg intravenously) administered for 5 minutes
      e. Systemic corticosteroids may be included, but use not supported with evidence
   3. Acute symptoms (but not emergency) may be treated with nonsedating antihistamines.
   4. Plasma-derived C1 INH (Berinert or Cinryze)

Patient Case

6. C.R. is a 13-year-old male adolescent with HAE. He was given the diagnosis at 6 years of age and has episodes of laryngeal edema and constriction about once a year. He has icatibant at home that he is supposed to take each time he begins to experience these symptoms. After the medication is administered, which is the next best step for him (and his family) to follow?
   A. Immediately seek emergency medical care.
   B. Take diphenhydramine 25–50 mg and closely monitor symptoms.
   C. Begin taking prednisone 40 mg and continue once daily for the next 14 days.
   D. If syncope occurs, lie down on a flat surface.

Table 26. Plasma-Derived C1 Inhibitor STEPS

Safety	Thrombosis/thrombotic event Severe hypersensitivity reactions during or after administration Donor screening required to reduce likelihood of bloodborne disease transmission	
Tolerability	Abdominal pain Dizziness Erythema	Headache Nausea
Efficacy	Used for the routine prophylaxis of HAE (Cinryze) or the acute management of angioedema (Berinert)	
Preference (Pearls)	Patients may self-administer both of these medications with training and instruction If the patient administers the medication for an acute episode of angioedema, he or she should then seek immediate medical attention	
Simplicity	Estimated to cost $5000 every 3–4 days for prophylaxis	

HAE = hereditary angioedema.

5. Selective bradykinin B2 receptor antagonist (Icatibant [Firazyr])

Table 27. Selective Bradykinin B2 Receptor Antagonist STEPS

Safety	Acute airway obstruction may occur during HAE May attenuate the antihypertensive effects of ACE inhibitors	
Tolerability	Injection-site reaction (97% of patients) Increased transaminase values	Pyrexia
Efficacy	Used in the treatment of HAE	
Preference (Pearls)	If the patient administers the medication for an acute episode of angioedema, he or she should then seek immediate medical attention	
Simplicity	Should be injected subcutaneously in the abdomen, 2–4 inches below the umbilicus, with a 25-gauge needle Inject for ≥ 30 seconds 30-mg dose costs around $8900	

ACE = angiotensin-converting enzyme.

6. Kallikrein inhibitor (Ecallantide [Kalbitor])

Table 28. Kallikrein Inhibitor STEPS

Safety	FDA black box warning: Serious hypersensitivity reactions, including anaphylaxis	
Tolerability	Diarrhea Fatigue Fever	Headache Nausea Upper respiratory tract infection
Efficacy	For use in the acute management of HAE attack	
Preference (Pearls)	Must be administered in the presence of a medical provider because of the risk of a hypersensitivity reaction	
Simplicity	Three doses (10 mg/mL/dose) given subcutaneously in the abdomen, upper arm, or thigh Separate injections by 2 inches; rotation of injection sites is not necessary About $4200 per 10-mg/mL dose	

7. Other considerations for patients who have more than one severe event per month include the following:
   a. 17-α-Alkylated androgens: Recommended only at the lowest dose that decreases attack frequency because the efficacy may be offset by the likelihood of adverse events
   b. Antifibrinolytics: Less efficacious than 17-α-alkylated androgens for long-term treatment
8. Recommend the hepatitis B vaccine series for any person who will be receiving human blood products to manage HAE.

F. Patient Information: U.S. Hereditary Angioedema Association (www.haea.org)

VIII. ACNE

A. Professional Treatment Guidelines *(Domain 3)*
   1. Guidelines of care for acne vulgaris management; American Academy of Dermatology (AAD) 2007
   2. Global Alliance to Improve Outcomes in Acne Group guideline on management of acne 2009

B. Types of Acneiform Presentation *(Domain 1)*
   1. Acne conglobata – Burrowing and interconnecting abscesses and irregular scars
   2. Acne mechanica – Lesions on areas of friction from protective sports gear
   3. Acne rosacea – Erythema and telangiectasias without comedones
   4. Comedogenic acne – Many comedones with minimal inflammation
   5. Common acne – Variety of pustules and comedones
   6. Cystic acne – Cystic presentation with infection, leading to scars

Table 29. Factors Associated with Developing Acne

Hormone Abnormalities or Fluctuations	Physical Occlusion or Damage	Medications
Excess androgen in men Menstruation Pregnancy Stress	Cosmetics Excessive exfoliation Occlusive dressings/bodyguards Pimple popping	Anabolic steroids Azathioprine Corticosteroids Cyclosporine Lithium Phenytoin Vitamin B_1, B_6, B_{12}

    C.   Presentation and Diagnosis *(Domain 1)*

        1.   Open (blackhead) and/or closed (whitehead) comedones

        2.   Pustules or papules at the core

        3.   Usually on upper torso, neck, face, and back

        4.   Distribution of comedones, physical presentation, and associated risk factors aid in acne classification.

    D.   Additional Testing *(Domain 1)*

        1.   Not necessary unless trying to rule out hyperandrogenism

        2.   Endocrinologic evaluations

            a.   Testosterone, free

            b.   Dehydroepiandrosterone sulfate

            c.   Luteinizing hormone

            d.   Follicle-stimulating hormone

    E.   Treatment *(Domains 1 and 2)*

        1.   Nonpharmacologic interventions

            a.   None has proved drastically effective for improving acne.

                i.   Avoid popping pimples.

                ii.   Face washing with non-comedogenic soap

                iii.   Sunlight exposure

            b.   Dietary changes (e.g., avoiding chocolate, fatty foods) have not been shown to improve or prevent acne.

            c.   Severity classification will guide therapy choices.

Table 30. Classification of Acne Severity

Severity	Definition
Mild	< 20 comedones OR < 15 inflammatory lesions OR < 30 total lesions
Moderate	20–100 comedones OR 15–50 inflammatory lesions OR 30–125 total lesions
Severe	> 5 cysts OR Total comedone count > 100 OR Total inflammatory lesion count > 50 OR > 125 total lesions

	Mild		Moderate		Severe
	Comedonal	Papular/Pustular	Papular/ Pustular	Nodular	Nodular/ Conglobate
First choice	TR	TR + TA	OA + TR ± BPO	OA + TR + BPO	OI
Alternatives	TR or AA or SA	TR + TA or AA	OA + TR ± BPO	OI or OA + TR ± BPO/AA	High-dose OA + TR + BPO
Alternatives for female individuals	(See First choice)	(See First choice)	OAAn + TR/AA ± TA	OAAn + TR ± OA ± TA	High-dose OA An + TR ± TA
Maintenance	TR	TR ± BPO			

Figure 4. Acne treatment algorithm.

AA = azelaic acid; BPO = benzoyl peroxide; OA = oral antibiotic; OAAn = oral antiandrogenic; OI = oral isotretinoin; SA = salicylic acid; TA = topical antimicrobial; TR = topical retinoid.

Reprinted with permission from: Gollnick H, Cunliffe W, Berson D, et al. Management of acne: a report from a Global Alliance to Improve Outcomes in Acne. J Am Acad Dermatol 2003;49(1 suppl):S1-37.

Additional graphic algorithm available in: Dreno B, Bettoli V, Ochsendorf F, et al. An expert view on the treatment of acne with systemic antibiotics and/or oral isotretinoin in the light of the new European recommendations. Eur J Dermatol 2006;16:565-71.

2. Pharmacologic interventions (mild to moderate acne)
   a. Retinoids, topical
      i. Adapalene (Differin, Differin XP)
      ii. Tazarotene (Tazorac)
      iii. Tretinoin (Avita, Retin-A)

Table 31. Topical Retinoids STEPS

Safety	Significant photosensitivity and sunburn risk Topical retinoids should be avoided in pregnancy, and women of childbearing age should use adequate contraception (two different methods are recommended [i.e., barrier and hormonal])
Tolerability	All versions are irritating to skin, but some preparations appear to be more tolerable because of formulation (microspheres) Use of other OTC medications may increase irritation (salicylic acid scrubs or astringents)
Efficacy	Reduce the presence of mild to moderate noninflammatory lesions Used in combination with topical antibiotics and benzoyl peroxide, considerably increases likelihood of lesion changes with no additional adverse events May take up to 3 months to see an effect, and therapy should be continued until no new lesions develop
Preference (Pearls)	Recommended as first-line therapy and the foundation for treatment of all forms/severity levels of acne except severe (nodular/conglobate) acne May see an initial worsening of symptoms, but they usually resolve in 2–4 weeks Patients should use at least SPF 15 sunscreen for outdoor activities Counsel patients that their skin may be more sensitive to weather extremes (wind, cold) Not recommended to be used as spot therapy; divide into four equal aliquots and smooth over entire face Tretinoin unstable in UV light and with benzoyl peroxide; non-issue with adapalene
Simplicity	Once-daily application, in the evening

SPF = sun protection factor.

      b.   Antimicrobials, topical
         i.   Clindamycin
         ii. Erythromycin

Table 32. Topical Antimicrobial STEPS

Safety	Pseudomembranous colitis and hypersensitivity reactions have rarely been reported (less than 1%) in patients using clindamycin
Tolerability	Dry skin Itching Erythema Scaling or peeling
Efficacy	Best efficacy when used in combination with topical retinoids and/or benzoyl peroxide
Preference (Pearls)	Used predominantly for the treatment of mild to moderate inflammatory or mixed acne If patients are using the topical clindamycin foam, dispense the dose into the cap or onto a cool surface and then administer small amounts to the affected area Because of concerns of Propionibacterium acnes resistance, should never be used as monotherapy
Simplicity	Available co-formulated with benzoyl peroxide May be applied once or twice daily after facial cleansing

      c.   Benzoyl peroxide, topical

Table 33. Benzoyl Peroxide STEPS

Safety	May disfigure skin with edema, blistering, and crusting Photosensitivity to UV light
Tolerability	Dry skin Scaling of skin Pruritus Skin bleaching
Efficacy	Bactericidal against Propionibacterium acnes and therefore provides benefit to individuals with both comedonal and inflammatory acne Efficacy comparable with that of tetracycline and minocycline without evidence of bacterial resistance
Preference (Pearls)	Used in combination with oral or topical antimicrobials because of concerns about resistance For patients experiencing skin irritation secondary to benzoyl peroxide use, decrease the frequency of application or temporarily discontinue until irritation resolves Counsel patients to wash away the drug after a few hours to help skin grow to tolerate its presence 10% lotion/gel is only minimally better than 2.5% and 5% preparations and is much less tolerated Will cause discoloration/bleaching of fabric (e.g., pillowcases, towels) that come in contact with the face or treated area
Simplicity	Twice-daily application Co-formulated with other topical acne treatment options, including adapalene, clindamycin, and erythromycin

d. Azelaic acid cream, 20% topical (Azelex) – (Azelaic acid 15% gel [Finacea] is FDA approved for treatment of rosacea.)

Table 34. Azelaic Acid STEPS

Safety	Avoid contact with eyes or other mucous membranes
Tolerability	Skin irritation (e.g., burning, stinging) is reported in a few individuals Isolated reports of hypopigmentation with use
Efficacy	Reported to possess comedolytic and antibacterial properties Effective for use in mild to moderate acne vulgaris Once-daily application is equal to twice-daily application for treatment response Adding it to topical antimicrobials and/or cleansers is more effective than using either component alone
Preference (Pearls)	Despite success in clinical trials, experts believe the drug has limited efficacy and applicability for treating acne If patients experience continual skin irritation with twice-daily use, decrease the dose to once daily or discontinue use until the irritation resolves May cause skin lightening in individuals with darker skin pigmentation or postinflammatory hyperpigmentation
Simplicity	Applied to skin once or twice daily

e. Oral contraceptives (estrogen containing)

Table 35. Oral Contraceptives for Acne STEPS

Safety	VTE risk Estrogen dose directly related to VTE (doses > 30 mcg associated with higher risk of VTE) Levonorgestrel appears to be a progestin least associated with VTE; levonorgestrel (second generation) < drospirenone (fourth generation) < desogestrel (third generation) Premenopausal breast cancer risk Cervical cancer risk Cerebrovascular disease risk Smoking after age 35 years increases risk of VTE
Tolerability	Abnormal vaginal bleeding Headaches Abdominal cramping
Efficacy	Reduced severity of inflammatory and noninflammatory acne
Preference (Pearls)	Recommended for use as an alternative agent for women with moderate to severe acne Low to moderate dose of ethinyl estradiol (20–35 mcg) appears to be the target dose Second- and third-generation progestins have the least androgenic activity Drospirenone (fourth generation) appears to have antiandrogenic activity Patient should have annual health evaluations while using oral contraceptives, including a Papanicolaou smear and a physical examination Smoking cessation counseling for patients who smoke or use cigarettes infrequently at bars, recreational events, or social gatherings May be used to treat other conditions, including dysmenorrhea and polycystic ovarian syndrome May be used to prevent pregnancy in patients using isotretinoin
Simplicity	Once-daily dosing

VTE = venous thromboembolism.

f. Dapsone 5% topical gel (Aczone)

Table 36. Topical Dapsone STEPS

Safety	Associated concerns are much less severe with topical dapsone therapy than with oral dapsone therapy Changes suggestive of mild hemolysis have been observed in some patients with G6PD deficiency who are using dapsone gel Photosensitivity
Tolerability	Oiliness/peeling Dryness Erythema
Efficacy	Significantly higher reductions in inflammatory lesions, noninflammatory lesions, and total lesions at 6 and 12 weeks than with placebo
Preference (Pearls)	Still undergoing studies that evaluate long-term efficacy as monotherapy and safety when combined with other anti-comedonal agents Localized discoloration of the skin and facial hair (yellow or orange) if benzoyl peroxide is used after dapsone gel
Simplicity	Apply only a small amount (pea size) to skin and gently rub in Patients may notice gritty appearance or particles after application

G6PD = glucose-6-phosphate dehydrogenase.

g. Salicylic acid, topical

Table 37. Salicylic Acid STEPS

Safety	Risk of salicylate toxicity when topical therapy is used for a long period on a large surface area of the body
Tolerability	Excessive erythema and/or peeling of the skin Scaling of skin Burning
Efficacy	Comedolytic properties are considered less potent than those of topical retinoids
Preference (Pearls)	Used when patient has skin irritation with a topical retinoid
Simplicity	Many topical application choices including gel, foam, pads, patches, and liquid cleansers Several times per day application (three or four times daily) Available to patients OTC

Patient Case

7. D.M. is a 17-year-old male adolescent with inflammatory nodular acne on his face, shoulders, and back that becomes increasingly irritated during football season secondary to friction from his helmet strap and shoulder pads. His current acne medications include an oral antibiotic, a topical retinoid, and benzoyl peroxide. He is beginning to develop scarring because of this irritation and would like something new. Which is the best alternative regimen for the patient to try?

    A. Oral isotretinoin.

    B. Topical retinoid plus azelaic acid.

    C. Oral antiandrogen (spironolactone).

    D. Topical retinoid plus topical antibiotic.

        h. Other topical agents to consider

            i. Spironolactone 50–200 mg orally

            ii. Gluconolactone (α-hydroxy fruit acid) 14%

    3. Pharmacologic interventions (moderate to severe acne)

        a. Combination treatment should be used to target as many of the pathophysiologic mechanisms of acne as possible.

            i. Improves acne resolution efficacy

            ii. Increases speed of lesion healing/resolution

            iii. Decreases the chance of antibiotic resistance

        b. Oral antibiotics should be used in combination with topical retinoids and/or benzoyl peroxide.

c. Oral antibiotics (tetracycline, doxycycline, minocycline)

Table 38. Oral Antibiotics for Acne STEPS

Safety	Tooth discoloration and enamel hypoplasia in children < 8 years (tetracyclines) Fetal and infant toxicity (tetracyclines and sulfamethoxazole/trimethoprim) Photosensitivity
Tolerability	Nausea Vomiting Diarrhea
Efficacy	Used for moderate to severe acne Minocycline, doxycycline, tetracycline, and erythromycin are all efficacious for acne symptoms The AAD recommends reserving oral antibiotics for moderate to severe acne and limiting the duration of use when possible Because of potential for bacterial resistance, benzoyl peroxide should be added to any regimen with an oral antibiotic
Preference (Pearls)	Minocycline appears most efficacious, followed by doxycycline and tetracycline, respectively Save erythromycin for patients who receive a recommendation against using tetracyclines (e.g., pregnancy, < 8 years); bacterial resistance most commonly reported with erythromycin Trimethoprim/sulfamethoxazole or trimethoprim alone may be used for individuals who cannot use the above-mentioned oral antibiotics Patients may try probiotics or yogurt to prevent vaginal candidiasis, but evidence for efficacy is inconclusive
Simplicity	Once- or twice-daily dosing Oral formulations Available agents are less expensive than other agents (non-contraceptives) for moderate to severe acne

d. Isotretinoin, oral (Claravis, Amnesteem, Sotret)

Table 39. Isotretinoin STEPS

Safety	Highly teratogenic (iPledge program) Suicidal ideations Pancreatitis
Tolerability	Hypertriglyceridemia Arthralgias, myalgias Possible scarring Excessive drying of skin and/or mucus membranes
Efficacy	Approved for the treatment of severe recalcitrant nodular acne Effectively reduces inflammatory lesions and acne cysts Reserved for severe acne, treatment-resistant acne, or acne resulting in physical or psychological scarring
Preference (Pearls)	iPledge program is for prescribers, distributors, patients, and pharmacists (see below) All pregnancies need to be referred to a reproductive toxicity specialist for evaluation Treat for up to 20 weeks and discontinue sooner if acne resolution is ≥ 70% Prescriptions should only be for a 1-month supply and should be filled within 7 days of prescription date Oral retinoids carry the same risk of sunburn as the topical retinoids, so recommend sunscreen (at least SPF 15) for all patients during outdoor activities Patients should be instructed not to donate blood during treatment and for 1 month after discontinuing treatment
Simplicity	Once- or twice-daily dosing Weight-based dosing (0.5–1 mg/kg divided) Requires monthly monitoring for complete blood cell count (with differential), glucose, lipids, creatine phosphokinase, liver function, and psychiatric/mood changes

SPF = sun protection factor.

F. iPledge Program (www.ipledgeprogram.com)
1. Single resource for all individuals and businesses involved with isotretinoin to document patient safety data
2. Wholesalers, pharmacies, prescribers, and patients must enroll in the program.
3. Creates a single resource to create a "verifiable link between the negative pregnancy test and the dispensing of the isotretinoin prescription to the female patient of childbearing potential"
4. Requires monthly provider documentation that a patient has been counseled on the risks of isotretinoin therapy
5. Before starting therapy, iPledge requires two consecutive blood or urine test results to be negative for pregnancy.
6. Patients commit to using two forms of contraception 1 month before, throughout, and 1 month after therapy with isotretinoin.
7. The above information must be documented monthly in the iPledge online recordkeeping program.

G. Supportive Therapy
   1. Discuss therapeutic expectations – Up to 6 weeks for decreased or resolved symptoms
   2. During the first 4–8 weeks of therapy, the patient's acne may worsen, but it will improve or resolve with time.
   3. Remind the patient of appropriate hygiene (though not a contributor to acne), moisturizers, and sunscreen.
   4. Psychological counseling has weak evidence for a possible benefit.

IX. PSORIASIS

A. Professional Treatment Guidelines – AAD Guidelines on Management of Psoriasis and Psoriatic Arthritis (J Am Acad Dermatol 2008;58:851-64) *(Domain 3)*

B. Types of Psoriasis *(Domain 1)*
   1. Plaque psoriasis (most common; about 80%–90% of cases)
   2. Pustular psoriasis (von Zumbusch variant)
   3. Guttate psoriasis
   4. Erythrodermic psoriasis (life-threatening emergency)
   5. Inverse psoriasis

Patient Case

8. J.W. presents to his primary care provider's office for his annual physical examination. He is a 25-year-old man with a medical history significant for bipolar disease with rapid cycling. His medications include quetiapine, valproic acid, sertraline, and lithium. Today, he presents with new, itchy, and painful skin lesions on his knees. He was involved in a car accident about 12 months ago, which resulted in several contusions on his upper legs from hitting the dashboard. Since then, lesions have developed, and he asks his primary care provider to identify them. The patient is given a diagnosis of psoriasis, and the provider believes the patient's mental health agents may be contributing to the development of these lesions. Which agent is most likely causing the psoriatic lesions?

   A. Quetiapine.
   B. Valproate.
   C. Sertraline.
   D. Lithium.

C. Factors Associated with Developing Psoriasis *(Domains 1 and 2)*
   1. Various genetic factors, as evidenced by the higher incidence reported between first- and second-degree relatives and monozygotic twins
   2. Skin trauma, concurrent skin disorders, and infection are environmental factors that affect the onset of psoriasis.
   3. Smoking is also a predisposing factor to developing psoriasis.
   4. Medication induced (NAILS)
      a. Nonsteroidal anti-inflammatory drugs
      b. Antimalarials or ACE inhibitors
      c. Inderal (and other β-blockers)
      d. Lithium
      e. Steroid withdrawal

D. Medical Comorbidities Associated with Psoriasis *(Domains 1 and 2)*
1. Autoimmune disease
2. Cardiovascular disease
3. Metabolic syndrome
4. Lymphoma, melanoma, and nonmelanoma skin cancer
5. Depression/suicide

E. Presentation and Diagnosis – Chronic Plaque Psoriasis *(Domain 1)*
1. Red, raised scaly patches with well-defined borders that are symmetric
2. Lesions may begin to form after an acute skin injury (Koebner phenomenon)
3. May occur anywhere on the skin, including the following:
   a. Arms and legs
   b. Buttocks
   c. Genitals
   d. Palms/soles
   e. Scalp
   f. Trunk
   g. Face
4. About 50% of patients will have evidence of fingernail involvement (and 35% will have toenail involvement).
5. Diagnosis is usually made by visualizing the lesions, and testing is rarely indicated.
6. PASI (Psoriasis Area Severity Index) commonly used in clinical trials to assess psoriasis, but not routinely used in clinical practice

F. Pretreatment Evaluation *(Domain 1)*
1. Classified as mild, moderate, or severe on the basis of percentage of body involvement
   a. Mild: Less than 3% of the body
   b. Moderate: 3%–10% of the body
   c. Severe: Greater than 10% of the body
2. Based on potential agents for treating, may consider the following:
   a. Metabolic profile
   b. Complete blood cell count
   c. Hepatic function panel
   d. Hepatitis and tuberculosis evaluation

G. Treatment Options – Nonpharmacologic *(Domains 1 and 2)*
1. Smoking cessation
2. Saline spa water therapy (limited efficacy)
3. UV radiation/phototherapy (UVB or UVA) for psoriasis cases that fail to respond to topical treatments
4. Moisturizers

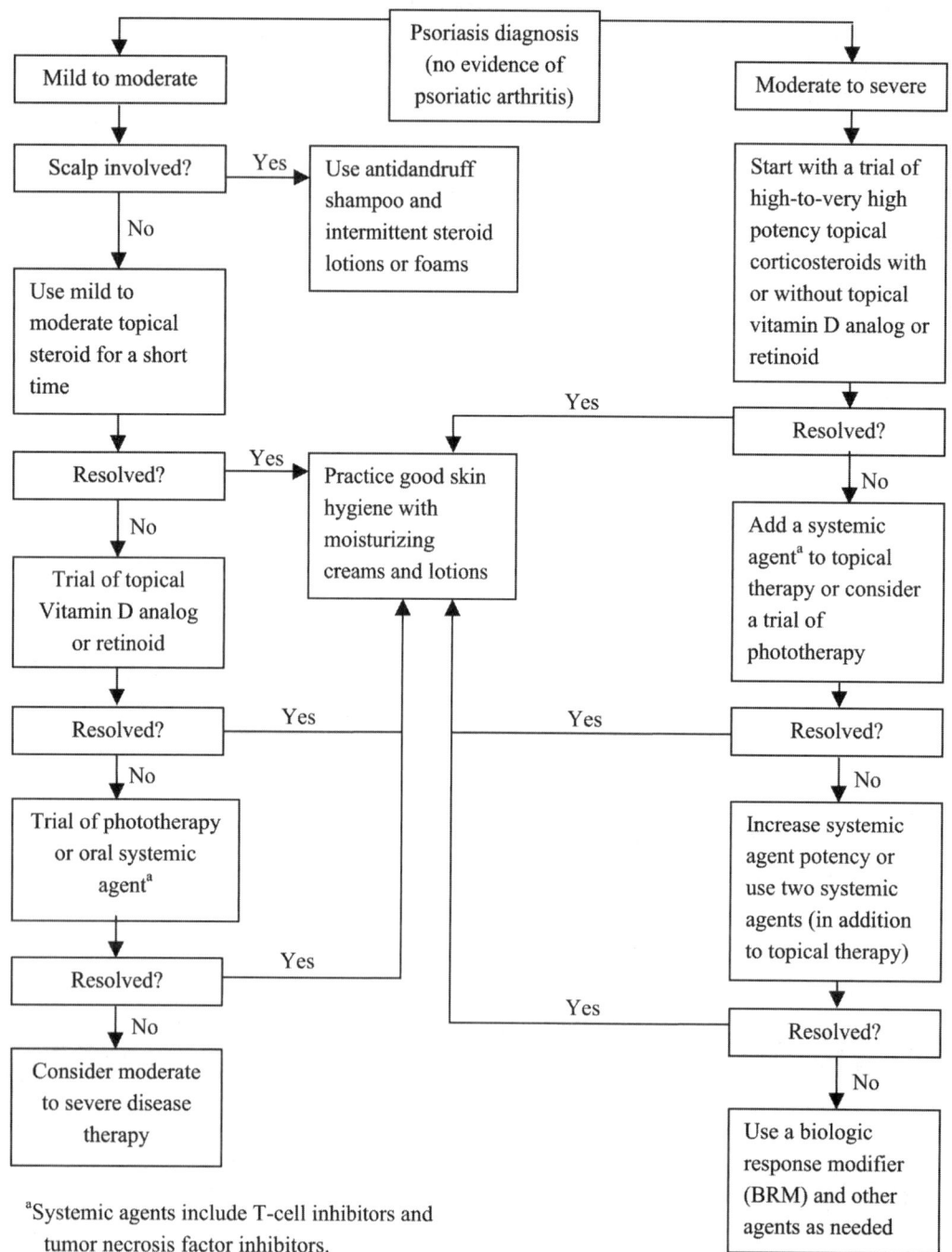

Figure 5. Psoriasis treatment algorithm.

BRM = biologic response modifier.

H. Pharmacologic Agents *(Domain 1)*
1. Topical therapy and targeted phototherapy are the first choice for mild to moderate disease (accounts for around 80% of cases).
2. For extensive, severe, disabling, or plaque psoriasis, systemic therapy may be necessary to control symptoms.
3. Consider biologic agents for moderate to severe disease or for patients whose response to topical or targeted phototherapy is insufficient.
4. Considerations with topical agents
   a. Choice of vehicle will alter medication penetration and relative efficacy – The optimal choice is usually the vehicle the individual patient will most likely use. Consider patient preference and limitations with each dosing vehicle.
      i. Hair-bearing areas may be best treated with foams, shampoos, gels, and sprays because they are less likely to leave a residue on the hair.
      ii. Creams are ideal for daytime application because they are less likely to glisten and/or stain clothes.
      iii. Consider ointments for nighttime application because they have less cosmetic appeal.
      iv. Dosing recommendations using "fingertip units" (ribbon of cream/ointment from tip of finger to distal-interphalangeal joint) – One fingertip unit is about 500 mg.

Table 40. FTU Needs to Various Anatomic Regions

Area	FTUs[a]	Area	FTUs[a]
Scalp	3	Leg (one)[b]	8
Face and neck	2.5	Buttocks	4
Hand (one)[b]	1	Knees	1
Arm (one)[b]	4	Trunk	8
Elbows	1	(anterior)	8
Both soles	1.5	Trunk	0.5
Foot (one)[b]	1.5	(posterior)	
		Genitalia	

[a]Two FTUs are about 1 g of topical agent.

[b]Includes anatomy peripheral to noted site (i.e., arm includes hands and fingers).

FTU = fingertip unit.

5. Corticosteroids, topical
   a. Cornerstone of treatment for most patients with psoriasis, particularly those with limited disease
   b. Many topical corticosteroids are classified as having several potencies, depending on their percentage concentration, application vehicle, and formulation.
   c. The AAD classifies corticosteroids from the Stoughton-Cornell classification system (1–7).
      i. 1 = superpotent and 7 = least potent
      ii. Potency is defined by vasoconstrictive, not anti-inflammatory, properties.

Table 41. Topical Corticosteroid STEPS

Safety	Skin atrophy Telangiectasia Striae distensae Exacerbation of dermatologic infections (rosacea, tinea infections)
Tolerability	Pustular or vesicular lesions Hyperesthesia Telangiectasia
Efficacy	Treatment of choice for patients with mild to moderate psoriatic disease Efficacy rates vary widely even among agents in the same potency class (41%–92%) Ultra–high-potency agents or ointment-based preparations are associated with greater efficacy
Preference (Pearls)	Corticosteroids are as effective as the vitamin D analogs, but with fewer adverse drug reactions To minimize adverse reactions and maximize adherence, application site needs to be considered in choosing the appropriate corticosteroid potency As clinical use continues, reduce potency or agent use to the minimal required for a clinical response Taper (do not abruptly discontinue) to avoid psoriasis rebound Limit ultra–high-potency topical steroids to 50 g weekly for up to 2–4 weeks
Simplicity	Once- or twice-daily local application May be used in conjunction with occlusive therapy to boost efficacy for low to medium potency Can be combined with other topical agents, UV light, and systemic agents

6. Vitamin D analog, topical (calcipotriene – Dovonex)

Table 42. Vitamin D Analog STEPS

Safety	Photosensitivity and an increased risk of UV-induced skin tumors Acute psoriatic eruptions of the scalp with direct application Topical solution and foam are flammable (51% isopropyl alcohol) Appears safe for pediatric use (studied in ages 2–14 years)
Tolerability	Hypercalcemia (applying > 100 g weekly) Worsening psoriasis Skin irritation
Efficacy	Calcipotriene is as effective as topical corticosteroids, but with more frequent adverse drug reactions Greatest efficacy when used in combination with betamethasone (combination product available)
Preference (Pearls)	Recommend use in combination with topical corticosteroid for added efficacy NOT contraindicated for use with UVB phototherapy; however, inactivated by UVA; apply after, not before, UVA exposure
Simplicity	Twice-daily application to affected areas; not to exceed 30% of body surface area

7. Retinoid, topical (tazarotene – Tazorac)

Table 43. Topical Retinoid STEPS

Safety	Pregnancy category X Photosensitivity
Tolerability	Increased sensitivity to environmental factors (wind, cold, heat) Skin burning, stinging, irritation
Efficacy	Achieves > 50% improvement in symptoms at 12 weeks in about half of treated patients
Preference (Pearls)	Recommended to use with topical corticosteroids for improved efficacy and improved tolerability To reduce the incidence of irritation: Use cream formulation Use the lower-concentration product Combine use with moisturizers Apply on alternating days Limit exposure (30–60 minutes) Apply with topical corticosteroids to reduce skin irritation and improve outcomes
Simplicity	Once-daily application

8. Additional topical agents to treat psoriasis
    a. Salicylic acid
        i. Usually used in addition to topical corticosteroid or immunosuppressive agents for additive effect
        ii. Avoid using topical salicylic acid in UVB phototherapy because it will decrease the efficacy of the phototherapy.
        iii. Contributes to total daily salicylate intake (potential toxicity)
    b. Anthralin (Dritho-Creme)
        i. Not as effective as topical corticosteroids or vitamin D analogs
        ii. Apply at increasing contact intervals (starting at 1 minute), and increase as tolerated.
        iii. Less cosmetically appealing secondary to staining of lesions, surrounding skin, hands, nails, clothing
    c. Coal tar
        i. 1% lotion is preferred to 5% extract for symptom improvement.
        ii. Often avoided secondary to cosmetic staining and undesirable odor
    d. Topical immunosuppressive agents (tacrolimus, pimecrolimus)
        i. No FDA-approved indications for psoriasis
        ii. Primary off-label use for facial symptoms or intertriginous (skinfold) areas
        iii. Black box warning issued by the FDA for increased risk of lymphoma
        iv. Approved for patients 2 years and older
    e. Nonmedicated topical moisturizers
        i. Accepted standard of care for patients with psoriasis
        ii. Limited evidence to support their benefit, but placebo has a 15%–47% response rate in clinical trials
        iii. Considered safe with few or no adverse events
    f. Less common topical agents
        i. Capsaicin
        ii. Indigo naturalis
        iii. Mahonia aquifolium bark extract

9. Combination topical therapy – Consider combination therapy for patients who do not achieve the desired effect with one agent.
   a. Topical corticosteroids plus salicylic acid
   b. Topical corticosteroids plus vitamin D analogs (co-formulated)
   c. Topical corticosteroids plus tazarotene
   d. Tacrolimus plus salicylic acid

I. Systemic (Biologic) Pharmacologic Agents
   1. T-cell inhibitors: Alefacept (Amevive) – No longer manufactured
   2. Tumor necrosis factor (TNF) inhibitors
      a. Adalimumab (Humira)
      b. Etanercept (Enbrel)
      c. Infliximab (Remicade)

Table 44. TNF Inhibitor STEPS

Safety	Increased risk of serious bacterial and/or fungal infections (contraindicated in patients with active, serious infections) Associated with reactivation of tuberculosis (NOTE: Recommendations for initial and periodic testing for tuberculosis with TNF inhibitors and other biologics can be found in the Bone/Joint and Rheumatology chapter) May increase risk of malignancy, including melanoma, leukemia, and lymphoma Linked with new or worsening heart failure and possibly death in patients with heart failure
Tolerability	Headache Abdominal pain Injection-site reactions Upper respiratory tract infection
Efficacy	A small percentage of patients may lose efficacy after 12 weeks of therapy with adalimumab Patients who decrease their etanercept dose from twice weekly to once weekly experience a decrease in therapeutic effect Infliximab appears to produce the greatest decrease in symptoms in the shortest time (10 weeks vs. 12 weeks)
Preference (Pearls)	Patients who discontinue adalimumab, etanercept, and/or infliximab abruptly are not at risk of rebound symptoms, but they may have a diminished effect when restarting therapy The TNF inhibitors have been combined with methotrexate to lessen the likelihood of patients developing resistance to therapy Highly effective, but very costly, therapeutic interventions Do not use with live vaccines; immune response of inactive vaccines may also be compromised
Simplicity	Adalimumab maintenance doses are administered subcutaneously every other week Etanercept maintenance doses are administered subcutaneously twice weekly x 12 weeks followed by once weekly thereafter Infliximab intravenous maintenance infusions are administered every 6–8 weeks

TNF = tumor necrosis factor.

J. Biologic Response Modifiers
1. Should be reserved for patients with moderate to severe disease or refractory disease because the risks associated with therapy may be greater than those associated with the disease
2. Questionable whether as efficacious as T-cell inhibitors or TNF inhibitors
3. Methotrexate

Table 45. Methotrexate STEPS

Safety	Contraindicated in pregnancy and breastfeeding; women who are planning to become pregnant should discontinue use 3 months before conception Significantly diminishes ability to generate an immune response Increased incidence of the following: • Any malignancy • Lung cancer • Melanoma • Non-Hodgkin lymphoma Avoid in patients with the following: • CrCl < 30 mL/minute • Platelet count < 50,000/mm^3 • White blood cell count < 3 x 10^3 cells/mm^3 • Liver transaminase values > 2 times the upper limit of normal	
Tolerability	Abdominal cramping Anorexia Bone marrow suppression Hypersensitivity pneumonitis	Increased aminotransferase values Infections Nausea Stomatitis
Efficacy	Effective for reducing symptoms of psoriasis, but may be less effective than cyclosporine	
Preference (Pearls)	Reserved for use in severe, intractable, and disabling psoriatic symptoms and/or psoriatic arthritis Reported as being slightly less effective than cyclosporine for psoriasis, but with fewer adverse events that require discontinuing therapy	
Simplicity	Administered with folic acid therapy (once daily)	

CrCl = creatinine clearance.

4. Cyclosporine

Table 46. Cyclosporine STEPS

Safety	Nephrotoxicity Do not use concurrently with UV phototherapy Cutaneous squamous cell carcinoma Avoid in patients receiving methotrexate, immunosuppressive agents, or coal tar Avoid use in patients with renal insufficiency, poorly controlled hypertension, malignancy, major infection, or poorly controlled diabetes Hypertriglyceridemia (triglycerides > 750 mg/dL) Increased risk of infections (bacterial, viral, fungal)
Tolerability	Flu-like symptoms Gingival hyperplasia Headaches
Efficacy	Despite being considered more efficacious than methotrexate, the greater number of serious adverse events limits its use
Preference (Pearls)	Reserved for patients whose condition does not respond to at least one systemic agent and who cannot use or tolerate biologic therapy Increase frequency of blood pressure monitoring after each dosage alteration
Simplicity	Twice-daily dosing for up to 1 year of therapy

5. Acitretin (Soriatane)

Table 47. Acitretin STEPS

Safety	Pregnancy category X Avoid using in individuals who plan, or are actively trying, to become pregnant Should continue oral contraceptive therapy for at least 3 years after discontinuing therapy Men or women using acitretin should not donate blood during, or up to 3 years after discontinuing, therapy because of the risk of a pregnant woman receiving the donation
Tolerability	Mucocutaneous reactions Unstable psoriasis-like reaction ("retinoid dermatitis") Dyslipidemia
Efficacy	Considered less effective than other systemic therapies for psoriasis Often used in combination with UVB or PUVA
Preference (Pearls)	Efficacy is dose-dependent, and optimal treatment dose is 50 mg daily Do Your PART Program (www.soriatane.com/patient/part.aspx)
Simplicity	Once-daily dosing

PART = Pregnancy Prevention Actively Required During and After Treatment; PUVA = psoralen plus ultraviolet light therapy.

6. Interleukin (IL) inhibitors
   a. Ustekinumab (Stelara) targets IL-12 and IL-23
   b. Secukinumab (Cosentyx) targets IL-17A

Table 48. Ustekinumab and Secukinumab STEPS

Safety	Pregnancy category B Increased risk of serious bacterial and/or fungal infections (contraindicated in patients with active, serious infections) Associated with reactivation of tuberculosis Risk of serious skin conditions, exfoliative dermatitis, and erythrodermic psoriasis
Tolerability	Nasopharyngitis Fatigue Headache Diarrhea Upper respiratory infections
Efficacy	May be used as first line for moderate to severe chronic plaque psoriasis Both agents have shown efficacy over etanercept

Preference (Pearls)	Secukinumab may exacerbate Crohn disease
	Ustekinumab has been associated with malignancies and reversible posterior
	  leukoencephalopathy syndrome (RPLS)
	Do not use with live vaccines; immune response of inactive vaccines may also
	  be compromised
	Highly effective, but very costly

Simplicity	Given subcutaneously into top of thigh, abdomen, upper arms, or buttocks; rotate sites Ustekinumab given at weeks 0, 4; then every 12 weeks thereafter Secukinumab dosed every 4 weeks after initial doses once weekly from weeks 0 through 4 Laboratory monitoring not necessary

7. Second-tier agents – Considered for patients whose condition does not respond to, or those who cannot tolerate, systemic therapy and who cannot afford or be treated with biologic agents
   a. Azathioprine
   b. Fumaric acid esters
   c. Hydroxyurea
   d. Leflunomide
   e. Mycophenolate mofetil
   f. Sulfasalazine
   g. Tacrolimus
   h. 6-Thioguanine
8. Other agents – Apremilast (Otezla)
   a. Phosphodiesterase type-4 inhibitor
   b. Oral medication approved for active psoriatic arthritis
9. After many treatment failures, patients and providers may consider the following:
   a. Goeckerman therapy (coal tar plus UVB for 3–5 weeks)
   b. Ingram regimen (dithranol/salicylic acid/zinc oxide paste [with or without coal tar] plus UVB for 3 weeks)

X. INFESTATIONS

A. Additional Resources *(Domain 3)*
1. Am J Clin Dermatol 2002;3:9-18
2. N Engl J Med 2006;354:1718-27
3. American Academy of Pediatrics Clinical Report on Head Lice 2010

B. Scabies *(Domain 1)*
1. Types
   a. Common scabies
   b. Crusted scabies (Norwegian scabies): Commonly found in immunocompromised, debilitated, or malnourished individuals
   c. Nodular scabies
2. Factors associated with contracting scabies *(Domain 2)*
   a. Person-to-person contact
      i. Higher likelihood in crowded communities
      ii. Hospitals, nursing homes, homeless shelters, jails/prisons, and schools have increased person-to-person contact and risk of mass infection.
   b. Impoverished areas
3. Presentation *(Domain 1)*
   a. Symptom onset
      i. May take 4–6 weeks for onset of symptoms in patients who have never had scabies
      ii. Symptoms may manifest as follows:
         (a) Be worse during evening hours and while sleeping
         (b) Worsen for 1–2 days after starting treatment
         (c) Persist for up to 1 week after resolving infestation
      iii. Subsequent re-infestations may present with symptoms as soon as 24 hours.
   b. Itching and lesions (common sites)
      i. Areola and nipples
      ii. Axillary folds
      iii. Extensor (outer) of elbows
      iv. Finger webs
      v. Flexor (inner) of wrists
      vi. Lower buttocks
      vii. Genitalia
   c. Primary lesions may develop into secondary lesions or bacterial infections.
      i. May persist for weeks or months after the infestation is eradicated
      ii. If crusted scabies develops, patients may appear to have psoriasis or seborrheic dermatitis.
4. Diagnostic studies *(Domains 1 and 3)*
   a. A definitive diagnosis can be made when a clinician identifies mites, eggs, mite pellets, or egg fragments under magnification (skin shaving).
   b. The Burrow Ink Test (BIT) may also be used to identify tracks left by the mite as it burrows under the skin.
   c. Epiluminescence microscopy is a newer in vivo technique that allows a detailed inspection of the superficial papillary dermis.
   d. Empiric therapy for generalized itching is not recommended and should only be used for a history of exposure with or without typical eruptions.

Patient Case

9. P.F. is the 26-year-old mother of two children (6 and 8 years old) who contracted scabies after spending the night at a neighborhood friend's house. The two daughters developed symptoms about 2 weeks after the exposure, and the family's primary care provider gave them a prescription for permethrin 5%. However, permethrin did not eradicate the infestation, and the symptoms recurred 1 month later. Which factor most likely caused the treatment failure?

    A. Increasing resistance patterns for scabies in the United States.

    B. The prescriber ordering an inappropriate dose of permethrin for the children (pediculosis dose).

    C. Not applying permethrin to areas such as the soles of feet or unexposed areas.

    D. Not evaluating infested/symptomatic areas and removing nits (eggs).

5. Treatment *(Domains 1 and 2)* – Infested patients and their close physical contacts should be treated at the same time, regardless of whether symptoms are present.
   a. Nonpharmacologic
      i. Evaluation of all close contacts within the past 30 days for symptoms of infestation
      ii. Identify all items in contact with the infested person for the past 72 hours.
         (a) Decontaminate all bedding, clothing, and toys using machine washer (at least 140°F water) and heated dryer.
         (b) Isolate items that cannot be put in a machine washer using an insecticide powder and sealed plastic bag for at least 72 hours.
         (c) Pesticide sprays and powders are not recommended; little evidence of benefit of vacuuming
      iii. In-hospital or nursing home situations
         (a) Isolate infested patients (may require prolonged isolation to ensure eradication).
         (b) Provide education and therapy for family, staff, and residents in contact with the person.
         (c) May require treatment of the entire at-risk population
      iv. Remove infested children from school until infestation is adequately treated.
   b. Family members, household contacts, and other close contacts
      i. All individuals who have had close personal contact with the patient in the past 30 days should be evaluated and treated for scabies.
      ii. Symptoms may take days to weeks to present, and transmission is possible during the initial asymptomatic period.

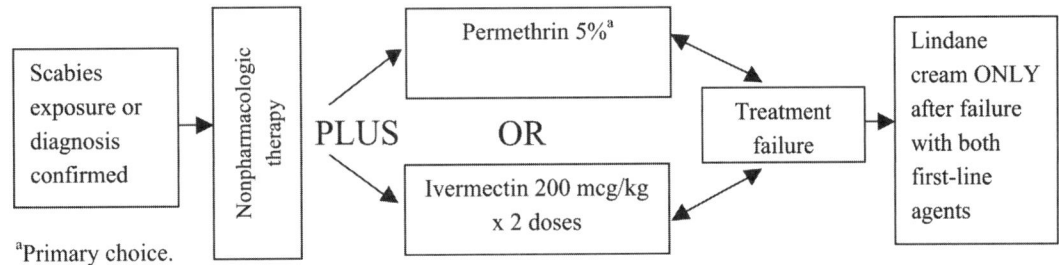

^aPrimary choice.

Figure 6. Scabies treatment algorithm.

c. Topical pharmacologic agents
  i. Permethrin 5%, topical (Elimite)

Table 49. Permethrin 5% STEPS

Safety	Photosensitivity
Tolerability	Burning and stinging Erythema and pruritus Numbness and tingling
Efficacy	5% cream is the efficacious dose (1% OTC formulation is ineffective) Most effective agent and first-line recommendation from the American Academy of Pediatrics and CDC Counsel patients to be sure to cover all areas of the body (e.g., soles of feet, hands, under nails) because missing these areas may allow a recurrence of infestation and symptoms
Preference (Pearls)	Total body (below head) application is required FDA approved for use in those ≥ 2 months Recommended as well-tolerated alternative treatment for those who cannot use lindane (infants and small children, patients with seizures or neurologic complications, therapeutic failure, or resistance to lindane) Pregnancy category B Reasonable cost: About $10 per bottle
Simplicity	Apply from head to toe, leave on for 8–14 hours before washing off with water; may reapply in 1 week if live mites appear

CDC = Centers for Disease Control and Prevention.

  ii. Ivermectin, oral (Stromectol)

Table 50. Ivermectin STEPS

Safety	Symptomatic postural hypotension Life-threatening dyspnea (three individuals) Association between 6-month mortality and ivermectin in long-term care residents
Tolerability	Peripheral edema Tachycardia Gastrointestinal effects Transaminase elevations Pruritus Fever Skin involvement (edema, urticarial rash)
Efficacy	Appears less effective than permethrin, but more effective than lindane
Preference (Pearls)	Not FDA approved for scabies treatment, but endorsed by the CDC May consider in patients whose infestations are not eradicated by permethrin Alternative for those who cannot completely cover body with topical treatments Administer on an empty stomach with water
Simplicity	Single oral dose 200 mcg/kg; may be repeated in 14 days

iii. Lindane, topical

Table 51. Lindane STEPS

Safety	Black box warning secondary to neurologic toxicity (seizures and death) with prolonged or repeated exposure
Tolerability	May cause pruritus lasting several weeks after infestation is eradicated
Efficacy	Appears to be less effective than permethrin for treating scabies
Preference (Pearls)	Not recommended as first-line therapy and should be used cautiously as a second-line agent for those who lack response to permethrin Total body (below head) application is required Apply to dry skin, leave on for 8–12 hours, and then wash off in warm shower or bath (do not exceed 12 hours) Be aware of thumb sucking in children Do not re-treat if infestation is not eradicated Must be dispensed with FDA-approved patient mediation guide
Simplicity	One application Conduct a 2- and 4-week follow-up to evaluate for new lesions High cost: About $125 per bottle

iv. Crotamiton, topical – Second-line topical agent because its efficacy is lower than that of other agents, high resistance, and increased reports of persistent itch after use

v. Malathion, topical – Use is discouraged because it contains 78% isopropyl alcohol, causing skin and genital irritation.

vi. "Natural" options (not proven effective in the United States)

   (a) Tea tree oils

   (b) Extracts of neem and turmeric

   (c) Bush tea

   (d) Coconut oil

   (e) Melaleuca oil plus lavender oil

C. Pediculosis ("Lice")

  1 Types *(Domain 1)*

    a. Pediculus capitis (head)

    b. Pediculus corporis (body)

    c. Phthirus pubis (pubic)

  2. Factors associated with contracting pediculosis *(Domain 2)*

    a. Adults with poor hygiene

    b. Direct hair-to-hair contact

    c. Sharing contaminated objects (toys, bedding, clothing, hats, hairbrushes)

    d. Overcrowded living conditions

  3. Presentation and diagnosis *(Domains 1 and 2)*

    a. Initially, patients may be asymptomatic, and diagnosis is based on physical findings (nits).

    b. Pruritus of the scalp and a feeling that something is "crawling" on the head

    c. Intense itching leads to scratching, with subsequent excoriations and secondary cellulitis.

  d. Usually asymptomatic, but may also see the following:
    i. Irritability
    ii. Rash
    iii. Malaise
    iv. Headache
  e. Nits (eggs) may be seen where hair exits scalp.
  f. Definitive diagnosis occurs by finding at least one live louse on visual inspection.
    i. Run a fine-toothed comb through wet hair, and identify lice on comb.
    ii. Lice are commonly found behind the ears and on the back of the neck.
    iii. Finding nits (louse eggs) on examination is not enough to indicate current infestation.
  g. Symptoms may persist for about 1 week after infestation is eradicated.

Patient Case

10. Y.M. is a 17-year-old female adolescent who contracted lice after sharing a hat with one of her softball team-mates. She was sent home from school after excessive scalp itching, and the school nurse identified nits at the proximal end of her hair follicles. She was treated with permethrin 1% at home but experienced pruritus and abnormal scalp tingling with the treatment. The lice infestation was not completely resolved with this treatment, and her family physician recommended a second course of therapy. Y.M. is extremely upset because her junior prom is only 2 weeks away, and she cannot have "lice" for her junior prom. Aside from manual removal of lice by fine-toothed combs, which would be the best addition to permethrin to enhance therapy and decrease the chance of another course of therapy?

 A. Add oral ivermectin 300 mcg/kg for two doses, separated by 7 days.

 B. Add topical malathion 0.5%, applied the day after treatment with permethrin.

 C. Apply a suffocation-based pediculicide after washing out permethrin.

 D. Add oral trimethoprim/sulfamethoxazole twice daily for 10 days.

---

  4. Treatment

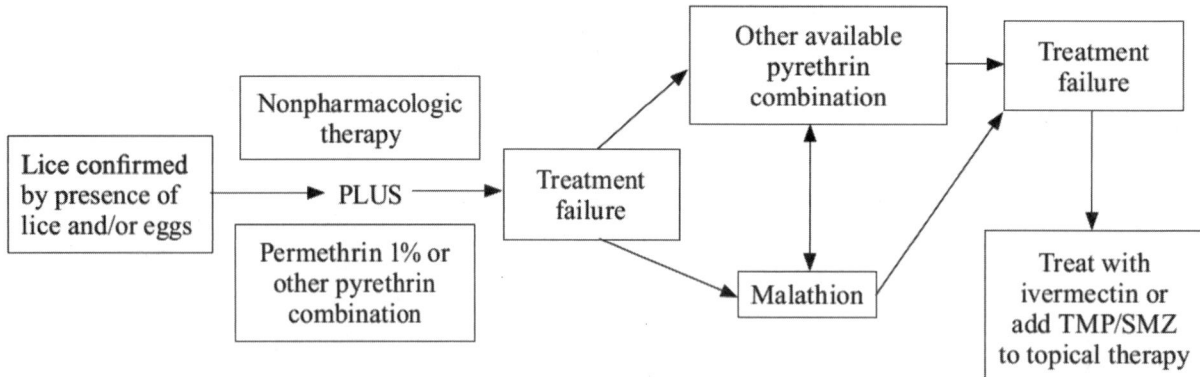

Figure 7. Lice treatment algorithm.

Note: Lindane no longer recommended; spinosad not included in treatment recommendations.

    a. Nonpharmacologic *(Domains 1 and 2)*
        i. Nit removal using a fine-toothed comb ("nit picking")
        ii. Use a conditioner or olive oil in hair to remove tangles.
        iii. Use a comb from a pediculicide product to comb hair, starting at the scalp.
        iv. Repeat every 2–3 days until no nits or eggs are found.
        v. Machine wash items (linens, clothing) in hot (140°F) water and high-heat dry.
        vi. Seal non-washable items in plastic bag for 14 days.
        vii. Centers for Disease Control and Prevention recommends against the use of lice bedding sprays.
        viii. Neon Nits is not recommended by the American Pediculosis Association.
        ix. The American Academy of Pediatrics does not recommend removing students from school because most children will have had lice for about 1 month before diagnosis.
            (a) Discourage close contact with other students.
            (b) Maintain patient privacy.
    b. Topical pharmacologic *(Domain 1)*
        i. Pyrethrins
            (a) Permethrin 1% (Nix) or pyrethrins 0.33% and piperonyl butoxide 3%–4% (RID; Pronto, Clear Lice System)
            (b) See STEPS analysis in Scabies.
            (c) Permethrin 1% formulation should be used for pediculosis (American Academy of Pediatrics).
            (d) May be used as prophylaxis in household contacts and areas where greater than 20% of the population is affected
            (e) Apply to washed and towel-dried hair and rinse after 10 minutes. May repeat in 7–10 days if nits still present
            (f) Resistance to permethrin and pyrethrins/piperonyl butoxide can be significant in various communities, necessitating the use of malathion.
        ii. Malathion 0.5% (Ovide)

Table 52. Malathion STEPS

Safety	0.5% lotion is flammable secondary to high isopropyl alcohol content (avoid use near source of ignition) Contraindicated in children < 24 months
Tolerability	Irritation of scalp and skin Avoid use for Phthirus pubis because of high alcohol content (irritation)
Efficacy	Evidence of resistance to malathion preparations in the United Kingdom, but malathion in the United States has a different formulation (terpineol, dipentene, and pine needle oil) without similar documentation of resistance
Preference (Pearls)	Use in individuals > 24 months when permethrin resistance is suspected Safety data are not reported for children < 6 years Pay attention to regional resistance patterns when selecting treatment High cost: About $125 per bottle
Simplicity	Apply to dry hair enough to sufficiently wet the hair and scalp, allow to dry, and remove after 8–12 hours One-time treatment (may be repeated in 7–9 days if live lice still present) Remove dead lice with a fine-toothed comb

iii. Spinosad 0.9% (Natroba)

Table 53. Spinosad STEPS

Safety	Not recommended for use in infants < 6 months secondary to benzyl alcohol (gasping syndrome)
Tolerability	Application site erythema and irritation Alopecia
Efficacy	Limited randomized controlled trial data suggest spinosad is markedly superior to permethrin for 14-day lice-free outcome
Preference (Pearls)	Not included in the 2010 American Academy of Pediatrics treatment recommendations because approved for use in the United States in January 2011
Simplicity	Single application Apply to dry hair, leave on for 10 minutes, and then rinse May repeat application in 7 days if nits are still present May be used without nit combing, although best results occur with nit combing

      iv. Other topical formulations
         (a) Lindane – See STEPS analysis in Scabies.
            (1) Is no longer recommended by the American Academy of Pediatrics and is banned in the state of California
            (2) Instruct patients to leave it on their scalp for no longer than 4 minutes.
         (b) Suffocation-based pediculicide
            (1) Petrolatum shampoo applied to scalp, dried with a hair dryer, left on overnight, and then washed out in the morning
            (2) Thorough hair washing for 7–10 days is required to remove the petrolatum residue.
            (3) Requires manual removal of lice and nits with fine-toothed comb
   c. Oral agents
      i. Trimethoprim and sulfamethoxazole (Bactrim, Septra)

Table 54. Trimethoprim/Sulfamethoxazole STEPS

Safety	Electrolyte (potassium) abnormalities Contraindicated in children < 2 months or pregnant/nursing women Contraindicated in patients with a history of anaphylaxis to sulfa-containing antibiotics
Tolerability	Nausea Vomiting Rash
Efficacy	Adding trimethoprim/sulfamethoxazole to permethrin has higher success rates than either agent alone
Preference (Pearls)	Add to traditional therapy (permethrin only) if nits and lice are found 2 weeks after first course of therapy
Simplicity	Twice daily for 10 days

   ii. Ivermectin, oral – See Ivermectin, oral in Scabies. As effective as malathion lotion

  d. "Natural" options

   i. Coconut oil plus anise spray

   ii. Coconut oil, anise oil, and ylang ylang oil (Hair-Clean 1-2-3)

   iii. Melaleuca oil plus lavender oil

 5. Follow-up (for scabies and pediculosis) *(Domain 2)*

  a. Confirm treatment success with patient and family.

  b. Re-treat with different agent if treatment is ineffective 1 month after final scheduled treatment.

  c. Identify causes of treatment failure.

   i. Nonadherence to or inappropriate treatment instructions

   ii. Not re-treating as recommended

   iii. Wrong product selected

   iv. Acquired resistance

XI. MINOR BURNS

 A. Professional Treatment Guidelines *(Domain 3)*

  1. No professional treatment guidelines are published for minor burn management.

  2. Review article: Am Fam Physician 2012;85:25-32

Table 55. Severity Classification for Burn Injuries

Degree	Characteristics and/or Criteria	Healing Times
First (superficial burn)	Involves only the epidermis Skin findings include red color, dry, and painful The burn rarely blisters	3–10 days
Second (partial-thickness burn)	Superficial, partial-thickness burn Involves all of the epidermis and part of the underlying dermis Skin findings include erythema, painful, and wet/weeping skin Blisters are clear Blanching when touched Deep partial-thickness burn Involves deeper layers of the dermis (reticular dermis) Skin findings include pale white or fixed red color and blanching absent with pressure Blisters present Patient has dull sensation or lack of pain with stimulation Often results in scarring and contractures	2 weeks
Third (full-thickness burn)	Destroys all skin layers, including underlying subcutaneous fat Skin findings include leathery feel; white, brown, or tan appearance; charred and dry or hard and waxy feel; and blanching absent with pressure No blistering Skin grafting is usually required	> 3 weeks
Fourth	Destroys all skin layers and extends into muscle, tendon, or bone	

Table 56. Common Causes of Minor Burns

Thermal Burns	Chemical Burns	Others	Medications[a]
Scalding (food/water)	Alkalis/acids	UV radiation	Amiodarone
Fire (flash/flame)	Petroleum	Particle radiation	Doxycycline
Hot surfaces	Phosphorus	Electrical burn/injury	Hydrochlorothiazide
	Airbags		Fluoroquinolones
	Hair dyes		NSAIDs
	Fabric detergents		Retinoids
	OTC pain products		Tetracycline
	(menthol related)		Voriconazole

[a]Note: Medications usually increase the risk of burn and are not the primary cause.

    B. Complications Are Usually Infectious, Resulting in Cellulitis. *(Domain 1)*
        1. Acinetobacter spp.
        2. Klebsiella spp.
        3. Pseudomonas aeruginosa
        4. Staphylococcus aureus
        5. Streptococcus pyogenes

    C. Treatment *(Domains 1 and 2)*
        1. Most minor burns (first degree and superficial, partial-thickness second degree) can be managed in the outpatient setting.
        2. Nonpharmacologic interventions
            a. Remove heat/burning source from skin (if safe to do so).
            b. Try to cool the burned area with cool, running water.
            c. Avoid using ice to cool burn because it can worsen the burn and symptoms.
            d. Wash (do not scrub) the burned area and loose skin.
            e. Do not remove blisters that are less than 6 mm and intact.
        3. Pain management
            a. NSAIDs may provide sufficient relief.
            b. Topical diclofenac (0.1%) reduced spontaneous pain and provoked pain and erythema with sunburn.
            c. If NSAIDs are insufficient, the patient may require a short course of opioid analgesia.
        4. Cover burns with moist dressing to promote healing (occlusive dressings for more serious burns).
        5. For first-degree burns, consider using topical agents such as the following:
            a. Aloe vera
            b. Antibiotic ointments
            c. Lotions
            d. Honey
        6. For second-degree burns, use topical antimicrobials or antiresorptive, occlusive dressings.
            a. Silver sulfadiazine (SSD)
                i. New occlusive dressings should be considered instead of SSD because of faster healing, decreased pain, fewer dressing changes, and improved patient satisfaction.
               ii. Use SSD cautiously in patients with sulfa allergy.

b. Non-silver treatment options include the following:
   i. Biobrane (biosynthetic dressings)
   ii. Silicone-coated nylon dressings (Mepitel)
   iii. Antimicrobial-releasing biosynthetic dressings (Hydron)
   iv. Hydrofiber dressing (Aquacel-Ag)
   v. Hydrocolloid dressing (DuoDERM)

7. Patients with more than a first-degree burn should be considered for a tetanus booster.

D. Education Tips for Households and Families *(Domain 2)*
1. Cook on rear burners when children are present.
2. Test bathwater temperature.
3. Do not hold a child while working with hot items.
4. Set water heaters to less than 130°F (54°C).
5. Use sunscreen with SPF (sun protection factor) 40 for prolonged exposure to UV light.

XII. DECUBITUS ULCERS

A. Professional Guidelines *(Domain 3)*
1. 2012 Institute for Clinical Systems Improvement pressure ulcer prevention and treatment protocol (2014 update, but no changes were made)
2. 2009 European Pressure Ulcer Advisory Panel and National Pressure Ulcer Advisory Panel international guidelines

B. Classification of Pressure Ulcers (National Pressure Ulcer Advisory Panel–European Pressure Ulcer Advisory Panel) *(Domain 1)*
1. Category/stage I: Nonblanchable erythema of intact skin
2. Category/stage II: Partial-thickness loss of dermis, appearing as open ulcer with red-pink wound bed without slough or bruising
3. Category/stage III: Full-thickness tissue loss, subcutaneous fat may be visible but bone, tendon, or muscle not exposed
4. Category/stage IV: Full-thickness tissue loss with exposed bone, tendon, or muscle visible or directly palpable
5. In the United States, two additional stages are used in classification.
   a. Unstageable/unclassified: Full-thickness tissue loss (with depth unknown) in which base of ulcer is covered by slough and/or eschar in the wound bed
   b. Suggestion of deep tissue injury, depth unknown – Purple or maroon localized area of discolored intact skin or blood-filled blister

C. Risk Factors for Developing Decubitus Ulcer *(Domain 2)*
1. Several risk assessment scales available; most commonly used is the Braden Scale for Predicting Pressure Sore Risk ("Braden Scale"). The Braden Q Scale is a modified Braden Scale for use in pediatric patients up to 18 years of age.
2. Levels or risk
   a. Mild risk: 15–18
   b. Moderate risk: 13–14
   c. High risk: 10–12
   d. Very high risk: 9 or less

3. The Braden Scale considers the following information:
    a. Sensory perception: Ability to respond meaningfully to pressure-related discomfort
    b. Moisture: Degree to which the skin is exposed to moisture
    c. Activity: Degree of physical activity
    d. Mobility: Ability to change and control body position
    e. Nutrition: Usual food intake pattern
    f. Friction and shear
4. Risk factors for developing decubitus ulcer
    a. Aging skin
    b. Comorbidities (type 1 or 2 diabetes, vasculitis, peripheral arterial disease, heart failure, malignancy, end-stage kidney disease, dementia or cognitive impairment, sensory disorder)
    c. Friction or pressure from any hard surface (bed, stretcher, wheelchair)
    d. Moist skin or environment in contact with skin
    e. Patients in long-term care facilities
    f. Patients with limited mobility, including those with coma/sedation, fractures, neurologic disorders, spinal cord injury, or stroke
    g. Poor nutrition (anorexia, dehydration, poor dentition)
    h. Previous ulcer

Table 57. Potential Complications of Decubitus Ulcer

Infectious	Noninfectious
Bacteremia Cellulitis Endocarditis Meningitis Osteomyelitis Sepsis	Amyloidosis (rare) Perineal-urethral fistula Pseudoaneurysm Squamous cell carcinoma (in the ulcer)

D. Patient Presentation and Diagnosis *(Domain 1)*
    1. Usually presents with significant pain radiating from the site of the ulcer and/or infection
    2. Evidence of any of the following on examination of the ulcer:
        a. Exudate
        b. Necrosis
        c. Foul odor
        d. Granulation or new skin formation
        e. Tunneling or undermining
    3. Blood tests (hemoglobin, albumin, iron studies) will help serve as markers for malnutrition.
    4. It is not necessary to swab and culture the wound. Aspiration may be necessary for wounds that do not heal with initial treatments.
    5. In certain instances, it may be necessary to conduct testing to rule out osteomyelitis (white blood cell count, erythrocyte sedimentation rate, blood culture, probe-to-bone test).

E. Nonpharmacologic Treatment *(Domains 1 and 2)*
    1. Minimize/eliminate friction and shear.
    2. Minimize pressure (offloading).
    3. Use specialty support surfaces.

4.   Reposition patient often.
   a.   Patients in bed
      i.   Use pillows or wedges to decrease pressure on bony prominences.
      ii. Turn patients every 2 hours (minimum).
   b.   Patients in sitting position
      i.   Encourage patients to weight shift every 15 minutes.
      ii. Avoid use of "donuts."

F.   Treatment *(Domain 1)*
   1.   Wound management
      a.   Surgical debridement of necrotic tissue
      b.   Hydrocolloid dressings
      c.   Evidence is insufficient to support wound cleaning with cleaners or antiseptics. These agents tend to destroy new tissue and are not helpful.
   2.   Dietary considerations
      a.   Recommended to take in 35–40 kcal/kg/day of energy and 1–1.5 g/kg/day of protein
      b.   The evidence is not robust for nutritional intervention, but this may contribute to faster wound healing.

Patient Case

11. Becaplermin is used to help accelerate the speed of ulcer healing in patients with pressure ulcers. The medication is applied topically, but it carries with it a high risk of mortality in certain patient populations. Which patient is most at risk of experiencing life-threatening adverse events when using becaplermin?

   A.   A 28-year-old woman using oral contraceptives for dysmenorrhea.
   B.   A 36-year-old man with a history of epilepsy.
   C.   A 48-year-old woman with a history of breast cancer.
   D.   A 56-year-old man treated with tiotropium for chronic obstructive pulmonary disease.

---

   3.   Becaplermin

Table 58. Becaplermin STEPS

Safety	Do not apply if there is a known neoplasm at the application site Increases risk of mortality because of malignancy with use of > 3 tubes of drug
Tolerability	Erythematous rash
Efficacy	Will accelerate the speed of ulcer healing, but must weigh risk of serious adverse events (malignancy) vs. decreased ulcer healing time
Preference (Pearls)	If not at least a 30% reduction in ulcer size at 10 weeks or complete resolution at 20 weeks, discontinue use of drug
Simplicity	To determine dose, measure the greatest width and length of the ulcer*: 15-g tube: (ulcer length [inches] x ulcer width [inches]) x 0.6 = length of gel (inches) 2-g tube: (ulcer length [inches] x ulcer width [inches]) x 1.3 = length of gel (inches) *Recalculate the dose every 1–2 weeks

4. Antibiotics are not considered first-line treatment options and should be reserved as follows:
    a. Oral antibiotics for patients with bacteremia, cellulitis, or osteomyelitis
    b. Topical antibiotics for patients without wound healing, despite 2 weeks of wound care
5. Pain management is especially important because of pain caused by cleaning, movement because of repositioning, and dressing changes after debridement.
    a. Topical agents such as lidocaine/prilocaine during debridement
    b. Topical morphine has shown efficacy for ulceration pain reduction.
6. Other interventions
    a. Pressure relief devices: Static or dynamic devices to reduce contact pressure
    b. Electrotherapy: Electrical stimulation has some evidence of increased wound healing.
    c. Negative pressure wound therapy: Weak evidence for efficacy, and the FDA issued an advisory for providers to be cautious and selective with candidates because of a high number of reported deaths and injuries

REFERENCES

Acne

1. Arowojulo AO, Gallo MF, Lopez LM, et al. Combined oral contraceptive pills for treatment of acne. Cochrane Database Syst Rev 2012;7:CD004425.

2. Dreno B, Bettoli V, Ochsendorf F, et al. An expert view on the treatment of acne with systemic antibiotics and/or oral isotretinoin in the light of the new European recommendations. Eur J Dermatol 2006;16:565-71.

3. Drugs for acne, rosacea and psoriasis. Treat Guidel Med Lett 2008;6:75-82.

4. DynaMed [Internet database]. Ipswich, MA: EBSCO Publishing. Available at www.ebscohost.com./dynamed. Accessed September 21, 2013.

5. Essential Evidence Plus [Internet database]. New York: John Wiley & Sons. Available at www.essentialevidenceplus.com. Accessed September 21, 2013.

6. Feldman S, Careccia RE, Braham KL, et al. Diagnosis and treatment of acne. Am Fam Physician 2004;69:2123-30.

7. Gollnick H, Cunliffe W, Berson D, et al. Management of acne: a report from a Global Alliance to Improve Outcomes in Acne. J Am Acad Dermatol 2003;49(1 suppl):S1-37.

8. Lehmann HL, Robinson KA, Andrews JS, et al. Acne therapy: a methodological review. J Am Acad Dermatol 2002;47:231-40.

9. Ozolins M, Eady EA, Avery AJ, et al. Comparison of five antimicrobial regimens for treatment of mild to moderate inflammatory facial acne vulgaris in the community: randomised controlled trial. Lancet 2004;364:2188-95.

10. Purdy S, de Berker D. Acne. BMJ 2006;333:949-53.

11. Strauss JS, Krowchuk DP, Leyden JJ, et al. Guidelines of care for acne vulgaris management. J Am Acad Dermatol 2007;56:651-63.

12. Thiboutot D, Gollnick H, Bettoli V, et al. New insights into the management of acne: an update from the Global Alliance to Improve Outcomes in Acne group. J Am Acad Dermatol 2009;60(5 suppl):S1-50.

Allergic Rhinitis

1. Angier E, Willington J, Scadding G, et al. Management of allergic and non-allergic rhinitis: a primary care summary of the BSACI guideline. Prim Care Respir J 2010;19:217-22.

2. DynaMed [Internet database]. Ipswich, MA: EBSCO Publishing. Available at www.ebscohost.com./dynamed. Accessed September 29, 2013.

3. Essential Evidence Plus [Internet database]. New York: John Wiley & Sons. Available at www.essentialevidenceplus.com. Accessed September 29, 2013.

4. Plaut M, Valentine MD. Clinical practice: allergic rhinitis. N Engl J Med 2005;353:1934-44.

5. Scadding GK, Durham SR, Mirakian R, et al. BSACI guidelines for the management of allergic and non-allergic rhinitis. Clin Exp Allergy 2008;38:19-42.

6. Wallace DV, Dykewicz MS, Bernstein DI, et al. The diagnosis and management of rhinitis: an updated practice parameter. J Allergy Clin Immunol 2008;122(2 suppl):S1-84.

Angioedema

1. Bowen T, Cicardi M, Farkas H, et al. 2010 International consensus algorithm for the diagnosis, therapy and management of hereditary angioedema. Allergy Asthma Clin Immunol 2010;6:24.

2. DynaMed [Internet database]. Ipswich, MA: EBSCO Publishing. Available at www.ebscohost.com./dynamed. Accessed September 28, 2013.

3. Joint Task Force on Practice Parameters. The diagnosis and management of urticaria: a practice parameter, part I: acute urticaria/angioedema; part II: chronic urticaria/angioedema. Ann Allergy Asthma Immunol 2000;85(6 pt 2):521-44.

4. Lang DM, Aberer W, Bernstein JA, et al. International consensus on hereditary and acquired angioedema. Ann Allergy Asthma Immunol 2012;109:395-402.

Burns

1. Drucker AM, Rosen CF. Drug-induced photosensitivity: culprit drugs, management and prevention. Drug Saf 2011;34:821-37.

2. DynaMed [Internet database]. Ipswich, MA: EBSCO Publishing. Available at www.ebscohost.com./dynamed. Accessed September 29, 2013.

3. Lloyd EC, Rodgers BC, Michener M, et al. Outpatient burns: prevention and care. Am Fam Physician 2012;85:25-32.

4. Storm-Versloot MN, Vos CG, Ubbink DT, et al. Topical silver for preventing wound infection. Cochrane Database Syst Rev 2010;3:CD006478.

5. Wasiak J, Cleland H, Campbell F, et al. Dressings for superficial and partial thickness burns. Cochrane Database Syst Rev 2013;3:CD002106.

Decubitus Ulcer

1. Berlowitz DR, Brandeis GH, Morris JN, et al. Deriving a risk-adjustment model for pressure ulcer development using the Minimum Data Set. J Am Geriatr Soc 2001;49:866-71.

2. DynaMed [Internet database]. Ipswich, MA: EBSCO Publishing. Available at www.ebscohost.com./dynamed. Accessed September 30, 2013.

3. European Pressure Ulcer Advisory Panel and National Pressure Ulcer Advisory Panel. Pressure Ulcer Prevention: Quick Reference Guide. Available at www.npuap.org/wp-content/uploads/2012/02/Final_Quick_Prevention_for_web_2010.pdf. Accessed on September 30, 2013.

4. Institute for Clinical Systems Improvement (ICSI). Pressure Ulcer Prevention and Treatment Protocol. Health Care Protocol. Bloomington, MN: Institute for Clinical Systems Improvement (ICSI), 2012. Available at https://www.icsi.org/guidelines__more/catalog_guidelines_and_more/catalog_guidelines/catalog_patient_safetyreliability_guidelines/pressure_ulcer. Accessed September 30, 2013.

Dry Eyes

1. American Academy of Ophthalmology Cornea/External Disease Panel. Dry Eye Syndrome. Limited Revision. San Francisco: American Academy of Ophthalmology (AAO), 2011. Available at www.guideline.gov/content.aspx?id=36094. Accessed on September 24, 2013.

2. DynaMed [Internet database]. Ipswich, MA: EBSCO Publishing. Available at www.ebscohost.com./dynamed. Accessed September 24, 2013.

Infestations

1. Barker SC, Altman PM. An ex vivo, assessor blind, randomized, parallel group, comparative efficacy trial of the ovicidal activity of three pediculosis after a single application – melaleuca oil and lavender oil, eucalyptus oil and lemon tea tree oil, and a "suffocation" pediculicide. BMC Dermatol 2011;11:14.

2. Chosidow O. Clinical practices. Scabies. N Engl J Med 2006;354:1718-27.

3. DynaMed [Internet database]. Ipswich, MA: EBSCO Publishing. Available at www.ebscohost.com./dynamed. Accessed September 20, 2013.

4. Essential Evidence Plus [Internet database]. New York: John Wiley & Sons. Available at www.essentialevidenceplus.com. Accessed September 19, 2012.

5. Flinders DC, De Schweinitz P. Pediculosis and scabies. Am Fam Physician 2004;69:341-8.

6. Frankowski BL, Bocchini JA Jr. Head lice. Pediatrics 2010;126:392-403.

7. Gunning K, Pippitt K, Kiraly B, et al. Pediculosis and scabies: a treatment update. Indian J Clin Pract 2013;24:211-6.

8. Jones KN, English JC III. Review of common therapeutic options in the United States for the treatment of pediculosis capitis. Clin Infect Dis 2003;36:1355-61.

9. UK National Guideline on the Management of Scabies Infestation. London: Clinical Effectiveness Group; British Association for Sexual Health and HIV (BASHH), 2008. Available at www.guideline.gov/content.aspx?id=12287. Accessed February 15, 2011.

10. Workowski KA, Berman S. Sexually transmitted diseases treatment guidelines, 2010. MMWR Recomm Rep 2010;59(RR12):1-110.

Macular Degeneration

1. Age-Related Eye Disease Study Research Group. A randomized, placebo-controlled, clinical trial of high-dose supplementation with vitamins C and E, beta carotene, and zinc for age-related macular degeneration and vision loss: AREDS Report No. 8. Arch Ophthalmol 2001;119:1417-36.

2. American Academy of Ophthalmology. Age-Related Macular Degeneration. San Francisco: American Academy of Ophthalmology Retina/Vitreous Panel (AAO), 2008. Available at http://one.aao.org/asset. axd?id=b1f95ead-7fd4-49e7-bcc9-b12249916069. Accessed September 20, 2013.

3. American Academy of Ophthalmology. Primary Open-Angle Glaucoma. San Francisco: American Academy of Ophthalmology (AAO) Glaucoma Panel, Preferred Practice Patterns Committee, 2010. Available at http://one.aao.org/asset. axd?id=a860f57a-0e6a-4c4f-b0f7-1a42e05073ff. Accessed September 19, 2012.

4. Arroyo JG. A 76-year-old man with macular degeneration. JAMA 2006;295:2394-406.

5. de Jong PT. Age-related macular degeneration. N Engl J Med 2006;355:1474-85.

6. DynaMed [Internet database]. Ipswich, MA: EBSCO Publishing. Available at www.ebscohost. com./dynamed. Accessed September 20, 2013.

7. Essential Evidence Plus [Internet database]. New York: John Wiley & Sons. Available at www.essentialevidenceplus.com. Accessed September 19, 2012.

8. Evans JR, Lawrenson JG. Antioxidant vitamin and mineral supplements for preventing age-related macular degeneration. Cochrane Database Syst Rev 2012;6:CD000253.

9. Tomany SC, Cruickshanks KJ, Klein R, et al. Sunlight and the 10-year incidence of age-related maculopathy: the Beaver Dam Eye Study. Arch Ophthalmol 2004;122:750-7.

Glaucoma

1. Arimoto A, Shimizu K, Shoji N, et al. Underestimation of intraocular pressure in eyes after laser in situ keratomileusis. Jpn J Ophthalmol 2002;46:645-9.

2. DynaMed [Internet database]. Ipswich, MA: EBSCO Publishing. Available at www.ebscohost.com./dynamed. Accessed September 20, 2013.

3. Essential Evidence Plus [Internet database]. New York: John Wiley & Sons. Available at www.essentialevidenceplus.com. Accessed September 20, 2013.

4. Fingeret M. Optometric Clinical Practice Guidelines: Care of the Patient with Open Angle Glaucoma. St. Louis: American Optometric Association, 2011.

5. Glaucoma: Diagnosis and Management of Chronic Open Angle Glaucoma and Ocular Hypertension. National Institute for Health and Clinical Excellence, April 2009. Available at www.nice.org.uk/guidance/CG85. Accessed September 20, 2013.

6. Screening for glaucoma: recommendation statement. Ann Fam Med 2005;3:171-2.

7. Vass C, Hirn C, Sycha T, et al. Medical interventions for primary open angle glaucoma and ocular hypertension. Cochrane Database Syst Rev 2007;4:CD003167.

Psoriasis

1. DynaMed [Internet database]. Ipswich, MA: EBSCO Publishing. Available at www.ebscohost.com./dynamed. Accessed September 22, 2013.

2. Essential Evidence Plus [Internet database]. New York: John Wiley & Sons. Available at www.essentialevidenceplus.com. Accessed September 22, 2013.

3. Kim GK, Del Rosso JQ. Drug-provoked psoriasis: is it drug induced or drug aggravated? J Clin Aesthetic Dermatol 2010;3:32-8.

4. Levine D, Gottlieb A. Evaluation and management of psoriasis: an internist's guide. Med Clin North Am 2009;93:1291-303.

5. Mason AR, Mason J, Cork M, et al. Topical treatments for chronic plaque psoriasis. Cochrane Database Syst Rev 2009;2:CD005028.

6. Menter A, Gottlieb A, Feldman SR, et al. Guidelines of care for the management of psoriasis and psoriatic arthritis, section 1: overview of psoriasis and guidelines of care for the treatment of psoriasis with biologics. J Am Acad Dermatol 2008;58:826-50.

7. Menter A, Korman NJ, Elmets CA, et al. Guidelines of care for the management of psoriasis and psoriatic arthritis, section 3: guidelines of care for the management and treatment of psoriasis with topical therapies. J Am Acad Dermatol 2009;60:643-59.

8. Menter A, Korman NJ, Elmets CA, et al. Guidelines of care for the management of psoriasis and psoriatic arthritis, section 4: guidelines of care for the management and treatment of psoriasis with traditional systemic agents. J Am Acad Dermatol 2009;61:451-85.

9. Nestle FO, Kaplan DH, Barker J. Psoriasis. N Engl J Med 2009;361:496-509.

10. Papp K, Cather JC, Rosoph L, et al. Efficacy of Apremilast in the treatment of moderate to severe psoriasis: a randomized controlled trial. Lancet 2012;380:738-46.

Urticaria

1. DynaMed [Internet database]. Ipswich, MA: EBSCO Publishing. Available at www.ebscohost.com./dynamed. Accessed September 29, 2013.

2. Essential Evidence Plus [Internet database]. New York: John Wiley & Sons. Available at www.essentialevidenceplus.com. Accessed September 29, 2013.

3. Grattan CE, Humphreys F. Guidelines for evaluation and management of urticaria in adults and children. Br J Dermatol 2007;157:1116-23.

4. Joint Task Force on Practice Parameters. The diagnosis and management of urticaria: a practice parameter part I: acute urticaria/angioedema, part II: chronic urticaria/angioedema; Joint Task Force on Practice Parameters. Ann Allergy Asthma Immunol 2000;85(6 pt 2):521-44.

5. Kanani A, Schellenberg R, Warrington R. Urticaria and angioedema. Allergy, Asthma Clin Immunol 2011;7(suppl 1):S9.

6. Poonawalla T, Kelly B. Urticaria: a review. Am J Clin Dermatol 2009;10:9-21.

7. Zuberbier T, Asero R, Bindslev-Jensen C, et al. EAACI/GA(2)LEN/EDF/WAO guideline: definition, classification and diagnosis of urticaria. Allergy 2009;64:1417-26.

Vertigo

1. American Academy of Otolaryngology-Head and Neck Foundation Committee on Hearing and Equilibrium guidelines for the diagnosis and evaluation of therapy in Menière's disease. Otolaryngol Head Neck Surg 1995;113:181-5.

2. Bhattacharyya N, Baugh RF, Orvidas L, et al. Clinical practice guideline: benign paroxysmal positional vertigo. Otolaryngol Head Neck Surg 2008;139(5 suppl 4):S47-81.

3. DynaMed [Internet database]. Ipswich, MA: EBSCO Publishing. Available at www.ebscohost.com./dynamed. Accessed September 26, 2013.

4. Hillier SL, McDonnell M. Vestibular rehabilitation for unilateral peripheral vestibular dysfunction. Cochrane Database Syst Rev 2011;2:CD005397.

5. Santos PM, Hall RA, Snyder JM, et al. Diuretic and diet effect on Menière's disease evaluated by the 1985 Committee on Hearing and Equilibrium guidelines. Otolaryngol Head Neck Surg 1993;109:680-9.

6. Thirlwall AS, Kundu S. Diuretics for Menière's disease or syndrome. Cochrane Database Syst Rev 2006;3:CD003599.

ANSWERS AND EXPLANATIONS TO PATIENT CASES

1. Answer: D

The antioxidant vitamin formulation should most closely match the combination from the AREDS study. This study evaluated the efficacy of vitamin C, vitamin E, beta-carotene, and zinc (choice D). However, this patient is a smoker, and beta-carotene use in patients who smoke increases the patient's risk of developing lung cancer. Hence, the patient should be taking a combination that does not include beta-carotene, such as choices B and C (Answer D is correct; Answers A–C are incorrect).

2. Answer: A

For this patient, initiating a prostaglandin analog such as travoprost (in choices A or B) is the best choice for therapy. In addition, she has to use only one drop in each eye every evening because the volume of one drop meets or exceeds the maximal volume the eye can retain topically (choice A). Extra drops would provide the patient no additional benefit (choice B). Although a β-blocker can be used as first-line therapy in patients with POAG, β-blockers are not as potent as prostaglandin analogs for lowering baseline IOPs (choices C and D) (Answer A is correct; Answers B-D are incorrect).

3. Answer: C

In patients with dry eyes, the indication to begin therapy with ophthalmologic cyclosporine is usually the occurrence of symptoms of dry eyes without relief from artificial tears (choice C). Despite the 54-year-old patient's daily symptoms (choice B) and the 63-year-old woman's once-weekly symptoms (choice A), both are receiving adequate relief from artificial tears. The 61-year-old patient in choice D with dry mouth, fatigue, and other dry mucus membranes as well as dry eyes appears to have symptoms more consistent with Sjögren disease and will require systemic cholinergic agents. The 58-year-old patient who is receiving no relief with artificial tears, and who is less productive as a result, is the best candidate for ophthalmologic cyclosporine (Answer C is correct; Answers A,B, and D are incorrect).

4. Answer: C

Steroid bursts are an appropriate intervention for acute moderate to severe exacerbations in patients with allergic rhinitis already treated with an oral antihistamine, allowing relatively quick symptom resolution (choice C). Doubling this patient's intranasal corticosteroid would probably provide no additional relief and would increase the chances of mucosal irritation and/or epistaxis (choice A). Although pseudoephedrine may be an acceptable alternative to some intranasal corticosteroids or intranasal/oral antihistamines, it is still an inferior intervention, and the goal is to provide maximal relief to this patient (choice B). Finally, montelukast use would not be beneficial because (1) it is not as efficacious as systemic corticosteroids and (2) the short duration of the intervention is not consistent with the appropriate use of montelukast for allergic rhinitis (choice D) (Answer C is correct; Answers A, B, and D are incorrect).

5. Answer: B

The nsAHs are the best first-line option for treating this patient's urticaria. The prednisone dose is too high for an acute urticarial rash in this child, and (if repeated events) it would not be the best choice for continued administration (choice C). Although famotidine affects histamine receptors, it targets the wrong receptor to make it acceptable for first-line therapy (choice D). Finally, loratadine would be the better choice because it is considered an nsAH with fewer central nervous system effects, and it would be safer for the child playing in and around water (Answer B is correct; Answers A, C, and D are incorrect).

6. Answer: A

After being administered a C1 inhibitor or a selective bradykinin B2 receptor antagonist, patients with HAE should seek immediate medical attention to manage their angioedema (choice A). These two classes of medications are approved for use in the outpatient management of acute HAE. The kallikrein inhibitors are only approved for in-hospital administration. Antihistamine or corticosteroid therapy may be warranted in these emergencies, but the patient should go directly to the emergency department for additional care. None of the plasma-derived products cause spontaneous syncope, so patients need not account for this adverse event (Answer A is correct; Answers C-D are incorrect).

7. Answer: A

The AAD treatment recommendations list oral isotretinoin as an alternative therapy, which, given the patient's nodular acne and lack of response to the first-line therapeutic combination, would be best for him (choice A). The other options listed for this question are appropriate drug combinations for treating acne, but none is potent enough or in a strong enough combination to be of use to the patient (choices B and D). Topical retinoid combinations are incorrect for this stage of acne because the pairing of agents is incorrect. Topical retinoids should be combined with an oral antibiotic, with or without benzoyl peroxide and/or azelaic acid. The listed combinations fail to meet these criteria. In addition, the use of antiandrogenic spironolactone (choice C) would not be beneficial to a male patient (Answer A is correct; Answers B-D are incorrect).

8. Answer: D

Lithium is probably contributing to this patient's psoriasis. It is not uncommon to see psoriasis first present after trauma to the skin. The acronym NAILS is a helpful reminder of the agents that may cause psoriasis: NSAIDs, antimalarials, ACE inhibitors, Inderal (β-receptor antagonist), lithium, and steroid withdrawal (answer D is correct; Answers A-C are incorrect).

9. Answer: C

Permethrin 5% is the appropriate dose for treating scabies infestations in most individuals. Although resistance patterns for permethrin 1% are developing in the United States for treating pediculosis, permethrin at this concentration is still highly effective for scabies (choice A). In addition, it is not necessary to "nit pick" when patients are using permethrin to eradicate scabies (choice D). For these two patients, treatment failure probably occurred because the children and/or their mother did not apply the agent to the entire body and missed some areas of infestation during application. Patients should be counseled to apply the agent to all surfaces of the body below the neck, including the palms of their hands and the soles of their feet (Answer C is correct; Answers A, B, and D are incorrect).

10. Answer: D

Adding trimethoprim/sulfamethoxazole to permethrin 1% for pediculosis is an appropriate choice (choice D). Although the other options are viable, the instructions for use are not appropriate. Ivermectin should be dosed only once, not twice (choice A). Malathion and suffocation-based pediculicide should be applied in place of (not in sequence with) permethrin 1% (Answer D is correct; Answers A-C are incorrect).

11. Answer: C

Becaplermin use has been associated with an increased risk of advanced malignancy and mortality in patients with an existing malignancy, such as the patient in choice C with breast cancer. Even though this medication is topical (locally applied), the malignant effects of the drug may be seen remotely from the application site. No negative outcomes are associated with becaplermin for patients who have seizure disorders (choice B) or who take oral contraceptives (choice A) or inhaled anticholinergics (choice D) (Answer C is correct; Answers A, B, and D are incorrect).

ANSWERS AND EXPLANATIONS TO SELF-ASSESSMENT QUESTIONS

1. Answer: A

In the AREDS study, the supplement combination shown to delay the progression from intermediate disease to advanced disease consisted of vitamin C 500 mg, vitamin E 400 international units, beta-carotene 15 mg, and zinc 80 mg. Certain situations warrant excluding a component of the combination (beta-carotene in patients with a history of lung cancer or in patients who smoke). The combination showed no benefit for patients without macular degeneration (Answer A is correct; Answers B-D are incorrect).

2. Answer: B

Answer B, the ophthalmologic β-blocker, is the best choice to add to this patient's therapy. The patient is already taking a prostaglandin analog (decreasing aqueous outflow resistance), and the dose increase is inappropriate because it does not enhance the IOP-lowering effect. According to recommendations from NICE, carbonic anhydrase inhibitors and adrenergic agents should be used after an ophthalmologic β-blocker fails to sufficiently decrease the IOP. Answers A, C, and D are options because their mechanism of action (decreased aqueous production) complements the prostaglandin analog, but only betaxolol has clear preference in the treatment recommendations.

3. Answer: A

There are several options for treating and relieving the symptoms of patients with mild to moderate dry eyes. First, be sure to assess for and remove any medications or factors that may be causing dry eyes. Next, apply artificial tears and evaluate response. This patient had a response, but not for a sufficient period. However, because she did receive some relief, she may need a different formulation that will remain present for a longer period. For this, an ointment application may be the best choice (answer A). Ophthalmologic cyclosporine would be the next step or should be used if the patient does not receive relief from artificial tears, 0.05%, not 0.1%, concentration (choices B and C, respectively). Systemic cholinergic agents (choice D) should be used in patients with other symptoms of dryness, including most mucus membranes, or in those whose condition does not respond to ophthalmologic cyclosporine (Answer A is correct; Answers B-D are incorrect).

4. Answer: C

In any patient with symptoms of vertigo, the goal is to identify the underlying cause of the disease, not just react to the symptom. For this patient, it appears that his primary care physician ruled out most causes of vertigo except for medication-induced symptoms. Of the four medications, carbamazepine (choice C) is the most likely cause of his symptoms. Although the antihypertensive hydrochlorothiazide (choice A) may be associated with vertigo because of electrolyte abnormalities or blood pressure changes, neither was present during this patient's physical and laboratory evaluations. Metformin (choice D) may also be a cause, but for hypoglycemia, the symptoms would most often be accompanied by tachycardia, diaphoresis, and possibly confusion (Answer C is correct; Answers A, B, and D are incorrect).

5. Answer: B

Although an intranasal corticosteroid is the best choice for this patient's symptoms (moderate to severe), her fear of epistaxis and reluctance to use the corticosteroid are a treatment barrier. Fexofenadine (choice B) should be used in this patient because it is an nsAH and will most likely provide better relief than the other available agents. Although most oral antihistamines are equally effective, clemastine (choice A) is a first-generation H_1 antihistamine with a greater chance of causing sedation than fexofenadine. According to treatment guidelines, montelukast (choice C) and other leukotriene inhibitors should be reserved for use until after a patient's treatment with an intranasal corticosteroid and an nsAH has been unsuccessful (Answer B is correct; Answers A, C, and D are incorrect).

6. Answer: C

Adding famotidine (answer C) may be the best choice for this patient because adding fexofenadine will ensure antagonism of both the H_1 and H_2 receptors. Agents such as diphenhydramine (choice B) or doxepin (choice D) may be effective, but they also cause fatigue, which could interfere with the patient's ability to work. In addition, diphenhydramine would work on the same receptors as fexofenadine, probably producing no additional effect. Adding famotidine will broaden histamine receptor antagonism and further decrease the presence and symptoms of urticaria. If given the option, the patient could also increase her oral antihistamine dose up to 4 times the suggested normal dose for up to 4 weeks to see whether the symptoms improve or resolve (Answer C is correct; Answers A, B, and D are incorrect).

7. Answer: D

In patients with HAE, one of the primary treatment strategies for preventing symptoms is using plasma-derived C1 INHs (such as Cinryze). Because this is a blood product and may be a vector for disease transmission, treatment guidelines recommend immunizing all patients for bloodborne pathogens, including hepatitis B (Answer D is correct; Answers A-C are incorrect).

8. Answer: A

Patients taking an oral retinoid should be enrolled in the iPledge program and be aware of the severe, increased risk of teratogenicity with pregnancy while actively taking the medication (answer A). Individuals enrolled in the iPledge program are extensively counseled on the risk of teratogenicity with pregnancy and are encouraged to be taking hormonal and barrier contraceptives. Even though routine monitoring of hepatic transaminase concentrations is recommended until patients reach an effective dose of oral retinoids, missed laboratory visits are not an indication to discontinue therapy (choice C). In addition, patients starting an oral retinoid should be counseled on the increased risk of mental health disorders (suicidality) with use, but they do not need a mental health provider to sign off on therapy (choice B). Finally, these analogs have no reported impact on night vision (choice D) (Answer A is correct; Answers B-D are incorrect).

9. Answer: B

Topical corticosteroids are the treatment of choice for individuals with mild to moderate psoriasis. Adding a vitamin D analog (calcipotriene, choice B) is the most reasonable choice because it is more effective in combination with a topical corticosteroid than is either agent alone. The oral corticosteroid burst in choice A is not indicated for a "flare-up" of psoriasis. Biologic agents (choice D) and methotrexate (choice C) should be reserved for individuals with severe or debilitating disease, those with greater than 10% of their body surface area covered with psoriatic lesions, and those with symptoms of psoriatic arthritis. For this patient, use of these agents would be excessive before trying other topical treatment options (Answer B is correct; Answers A, C, and D are incorrect).

10. Answer: D

The best agent for this patient would be etanercept (choice D). Cyclosporine (choice B) would not be a good choice for her because of poorly controlled hypertension and poor efficacy compared with biologic therapy. Acitretin, etanercept, and the TNF inhibitors are superior agents for treating psoriasis and accompanying psoriatic arthritis. Methotrexate is an acceptable agent because it can be used in severe disease with or without the presence of arthritis. However, given that methotrexate's efficacy for controlling symptoms in psoriasis is less than that of the TNF inhibitors, it should be reserved for second-line therapy. Methotrexate should be considered to treat psoriasis only in patients whose condition does not respond to a T-cell inhibitor or TNF inhibitor or who are unable to afford biologic therapy (Answer D is correct; Answers A-C are incorrect).

11. Answer: B

Permethrin 5% (answer B) would be the treatment of choice for this patient. Permethrin 1% lotion (choice A) is too low in concentration to work for a scabies infestation. It may be used for pediculosis (lice), but it would not be effective for this patient's condition. In addition, the degree of resistance to permethrin 5% for scabies is not yet sufficient to warrant a change to malathion (choice C), given its inferiority to permethrin and high likelihood for dermatologic drying and irritation. The neurotoxicity associated with lindane (choice D) makes it a less desirable first-line treatment option for the first symptoms of untreated scabies; it should be reserved for patients who cannot be treated with less potentially harmful therapies (Answer B is correct; Answers A, C, and D are incorrect).

12. Answer: A

All individuals in the household and in close contact with the infested person should be examined and most likely treated for a scabies infestation, even if he or she is asymptomatic (answer A). Household and close contacts within the past 30 days need to be evaluated and treated. Given the long period between initial infestation and presence of symptoms, it is unreasonable to wait for individuals to develop symptoms. During the asymptomatic period, these contacts could possibly contaminate those around them (sometimes for a second or third time). An "on-call" prescription for a scabicide is also not feasible because it still requires individuals to be symptomatic and possibly transmit/retransmit the infestation (Answer A is correct; Answers B-D are incorrect).

13. Answer: C

The patient's symptoms are consistent with a first-degree UV light burn. This will probably take 5–10 days to completely heal and does not require any therapy beyond miniaturization and pain management (answer C). Silver-based creams such as silver sulfadiazine (choice A) are not recommended for burns because they delay healing time and (in more serious burns) may result in an increased risk of infection. Topical aloe is an option, but occlusive and wet dressings should be reserved for second-degree and more serious burns (choice B). The same reasoning is also applicable for not choosing the hydrocolloid dressing (choice D). This patient should receive sufficient relief from an NSAID such as ibuprofen (Answer C is correct; Answers A, B, and D are incorrect).

14. Answer: C

The continued use of becaplermin is based on the percentage of wound healing in the first 10 weeks and the resolution at 20 weeks. Although he must continue taking becaplermin, the same dose should not be used; instead, a new dose should be calculated according to his wound size reduction. Patients who have at least a 30% reduction in wound size after the first 10 weeks of therapy should continue the medication for 20 weeks. In patients without much wound resolution, the medication should be discontinued. The becaplermin dose is based on a calculation that considers ulcer length and width and should not arbitrarily be increased or decreased on the basis of impression. For this patient, continuing at the same dose or increasing the dose would be excessive. A 35% reduction in wound size would necessitate a new dose of around 75% of his original dose (as the new dose). Doses should be recalculated every 1–2 weeks according to the ulcer size (Answer C is correct; Answers A, B, and D are incorrect).

Oncology Supportive Care

LeAnn B. Norris, Pharm.D., BCPS, BCOP

South Carolina College of Pharmacy
Columbia, South Carolina

ONCOLOGY SUPPORTIVE CARE

LeAnn B. Norris, Pharm.D., BCPS, BCOP

South Carolina College of Pharmacy
Columbia, South Carolina

Learning Objectives

1. Identify, assess, and recommend appropriate pharmacotherapy for managing common complications of cancer chemotherapy, including nausea and vomiting, myelosuppression and the appropriate use of growth factors, infection, anemia and fatigue, cardiotoxicity, and extravasation injury.
2. Assess and recommend appropriate pharmacotherapy for managing cancer-related pain.
3. Assess and recommend appropriate pharmacotherapy for managing oncologic emergencies, including hypercalcemia, tumor lysis syndrome, and spinal cord compression.

Self-Assessment Questions

Answers and explanations to these questions can be found at the end of this chapter.

1. A 50-year-old man is in the clinic to receive his third cycle of R-CHOP (rituximab, cyclophosphamide, doxorubicin, vincristine, and prednisone) for non-Hodgkin lymphoma. He is very anxious, with nausea and vomiting lasting for about 12 hours after his previous cycle of chemotherapy. The antiemetic regimen he received for his previous cycle of chemotherapy was granisetron 1 dose plus dexamethasone 1 dose administered 30 minutes before chemotherapy. Which regimen is most appropriate for the patient to receive on day 1 of the next cycle of chemotherapy?

   A. Granisetron 1 dose plus dexamethasone 1 dose administered 30 minutes before chemotherapy.
   B. Dolasetron 1 dose plus dexamethasone 1 dose plus aprepitant 1 dose administered 30 minutes before chemotherapy.
   C. Palonosetron 1 dose plus dexamethasone 1 dose plus lorazepam 1 dose administered 30 minutes before chemotherapy.
   D. Metoclopramide 1 dose plus dexamethasone 1 dose plus aprepitant 1 dose administered 30 minutes before chemotherapy.

2. A 65-year-old man with metastatic non–small cell lung cancer is brought to the clinic by his family because of alterations in his mental status. Pertinent laboratory values include a serum calcium concentration of 12 mg/dL and an albumin concentration of 2 g/dL. Which therapy is best for this patient's altered mental status due to hypercalcemia of malignancy?

   A. Calcitonin 4 units/kg every 12 hours.
   B. Furosemide 20 mg orally.
   C. Dexamethasone 10 mg orally two times a day.
   D. Zoledronic acid 4 mg intravenously.

3. A 20-year-old man was recently given a diagnosis of acute myeloid leukemia. He has an elevated white blood cell count (WBC), and he will receive chemotherapy tomorrow. Which is the best prevention strategy for tumor lysis syndrome (TLS)?

   A. Hydration with 5% dextrose (D_5W), 1 L before chemotherapy, plus allopurinol 300 mg/day.
   B. Hydration with D_5W, 100 mL/hour starting at least 24 hours before chemotherapy, plus allopurinol 300 mg/day.
   C. Hydration with normal saline 250 mL/hour starting at least 24 hours before chemotherapy plus allopurinol 300 mg/day.
   D. Hydration with normal saline 100 mL/hour starting at least 24 hours before chemotherapy plus sodium bicarbonate 500 mg orally every 6 hours.

4. An 18-year-old man is about to begin chemotherapy for acute lymphoblastic leukemia. On today's complete blood cell count (CBC), his hemoglobin is 7g/dL, and he is experiencing fatigue. Which is the best treatment recommendation?

   A. Initiate epoetin.
   B. Administer transfusion of packed red blood cells (RBCs).
   C. Delay chemotherapy treatment until hemoglobin recovers.
   D. Reduce chemotherapy dosages to prevent further decreases in hemoglobin.

5. A patient received her fourth cycle of chemotherapy with paclitaxel/carboplatin for ovarian cancer 12 days ago. She reports to the clinic this morning with a temperature of 103°F. Her CBC is WBC 500 cells/mm³, segmented neutrophils 55%, band neutrophils 5%, basophils 15%, eosinophils 5%, monocytes 15%, and platelet count 99,000 cells/mm³. She denies any signs or symptoms of infection. Her blood pressure (BP) is 115/60 mm Hg, heart rate is 80 beats/minute, and respiratory rate is 15 breaths/minute. Which best represents the patient's absolute neutrophil count (ANC)?

A. 275 cells/mm³.
B. 300 cells/mm³.
C. 25 cells/mm³.
D. 500 cells/mm³.

6. Which is the best course of action for the patient in the previous question?

A. Admit to the hospital for intravenous antibiotic drugs.
B. Treat as an outpatient with antibiotic drugs.
C. Initiate a colony-stimulating factor (CSF).
D. Discontinue chemotherapy.

7. Which statement about the above patient is most accurate?

A. Given her monocyte count, her neutropenia is expected to last for another week.
B. This is a nadir neutrophil count, and neutrophils would be expected to start increasing soon.
C. The elevated absolute eosinophil count indicates an allergic reaction to carboplatin.
D. It is unusual for the ANC to be this low in the setting of an elevated platelet count.

8. A 60-year-old man has head and neck cancer with extensive involvement of facial nerves. His pain medications include transdermal fentanyl 100 mcg/hour every 72 hours and oral morphine solution 40 mg every 4 hours as needed. He is still having problems with neuropathic pain. Which treatment is best to recommend?

A. Begin gabapentin and decrease the dosage of fentanyl.
B. Increase the dosages of fentanyl and morphine.
C. Begin diazepam and increase the dosage of fentanyl.
D. Begin gabapentin and continue fentanyl and morphine at the same dosage.

9. A patient is receiving chemotherapy for limited-stage small cell lung carcinoma. After the third cycle of chemotherapy, she is hospitalized with febrile neutropenia. She recovers, and today she is scheduled to receive the fourth cycle of chemotherapy. Which statement is the best treatment course for this patient?

A. The patient should receive filgrastim 250 mcg/m²/day subcutaneously for 10 days, given at least 24 hours after chemotherapy.
B. The patient should receive filgrastim 5 mcg/kg/day subcutaneously, starting today.
C. The patient should receive pegfilgrastim 1 mg/day subcutaneously for 6 days, given at least 24 hours after chemotherapy.
D. The patient should receive filgrastim 5 mcg/kg/day subcutaneously for 7 days, given at least 24 hours after chemotherapy.

10. A 60-year-old woman with breast cancer is to begin chemotherapy with AC (doxorubicin and cyclophosphamide). Laboratory values today include sodium 140 mEq/L, potassium 3.8 mEq/L, glucose 100 mg/dL, serum creatinine 1.1 mg/dL, aspartate aminotransferase 6 IU/L, alanine aminotransferase 35 IU/L, and total bilirubin 2 mg/dL. Which statement is most appropriate?

A. The dosage of doxorubicin should be decreased.
B. The dosage of cyclophosphamide should be decreased.
C. Both chemotherapy drugs should be given at standard dosages.
D. Both chemotherapy drugs should be given at decreased dosages.

11. Large cell lymphoma is considered intermediate (between indolent and highly aggressive) in tumor growth and biology. Large cell lymphoma is sensitive to chemotherapy and potentially curable. Metastatic colorectal cancer is considered slow growing. Although responses to chemotherapy commonly occur and chemotherapy can prolong survival (by months), metastatic colorectal cancer is not generally considered curable with chemotherapy. Given these differences between large cell lymphoma and metastatic colorectal cancer, which one of the following statements is correct?

A. Patients with large cell lymphoma should receive allopurinol before the first cycle of chemotherapy because they are at an elevated risk of developing TLS.

B. Patients with metastatic colorectal cancer should receive allopurinol before the first cycle of chemotherapy because they are at an elevated risk of developing TLS.

C. Patients with large cell lymphoma should receive pamidronate before the first cycle of chemotherapy because they are at an elevated risk of developing hypercalcemia.

D. Patients with metastatic colorectal cancer should receive pamidronate before the first cycle of chemotherapy because they are at an elevated risk of developing hypercalcemia.

12. Consider the information provided above about large cell lymphoma and metastatic colorectal cancer. Patient 1 with large cell lymphoma is receiving CHOP-R (cyclophosphamide, doxorubicin [hydroxydaunomycin], vincristine [Oncovin], prednisone, and rituximab) chemotherapy. Patient 2 with metastatic colorectal cancer is receiving FOLFIRI (5-fluorouracil-leucovorin, irinotecan) chemotherapy. On the day cycle 2 is due, both patients have an ANC of 800 cells/mm³. Which statement is most appropriate given the ANC?

A. Patient 1 should get chemotherapy to keep him on schedule because he has a curable disease.

B. Patient 2 should get chemotherapy to keep him on schedule because he has a curable disease.

C. The chemotherapy for patient 1 should be held for now, and he should receive filgrastim after the next time he has chemotherapy.

D. The chemotherapy for patient 2 should be held for now, and he should receive filgrastim after the next time he has chemotherapy.

13. Sometimes, extravasation is not immediately evident when it occurs. Immediately after patient 1 receives CHOP-R, an extravasation is suspected. Which is the best treatment recommendation for the patient's extravasation?

A. Application of a warm pack for suspected extravasation of doxorubicin.

B. Application of a cold pack for suspected extravasation of vincristine.

C. Application of dimethyl sulfoxide and intravenous dexrazoxane for suspected extravasation of doxorubicin.

D. Application of sodium thiosulfate for suspected extravasation of vincristine.

BPS Pharmacotherapy Specialty Examination Content Outline

This chapter covers the following sections of the Pharmacotherapy Specialty Examination Content Outline:

1. Domain 1: Patient-Centered Pharmacotherapy
   a. Tasks 1, 4
   b. Systems and Patient-Care Problems:
      i. Antiemetics
      ii. Pain Management
      iii. Treatment of Febrile Neutropenia
      iv. Use of CSFs in Neutropenia and Febrile Neutropenia
      v. Thrombocytopenia
      vi. Anemia/Fatigue
      vii. Chemoprotectants
      viii. Oncology Emergencies
      ix. Miscellaneous Antineoplastic Pharmacotherapy
      x. Parathyroid disorders
2. Domain 3: System-Based Standards and Population-Based Pharmacotherapy
   a. Tasks 1, 3, 6

I. ANTIEMETICS

A. Important Definitions Pertaining to Chemotherapy-Induced Nausea and Vomiting (CINV)
   1. Nausea is described as an awareness of discomfort that may or may not precede vomiting; nausea is accompanied by decreased gastric tone and decreased peristalsis.
   2. Retching is the labored movement of abdominal and thoracic muscles associated with vomiting without the expulsion of vomitus and is also called dry heaves.
   3. Vomiting (emesis) is the ejection or expulsion of gastric contents through the mouth.
      a. Acute onset: Occurs 0–24 hours after chemotherapy administration and commonly resolves within 24 hours (intensity peaks after 5–6 hours)
      b. Delayed onset: Occurs more than 24 hours after chemotherapy administration
         i. Delayed symptoms are best described with cisplatin, although they are commonly reported in association with other agents as well (carboplatin or doxorubicin).
         ii. The distinction between acute and delayed symptoms with respect to time of onset is somewhat arbitrary, and it becomes blurred when chemotherapy is administered for many days.
         iii. The importance of the distinction between acute and delayed (and anticipatory) symptoms is that they probably have different mechanisms and therefore different management strategies.
   4. Anticipatory vomiting (or nausea) is triggered by sights, smells, or sounds and is a conditioned response; it is more likely to occur in patients whose previous postchemotherapy nausea and vomiting was not well controlled.
   5. Breakthrough emesis occurs despite prophylactic treatment or necessitates additional rescue medications.
   6. Refractory emesis is emesis that occurs during treatment cycles when antiemetic prophylaxis or rescue therapy has failed in previous cycles.

B. Risk Factors for CINV
   1. Patient-related risk factors
      a. Patient's age (younger than 50 years)
      b. Female sex
      c. History of motion sickness
      d. History of nausea or vomiting during pregnancy
      e. Poor control of nausea or vomiting in previous chemotherapy cycles
      f. History of chronic alcoholism (decreases incidence of emesis)
   2. Emetogenicity of chemotherapy agents: Several schemes for assessing emetogenicity have been proposed.
      a. Originally, emetogenic risk was classified as "none," "mild," "moderate," or "severe."
      b. The Hesketh model, proposed in 1997, classified emetogenic risk as levels ranging from level 1 (less than 10% frequency of emesis) to level 5 (more than 90% frequency of emesis).
      c. Current model includes four levels for intravenous chemotherapy and two levels for oral chemotherapy.
      d. Levels for intravenous chemotherapy (e.g., minimal, low, moderate, high emetogenic risk) are defined by the percentage of patients expected to experience emesis when not receiving antiemetic prophylaxis.
      e. Levels for oral chemotherapy (prophylaxis recommended and as needed)
   3. Radiation therapy can also cause nausea and vomiting. The incidence and severity of radiation-induced nausea and vomiting vary by site of radiation and size of radiation field.
      a. Mildly emetogenic: Radiation to the head and neck or to the extremities
      b. Moderately emetogenic: Radiation to the upper abdomen or pelvis or craniospinal radiation
      c. Highly emetogenic: Total body irradiation, total nodal irradiation, and upper-half-body irradiation

C. General Principles for Managing CINV and Radiation-Induced Nausea and Vomiting

1. Prevention is the key. Prophylactic antiemetics should be administered before moderately or highly emetogenic agents and before moderately and highly emetogenic radiation.

2. Antiemetics should be scheduled for delayed nausea and vomiting for select chemotherapy regimens (e.g., cisplatin, doxorubicin/cyclophosphamide (AC)), and rescue antiemetics should be available if prolonged acute symptoms or ineffective antiemetic prophylaxis occurs.

3. Begin with an appropriate antiemetic regimen based on the emetogenicity of the chemotherapy drugs.

   a. The most common antiemetic regimen for highly emetogenic chemotherapy and radiation is the combination of a neurokinin 1 (NK1) receptor antagonist, a serotonin receptor antagonist, and dexamethasone. Adding a corticosteroid to a serotonin receptor antagonist for highly (or moderately) emetogenic anticancer therapy increases efficacy by 10%–20%. Based on randomized clinical trial data, the AC regimen (see Table 1) should always include a three-drug regimen with an NK1 receptor antagonist, a serotonin receptor antagonist, and dexamethasone.

   b. For moderately emetogenic chemotherapy, the most common antiemetic regimen now includes a serotonin receptor antagonist and dexamethasone. The use of an NK1 receptor antagonist may be considered after risk stratification.

   c. The combination of high-dose metoclopramide and dexamethasone was the most common regimen to prevent delayed nausea and vomiting before the availability of aprepitant. This combination is still used when aprepitant has not been incorporated into the initial regimen for CINV.

   d. Single-agent phenothiazine, butyrophenone, or steroids are used for mildly to moderately emetogenic regimens and are given on either a scheduled or an as-needed basis for prolonged symptoms (i.e., breakthrough symptoms).

   e. Consider using a histamine-2 blocker or proton pump inhibitor (PPI) for dyspepsia (which can mimic nausea).

   f. Cannabinoids are generally used after other regimens have failed or to stimulate appetite.

   g. Agents whose primary indication is other than treatment of nausea and vomiting are being investigated (e.g., olanzapine). Clinically, these agents may be used for patients whose symptoms do not respond to standard antiemetics.

   h. Potential drug interactions between antineoplastic agents or antiemetics and other drugs should always be considered.

   i. Follow-up is essential. The response to the emetogenic regimen should always guide the choice of antiemetic regimen for subsequent therapy courses.

D. Emetogenic Potential of Intravenous Chemotherapy Agents

Table 1. Emetogenic Potential of Intravenous Chemotherapy Agents

High Emetic Risk (>90% frequency of emesis)	
AC (combination defined as either doxorubicin or epirubicin with cyclophosphamide) Carmustine >250 mg/m^2 Cisplatin^a Cyclophosphamide >1500 mg/m^2 Dacarbazine	Doxorubicin >60 mg/m^2 Epirubicin >90 mg/m^2 Ifosfamide ≥2 g/m^2/dose Mechlorethamine Streptozocin
Moderate Emetic Risk (30%–90% frequency of emesis)	
Aldesleukin >12–15 million IU/m^2 Amifostine >300 mg/m^2 Arsenic trioxide Azacitidine Bendamustine Busulfan Carboplatin Carmustine ≤250 mg/m^2 Clofarabine Cyclophosphamide ≤1500 mg/m^{2a} Cytarabine >200 mg/m^2	Dactinomycin Daunorubicin Doxorubicin <60 mg/m^2 Epirubicin ≤90 mg/m^2 Idarubicin Ifosfamide <2 g/m^2/dose Interferon alfa ≥10 million IU/m^2 Irinotecan Melphalan Methotrexate ≥250 mg/m^2 Oxaliplatin Temozolomide
Low Emetic Risk (10%–30% frequency of emesis)	
Ado-trastuzumab emtansine Aldesleukin ≤12 million IU/m^2 Amifostine ≤300 mg/m^2 Belinostat Blinatumomab Brentuximab vedotin Cabazitaxel Carfilzomib Cytarabine (low dose) 100–200 mg/m^2 Docetaxel Doxorubicin (liposomal) Eribulin Etoposide Floxuridine Fluorouracil Gemcitabine	Interferon alfa >5 million IU/m^2 to <10 million IU/m^2 Ixabepilone Methotrexate >50 mg/m^2 to <250 mg/m^2 Mitomycin Mitoxantrone Omacetaxine Paclitaxel Paclitaxel/albumin Pemetrexed Pentostatin Pralatrexate Romidepsin Thiotepa Topotecan Ziv-aflibercept

Table 1. Emetogenic Potential of Intravenous Chemotherapy Agents *(continued)*

Minimal Emetic Risk (<10% frequency of emesis)	
Alemtuzumab	Obinutuzumab
Asparaginase	Ofatumumab
Bevacizumab	Panitumumab
Bleomycin	Pegaspargase
Bortezomib	Peginterferon
Cetuximab	Pembrolizumab
Cladribine (2-chlorodeoxyadenosine)	Pertuzumab
Cytarabine <100 mg/m²	Ramucirumab
Decitabine	Rituximab
Denileukin diftitox	Siltuximab
Dexrazoxane	Temsirolimus
Fludarabine	Trastuzumab
Interferon alfa ≤5 million IU/m²	Valrubicin
Ipilimumab	Vinblastine
Methotrexate ≤50 mg/m²	Vincristine
Nelarabine	Vincristine (liposomal)
Nivolumab	Vinorelbine

ᵃCauses delayed emesis.

E. Emetogenic Potential of Oral Chemotherapy Agents (Table 2)

Table 2. Emetogenic Potential of Oral Chemotherapy Agents

Moderate to High Emetic Risk; Prophylaxis Recommended	
Altretamine	Lomustine (single day)
Busulfan ≥4 mg/day	Mitotane
Ceritinib	Olaparib
Crizotinib	Panobinostat
Cyclophosphamide ≥100 mg/m²/day	Procarbazine
Estramustine	Temozolomide >75 mg/m²/day
Etoposide	Vismodegib
Lenvatinib	

Table 2. Emetogenic Potential of Oral Chemotherapy Agents *(continued)*

Moderate to Low Emetic Risk; As Needed	
Afatinib	Melphalan
Axitinib	Mercaptopurine
Bexarotene	Methotrexate
Bosutinib	Nilotinib
Busulfan <4 mg/day	Palbociclib
Cabozantinib	Pazopanib
Capecitabine	Pomalidomide
Chlorambucil	Ponatinib
Cyclophosphamide <100 mg/m²/day	Regorafenib
Dabrafenib	Ruxolitinib
Dasatinib	Sorafenib
Erlotinib	Sunitinib
Everolimus	Temozolomide ≤75 mg/m²/day
Fludarabine	Thalidomide
Gefitinib	Thioguanine
Hydroxyurea	Topotecan
Ibrutinib	Trametinib
Idelalisib	Tretinoin
Imatinib	Vandetanib
Lapatinib	Vemurafenib
Lenalidomide	Vorinostat

F. Antiemetics
1. Serotonin-3 (5-HT3) receptor antagonists (dolasetron, granisetron, ondansetron, and palonosetron)
   a. Mechanism of action (MOA): Block serotonin receptors peripherally in the gastrointestinal tract and centrally in the medulla
   b. Adverse events: Headache and constipation, occurring in 10%–15% of patients. May increase liver function tests and cause QT prolongation (especially with high dosages or intravenous push administration).
   c. Dolasetron, granisetron, ondansetron, and palonosetron are considered equally efficacious at equivalent dosages. Therefore, the antiemetic drug of choice is often based on cost and organizational contract.
   d. Dosage forms: Granisetron and ondansetron are available in oral and intravenous forms (including an orally disintegrating tablet for ondansetron). Dolasetron is now indicated only in CINV in its oral form. Granisetron is also available in a transdermal patch (34.3 mg applied about 24–48 hours before the first dose of chemotherapy; maximal duration of patch is 7 days).
   e. Palonosetron is indicated to prevent acute CINV for highly emetogenic chemotherapy and acute and delayed CINV for moderately emetogenic chemotherapy.
      i. Half-life: About 40 hours (longer compared with other serotonin antagonists)
      ii. Dosage: 0.25 mg intravenous push 30 minutes before chemotherapy administration
      iii. May be used before the start of a 3-day chemotherapy regimen instead of several daily doses of oral or intravenous serotonin-3 receptor antagonists
      iv. Adverse events: Headache and constipation (same as other serotonin antagonists)

2. Corticosteroids (dexamethasone, methylprednisolone)
   a. MOA: Unknown; thought to act by inhibiting prostaglandin synthesis in the cortex
   b. Adverse effects associated with single doses and short courses of steroids are infrequent; they may include euphoria, anxiety, insomnia, increased appetite, and mild fluid retention; rapid intravenous administration may be associated with transient and intense perineal, vaginal, or anal burning.
   c. Dexamethasone has been studied more often in clinical trials than methylprednisolone.
3. NK1 receptor antagonists (aprepitant, fosaprepitant, rolapitant)
   a. MOA: Aprepitant is a selective high-affinity antagonist of human substance P/NK1.
   b. Aprepitant is approved for use in combination with other antiemetic drugs for preventing acute and delayed nausea and vomiting associated with initial and repeat courses of chemotherapy known to cause these problems, including high-dose cisplatin.
   c. Aprepitant improved the overall complete response (defined as no emetic episodes and no use of rescue therapy) by about 20% when added to a serotonin receptor antagonist and dexamethasone.
   d. Aprepitant dosage: 125 mg on day 1, then 80 mg on day 2 and 80 mg on day 3
   e. Fosaprepitant dosage (prodrug): 150 mg intravenously on day 1 only (intravenous formulation)
   f. Metabolized primarily by cytochrome P450 (CYP) 3A4 with minor metabolism by CYP1A2 and CYP2C19
       i. Oral contraceptives: May reduce the effectiveness of oral contraceptives. Would recommend another form of birth control for women of childbearing age when taking with aprepitant
       ii. Warfarin: May decrease international normalized ratio (clinically significant). After completing a 3-day course of aprepitant, patients should have their international normalized ratios checked within 7–10 days.
       iii. Dexamethasone: May increase area under the curve of dexamethasone. Decrease dosage by about 40% on day 2 or 3 if dexamethasone given orally (not necessary if given intravenously because of first-pass metabolism).
       iv. Caution use in patients with lymphoma: Studies suggest neuropathy is more common in patients on R-CHOP receiving aprepitant, because of aprepitant's CYP3A4 inhibition.
   g. Adverse events: Asthenia, dizziness, and hiccups
   h. MOA: Rolapitant substance P/NK1 receptor antagonist indicated in combination with other antiemetic agents in adults with cancer for the prevention of delayed nausea and vomiting associated with initial and repeat courses of emetogenic cancer chemotherapy, including highly emetogenic chemotherapy.
   i. Rolapitant dosage: 180 mg orally on day 1 only in combination with dexamethasone on days 2 and 3
   j. Adverse events: Loss of appetite, neutropenia, and hiccups
4. NK1 receptor antagonist/serotonin 5-HT3 combination netupitant/palonosetron
   a. MOA: Fixed combination of netupitant, a substance P/NK1 receptor antagonist, and palonosetron, a serotonin-3 (5-HT3) receptor antagonist indicated for the prevention of acute and delayed nausea and vomiting associated with initial and repeat courses of cancer chemotherapy, including highly emetogenic chemotherapy. Oral palonosetron prevents nausea and vomiting during the acute phase, and netupitant prevents nausea and vomiting during both the acute and delayed phases after cancer chemotherapy.
   b. Netupitant/palonosetron dosage: 1 capsule once on day 1 (capsule contains 300 mg of netupitant/palonosetron 0.5 mg)
   c. Adverse effects: Headache, asthenia, dyspepsia, fatigue, constipation, and erythema
   d. Caution in patients with hepatic dysfunction, severe renal impairment, or end-stage renal disease

5. Benzamide analogs (metoclopramide)
   a. MOA: Blockade of dopamine receptors in the chemoreceptor trigger zone; stimulation of cholinergic activity in the gut, increasing (forward) gut motility; and antagonism of peripheral serotonin receptors in the intestines. These effects are dose related.
   b. Adverse events: Mild sedation and diarrhea, as well as extrapyramidal reactions (e.g., dystonia, akathisia), which may be mitigated by diphenhydramine or lorazepam.
   c. High dosages of metoclopramide are used for desired results (1–2 mg/kg intravenously)
6. Phenothiazines (prochlorperazine, chlorpromazine, promethazine)
   a. MOA: Block dopamine receptors in the chemoreceptor trigger zone
   b. Adverse events: Drowsiness, hypotension, akathisia, and dystonia
   c. Chlorpromazine is often preferred in children because it is associated with fewer extrapyramidal reactions than prochlorperazine.
7. Butyrophenones (haloperidol, droperidol)
   a. MOA: Similar to phenothiazines
   b. They are at least as effective as the phenothiazines, and some studies indicate they are superior; they offer a different chemical structure that may bind differently to the dopamine receptor and offer an initial alternative when a phenothiazine fails.
   c. Adverse events: Sedation; hypotension is less common than with phenothiazines; extrapyramidal symptoms are also seen.
   d. The use of droperidol as an antiemetic has fallen out of favor because of the risk of QT prolongation or torsades de pointes.
8. Benzodiazepines (lorazepam)
   a. Lorazepam as a single agent has minimal antiemetic activity. However, several properties make lorazepam useful in combination with or as an adjunct to other antiemetics.
      i. Anterograde amnesia helps prevent anticipatory nausea and vomiting.
      ii. Relief of anxiety
      iii. Management of akathisia caused by phenothiazines, butyrophenones, or metoclopramide
   b. Adverse events: Amnesia, sedation, hypotension, perceptual disturbances, and urinary incontinence. Note that amnesia and sedation may, in fact, be desirable.
9. Atypical antipsychotic (olanzapine)
   a. Approved by the U.S. Food and Drug Administration (FDA) to treat schizophrenia and bipolar disorder, this thienobenzodiazepine is used off label as an alternative agent for preventing nausea and vomiting in highly emetogenic regimens and may be used as an option for breakthrough nausea and vomiting.
   b. MOA: Blocks multiple neurotransmitters, including dopamine, serotonin, catecholamines, acetylcholine, and histamine
   c. Adverse effects: Sedation, dry mouth, increased appetite, weight gain, postural hypotension, QTc prolongation, and dizziness
   d. Olanzapine has been associated with an elevated risk of hyperlipidemia, hyperglycemia, and new-onset diabetes. Use with caution in older adults because olanzapine use in this patient population has been associated with an elevated risk of death and an elevated incidence of cerebrovascular adverse events in patients with dementia-related psychosis (black box warning)
   e. Recently, a phase III study was conducted comparing olanzapine with aprepitant in highly emetogenic chemotherapy regimens. Overall response rates were similar in both groups for acute and delayed nausea and vomiting. The proportion of patients without nausea was similar between the two groups in the acute period but was higher in the olanzapine arm in the delay period, resulting in a higher rate of nausea control. As an alternative to aprepitant, an olanzapine-based regimen may be an option in highly or moderately emetogenic regimens according to the most recent National Comprehensive Cancer Network (NCCN) guidelines.

10. Cannabinoids (dronabinol, nabilone)
   a. MOA: Cannabinoid receptors may mediate at least some of the antiemetic activity of this class of agents. Additional antiemetic mechanisms that have been proposed include inhibition of prostaglandins and blockade of adrenergic activity.
   b. Adverse events: Drowsiness, dizziness, euphoria, dysphoria, orthostatic hypotension, ataxia, hallucinations, and time disorientation. Appetite stimulation is also seen with cannabinoids and may, in fact, be desirable.

G. Emesis Prevention Algorithms (Tables 3 and 4)

Table 3. Emesis Prevention Algorithm for Intravenous Chemotherapy (per NCCN Guidelines)

Level of Emetogenicity	Emesis Treatment Day 1	Emesis Treatment Days 2, 3, and 4
High	Neurokinin-1 antagonist - Aprepitant 125 mg PO - Fosaprepitant 150 mg IV once - Rolapitent 180 mg PO AND Serotonin 5-HT3 antagonist AND Steroid ± Lorazepam ± Histamine-2 blocker or proton pump inhibitor	- If aprepitant PO given day 1, aprepitant 80 mg PO daily on days 2 and 3 - If fosaprepitant given on day 1, no further aprepitant needed on days 2 and 3. Dexamethasone dosage is twice daily on days 3 and 4. AND steroid until day 4
	OR Netupitant-containing regimen - Netupitant 300 mg/palonosetron 0.5 mg PO once - Dexamethasone 12 mg PO/IV ± Lorazepam ± Histamine-2 blocker or proton pump inhibitor	OR Dexamethasone 8 mg PO/IV daily on days 2 and 3
	OR Olanzapine-containing regimen: 1. Olanzapine 10 mg PO day 1 2. Palonosetron 0.25 mg IV day 1 3. Dexamethasone 20 mg IV day 1 ± Lorazepam ± Histamine-2 blocker or proton pump inhibitor	OR Olanzapine-containing regimen: Olanzapine 10 mg PO days 2–4 (if given day 1)

Table 3. Emesis Prevention Algorithm for Intravenous Chemotherapy (per NCCN Guidelines) *(continued)*

Level of Emetogenicity	Emesis Treatment Day 1	Emesis Treatment Days 2, 3, and 4

Moderate	Serotonin 5-HT3 antagonist
	
	AND
	
	Steroid
	
	WITH/WITHOUT
	
	Neurokinin-1 antagonist
	± Lorazepam
	± Histamine-2 blocker or proton pump inhibitor
	
	OR
	
	Netupitant-containing regimen
	  - Netupitant 300 mg/palonosetron 0.5 mg PO once
	  - Dexamethasone 12 mg PO/IV
	± Lorazepam
	± Histamine-2 blocker or proton pump inhibitor
	
	OR
	
	Olanzapine-containing regimen:
	  1. Olanzapine 10 mg PO day 1
	  2. Palonosetron 0.25 mg IV day 1
	  3. Dexamethasone 20 mg IV day 1
	± Lorazepam
	± Histamine-2 blocker or proton pump inhibitor
		Serotonin 5-HT3 antagonist
		
		OR
		
		Steroid monotherapy daily on days 2 and 3
		
		OR
		
		Neurokinin-1 antagonist
		
		OR
		
		Dexamethasone 8 mg PO/IV daily on days 2 and 3
		
		OR
		
		Olanzapine-containing regimen:
		Olanzapine 10 mg PO days 2–4 (if given day 1)

Level of Emetogenicity	Emesis Treatment Day 1	Emesis Treatment Days 2–3
Low	Steroid OR Metoclopramide as needed OR Prochlorperazine as needed OR Serotonin-3 antagonists (oral therapy) daily ± Lorazepam ± Histamine-2 blocker or proton pump inhibitor	Steroid OR Metoclopramide as needed OR Prochlorperazine as needed OR Serotonin-3 antagonists (oral therapy) daily ± Lorazepam ± Histamine-2 blocker or proton pump inhibitor
Minimal	No routine prophylaxis	No routine prophylaxis

IV = intravenous(ly); PO = by mouth

Table 4. Emesis Prevention Algorithm for Oral Chemotherapy per NCCN Guidelines

Level of Emetogenicity	Emesis Treatment (start before chemotherapy and continue daily)
High to moderate emetic risk	Serotonin-3 antagonist (choose one): Dolasetron 100 mg daily Granisetron 2 mg PO daily or 1 mg PO BID Ondansetron 16–24 mg PO daily ± Lorazepam ± Histamine-2 blocker or proton pump inhibitor
Low to minimal emetic risk	Metoclopramide 10–40 mg PO and then q4h or q6h PRN Prochlorperazine 10 mg PO or IV and then q6h PRN (maximum 40 mg/day) OR Haloperidol 1–2 mg PO and then q4h or q6h PRN OR Serotonin-3 antagonist (choose one): Dolasetron 100 mg daily Granisetron 2 mg PO daily or 1 mg PO BID Ondansetron 16–24 mg PO daily ± Lorazepam ± Histamine-2 blocker or proton pump inhibitor

BID = twice daily; h = hours; IV = intravenous; PO = by mouth; PRN = as needed; q4h = every 4 hours; q6h = every 6 hours.

Patient Cases

1. A 60-year-old woman was recently given a diagnosis of advanced non–small cell lung cancer. She will begin treatment with cisplatin 100 mg/m² plus vinorelbine 30 mg/m². Which is the most appropriate antiemetic regimen for preventing acute emesis?

    A. Aprepitant plus palonosetron plus dexamethasone.

    B. Aprepitant plus prochlorperazine plus dexamethasone.

    C. Aprepitant plus granisetron plus ondansetron.

    D. Lorazepam plus ondansetron plus metoclopramide.

2. Which is the most appropriate regimen for anticipatory nausea and vomiting?

    A. Aprepitant plus dexamethasone.

    B. Aprepitant plus metoclopramide.

    C. Ondansetron plus dexamethasone.

    D. Aprepitant plus ondansetron plus dexamethasone plus lorazepam.

II. PAIN MANAGEMENT

A. Principles of Cancer Pain Management
1. The most important step in treating pain is the assessment.
2. The oral route is preferred when available. Although the ratio of oral to parenteral potency of morphine is commonly noted to be 6:1, clinical observation of chronic morphine use indicates that this ratio is closer to 3:1.
3. Choose the analgesic drug and dosage to match the patient's degree of pain.
4. For persistent severe pain, use a product with a long duration of action. Pain medications should always be administered on a scheduled basis or around the clock, not as needed.
    a. It is always easier to prevent pain from recurring than to treat it once it has recurred.
    b. As-needed dosing should be used for breakthrough pain, which is pain that "breaks through" the regularly scheduled opioid; an immediate-release, short-acting opioid should always accompany a long-acting opioid.
5. Reevaluate pain and pain relief often, especially when initiating pain therapy; if more than two as-needed doses are necessary for breakthrough pain in a 24-hour period, consider modifying the regimen. Before adding or changing to another drug, maximize the dosage and schedule of the current analgesic drug.
6. Provide medications to prevent other potential side effects from opioid therapy (e.g., constipation).
7. Use appropriate adjuvant analgesics and nondrug measures to maximize pain control.

B. Diagnosis and Assessment of Pain
1. Best addressed by proper pain assessment including comprehensive history and physical examination
2. Evaluation of pain management: Pain intensity, pain relief, and medication adverse effects or allergies must be assessed and reassessed.
3. Objective observations such as grimacing, limping, or tachycardia may be helpful in assessment.
4. Clinicians must accept the patient's report of pain.

C. Pain Rating Scales
1. Use pain assessment tools to evaluate pain intensity at baseline and to assess how well a pain medication regimen is working.
    a. Numeric rating scale of 0–10, with 0 = no pain and 10 = worst pain imaginable
    b. Pediatric patients: Faces-of-Pain Scale, poker chip method
2. Because pain is subjective, it is best evaluated by the patient (i.e., not a caregiver and not the health professional).

D. Treatment of Pain: The Analgesic Ladder
1. For mild to moderate pain (pain rating of 1–3 on a 10-point scale), the first step is a nonopioid analgesic drug: Nonsteroidal anti-inflammatory drug (NSAID), aspirin, or acetaminophen (APAP), or consider slow titration of short-acting opioids either as needed or as scheduled.
2. For persistent or moderate to severe pain (pain rating of 4–6 on a 10-point scale), add a weak opioid: Codeine or hydrocodone, available in combination with nonopioid analgesic drugs. Slow titration of a short-acting opioid may also be considered.
3. For persistent or for severe pain (pain rating of 7–10 on a 10-point scale), replace the weak opioid with a strong opioid: Morphine, oxycodone, or similar drug. In opioid-naive patients experiencing severe pain, short-acting opioids should be rapidly titrated. Once a patient with persistent pain is taking stable dosages of short-acting opioids, the drug should be changed to an extended-release or long-acting formulation with breakthrough short-acting opioids.

E. Nonopioid Analgesics: NSAIDs
   1. MOA: Act peripherally to inhibit the activity of prostaglandins in the pain pathway
   2. There is a ceiling effect to the analgesia provided by NSAIDs.
   3. Adverse events: Consider inhibition of platelet aggregation and the effects of inhibition of renal prostaglandins. NSAIDs in patients with hematologic disorders are not recommended because of platelet inhibition. In addition, there are concerns about the possibility that NSAIDs will mask fever in a patient with neutropenia who is potentially febrile.
   4. Remember, NSAIDs are generally used in addition to, not instead of, opioids.
   5. NSAIDs are often used for patients with cancer and metastatic bone pain.

F. Nonopioid/Opioid Combinations
   1. Aspirin or APAP or ibuprofen plus codeine or hydrocodone or oxycodone is the most commonly used combination.
   2. Be aware of the risk of APAP overdose with these products. As with any combination product, dosage escalation of one component necessitates escalation of the others. For patients needing high dosages, pure opioids are preferred.
   3. Oxycodone/APAP is available in several strengths; however, the amount of APAP increases with increasing oxycodone.

G. Opioid Analgesics
   1. Mechanism: Opioids act centrally in the brain (periaqueductal gray region) and at the level of the spinal cord (dorsal horn) at specific opioid receptors.
   2. The opioids have no analgesic ceiling.
   3. Morphine
      a. Morphine is the standard with which all other drugs are compared; opioids may differ in duration of action, relative potency, oral effectiveness, and adverse event profiles, but none is clinically superior to morphine.
      b. Flexibility in dosage forms and administration routes: Oral (sustained release, immediate release), sublingual, intravenous, intrathecal/epidural, subcutaneous, and rectal
      c. Long duration of action: Sustained-release products last 8–12 hours or, for some preparations, 24 hours.
      d. Morphine is one of the least expensive opioids but should be used with caution in patients with renal dysfunction because of the metabolite.
   4. Oxycodone
      a. Available in oral formulation only
      b. Available as a single drug (i.e., not in combination) in both long- and short-acting formulations
      c. Alternative to morphine in the setting of renal dysfunction
   5. Fentanyl
      a. Fentanyl is available as an intravenous formulation; a sublingual, intranasal, or transdermal preparation; an oral transmucosal preparation; and a buccal tablet. Transmucosal and buccal fentanyl are used for breakthrough pain.
      b. Each transdermal patch provides sustained release of drug and can provide pain relief for 48–72 hours. These should not be used in opioid-naive patients.
      c. Consider the implications for dosing transdermal fentanyl in cachectic patients: Fentanyl initially forms a depot in subcutaneous tissue, and patients with little or no fat may not achieve pain relief.
      d. Slow onset and long elimination after patch application and removal, respectively
      e. Bioavailability is greater with buccal tablets than with the transmucosal preparation; thus, equivalent dosages are higher for transmucosal and lower for buccal tablets.

6. Hydromorphone
   a. Available in intravenous and oral formulations (short- and long-acting)
   b. Considered a semisynthetic compound
   c. Alternative to morphine with higher potency
   d. Alterative option in patients with renal dysfunction
7. Oxymorphone
   a. Semisynthetic opioid analgesic
   b. Most commonly seen as immediate- and extended-release tablets
   c. Used for moderate to severe pain
   d. Should not be implemented in patients who are not currently on an opioid regimen
8. Methadone
   a. Semisynthetic used in maintenance treatment for opioid-dependent patients and as an effective analgesic in patients taking opioids long term for moderate to severe pain
   b. Has activity not only at the opioid receptors but also at the N-methyl-D-aspartate receptor, which may confer benefit to patients with neuropathic pain
   c. Complex pharmacokinetics with extended half-life (8–59 hours), which creates difficulties in dosing and transitioning from one opioid to another
   d. Associated with QT prolongation and torsades de pointes
   e. Effective long-acting agent also used for neuropathic pain
   f. Start low and titrate slowly (only escalating after 3–5 days) because of the changing conversion ratios with increasing morphine equivalents.

H. Adverse Events
   1. Sedation: Tolerance usually develops within several days; remember that more sedation may be expected in a patient who has been unable to sleep because of uncontrolled pain. For patients who do not develop tolerance to sedation and have good pain control, a dosage reduction may be considered. If dosage reduction compromises pain control, adding a stimulant (e.g., dextroamphetamine, methylphenidate) may be considered. Other central nervous system adverse events include dysphoria and hallucinations.
   2. Constipation is very common, and tolerance does not develop to this effect. Decreased intestinal peristalsis is caused by decreased intestinal tone; delayed gastric emptying may also occur. Regular use of stool softeners in addition to a stimulant laxatives is imperative to manage constipation.
   3. Nausea and vomiting are common. As seen with sedation, tolerance develops within about a week. Nausea and vomiting may have a vestibular component, developing as pain relief promotes increased mobility. Antivertigo agents (e.g., meclizine, dimenhydrate) may be useful in managing the vestibular component, although these agents should be used with caution because combination use with opioids may increase sedation. Nausea and vomiting may also occur because of stimulation of the chemoreceptor trigger zone. Drugs that block dopamine receptors (e.g., phenothiazines) provide relief of this component of nausea and vomiting until tolerance develops.
   4. Urinary retention and bladder spasm are more common in older adults and in patients taking long-acting formulations.

I. Bisphosphonates
   1. Bisphosphonates decrease the worsening of pain by preventing disease progression in the bone and the number of skeletal-related events in patients with breast cancer and multiple myeloma when given for 1 year. Skeletal-related events include pathologic fracture, need for radiation therapy to bone, surgery to bone, and spinal cord compression.

2. In 2000, the American Society of Clinical Oncology published initial guidelines for the use of bisphosphonates in breast cancer (updated in November 2003).

    a. It is recommended that patients with breast cancer who have evidence of bone metastases on plain radiographs receive either pamidronate 90 mg delivered over 2 hours or zoledronic acid 4 mg over 15 minutes every 3–4 weeks. Dosage adjustments for renal dysfunction are necessary according to package insert recommendations.

    b. Women with abnormal bone scan and abnormal computed tomographic scan or magnetic resonance imaging showing bone destruction but a normal radiograph should also receive the above-recommended bisphosphonates.

    c. Therapy should continue until there is evidence of a substantial decline in a patient's performance status.

    d. Bisphosphonates may be used in combination with other pain therapies in patients with pain caused by osteolytic disease.

3. In 2002, the American Society of Clinical Oncology published guidelines for the use of bisphosphonates in multiple myeloma.

    a. Patients with lytic bone destruction seen on plain radiographs should receive either pamidronate 90 mg intravenously over at least 2 hours or zoledronic acid 4 mg over 15 minutes every 3–4 weeks.

    b. Therapy should continue until there is evidence of substantial decline in a patient's performance status.

    c. Patients with osteopenia but no radiologic evidence of bone metastases can receive bisphosphonates.

    d. Bisphosphonates are not recommended for patients with solitary plasmacytoma, smoldering or indolent myeloma, or monoclonal gammopathy of undetermined significance.

    e. Bisphosphonates may be used in patients with pain caused by osteolytic disease.

4. Adverse events: Low-grade fevers, nausea, anorexia, vomiting, hypomagnesemia, hypocalcemia, hypokalemia, and nephrotoxicity

    a. Serum creatinine should be monitored before each dose (see package insert for specific recommendations).

    b. Package insert recommends initiating patients on oral calcium 500 mg plus vitamin D 400 IU/day to prevent hypocalcemia.

    c. Several reports of osteonecrosis of the jaw occurring in patients receiving bisphosphonates have appeared in the literature. Osteonecrosis of the jaw usually follows a dental or dental disorder. The long half-life of bisphosphonates in bone makes this adverse event difficult to prevent and manage. Patient education and education of dentists are important. Patients should have a dental examination with preventive dentistry before treatment with bisphosphonates.

J. Receptor Activator of NF-κB Ligand (RANKL) Inhibitor

    1. Denosumab: Fully human monoclonal antibody that targets and inhibits RANKL, a protein that acts as the primary signal to promote bone removal

    2. Indication: Prevention of skeletal-related events in patients with bone metastases from solid tumors

    3. Dosage: 120 mg subcutaneously every 4 weeks

    4. Adverse events: Urinary and respiratory tract infections, cataracts, constipation, rashes, hypocalcemia (especially in patients with CrCl less than 30 mL/minute), and joint pain

    5. Contraindications: Hypocalcemia. Patients should be taking calcium and vitamin D.

    6. No adjustment for hepatic or renal dysfunction is needed.

K. Adjuvant analgesics are drugs whose primary indication is other than pain; they are used to manage specific pain syndromes. Most often, adjuvant analgesics are used in addition to, rather than instead of, opioids.
1. Antidepressants (e.g., amitriptyline, duloxetine) and anticonvulsants (e.g., gabapentin, carbamazepine, pregabalin) are used for neuropathic pain (e.g., phantom limb pain, nerve compression caused by tumor).
2. Transdermal lidocaine is useful in localized neuropathic pain.
3. Corticosteroids are useful in pain caused by nerve compression or inflammation, lymphedema, bone pain, or elevated intracranial pressure.
4. Benzodiazepines: Diazepam, lorazepam. Useful for muscle spasms; baclofen is another alternative for intractable muscle spasms.
5. Strontium-89: Radionuclide for treatment of bone pain caused by osteoblastic lesions; a single dose may provide relief for several weeks or even months; however, it is myelosuppressive.
6. NSAIDs are recommended for treating pain caused by bone metastases. Prostaglandins sensitize nociceptors (pain receptors) to painful stimuli, thus providing a rationale for using NSAIDs.

L. Risk Evaluation and Mitigation Strategy (REMS) for Extended-Release/Long-Acting Opioid Analgesics
1. On June 9, 2012, the FDA announced it would require manufacturers of extended-release and long-acting opioid analgesics to provide training for health care professionals who prescribe these agents.
2. Components of the REMS program
    a. Prescriber education: Information on extended-release or long-acting opioid analgesics; information on assessing patients for treatment with these drugs; initiating therapy, modifying dosing, and discontinuing use of extended-release or long-acting opioid analgesics; managing therapy and monitoring patients; and counseling patients and caregivers about the safe use of these drugs. Prescribers will also learn how to recognize evidence of potential opioid misuse, abuse, and addiction.
    b. Patient counseling: Patient counseling documents for providers will be developed to assist prescribers in counseling patients about their responsibilities for using these medications safely. Patients will receive an updated medication guide, together with their prescription, that contains information on the safe use and disposal of extended-release or long-acting opioid analgesics from their pharmacist. Guide will include instructions for patients to consult their health care professional before changing dosages, signs of potential overdose and emergency contact instructions, and advice on safe storage to prevent accidental exposure of family members.
    c. Short-acting opioid products are not included in this program.

Patient Cases

3. A 75-year-old man has metastatic prostate cancer. The main sites of metastatic disease are regional lymph nodes and bone (several hip lesions). He experiences aching pain with occasional shooting pains. The latter are thought to be the result of nerve compression by enlarged lymph nodes. He has been taking oxycodone/APAP 5 mg 2 tablets every 4 hours and ibuprofen 400 mg every 8 hours. His current pain rating is 8/10, and he states that his pain cannot be controlled. Which is the best recommendation to manage his pain at this time?

    A. Increase oxycodone/APAP to 7.5 mg/325 mg, 2 tablets every 4 hours.

    B. Increase oxycodone/APAP to 10 mg/325 mg, 2 tablets every 4 hours.

    C. Discontinue oxycodone/APAP, discontinue ibuprofen, and add morphine sustained release every 12 hours.

    D. Discontinue oxycodone/APAP and add morphine sustained release every 12 hours.

4. Which is the most appropriate adjunctive medication for this patient's pain?

    A. Naproxen.

    B. Single-agent (single ingredient) APAP.

    C. Gabapentin.

    D. Baclofen.

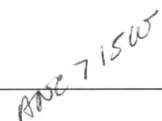

III. TREATMENT OF FEBRILE NEUTROPENIA

    A. Principles of Chemotherapy-Induced Bone Marrow Suppression

      1. Bone marrow suppression is the most common dose-limiting toxicity associated with traditional cytotoxic chemotherapy.

      2. WBC = a normal range of 4.8–10.8 × 100 cells/mm³ with a circulating life span of 6–12 hours; decreased WBC = neutropenia, leucopenia, or granulocytopenia; the risk is life-threatening infections; the risk increases with absolute neutrophil count (ANC) less than 500 cells/mm³, and the risk is greatest with ANC less than 100 cells/mm³. Because neutrophils have the fastest turnover, the effects of cytotoxic chemotherapy are greatest on neutrophils (compared with platelets or red blood cells [RBCs]).

        a. The nadir (usually described by the ANC) is the lowest value to which the blood count falls after cytotoxic chemotherapy. Usually occurs 10–14 days after chemotherapy administration, with counts usually recovering by 3–4 weeks after chemotherapy; exceptions include mitomycin, decitabine, and nitrosoureas (carmustine and lomustine), which have nadirs of 28–42 days after chemotherapy and recovery of neutrophils 6–8 weeks after treatment

        b. ANC = WBC × percentage granulocytes or neutrophils (segmented neutrophils plus band neutrophils). Example: A patient's WBC = 4500 cells/mm³ with 10% segmented neutrophils and 5% band neutrophils. What is the ANC? 4500 × (0.1 + 0.05) = 675 cells/m³.

        c. To receive chemotherapy, a patient should have a WBC greater than 3000 cells/mm³ or an ANC greater than 1500 cells/mm³ and a platelet count of 100,000 cells/mm³ or more. These are general guidelines; some protocols and FDA labels or package inserts specify different (lower) thresholds for administering chemotherapy; if cytopenia is attributable to disease in the bone marrow, chemotherapy (full dose) may cause improvement; some drugs are nonmyelosuppressive (e.g., vincristine, bleomycin, monoclonal antibodies).

        d. The potential curability of the disease influences what action will be taken during the next cycle of chemotherapy, either dosage reduction of myelosuppressive chemotherapy or support with a CSF.

      3. Other factors affecting myelosuppression include previous chemotherapy, previous radiation therapy, and direct bone marrow involvement by tumor.

B. Neutropenia and Febrile Neutropenia
1. Infectious Diseases Society of America guidelines for antibiotic use were updated in 2010.
2. Neutropenia is defined as an ANC of 500 cells/mm³ or less or a count of less than 1000 cells/mm³, with a predicted decrease to less than 500 cells/mm³ during the next 48 hours.
3. Febrile neutropenia is defined as neutropenia and a single oral temperature of 101°F or more or a temperature of 100.4°F or more for at least 1 hour.
4. Neutropenic patients are at an elevated risk of developing serious and life-threatening infections.
5. The usual signs and symptoms of infection (e.g., abscess, pus, infiltrates on chest radiograph) are absent, with fever often being the only indicator. In addition, cultures are negative more often than not. Therefore, prompt investigation and treatment of febrile neutropenia are essential.
6. The initial assessment of patients with febrile neutropenia includes a risk assessment for complications and severe infection.
    a. Characteristics of low-risk neutropenia include the following: ANC of 100 cells/mm³ or more and absolute monocyte count of 100 cells/mm³ or more, normal chest radiograph, almost normal renal and hepatic function, neutropenia for less than 7 days and resolution expected in less than 10 days, no intravenous access site or catheter site infection, early evidence of bone marrow recovery, malignancy in remission, peak oral temperature of less than 102°F, no neurologic or mental status changes, no appearance of illness, absence of abdominal pain, and no comorbid complications (e.g., shock, hypoxia, pneumonia, other deep organ infection, vomiting, diarrhea).
    b. The Multinational Association for Supportive Care in Cancer has developed a scoring index to help identify patients with low-risk febrile neutropenia. Scores are assessed on the basis of factors such as those listed above.
    c. Febrile neutropenia that is considered to carry a low risk of complications may be treated with either oral or intravenous antibiotics in an outpatient or inpatient setting.
    d. Patients with high-risk febrile neutropenia (i.e., patients who do not have low-risk characteristics as noted above) should receive intravenous antibiotics in the hospital.
7. Considerations in the initial selection of an antibiotic include the potential infecting organism, potential sites and source of infection, local antimicrobial susceptibilities, organ dysfunction potentially affecting antibiotic clearance or toxicity, and drug allergy. The most common source of infection is endogenous flora, which could be gram-negative or gram-positive bacteria; the more prolonged the neutropenia (and the more prolonged the administration of antibacterial antibiotics), the greater chance of fungi playing a role in the infection.
8. All patients should be reassessed after 3–5 days of antibiotic therapy, and antibiotics should be adjusted accordingly.
9. Prophylactic antibiotics (fluoroquinolones, TMP/SMX) may be considered for patients who are receiving chemotherapy who are expected to be profoundly neutropenic for more than 7 days.

IV. USE OF COLONY-STIMULATING FACTORS IN NEUTROPENIA AND FEBRILE NEUTROPENIA

A. CSFs improve both the production and function of their target cells. Four products and one biosimilar are currently available in the United States: Granulocyte colony-stimulating factor (G-CSF, or filgrastim [Neupogen]) or tbo-filgrastim (Granix), pegylated granulocyte colony-stimulating factor (pegfilgrastim, or PEG G-CSF) granulocyte-macrophage colony-stimulating factor (GM-CSF, sargramostim [Leukine]), and filgrastim-sndz (Zarxio).

B. Pegfilgrastim, the long-acting agent, is approved for use in patients with nonmyeloid malignancies who are receiving myelosuppressive chemotherapy associated with a high incidence of febrile neutropenia.

C. Studies have shown that G-CSF and GM-CSF reduce the incidence, magnitude, and duration of neutropenia after chemotherapy and bone marrow transplantation.

D. Guidelines for the use of CSFs were established by the American Society of Clinical Oncology in 1994; the most recent update was published in 2006.

E. CSFs are recommended with chemotherapy regimens associated with a 20% or greater risk of febrile neutropenia.
   1. G-CSF, tbo-filgrastim, GM-CSF, and filgrastim-sndz are given by daily subcutaneous injection.
   2. To date, no large trials have compared G-CSF and GM-CSF. Therefore, although it cannot be stated unequivocally that the two are therapeutically equivalent, they are often used interchangeably. However, they have varying adverse effect profiles (increased in fluid retention and fevers with GM-CSF).
   3. A meta-analysis of tbo-filgrastim and filgrastim resulted in tbo-filgrastim being noninferior to filgrastim for reducing the incidence of febrile neutropenia. Toxicities are considered similar between the two agents.
   4. Pegfilgrastim is given as a single 6-mg subcutaneous dose, generally administered 24 hours after chemotherapy. Pegfilgrastim on-body injector is also available for administration in the outpatient setting.
   5. A single dose of pegfilgrastim is as effective as 11 daily doses of G-CSF 5 mcg/kg in reducing the frequency and duration of severe neutropenia, promoting neutrophil recovery, and reducing the frequency of febrile neutropenia.
   6. Tbo-filgrastim was approved in an original biologics license application by the FDA in 2012. The FDA has not approved tbo-filgrastim as a biosimilar to Neupogen (filgrastim). Tbo-filgrastim is administered at 5 mcg/kg daily.
   7. Filgrastim-sndz was the first biosimilar approved by the FDA (March 2015). Filgrastim-sndz is also administered at 5 mcg/kg daily.
   8. The choice of CSF (pegfilgrastim vs. filgrastim) should be based on the expected duration of neutropenia and the specific anticancer regimen (e.g., short courses of a daily CSF rather than one dose of pegfilgrastim) with chemotherapy administration on a weekly schedule.
   9. Adverse events associated with all three preparations appear similar; they include bone pain (most common) and fever.
   10. The CSF should be initiated between 24 and 72 hours after the completion of chemotherapy.
   11. The package literature recommends continued administration of G-CSF until the postnadir ANC is greater than 10,000 cells/mm^3; however, both G-CSF and GM-CSF are usually discontinued when adequate neutrophil recovery is evident. To decrease cost without compromising patient outcome, many centers continue the CSF until ANC is greater than 2000–5000 cells/mm^3. Note that the ANC will decrease about 50% per day after the CSF is discontinued if the marrow has not recovered (i.e., if the CSF is discontinued before the ANC nadir is reached).
   12. Avoid the concomitant use of CSF in patients receiving chemotherapy and radiation therapy; the potential exists for worsening myelosuppression.

F. Refer to the American Society of Clinical Oncology Guidelines for the following indications: increasing chemotherapy dosage intensity, using as adjuncts to progenitor cell transplantation, administering to patients with myeloid malignancies, and using in pediatric populations.

G. American Society of Clinical Oncology Guidelines for Secondary CSF Administration
1. If chemotherapy administration has been delayed or the dosage reduced because of prolonged neutropenia, then CSF use can be considered for subsequent chemotherapy cycles; administering CSF in this setting is considered secondary prophylaxis.
2. Dosage reduction of chemotherapy should be considered the first option (i.e., instead of a CSF) after an episode of neutropenia in patients being treated with the intent to palliate (i.e., not a curative intent).

H. Use of CSFs for Treatment of Established Neutropenia
1. Administering CSFs in patients who are neutropenic but not febrile is not recommended.
2. Administering CSFs in patients who are neutropenic and febrile may be considered in the presence of risk factors for complications (e.g., ANC less than 100 cells/mm^3, pneumonia, hypotension, multi-organ dysfunction, invasive fungal infection); CSFs may be used in addition to antibiotics to treat neutropenia in patients with these risk factors.

Patient Cases

5. A 50-year-old woman is receiving adjuvant chemotherapy for stage II breast cancer. She received her third cycle of AC 10 days ago. Her CBC today includes WBC 600 cells/mm^3, segmented neutrophils 60%, band neutrophils 10%, monocytes 12%, basophils 8%, and eosinophils 10%. She is afebrile. Which best represents this patient's ANC?

   A. 600 cells/mm^3.

   B. 360 cells/mm^3.

   C. 240 cells/mm^3.

   D. 420 cells/mm^3.

6. Given this ANC, which statement is most appropriate?

   A. The patient should be initiated on a CSF.

   B. The patient should begin prophylactic treatment with either a quinolone antibiotic or trimethoprim/sulfamethoxazole.

   C. The patient, who is neutropenic, should be monitored closely for signs and symptoms of infection.

   D. Decrease the dosages of AC with the next cycle of treatment.

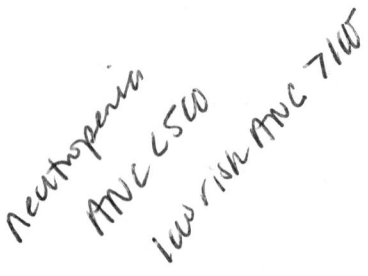

V. THROMBOCYTOPENIA

A. Megakaryocytes (platelets) = a normal range of 140,000–440,000 cells/mm³ with a circulating life span of 5–10 days.

B. Thrombocytopenia is defined as a platelet count less than 100,000 cells/mm³; however, the risk of bleeding is not substantially elevated until the platelet count is 20,000 cells/mm³ or less. Practices for platelet transfusion vary widely from institution to institution. Many institutions do not transfuse platelets until the patient becomes symptomatic (ecchymosis, petechiae, hemoptysis, or hematemesis). Other institutions transfuse when the platelet count is 10,000 cells/mm³ or less, even in the absence of bleeding.

C. Oprelvekin (interleukin-11) is approved to prevent severe thrombocytopenia in patients undergoing chemotherapy for nonmyeloid malignancies.
   1. Oprelvekin is administered as a daily subcutaneous injection, beginning 6–24 hours after completion of myelosuppressive chemotherapy.
   2. Treatment is continued until a postnadir platelet count of 50,000 cells/mm³ or greater is achieved; dosing beyond 21 days is not recommended, and oprelvekin must be discontinued at least 2 days before (the next cycle of) chemotherapy.
   3. The current role of oprelvekin is to maintain the dosage intensity of chemotherapy, although it is not nearly as widely used as the CSFs for neutrophils. A pharmacoeconomic analysis (from the payer's perspective) did not show oprelvekin to be a cost-saving strategy compared with routine platelet transfusions for patients with severe chemotherapy-induced thrombocytopenia.
   4. Common adverse events associated with oprelvekin include edema, shortness of breath, tachycardia or arrhythmias, and conjunctival redness.
   5. Although commercially available, oprelvekin is not currently used in clinical practice.

VI. ANEMIA AND FATIGUE

A. Overview of Anemia
   1. Occurs in 3.4 million Americans each year and most common in women, African Americans, and older adults
   2. Defined as hemoglobin (Hgb) less than 13 g/dL in men or 12 g/dL in women
   3. Anemia defined as a reduction of RBC mass, number of RBCs, and Hgb concentration of RBCs
   4. Caused by a deficiency, impaired bone marrow function, and peripheral causes.
   5. Signs and symptoms of anemia include weakness and fatigue, irritability, tachycardia and palpitations, shortness of breath, chest pain, pale appearance, dizziness, decreased mental acuity, ecchymoses, blood in urine or stool, and hematomas.
   6. There are several types of anemia, including microcytic (iron deficiency anemia), macrocytic/megaloblastic anemia (vitamin B_{12} deficiency, folic acid deficiency), anemia of chronic disease (including chemotherapy-induced anemia), anemia of critical illness, hemolytic anemias, and drug-induced anemias.
   7. Hematologic laboratory values:

Table 5. Hematologic Laboratory Values

Test	Reference Range	Definition
Hgb	M 13.5 - 17.5 g/dL F 12 - 16 g/dL	Hemoglobin per volume of whole blood
Hct	M 41%–53% F 36%–46%	Percentage of total blood volume composed of RBCs (3 × Hgb)
MCV	80–96 fL	Average volume of RBCs (Hct/RBC)
MCHC	31%–37%	Weight of Hgb per volume (Hgb/Hct)
MCH	26–34 pg	Percentage volume of Hgb in RBC (Hgb/RBC)
RBC	4.5–5.9 million/m3	RBCs per unit blood
Reticulocyte count	0.5%–1.5%	Immature RBCs
RDW	11%–16%	RBC distribution width
EPO	0–19 mU/mL	Endogenous erythropoietin
Serum iron	M 50–160 mcg/dL F 12–150 mcg/dL	Concentration of iron bound to transferrin
TIBC	250–400 mcg/dL	Iron binding capacity of transferrin
Ferritin	M 15–200 ng/mL F 12–150 ng/mL	Stored iron concentration
Folate	1.8–1.6 ng/mL	Serum folic acid
Vitamin B12	100–900 pg/mL	Serum vitamin B12
Transferrin saturation	>30%	Serum iron divided by TIBC

EPO = erythropoietin; F = female; Hct = hematocrit; Hgb = hemoglobin; M = male; MCH = mean corpuscular hemoglobin; MCHC = mean corpuscular hemoglobin concentration; MCV = mean corpuscular volume; RBC = red blood cells; RDW = RBC distribution width; TIBC = iron binding capacity of transferrin.

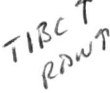

B. Microcytic Anemia

1. Iron deficiency is the most common nutritional deficiency, with laboratory values reflecting a decreased RBC, Hgb/Hct, mean corpuscular volume (MCV), mean corpuscular hemoglobin concentration (MCHC), iron, ferritin, and transferrin. Total iron binding capacity (TIBC) and RBC distribution width (RDW) are increased.

2. Treatment includes oral iron supplementation: 200 mg elemental iron divided twice daily or three times daily for 3–6 months.

3. Available oral iron products (multiple branded agents):

Table 6. Available Oral Iron Products (multiple branded agents):

Product	% Elemental	Elemental Iron
Ferrous sulfate 325 mg tablet	20%	65 mg
Ferrous gluconate 325 mg tablet	12%	39 mg
Ferrous fumarate 100 mg tablet	33%	33 mg
Polysaccharide iron complex 150 mg capsule	100%	150 mg
Carbonyl iron 50 mg caplet	100%	50 mg

4. Iron side effects include constipation and nausea or vomiting.

5. Iron products should be taken with food to avoid gastrointestinal discomfort (but absorption will be decreased). Vitamin C may increase the absorption of iron and is often used to increase the efficacy of iron products. Iron therapy may cause dark stools.

6. Parental iron products:

Table 7. Parental Iron Products

	Iron Dextran	**Sodium Ferric Gluconate**	**Iron Sucrose**	**Ferumoxytol**
Elemental iron	50 mg/mL	62.5 mg/5 mL	20 mg/mL	30 mg/mL
Preservative	None	Benzyl alcohol 9 mg/5 mL 20%	None	None
Indication	IDA where PO not an option	IDA in patients on chronic HD receiving EPO	IDA in patients on chronic HD receiving EPO	IDA with CKD
Warning	Boxed warning: anaphylactic type reactions	Hypersensitivity reactions	Boxed warning: anaphylactic type reactions	Hypersensitivity reactions
IM injection	Yes	No	Yes	No
Usual dosage	100 mg IV push (no faster than 50 mg/min)	125 mg diluted in 100 ml NS over 60 min (IV injection at 12.5 mg/min)	100 mg at 1 mL undiluted solution/min into dialysis line	510 mg IV injection repeated 3–8 days later
Test dose	Yes	No	No	No
Common adverse events	Pain, stinging at injection site (brown), hypotension, flushing, chills, fever, myalgia, anaphylaxis	Cramps, nausea or vomiting, flushing, hypotension, rash, pruritus	Leg cramps and hypotension	Diarrhea, constipation, nausea, dizziness, hypotension, peripheral edema

CKD = chronic kidney disease; EPO = erythropoietin; HD = hemodialysis; IDA = iron deficiency anemia; IM = intramuscular; IV = intravenous; NS = normal saline; PO = by mouth.

C. Macrocytic Anemia

1. Vitamin B_{12} and folate deficiency are the most common causes of macrocytic anemia. Causes of B_{12} deficiency include inadequate intake, malabsorption, and inadequate utilization. Folate deficiency is caused by inadequate intake, decreased absorption, hyperutilization, and inadequate utilization.

2. In B_{12} deficiency RBC, Hgb and Hct, and serum B_{12} are decreased, with an increase in MCV, MCH, methylmalonic acid, and homocysteine. Hypersegmented polymorphonuclear leukocytes may also be present on the peripheral smear.

3. In folate deficiency, RBC, Hgb and Hct, and serum folic acid are decreased, with an increase in MCV and MCH. B_{12} will be normal (will need to rule out this deficiency).

4. In B_{12} deficiency, patients may experience neurological changes, glossitis, weakness, loss of appetite, and possibly thrombocytopenia, leucopenia, and pancytopenia. Folate deficiency also presents with glossitis and other central nervous system symptoms including weakness, forgetfulness, headache, syncope, and loss of appetite.

5. Treatment options for vitamin B_{12} deficiency include oral replacement daily or intramuscular replacement weekly for 1 month, then monthly.

6. Folate deficiency anemia should be treated with 1 mg of folate daily for 4 months. Women who are pregnant should take supplements to prevent neural tube defects in the fetus.

D. Anemia of Chronic Disease (Specifically Chemotherapy-Induced Anemia): Causes of Anemia and Fatigue in Adult Patients with Cancer

1. Unmanaged pain or other symptoms can increase fatigue.

2. Decreased RBC production because of anticancer therapy, either radiation or chemotherapy

3. Decreased or inappropriate endogenous erythropoietin production or decreased responsiveness to endogenous erythropoietin

4. Decreased body stores of vitamin B_{12}, iron, or folic acid

5. Increased destruction of RBCs

6. Blood loss

7. Although anemia can certainly contribute to or worsen fatigue, there are probably other (perhaps many) mechanisms of fatigue (e.g., cytokines) that are independent of hemoglobin concentration.

E. Principles of Anemia and Fatigue

1. Fatigue is estimated to affect 60%–80% of all patients with cancer.

2. Fatigue may be caused by the disease or treatment.

3. Fatigue can be assessed with a numeric rating scale, 0 = no fatigue and 10 = worst fatigue imaginable, or with any of several questionnaires (e.g., FACT-An).

4. Drugs used in the treatment of anemia and fatigue

   a. Epoetin and darbepoetin alfa (erythropoiesis-stimulating agents [ESAs]) are approved for treating chemotherapy-induced anemia, the end point of treatment being a decreased need for transfusion. Darbepoetin has additional carboxy chains, resulting in a longer half-life compared with epoetin.

   b. In recent years, reports of a detrimental effect of ESAs (e.g., increased deaths, poorer chemotherapy outcomes) have led to changes in practice guidelines and reimbursement for these agents. Hemoglobin targets are lower than they were previously, and hemoglobin is carefully monitored. According to the most recent guidelines, ESAs are initiated once a patient's hemoglobin drops below 10 g/dL.

   c. It is important to distinguish between the use of these agents for chemotherapy-associated anemia and cancer-associated anemia. The latter is not an approved use. These agents should be used only in the noncurative setting.

   d. Adverse events: Hypertension and seizures, venous thromboembolism, and pure red cell aplasia (rare)

   e. The use of these agents requires baseline and follow-up monitoring to determine whether agents need titration or discontinuation.

5. Transfusions are an option if patients are symptomatic. Transfusion goal is to maintain hemoglobin between 8 g/dL and 10 g/dL.

F. Dosing of Erythropoiesis-Stimulating Agents

Table 8. Dosing of Erythropoiesis-Stimulating Agents

Agent	Starting Dosage	Dosage Increase	Dosing Parameters
Erythropoietin (Procrit, Epogen)	150 units/kg subcutaneously 3 times/week 40,000 units subcutaneously weekly	300 units/kg subcutaneously 3 times/week 60,000 units subcutaneously weekly	Hemoglobin must be <10 to initiate and continue therapy Evaluate after 4 weeks and increase dosage if rise is <1 g/dL Decrease by ~25% if rapid rise in hemoglobin Discontinue therapy if no response after 8 weeks
Darbepoetin (Aranesp)	2.25 mcg/kg subcutaneously weekly 500 mcg every 3 weeks	4.5 mcg/kg subcutaneously weekly Not applicable	Hemoglobin must be <10 to initiate and continue therapy Evaluate after 6 weeks and increase dosage if rise is <1 g/dL Decrease by ~40% if rapid rise in hemoglobin Discontinue therapy if no response after 8 weeks

G. REMS for ESAs
   1. The FDA requires these agents to be prescribed and monitored under a risk management program to ensure their safety.
   2. Requirements of the REMS program
      a. All patients who are prescribed and receive ESAs must be provided with a medication guide on therapy initiation and with each dose, explaining the risks and benefits of these agents. Patients will also be asked to sign an acknowledgment form that confirms they have talked with their health care professional about the risks of ESAs (may cause tumors to grow faster, may cause patients to die sooner, and may cause patients to develop blood clots or heart problems).
      b. Health care providers prescribing ESAs to patients with cancer must be enrolled in the ESA APPRISE (Assisting Providers and Cancer Patients with Risk Information for the Safe Use of ESAs).

Patient Case

7. A 45-year-old woman is beginning her third cycle of chemotherapy for the adjuvant treatment of breast cancer. At diagnosis, her hemoglobin was 10 g/dL; however, today her hemoglobin is less than 10 g/dL. The patient has fatigue that is interfering with her activities of daily living. Which is the most appropriate treatment option?

   A. Treatment with epoetin should be considered.

   B. Treatment with darbepoetin should be considered when hemoglobin decreases to less than 9 g/dL.

   C. The patient is being treated in the curative setting and therefore is not eligible to receive an ESA.

   D. The patient should not receive RBC transfusions because she is symptomatic.

VII. CHEMOPROTECTANTS

A. Properties of an Ideal Protectant Drug for Chemotherapy- and Radiation-Induced Toxicities
   1. Easy to administer
   2. No adverse events
   3. Prevents all toxicities, including non–life-threatening (alopecia) toxicities, irreversible morbidities (neuropathies, ototoxicity), and mortality (severe myelosuppression, cardiotoxicity)
   4. Does not interfere with the efficacy of the cancer treatment
   5. To date, no such drug has been identified.

B. Dexrazoxane
   1. The anthracyclines (daunorubicin, doxorubicin, idarubicin, and epirubicin), anthracenedione, and mitoxantrone can cause cardiomyopathy that is related to the total lifetime cumulative dosage.
   2. Dexrazoxane acts as an intracellular chelating agent; iron chelation leads to a decrease in anthracycline-induced free radical damage.
      a. Dexrazoxane is approved for use in patients with metastatic breast cancer. It may be considered for patients who have received doxorubicin 300 mg/m^2 or more and who may benefit from continued doxorubicin, considering the patient's risk of cardiotoxicity with continued doxorubicin use.
      b. Dexrazoxane may increase the hematologic toxicity of chemotherapy.
      c. An early study suggested that dexrazoxane decreases the response rate to chemotherapy. More recent data suggest this is not the case, but dexrazoxane is still not indicated for patients with early (curable) breast cancer.
   3. Dexrazoxane is also approved for use as an antidote for the extravasation of anthracycline chemotherapy.

C. Amifostine
   1. Amifostine is used to prevent nephrotoxicity from cisplatin.
   2. It is also used to decrease the incidence of both acute and late xerostomia in patients with head and neck cancer who are undergoing fractionated radiation therapy.
   3. Adverse events associated with amifostine include sneezing, allergic reactions, warm or flushed feeling, metallic taste in mouth during infusion, nausea and vomiting, and hypotension. The latter is the most clinically significant toxicity. Prevention of hypotension includes withholding antihypertensive medications, using hydration, and close monitoring of BP. Because of the problems with nausea and vomiting and the incidence of hypotension, this agent is not used very often.

D. Mesna (sodium-2-mercaptoethane sulfonate)
   1. The metabolite acrolein is produced from both cyclophosphamide and ifosfamide, and it has been implicated in sterile hemorrhagic cystitis.
   2. Mesna detoxifies acrolein by binding to the compound and preventing its interaction with host cells.
   3. Mesna is always used with ifosfamide and may be used with cyclophosphamide (in dosages of 1500 mg/m^2 or greater), although this is not a label indication.
   4. Mesna may be given intravenously or orally. Several dosing schedules may be used. With any schedule, mesna must begin concurrently with or before ifosfamide or cyclophosphamide and end after ifosfamide or cyclophosphamide because of its short half-life (i.e., mesna must be present in the bladder when acrolein is present in the bladder).

Patient Cases

8. A 38-year-old woman has a history of Hodgkin lymphoma. Two years ago, she completed six cycles of ABVD chemotherapy (i.e., doxorubicin, bleomycin, vinblastine, and dacarbazine). Each cycle included doxorubicin 50 mg/m². Recently, she was given a diagnosis of stage IV breast cancer. She will be initiated on doxorubicin 50 mg/m² and cyclophosphamide 500 mg/m² for four cycles. Which statement is most applicable?

    A. The patient has not reached the appropriate cumulative dosage of doxorubicin to consider dexrazoxane.

    B. The patient has reached the appropriate cumulative dosage of doxorubicin to consider dexrazoxane.

    C. The patient should not receive any more doxorubicin because she is at an elevated risk of cardiotoxicity.

    D. The patient should not receive dexrazoxane because of the possibility of increased myelosuppression.

9. Which is the best sequence for administering mesna and ifosfamide?

    A. Mesna before ifosfamide and then at 4 and 8 hours after ifosfamide.

    B. Ifosfamide before mesna and then at 4 and 8 hours after mesna.

    C. Mesna and ifosfamide beginning and ending at the same time.

    D. Mesna on day 1 and ifosfamide on days 2–5.

VIII. ONCOLOGIC EMERGENCIES

A. Hypercalcemia

1. The most common tumors associated with hypercalcemia are lung (metastatic non–small cell lung cancer more than small cell lung cancer), breast, multiple myeloma, head and neck, renal cell, and non-Hodgkin lymphoma.

2. Cancer-associated hypercalcemia results from increased bone resorption with calcium release into the extracellular fluid; in addition, renal clearance of calcium is decreased.

    a. Some tumors cause direct bone destruction, resulting in osteolytic hypercalcemia.

    b. Other tumors release parathyroid hormone–related protein (i.e., humoral hypercalcemia).

    c. Immobile patients are also at an elevated risk of hypercalcemia because of increased resorption of calcium.

    d. Medications (e.g., hormonal therapy, thiazide diuretics) may precipitate or exacerbate hypercalcemia.

    e. Corrected Ca (mg/dL) = (4 – plasma albumin in g/dL) × 0.8 + serum calcium.

    f. Symptoms of hypercalcemia: Lethargy, confusion, anorexia, nausea, constipation, polyuria, and polydipsia

3. Management of hypercalcemia

    a. Mild hypercalcemia (corrected calcium less than 12 mg/dL) may not warrant aggressive treatment. Hydration with normal saline followed by observation is an option in asymptomatic patients with chemotherapy-sensitive tumors (e.g., lymphoma, breast cancer).

    b. Moderate hypercalcemia (corrected calcium 12–14 mg/dL) requires basic treatment of clinical symptoms with aggressive hydration.

    c. Severe hypercalcemia (corrected calcium greater than 14 mg/dL; symptomatic) requires aggressive inpatient treatment.

        i. Hydration with normal saline about 3–6 L in 24 hours

        ii. Loop diuretics may be administered after volume status has been corrected or to prevent fluid overload during hydration.

        iii. Thiazide diuretics are contraindicated in hypercalcemia because of the increase in renal tubular calcium absorption.

        iv. Bisphosphonates bind to hydroxyapatite in calcified bone, which prevents dissolution by phosphatases and inhibits both normal and abnormal bone resorption. The onset of action is 3–4 days.

        v. Calcitonin (intramuscular formulation) inhibits the effects of parathyroid hormone and has a rapid-onset (though short-lived) hypocalcemic effect.

        vi. Steroids may be used to lower calcium in patients with steroid-responsive tumors (lymphoma and myeloma).

        vii. Phosphate is reserved for patients who are both hypophosphatemic and hypercalcemic. Phosphate is seldom used because of the possibility of calcium and phosphate precipitation in soft tissue.

        viii. Dialysis may be needed in patients with hypercalcemia and renal failure.

B. Spinal Cord Compression

  1. Signs and symptoms include back pain, weakness, paresthesias, and loss of bowel and bladder function.

  2. Treatment consists of dexamethasone and radiation therapy or surgery.

C. Tumor Lysis Syndrome

  1. Occurs secondary to the rapid cell death that follows the administration of chemotherapy in patients with leukemia or lymphoma or in patients with high tumor burdens from other diseases that are also highly chemosensitive. Tumor lysis syndrome (TLS) can occur spontaneously in hematologic malignancies, without being triggered by the administration of chemotherapy (i.e., some patients present in tumor lysis).

  2. Manifestations include hyperuricemia, hyperkalemia, hyperphosphatemia, and secondary hypocalcemia. Uric acid and calcium/phosphorus may precipitate in the kidney and can lead to renal failure.

  3. The primary management strategy is prevention with intravenous hydration (with normal saline) and allopurinol.

  4. Rasburicase is a recombinant urate oxidase that converts uric acid into allantoin, which is 5–10 times more soluble in urine than uric acid. Rasburicase should be considered for patients at high risk of developing TLS, such as those with a serum uric acid concentration greater than 8 mg/dL, a large tumor burden, preexisting renal dysfunction, or an inability to take allopurinol. The drug is expensive, and currently it is not recommended for prophylaxis in all patients but may be used together with hydration for treatment of TLS. The approved dosage is 0.2 mg/kg intravenously for 5 doses. There is now increasing evidence for the use of an off-label, low, fixed, single dose of rasburicase for chemotherapy-induced hyperuricemia in adults. The FDA indication is management of uric acid levels. Rasburicase causes enzymatic degradation of the uric acid in blood, plasma, and serum samples, potentially resulting in spuriously low plasma uric acid assay readings. Blood must be collected in prechilled tubes containing heparin anticoagulant; immediately immerse plasma samples for uric acid measurement in an ice water bath.

IX. MISCELLANEOUS ANTINEOPLASTIC PHARMACOTHERAPY

A. Leucovorin rescue may be used after methotrexate doses greater than 100 mg/m²; in general, methotrexate doses greater than 500 mg/m² require leucovorin rescue.

B. Factors that increase the likelihood of methotrexate toxicity include renal dysfunction (causing delayed elimination), third-space fluid (e.g., pleural effusion, ascites), and administration of other drugs that may delay methotrexate elimination (penicillin, NSAIDs, PPIs). Toxic reactions include mucous membrane toxicity (e.g., oral mucositis), renal and hepatic toxicity, central nervous system toxicity, and myelosuppression.

C. The dosage of leucovorin depends on the methotrexate dosage or level and the time since the completion of methotrexate. Methotrexate levels are usually obtained 24–48 hours after intermediate- or high-dose methotrexate, and leucovorin is continued until the methotrexate level falls to less than 0.1 mM (less than 1×10^{-7} M). This regimen is typically protocol driven.

D. In contrast to its use with methotrexate, leucovorin is given in combination with fluorouracil in colorectal cancer to improve activity, not to rescue normal cells.

E. Glucarpidase, a carboxypeptidase enzyme, is now approved and indicated for treating toxic methotrexate concentrations (greater than 1 µmol/L) in patients with delayed methotrexate clearance due to renal function. Administered as a single intravenous dose of 50 units/kg. Continue leucovorin until the methotrexate concentration has been maintained below the leucovorin treatment threshold for a minimum of 3 days. However, caution must be used with administering leucovorin in conjunction with glucarpidase. Leucovorin should not be administered within 2 hours before or after a dose of glucarpidase.

F. Extravasation Injuries
1. A vesicant is an agent that, on extravasation, can cause tissue necrosis. Vesicant antineoplastic drugs include doxorubicin, daunorubicin, epirubicin, mechlorethamine, mitomycin, vincristine, vinblastine, vinorelbine, and streptozocin.
2. Anthracyclines cause the most severe tissue damage on extravasation.
3. The literature generally recommends administering vesicants by intravenous injection rather than infusion, but some exceptions exist.
   a. Some institutional policies require infusions for every drug or approved protocols.
   b. Vincristine has been incorrectly administered by intrathecal injection, with fatal consequences. Dilution of vincristine for administration as a short intravenous infusion has been recommended to prevent this error from occurring.
   c. Paclitaxel is administered as an infusion (1, 3, or 24 hours, depending on the protocol).
4. Management of extravasation
   a. Cold for doxorubicin, daunorubicin, and epirubicin
   b. Heat for vincristine, vinblastine, and vinorelbine
   c. Sodium thiosulfate for mechlorethamine
   d. Topical dimethyl sulfoxide has been recommended for anthracyclines. Its use is not as well established as that of the antidotes above. Hyaluronidase is recommended for vinca alkaloids, but hyaluronidase is of limited availability. Antidotes for mitomycin, streptozocin, paclitaxel, and oxaliplatin are not well documented in the literature.

e. Dexrazoxane (Totect) for doxorubicin, daunorubicin, idarubicin, and epirubicin. Cold compress should be removed 15 minutes before dexrazoxane treatment.

f. Many institutions do not allow the administration of vesicants through a peripheral vein but instead require that vesicants be administered through a central line with a venous access device. Although administering vesicants through a central line minimizes the likelihood of an extravasation injury, extravasation may still occur. Management of extravasation is intended for suspected or actual extravasation from a peripheral or central vein.

G. Management of Diarrhea
1. Intensive loperamide therapy using dosages higher than recommended was initially described for irinotecan-induced diarrhea. Atropine is used to prevent cholinergic activity of acute irinotecan-induced diarrhea. There is no maximal dosage of loperamide when used for delayed diarrhea in this setting. The recommended dosing regimen of loperamide is 4 mg by mouth, followed by 2 mg every 2 hours until diarrhea free.
2. Intensive antidiarrhea treatment is also used for other agents (e.g., fluorouracil, epidermal growth factor receptor inhibitors).

H. Dosage Adjustment for Organ Dysfunction
1. Conflicting recommendations for dosage adjustment have been reported. Many drugs have not been studied in patients with organ dysfunction. Consultation of oncology-specific drug information resources may be useful.
2. Dosage adjustment for renal dysfunction may be considered for methotrexate, carboplatin, cisplatin, etoposide, bleomycin, topotecan, capecitabine, and lenalidomide.
3. Dosage adjustment for hepatic dysfunction is often based on total bilirubin concentrations.

REFERENCES

Antiemetics

1. Gralla RJ, Raftopoulos H. Progress in the control of chemotherapy-induced emesis: new agents and new studies. J Oncol Pract 2009;5:130-3.

2. Grunberg SM, Warr D, Gralla RJ, et al. Evaluation of new antiemetic agents and definition of antineoplastic agent emetogenicity: state of the art. Support Care Cancer 2010;19:S43-47.

3. Herrstedt J, Dombernowsky P. Anti-emetic therapy in cancer chemotherapy: current status. Basic Clin Pharmacol Toxicol 2007;101:143-50.

4. Hesketh PJ, Kris MG, Grunberg SM, et al. Proposal for classifying the acute emetogenicity of cancer chemotherapy. J Clin Oncol 1997;15:103-9.

5. Multinational Association for Supportive Care in Cancer. MASCC/ESMO Antiemetic Guideline 2010. Available at www.mascc.org. Accessed October 10, 2012.

6. Naeim A, Dy SM, Lorenz KA, et al. Evidence-based recommendations for cancer nausea and vomiting. J Clin Oncol 2008;26:3903-10.

7. National Comprehensive Cancer Network (NCCN). Clinical Practice Guidelines in Oncology: Antiemesis, version 2. 2015. Available at www.nccn.org/professionals/physician_gls/pdf/antiemesis.pdr. Accessed October 12, 2015.

8. Navari RM, Gray SE, Kerr AC. Olanzapine versus aprepitant for the prevention of chemotherapy-induced nausea and vomiting: a randomized phase III trial. J Support Oncol 2011;9:188-95.

9. Navari RM, Nagy CK, Gray SE. Olanzapine versus metoclopramide for the treatment of breakthrough chemotherapy-induced nausea and vomiting in patients receiving highly emetogenic chemotherapy. Support Care Cancer 2013;21:1655-63.

Pain Management

1. Berenson JR, Hillner BE, Kyle RA, et al. American Society of Clinical Oncology clinical practice guidelines: the role of bisphosphonates in multiple myeloma. J Clin Oncol 2002;20:3719-36.

2. Foley KM. The treatment of cancer pain. N Engl J Med 1985;313:84-95.

3. Hillner BE, Ingle JN, Chlebowski RT, et al. American Society of Clinical Oncology 2003 update on the role of bisphosphonates and bone health issues in women with breast cancer. J Clin Oncol 2003;21:4042-57.

4. National Comprehensive Cancer Network (NCCN). Clinical Practice Guidelines in Oncology: Adult Cancer Pain, version 2.2015. Available at www.nccn.org/professionals/physician_gls/f_guidelines.asp. Accessed October 10, 2015.

5. U.S. Department of Health and Human Services (DHHS). Public Health Service Agency for Health Care Policy and Research (AHCPR). Clinical Practice Guideline, No. 9. Management of Cancer Pain. AHCPR Publication 94-0592, March 1994. Washington, DC: DHHS, 1994.

6. U.S. Food and Drug Administration Web site. FDA Approves a Risk Evaluation and Mitigation Strategy (REMS). Available at www.fda.gov/Drugs/DrugSafety/InformationbyDrugClass/ucm309742.htm#Q7. Accessed October 10, 2012.

Febrile Neutropenia and CSFs

1. Freifeld AG, Bow EJ, Sepkowitz KA, et al. The Infectious Diseases Society of America 2010 guidelines for the use of antimicrobial agents in patients with cancer and neutropenia: salient features and comments. Clin Infect Dis 2011;52:e56-93.

2. Hughes WT, Armstrong D, Bodey GP, et al. 2002 guidelines for the use of antimicrobial agents in neutropenic patients with unexplained fever. Clin Infect Dis 2002;34:730-51.

3. Klastersky J, Paesmans M. Risk-adapted strategy for the management of febrile neutropenia in cancer patients. Support Care Cancer 2007;15:477-82.

4. National Comprehensive Cancer Network (NCCN). Clinical Practice Guidelines in Oncology: Myeloid Growth Factors, version 1.2015. Available at www.nccn.org/professionals/physician_gls/f_guidelines.asp. Accessed October 12, 2015.

5. National Comprehensive Cancer Network (NCCN). Clinical Practice Guidelines in Oncology: Prevention and Treatment of Cancer-Related Infections, version 2.2015. Available at www.nccn.org/professionals/physician_gls/f_guidelines.asp. Accessed October 10, 2015.

6. Smith TJ, Khatcheressian J, Lyman GH, et al. 2006 Update of recommendations for the use of white blood cell growth factors: an evidence-based clinical practice guideline. J Clin Oncol 2006;24:1-19.

Thrombocytopenia

1. Adams VR, Brenner TL. Oprelvekin (Neumega). J Oncol Pharm Pract 1999;5:117-24.

2. Cantor SB, Elting LS, Hudson DV, et al. Pharmacoeconomic analysis of oprelvekin for secondary prophylaxis of thrombocytopenia for solid tumor patients receiving chemotherapy. Cancer 2003;97:3099-106.

3. Schiffer CA, Anderson KC, Bennett CL, et al. Platelet transfusions for patients with cancer: clinical practice guidelines of the American Society of Clinical Oncology. J Clin Oncol 2001;19:1519-38.

Anemia and Fatigue

1. National Comprehensive Cancer Network (NCCN). Practice Guidelines in Oncology: Cancer- and Chemotherapy-Induced Anemia, version 1.2016. Available at www.nccn.org/professionals/physician_gls/f_guidelines.asp. Accessed October 12, 2015.

2. Rizzo JD, Somerfield MR, Hagerty KL, et al. Use of epoetin and darbepoetin inpatients with cancer: 2007 American Society of Clinical Oncology/American Society of Hematology clinical practice guideline update [published correction appears in J Clin Oncol 2008;26:1192]. J Clin Oncol 2008;26:132-49.

Chemoprotectants

1. Bukowsi R. Cytoprotection in the treatment of pediatric cancer: review of current strategies in adults and their application to children. Med Pediatr Oncol 1999;32:124-34.

2. Hensley ML, Hagerty KL, Kewalramani T, et al. American Society of Clinical Oncology 2008 clinical practice guideline update: use of chemotherapy and radiation therapy protectants. J Clin Oncol 2009;27:127-45.

3. Links M, Lewis C. Chemoprotectants: a review of their clinical pharmacology and therapeutic efficacy. Drugs 1999;57:293-308.

4. Schuchter LM, Hensley ML, Meropol NJ, et al. 2002 update of recommendations for the use of chemotherapy and radiotherapy protectants: clinical practice guidelines of the American Society of Clinical Oncology. J Clin Oncol 2002;20:2895-903.

Oncologic Emergencies

1. Abrahm JL. Management of pain and spinal cord compression in patients with advanced cancer. Ann Intern Med 1999;131:37-46.

2. Brigden ML. Hematologic and oncologic emergencies. Doing the most good in the least time. Postgrad Med 2001;109:143-63.

3. Coiffler B, Altman A, Pui CH, et al. Guidelines for the management of pediatric and adult tumor lysis syndrome: an evidence-based review. J Clin Oncol 2008;26:2767-78.

4. Holdsworth MT, Nguyen P. Role of i.v. allopurinol and rasburicase in tumor lysis syndrome. Am J Health Syst Pharm 2003;60:2213-24.

5. Krimsky WS, Behrens RJ, Kerkvliet GJ. Oncology emergencies for the internist. Cleve Clin J Med 2002;69:209-22.

6. Nakshima L. Guidelines for the treatment of hypercalcemia associated with malignancy. J Oncol Pharm Pract 1997;3:31-7.

7. Nicolin G. Paediatric update. Emergencies and their management. Eur J Cancer 2002;38:1365-77.

8. Vadhan-Raj S, Fayad LE, Fanale MA, et al. A randomized trial of single-dose rasburicase versus five-daily doses in patients at risk for tumor lysis syndrome. Ann Oncol 2012;23:1640-5.

9. Yim BT, Sims-McCallum RP, Chong PH. Rasburicase for the treatment and prevention of hyperuricemia. Ann Pharmacother 2003;37:1047-54.

ANSWERS AND EXPLANATIONS TO PATIENT CASES

1. Answer: A

This is a highly emetogenic regimen that is associated with delayed nausea and vomiting. The best choice is a serotonin receptor antagonist with dexamethasone and aprepitant for prophylaxis against nausea and vomiting. Prochlorperazine is not effective against a highly emetogenic stimulus. Granisetron and ondansetron are both serotonin receptor antagonists, and no rationale exists for combining them. Lorazepam may be a useful addition, but it does not replace dexamethasone or aprepitant for highly emetogenic chemotherapy.

2. Answer: D

Lorazepam is recommended for use in combination with the standard antiemetic regimen based on chemotherapy emetogenicity to prevent anticipatory nausea and vomiting. Aprepitant and dexamethasone should and can be used together to prevent acute and delayed emesis. Metoclopramide would not be appropriate for anticipatory nausea and vomiting. Serotonin receptor antagonists are generally thought not to be effective alone in preventing anticipatory nausea and vomiting.

3. Answer: D

The patient is taking oxycodone/APAP 5 mg/325 mg, which provides 60 mg of oxycodone per day and 3900 mg of APAP. We should not increase his current drugs because of concerns about APAP toxicity. If he is changed to a higher strength of the combination product, APAP toxicity is still a concern, which eliminates the choices of increasing to oxycodone/APAP 7.5 mg 2 tablets every 4 hours. Adding sustained-release morphine is a good option. Continuing the ibuprofen might be helpful for bone pain. Oxycodone/APAP, which is short acting, could be continued for breakthrough pain, but he is already getting a lot of APAP without good pain relief.

4. Answer: C

Gabapentin might help the neuropathic component (i.e., the shooting pains) of his pain. He is already receiving an NSAID, so there is no need to add naproxen. There is no point to adding APAP, and the case does not mention muscle spasms.

5. Answer: D

To calculate the ANC, multiply the WBC by the segmented neutrophils and the band neutrophils: 600 cells/mm^3 × (0.6 + 0.1) = 420 cells/mm^3.

6. Answer: C

The patient is neutropenic; however, she should not begin a CSF. Her ANC is greater than 100 cells/mm^3, and she has no signs or symptoms of active infection. Prophylactic treatment with antibiotic drugs is not necessary and can increase the risk of resistant organisms. At this time, the patient should be monitored for evidence of infection (e.g., she should be instructed to take her temperature and return to the clinic or emergency department if she has a single oral temperature of 101°F or more or of 100.4°F or more for at least 1 hour or if she develops any signs or symptoms of infection). Because the disease is potentially curable, dosages should not be reduced on the next cycle.

7. Answer: C

Recent literature and subsequent changes in guidelines and Centers for Medicare & Medicaid Services reimbursement suggest that an erythropoiesis-stimulating protein be considered when hemoglobin is less than 10 g/dL. However, this patient is being treated potentially for a cure; therefore, she would not be eligible for an ESA. Transfusions are an option if patients are symptomatic. Transfusion goal is to maintain hemoglobin between 8 and 10 g/dL.

8. Answer: B

The patient has received a cumulative dose of 300 mg/m^2 of doxorubicin (50 mg/m^2 × 6 cycles). This is the appropriate cumulative dosage of doxorubicin to consider dexrazoxane. She is at an elevated risk of cardiotoxicity; however, dexrazoxane protects the heart from this toxicity. Dexrazoxane may increase the myelosuppression from chemotherapy, but that does not represent a contraindication.

9. Answer: A

Several different schedules of ifosfamide and mesna administration exist (e.g., ifosfamide short infusion, followed by intermittent infusions of mesna and continuous infusion of both ifosfamide and mesna). But mesna should always be continued longer than ifosfamide.

ANSWERS AND EXPLANATIONS TO SELF-ASSESSMENT QUESTIONS

1. Answer: C

Patients who have had poor control of nausea and vomiting on previous cycles of chemotherapy are at an elevated risk of anticipatory emesis. Anxious patients are also at an elevated risk of CINV. Benzodiazepines help decrease anxiety and, by causing anterograde amnesia, may minimize anticipatory symptoms. Although it is unclear whether patients who do not respond to one serotonin receptor antagonist will respond to another, a change in regimen is needed. Substituting dolasetron for granisetron would be acceptable, but adding lorazepam is essential. Palonosetron is the preferred serotonin receptor antagonist in some guidelines, but this is not universally agreed on. For this patient, the palonosetron option also includes lorazepam. Metoclopramide is another option, but an effective dose might be difficult to administer orally (especially as tablets), and again, adding lorazepam would be preferred over adding aprepitant in this patient.

2. Answer: D

This patient's altered mental status is probably caused by hypercalcemia. The corrected calcium is 13.6 mg/dL. Corrected calcium concentrations greater than 12 g/dL should be treated with a bisphosphonate (either pamidronate or zoledronic acid) in addition to hydration with normal saline. Furosemide may be needed during hydration but not before hydration because the patient is probably dehydrated. This patient does not need rapid reversal of hypercalcemia; therefore, calcitonin is not needed. Dexamethasone may be used in patients with lymphoma or myeloma, but it will have no effect on metastatic non–small cell lung cancer.

3. Answer: C

The patient is at risk of TLS because he has a chemosensitive tumor and a high tumor burden (elevated WBC). Prevention is the key in TLS, which includes adequate saline hydration and the use of allopurinol. Dextrose 5% is not an appropriate intravenous fluid for hydration because it does not contain saline. The value of alkalinization with sodium bicarbonate is somewhat controversial, and alkalinization is not a replacement for allopurinol.

4. Answer: B

This anemia is not attributable to treatment because chemotherapy has not yet begun. Epoetin and darbepoetin are indicated only for noncurative chemotherapy-associated anemia. Chemotherapy should not be delayed, nor should chemotherapy dosages be reduced in the setting of a potentially curable malignancy. Therefore, the patient should receive a transfusion of packed RBCs.

5. Answer: B

$(55\% + 5\%) \times 500 = 300$.

6. Answer: A

The patient is neutropenic (ANC 300 cells/mm³). Temperature of 103°F places the febrile neutropenia outside the definition of low-risk febrile neutropenia. Therefore, the patient should be hospitalized for intravenous antibiotics and an infection workup. She does not have any of the appropriate reasons to administer CSFs (i.e., documented pneumonia, hypotension, sepsis syndrome, or fungal infection). Her chemotherapy may need to be delayed, but it should be continued. She should receive a CSF with the next cycle of chemotherapy.

7. Answer: B

Febrile neutropenia developed at the time of the expected neutrophil nadir, 12 days after chemotherapy. Marrow recovery would be expected to follow. The percentage of eosinophils may be slightly elevated, but the absolute count is low. The platelet count is also low, not elevated. Neutrophils are often affected by myelosuppressive chemotherapy to a greater degree than platelets.

8. Answer: D

Opioids may provide some relief from neuropathic pain, but often the response to opioids is less than optimal. In general, higher dosages of opioids provide greater pain relief; therefore, increasing the dosage of fentanyl and morphine is an option for this patient. Nothing in the history suggests that the patient is deriving much, if any, benefit at the present opioid dosages. Adjuvant analgesic drugs, including tricyclic antidepressants and anticonvulsants, are used to help manage neuropathic pain. Gabapentin, with a good adverse event profile, is a reasonable option. However, adjuvant analgesic drugs should not be given to decrease the opioid dosage or discontinue the use of opioid drugs. (It may be possible to decrease the dosage later if gabapentin provides adequate pain relief.) Diazepam is more effective for muscle spasms than for neuropathic pain, and this option includes decreasing the fentanyl dosage at the same time the new drug is initiated.

9. Answer: D

Limited-stage small cell lung cancer is potentially curable; therefore, the patient should continue on the planned dosages of chemotherapy. The correct dosage of filgrastim is 5 mcg/kg/day subcutaneously, not 250 mcg/m^2 (this is the dose for sargramostim). The correct dosage for pegfilgrastim is a single 6-mg injection. Filgrastim should not be given on the same day as chemotherapy; therefore, Answer D is correct.

10. Answer: A

Doxorubicin undergoes hepatic clearance, and there are recommendations for dosage reduction based on bilirubin. There is no reason to reduce the dosage of cyclophosphamide.

11. Answer: A

Large cell lymphoma is faster growing and more chemosensitive than metastatic colorectal cancer. Therefore, patients with large cell lymphoma are more likely to develop hyperuricemia or TLS from rapid cell turnover, both before treatment and after chemotherapy. Hypercalcemia is not a common complication of either of these diseases. Some aggressive lymphomas may be associated with hypercalcemia, but pamidronate is used to treat, not prevent, this complication.

12. Answer: C

Neither patient should undergo chemotherapy with an ANC of 800 cells/mm^3. Both can be treated when neutropenia resolves (probably within 1 week). It is important to keep patient 1 on schedule because his disease is potentially curable; therefore, patient 1 should receive filgrastim after the next chemotherapy treatment to prevent another dose delay. When patient 2 resumes chemotherapy, his dosages can be decreased to prevent a recurrence of neutropenia. The dosage decrease is not likely to have a substantially negative effect on the treatment outcome because the treatment goal is usually not cure.

13. Answer: C

Injury after extravasation of an anthracycline is potentially the most severe. Therefore, when the recommended antidotes for different vesicants conflict (e.g., heat vs. cold), treatment should be directed at the anthracycline. Dexrazoxane is now indicated for doxorubicin extravasation. Cold rather than heat would also be appropriate. Although vincristine is considered a vesicant, sodium thiosulfate is not the recommended antidote..

Drug Information, Evidence-Based Medicine, Research, and HIPAA

Kevin M. Sowinski, Pharm.D., FCCP

Purdue University
West Lafayette and Indianapolis, Indiana
Indiana University
Indianapolis, Indiana

Drug Information, Evidence-Based Medicine, Research, and HIPAA

Kevin M. Sowinski, Pharm.D., FCCP

Purdue University
West Lafayette and Indianapolis, Indiana
Indiana University
Indianapolis, Indiana

Learning Objectives

1. Differentiate between primary, secondary, and tertiary sources of information, and analyze these resources to answer questions related to clinical practice.
2. List the pros and cons associated with primary, secondary, and tertiary sources of information.
3. Identify commonly used primary, secondary, and tertiary literature sources.
4. Describe the steps involved in a top-down and bottom-up evidence-based medicine (EBM) approach.
5. Critically evaluate EBM resources.
6. Critically evaluate clinical guidelines.
7. Identify strategies available for seeking drug information resources on the Internet.
8. List appropriate questions for evaluating Internet drug information websites and electronic applications.
9. Define research and differentiate it from quality improvement activities.
10. Define the composition, functions, and roles of the institutional review board (IRB).
11. Define HIPAA (Health Insurance Portability and Accountability Act of 1996) regulations and their impact on clinical practice and research.
12. Describe the various steps of the professional writing and peer-review processes.

Self-Assessment Questions

Answers and explanations to these questions may be found at the end of the chapter.

1. Which statement best describes an example of primary literature?

   A. A review article in Pharmacotherapy.
   B. Dosing information from Lexicomp.
   C. A study evaluating clopidogrel for the treatment of acute venous thromboembolism.
   D. A PubMed search using the key words fluticasone furoate, vilanterol, and chronic obstructive pulmonary disease (COPD).

2. Which would NOT help you determine whether an Internet site likely contains reliable online health information?

   A. Advertisements on the page.
   B. Publication date.
   C. Credentials of the author.
   D. Publisher background.

3. An ambulatory care pharmacist is searching the Internet for appropriate diabetes education resources for one of her patients. Which is the best indicator that the website is reliable?

   A. Health On the Net Foundation stamp of approval.
   B. Does not give the most recent update or the authors of the articles.
   C. References that include Wikipedia and www.paulsdiabetesadvice.com.
   D. Article that states personal opinions regarding diabetes treatment.

4. A resident pharmacist in ambulatory care practice is asked by the attending physician whether any new studies have been published relative to the use of diuretics in heart failure since the most recent Cochrane review. Which is the best resource for the resident to use?

   A. www.guideline.gov.
   B. UpToDate.
   C. DiPiro's Pharmacotherapy.
   D. PubMed.

5. Which best describes the step in the process of evidence-based medicine (EBM) practice that includes use of the PICO (the patient problem or population, intervention, comparison, and outcome[s]) format?

   A. Appraise.
   B. Acquire.
   C. Apply.
   D. Ask.

6. Which best describes an individual who is required to be part of an institutional review board (IRB)?

   A. Lawyer.
   B Individual with scientific expertise.
   C. Patient advocate employed by the Institution.
   D. Spiritual advisor.

7. Which best describes information that is considered protected health information (PHI)?

   A. Town of residence.
   B. Certificate and license numbers.
   C. Age of a patient who is 46 years old.
   D. State of residence.

I. INTRODUCTION

A. Why Do Pharmacists Need to Know About These Topics?

B. As These Topics Pertain to You, Ambulatory Care Pharmacy Specialty Examination Content Outline

1. *Domain 3:* Translation of evidence into practice (14%)
2. Task statements:
   a. Retrieve biomedical literature applicable to ambulatory care pharmacy practice
   b. Interpret biomedical literature with respect to study design methodology, statistical analysis, and significance and applicability of reported data and conclusions
   c. Respond to requests for information from patients and health care professionals using evidence-based literature
   d. Use the principles and strategies of project and research design to generate and disseminate information in ambulatory care
   e. Enlist evidence-based strategies to effectively teach students, residents, pharmacists, and other health care professionals

II. OVERVIEW OF DRUG INFORMATION RESOURCES

A. Tertiary Literature
   1. Established knowledge or consensus of opinion; works that summarize, discuss, criticize, etc., the primary literature
   2. Pros
      a. Provides an analysis and summary of the primary literature
      b. Provides a discussion of studies that are thought to be well conceived and significant to the field
      c. Usually easy to use; more concise, accessible, and convenient
   3. Cons
      a. Significant lag time for updates – Primary literature publication outpaces tertiary literature.
      b. Interpretation is dependent on the author's opinion, which may lead to incorrect interpretation of primary literature.
      c. Incomplete; space limitations may exist
   4. Formats
      a. Available as paper text, as CD/DVD-ROM, online, or as mobile applications (PDA [personal digital assistant], tablet, smartphone)
      b. Electronic access online is generally considered the easiest to use, the most up to date, and the most accessible format to use from several locations.
      c. The content of information in each format is not necessarily the same.
      d. Mobile applications are a rapidly expanding area. The content of information for mobile applications is likely to be different from that in other formats of the same title because of storage and memory limitations.
   5. Evaluation of tertiary resources
      a. Authors' experience/expertise relative to the topic; are they experts, with appropriate experience?
      b. Is the information timely on the basis of its publication date, or is this a rapidly changing topic?
      c. Is the conclusion of the author supported by the primary literature? And is the work properly cited?
      d. Is the resource relevant and free of bias or blatant errors?
      e. Quality of references used

6. Selected tertiary drug information resources for the ambulatory care clinical pharmacist
   a. References selected are available electronically, are geared toward the health care professional, provide drug and alternative treatment monographs, and provide patient-oriented information. Many other appropriate references are available; this is only a partial list.
   b. Clinical Pharmacology (www.clinicalpharmacology.com)
   c. Drug Facts and Comparisons (www.factsandcomparisons.com)
   d. Lexicomp online (www.lexi.com)
   e. Micromedex Healthcare Series (www.micromedex.com)
      i. Detailed Drug Information for the Consumer
      ii. CareNotes System

B. Secondary Literature
   1. Index or abstract of the primary literature and tertiary literature found in journals, with the goal of directing the user to the primary literature. Its primary purpose is to provide a rapid method for searching the primary literature and keep readers well informed on primary literature publications.
   2. Pros: Provides efficient and accessible access to the primary literature
   3. Cons
      a. Different databases use different "vocabulary" or search strategies.
      b. Only abstracts or citations are available; primary literature from the search must be obtained from alternative sources and is costly.
   4. Formats
      a. Most secondary literature is electronic or in online databases.
      b. Indexing system: Provides biographic citation information (e.g., title, author, citation)
      c. Abstracting system: Provides biographic citation information and an abstract

C. Primary Literature
   1. Original articles that have not been interpreted, condensed, or evaluated (except by peer review) by others
      a. Research studies and reports; case studies/series published and unpublished
      b. Review articles or editorials are not primary literature.
   2. Pros
      a. Detailed, original articles
      b. Direct access to the research reports and conclusions
   3. Cons
      a. The reader must sift through methods, interpret the data and conclusions, and make decisions about the author's conclusion.
      b. The reader must have strong literature evaluation (e.g., statistics, clinical study) skills.
      c. Time-consuming, both in the searching and in the evaluating

Table 1. Examples of Primary, Secondary, and Tertiary Literature

Primary Literature	Secondary Literature	Tertiary Literature
Original articles (randomized controlled clinical trials; nonrandomized, prospective, clinical trials; cohort studies; case-control studies; case series; and case reports)	MEDLINE EMBASE PubMed Google Scholar IDIS Journal watch LexisNexis BIOSIS IPA Cochrane Library Current Contents CINAHL	General textbooks (e.g., Pharmacotherapy, Applied Therapeutics, Briggs' Drugs in Pregnancy and Lactation, Meyler's Side Effects of Drugs) General product information (e.g., American Hospital Formulary Service, Drug Facts and Comparisons, Physicians' Desk Reference, Drug Information Handbook, Clinical Pharmacology, UpToDate) Review articles Treatment guidelines Electronic textbooks and databases (McGraw-Hill ACCESS Pharmacy, STAT!Ref, Lippincott Health Sciences Library)

CINAHL = Cumulative Index to Nursing and Allied Health Literature; IDIS = Iowa Drug Information System; IPA = International Pharmaceutical Abstracts.

III. INTERNET SOURCES OF DRUG INFORMATION

A. Introduction: Use of the Internet for Drug Information
1. Currently used as a drug information tool by most U.S. adults
2. In the past decade, an increased number of U.S. adults have used the Internet for drug information.
3. Institute of Medicine: "The Internet is a bit like the Wild West: It has vast amounts of unregulated territory and no one in charge."

B. Search Engines
1. Basic search engines (e.g., Google, Yahoo, Bing)
   a. Search tool that sends the user's search request to a single search engine
   b. Examples: Google, Yahoo, Bing, ASK.com
2. Metasearch engines
   a. A search tool that sends the user's search request to several search engines and/or databases
   b. Examples: Dogpile, MetaCrawler, WebCrawler
3. Boolean logic: Use of Boolean operators such as and, or, and not to help narrow searches
4. MEDLINE MeSH (Medical Subject Headings) terms
   a. Standardized vocabulary used for indexing in MEDLINE
   b. Content filters: Specific for a drug or disease being searched. Ensures that the searcher is looking for the most appropriate content (e.g., heart failure)
   c. Validity filters: Use to narrow the search to only the highest-quality studies (e.g., randomized controlled trials, double-blind studies).

C. Evaluating Information on the Internet
1. Evaluation instruments
   a. Medication Website Assessment Tool
   b. Health On the Net Foundation Code of Conduct
   c. Healthcare Website Assessment Tool (HWAT 3.0)

2. National Institutes of Health tutorial: Tutorial geared toward patients

Table 2. Questions to Ask When Evaluating Websites

Variable	Questions
Source of information	What and who is responsible for the site, and is this information readily available on the site?
	What is the purpose of the site? Why was the website created, and what is the mission in providing the information?
Cost of access	Does the site want anything from you in return? If so, what and why? Does the site want your personal information, and if so, what will the site do with it? What personal information is required?
	Who is funding the site? Is there a site sponsor? Is the sponsorship readily available on the website and openly displayed? Does the sponsor gain any benefit?
Quality of information	Is the information current? Is the information correct? Has it been written and/or reviewed by appropriately trained health care professionals? Is the information based on opinion or high-quality controlled clinical trials? What is the editorial policy for the site?
Usability	Does the site provide information such as a site map, contact information, a mission/purpose statement, or the best way to use the site?
	Does the website make unbelievable claims or claim to be the answer to all questions or problems? Does it claim to be the only one to have true insight into the issues?

Adapted from: Murphy JE, Lee MW-N, eds. Pharmacotherapy Self-Assessment Program, 8th ed. Lenexa, KS: ACCP, 2013 [information abstracted from National Library of Medicine].

IV. EVIDENCE-BASED CLINICAL PRACTICE

A. Introduction to Evidence-Based Pharmacy/Medicine (EBM)
   1. EBM uses the scientific method as an important source of knowledge. In addition to the scientific method, other sources of knowledge are listed below.
      a. Reference to tradition: Accepting certain truths or facts as givens
      b. Reference to authority: Placing trust in those who are experts in a given area
      c. Trial and error: Making several attempts to solve a problem by chance. Used when no other basis for making a decision is possible
      d. Logical reasoning: Deductive reasoning
      e. Scientific method: Applying a logical process to identify a problem, collecting data, and developing a conclusion
   2. Definitions
      a. "The conscientious, explicit, and judicious use of current best evidence in making decisions about the care of individual patients while integrating clinical experience with the best available evidence from a systemic search" (BMJ 1996;213:71-2)

    b.   EBM is the integration of clinical expertise, patient values, and the best research evidence into the decision-making process for patient care. Clinical expertise refers to the clinician's cumulated experience, education, and clinical skills. The patient brings to the encounter his or her own personal preferences and specific concerns, expectations, and values. The best research evidence is usually found in clinically relevant research that has been conducted using sound methodology (Sackett 2000).

    c.   Process of making disease management decisions by evaluating and rating the quality of studies

    d.   Criticisms of EBM

        i.   "Cookbook" or reduced clinician autonomy

        ii.   Too difficult to apply to individual patients

        iii.   Limited data to suggest that evidence-based guidelines translate to improved care

3.   Summary of factors that influence the medical decision

    a.   Clinical evidence

    b.   Clinical experience

    c.   Patient circumstance

    d.   Patient desires

4.   Five-step process of EBM practice

    a.   Assess the patient: Start with a question that comes from the clinical care of a patient.

    b.   Ask the question: Develop an answerable question that reflects the clinical dilemma posed. PICO format:

        i.   (P)roblem/patient/population

        ii.   (I)ntervention

        iii.   (C)omparison

        iv.   (O)utcome

    c.   Acquire the evidence: Gather and assemble the data needed to make a conclusion.

    d.   Appraise the evidence: Use literature evaluation skills to assess the quality, quantity, and applicability of the data collected.

    e.   Apply to the patient: Incorporate the evidence into clinical practice.

    f.   Act on and assess your decision.

5.   EBM approaches

    a.   Top-down: Describes the EBM process, which requires resources and time. This approach is best suited for situations in which decisions are made about groups of patients (e.g., evidence-based guidelines).

    b.   Bottom-up: Describes the EBM process with fewer resources and limited time. This approach is best suited for individual patient decisions when resources and time are limited (e.g., day-to-day decisions that clinicians must make).

Table 3. Levels of Evidence Based on Several Evaluation Scales

Ranking	Type of Evidence	CEBM Scale	USPSTF Scale	ACC Scale
Highest	RCT	1[a]	I	A
	Nonrandomized, prospective, CT	—	II-1	B
	Cohort studies	2[a]	II-2	C
	Case-control studies	3[a]	II-2	C
	Case series	4	II-3	C
Lowest	Expert opinion	5	III	—

[a]A systematic review of these study types ranks higher than individual studies.

ACC = American College of Cardiology; CEBM = Centre for Evidence-Based Medicine; CT = clinical trial; RCT = randomized controlled trial; USPSTF = United States Preventive Services Task Force.

From: Shumock G, Brundage DM, Chapman MM, et al., eds. Pharmacotherapy Self-Assessment Program, 5th ed. Kansas City, MO: ACCP, 2005.

B. Evaluating Clinical Guidelines
1. Agency for Healthcare Research and Quality
    a. National Guidelines Clearinghouse (www.guidelines.gov)
    b. Allows a comparison of guidelines
2. Appraisal of Guidelines for Research and Evaluation (AGREE)
    a. Evaluates the process of practice guideline development and the quality of reporting
    b. www.agreetrust.org/
3. Bandolier
    a. "Evidence-based thinking about healthcare"
    b. Independent group based in Oxford, UK
    c. www.medicine.ox.ac.uk/bandolier/index.html

C. Sources of Clinical Guidelines (Note: These are only examples, not a complete list.)
1. National Library of Medicine (PubMed) (www.pubmed.gov)
2. Agency for Healthcare Research and Quality (www.ahrq.gov)
3. National Institute for Clinical Evidence
    a. www.nice.org.uk/
    b. UK National Health Service
4. Cochrane Collaboration (www.cochrane.org/)
5. Association websites
    a. American Heart Association (www.heart.org)
    b. American College of Cardiology Foundation (www.acc.org)
    c. American Society of Clinical Oncology (www.asco.org)
    d. American Academy of Family Physicians (www.aafp.org)
    e. The American Society of Health-System Pharmacists (www.ashp.org/bestpractices) provides links to best practice policies and guidelines.

V. INSTITUTIONAL REVIEW BOARD/HUMAN SUBJECTS' RESEARCH

A. Definitions
1. Research: "Systematic investigation (i.e., research development, testing, and evaluation) designed to develop or contribute to generalizable knowledge"
2. Human subject: "Living individual about whom an investigator obtains data through intervention or interaction with the individual OR identifiable private information"
3. Quality improvement versus research
    a. In general, if the results of a project are presented outside an organization (i.e., contributes to generalized knowledge), either as a publication or a presentation, it is defined as research.
    b. If the results of a project are to be used internally, and not meant to contribute to generalized knowledge, the activities will fall under quality improvement. Ideally, the IRB makes this decision.

B. History and Development of Research Ethics
1. Nuremberg Code (1948)
    a. Subjects should give informed voluntary consent.
    b. The benefits of research must outweigh the risks.
2. Declaration of Helsinki (1964)
    a. Governs international research ethics
    b. Defines rules for "research combined with clinical care" and "nontherapeutic research"
    c. Basis for good clinical practices used today

3. Tuskegee Syphilis Study (1972)
   a. The study did not minimize risks to human subjects. In fact, it increased their risks.
   b. These issues heightened awareness of the need to protect human subjects and to ensure their informed voluntary consent.
4. Belmont Report (1978): Prepared by the National Commission for the Protection of Human Subjects of Biomedical and Behavioral Research
   a. Summarizes the basic ethical principles identified in its deliberations
   b. Serves as a statement of basic ethical principles and guidelines that assist in resolving the ethical problems that surround the conduct of research with human subjects
5. Code of Federal Regulations (CFR) (1981): The Department of Health and Human Services (DHHS) and the U.S. Food and Drug Administration (FDA) issued regulations according to the Belmont Report:
   a. DHHS: CFR Title 45 (public welfare), Part 46 (protection of human subjects)
   b. FDA: CFR Title 21 (food and drugs), Parts 50 (protection of human subjects) and 56 (IRBs)
6. Common Rule (1991)
   a. Obtaining and documenting informed consent
   b. IRB membership, function, operations, review of research, and recordkeeping
   c. Additional protections for certain vulnerable research subjects: Pregnant women, prisoners, children, individuals with impaired capacity
   d. Ensuring compliance by research institutions
      i. All institutions that conduct federally sponsored research must provide the federal government an "assurance" that states the institution's principles for protecting the rights and welfare of human subjects.
      ii. Multiple project assurance is the most common approach to this.
7. IRB review of studies: Reviewed at one of three levels, depending on the level of risk to the human subjects. These are the federal guidelines that define the categories of review, which are as follows:
   a. Exemption from full IRB review
      i. Categories
         (a) Research conducted in established or commonly accepted educational settings
         (b) Research involving the use of educational tests (cognitive, diagnostic, aptitude, achievement), survey procedures, interview procedures, or observation of public behavior
         (c) Research involving the collection or study of existing data, documents, records, pathologic specimens, or diagnostic specimens if these sources are publicly available or if the information is recorded by the investigator in such a manner that subjects cannot be identified, directly or through identifiers linked to the subjects
         (d) Research and demonstration projects that are conducted by or subject to the approval of department or agency heads
      ii. Projects are not assigned an expiration date.
      iii. The IRB makes the final decision on exemption; a staff member usually reviews the proposal.
      iv. Review usually takes a few days.
   b. Expedited IRB review
      i. Minimal risk to participant
      ii. Minor change to previously approved study
      iii. Chairperson or designee reviews the proposal.
      iv. Review usually takes a few weeks.

    c. Full IRB review: More than minimal risk
       i. Review protocol and supporting documents.
       ii. Lengthy process, usually months
       iii. Full IRB reviews the proposal.

Table 4. Examples of IRB Review Categories

Type of Review	Examples
Exemption from review	Epidemiologic study with NHANES data Study of changes in the number of days requiring antibiotics, using de-identified institutional data
Expedited review	Cross-sectional study of patients with heart failure measuring a biomarker, requiring a single blood sample Case-control study of the relationship between admission to the hospital and drug use
Full review	Randomized controlled trial of a new drug or device for heart failure therapy Cross-sectional study requiring bronchoscopy after administration of methacholine

IRB = institutional review board; NHANES = National Health and Nutrition Examination Survey.

  8. IRB composition
    a. At least five members
       i. Chairperson
       ii. Scientific member
       iii. Nonscientific member
       iv. Layperson unaffiliated with the institution
       v. Practitioner
    b. Sufficient qualifications through the experience, expertise, and diversity of its members and backgrounds, including considerations of their racial and cultural heritage and their sensitivity to issues such as community attitudes, to promote respect for its advice and counsel in safeguarding the rights and welfare of human subjects
    c. Membership must be able to ensure protection of vulnerable populations.
    d. Membership must come from more than one profession.
  9. Informed consent
    a. Informed consent is a process, not a form. Information must be presented to the individual (or representative) to enable that person to make a voluntary decision to participate as a research subject.
    b. Components
       i. Description of any reasonably foreseeable risks or discomforts
       ii. Description of any benefits to the subject or to others that may reasonably be expected
       iii. Disclosure of appropriate alternative procedures or courses of treatment, if any
       iv. Statement describing the extent, if any, to which confidentiality of records identifying the subject will be maintained
       v. For research involving more than minimal risk, an explanation about whether any compensation, and an explanation about whether any medical treatments, will be available if injury occurs
       vi. Contact information for answers to questions about the research and research subjects' rights; whom to contact if the subject has a research-related injury
       vii. A statement that participation is voluntary; refusal to participate will involve no penalty or loss of benefits, and the subject may discontinue participation at any time without penalty

    c. Waiver or alteration of consent: An IRB may waive/alter informed consent if the following are met:
        i. No more than minimal risk
        ii. Will not adversely affect the rights and welfare of the subjects
        iii. The research could not practicably be carried out without waiver.
        iv. Subjects will be provided additional pertinent information after participation.
    d. An IRB may also waive informed consent in a limited class of research in emergency settings.

VI. HEALTH INSURANCE PORTABILITY AND ACCOUNTABILITY ACT OF 1996 (HIPAA)

A. Health Care Access, Portability, and Renewability (Title I): Ensures that individuals moving from one health plan to another or to another type of health plan (individual vs. group) will have continuity of coverage and will not be denied coverage under preexisting condition clauses or other reasons

B. Preventing Health Care Fraud and Abuse; Administrative Simplification; Medical Liability Reform (Title II)
    1. Privacy rule
    2. Transactions and code set rules: Simplify transactions.
    3. Security rule: Administrative, physical, and technical standards
    4. Enforcement rule: Increases the federal government's fraud enforcement authority in many areas
    5. Unique Identifiers Rule (National Provider Identifier)

C. Sets a National Standard for Accessing and Handling Medical Information. Privacy is now the law rather than an ethical issue.

D. Covered Entities
    1. Health care providers who conduct certain financial and administrative transactions (billing, fund transfers) electronically
    2. Health plans and health care clearinghouses

E. Protected Health Information (PHI): 18 identifiers
    1. Name
    2. All geographic subdivisions smaller than a state, including street address, city, county, precinct, and zip code, and their equivalent geocodes, except for the initial three digits of a zip code, if one of the following applies according to the current publicly available data from the Bureau of the Census:
        a. The geographic unit formed by combining all zip codes with the same three initial digits contains more than 20,000 people, and
        b. The initial three digits of a zip code for all such geographic units containing 20,000 or fewer people is changed to 000.
    3. All elements of dates (except year) for dates directly related to an individual, including birth date, admission date, discharge date, and date of death; and all ages older than 89 years and all elements of dates (including year) indicative of such age, except that such ages and elements may be aggregated into a single category of age 90 years or older
    4. Telephone numbers
    5. Fax numbers
    6. Electronic mail addresses
    7. Social Security numbers
    8. Medical record numbers
    9. Health plan beneficiary numbers
    10. Account numbers

11. Certificate and license numbers

12. Vehicle identifiers and serial numbers, including license plate numbers

13. Medical device identifiers and serial numbers

14. Internet universal resource locators

15. Internet protocol (IP) addresses

16. Biometric identifiers (fingerprints and voiceprints)

17. Full-face photographic images and comparable images

18. Any other unique identifying number, characteristic, or code (may assign a code for de-identified information to be re-identified)

F. Business Associates Agreement
   1. PHI belongs to the covered entity, but another person (nonemployee hospital health care personnel providing service to the covered entity) is using or disclosing the PHI to perform a function or activity on behalf of the covered entity
   2. Providing services to the covered entity if the provision of the service involves the disclosure of PHI to the service provider

G. Patient Information
   1. Patients must be notified if their health information is used and disclosed, and they must be notified of their right to privacy under HIPAA.
   2. Usually, by a Notice of Privacy Practices (letter or brochure)

H. Responsibilities as a Health Care Provider
   1. If you use or share health information that is not work related, you could be subject to disciplinary action (loss of privileges, dismissal) or civil and/or criminal penalties.
   2. You can share patient information for work-related reasons.
      a. Treatment: Provide, coordinate, manage health or related services; consultations; referral
      b. Payment: Obtain payment or reimbursement for providing health care services: Determining eligibility, adjusting insurance rates, handling billing and claims management, handling collections, handling preauthorizations, and determining medical necessity
      c. Health care operations – Things that we do to run and that improve our business
      d. Authorized by the patient: If patients give permission to use or disclose their PHI, we can share the minimum amount of information necessary to accomplish our purpose.
   3. Day-to-day activities
      a. Be mindful of bulletin boards, white boards, desks, computer monitors without privacy screens, etc.
      b. Discussions with patients/families: Draw curtain, speak quietly; find an empty room or other private area.
      c. Do not discuss what you see and hear at work or in places such as hallways or elevators.
      d. Use shredders or place in HIPAA-compliant locked recycling bins. Do not place in garbage or unlocked bins.
      e. Printers and fax machines should be in appropriate locations. Many fax machines and copiers have hard drives.
      f. Do not share user accounts when PHI is accessible (or ever).
      g. Electronic mail is usually not secure; encryption and password protection varies by organization.
      h. Cloud-based storage locations: Dropbox, Dox, Google, etc. Check with your institution. Smartphones, USB storage drives, laptops, and tablets: Major concerns for privacy

I. Research/Quality Improvement Under HIPAA
   1. Research: Approved by the IRB
      a. HIPAA authorization: Permission from individuals to use their PHI. Certain statements are required on the informed consent. Some statements depend on local IRB requirements.
      b. De-identified data
      c. Limited data sets
   2. If you are reviewing a patient record for anything other than a need to know the basis for the care of a patient, you need to determine whether it is quality improvement or research and take the appropriate action.
   3. Quality improvement: Work with internal committees. For example, a review of adverse drug reactions usually takes place under the authority of the pharmacy and therapeutics committee (a medical staff–authorized quality improvement activity).

J. Penalties for Violations
   1. Civil penalties: Accidental disclosure: $100/person/violation, up to $25,000 per year
   2. Criminal penalties
      a. Knowing misuse of information: $50,000 and 1 year in jail
      b. False pretenses: $100,000 and 5 years in jail
      c. Harmful intent, sell information: $250,000 and 10 years in jail

K. Health Information Technology for Economic and Clinical Health Act (HITECH Act)
   1. Title XIII of the American Recovery and Reinvestment Act of 2009
   2. Purpose is to promote and expand the adoption of health information technology.
   3. Anticipates the increase in electronic transactions of PHI, thus increasing the scope of privacy and security protections
   4. Civil penalties for willful neglect up to $250,000 with repeat or uncorrected up to $1.5 million
      a. Breach notification: Notify patient of all breaches.
      b. Breach notification: Notify DHHS and the media if there are greater than 500 patients.
   5. If provider has an electronic health record system, individuals may obtain their PHI electronically (ePHI); the individual can also designate a third party to receive the ePHI.

VII. PROFESSIONAL WRITING: THE PUBLICATION PROCESS

A. Primary Literature
   1. Experimental studies
   2. Observational studies
   3. Descriptive reports

B. Publication Process
   1. Journal selection
      a. Topic
      b. Journal quality
         i. Impact factor
         ii. Immediacy index
      c. Open access
   2. Preparation of submission: Paper parts
      a. Title page

    b. Abstract

    c. Introduction/background

    d. Methods

    e. Results

    f. Discussion

3. Editorial and peer review

    a. Types of reviews

        i. Single-blind review: The reviewer's identity is hidden from the author, but the reviewer knows the author.

        ii. Double-blind review: Both reviewer and author are blinded.

        iii. Open review: Reviewer and author are known to each other.

        iv. Published review: Reviewers' comments are published together with the paper.

    b. Role of reviewer

        i. Does the scientific content have value and originality?

        ii. Is the paper consistent with journal guidelines?

        iii. Are the methods appropriate?

        iv. What changes should be made or additional experiments conducted?

        v. Make a recommendation (accept, revise, reject) to the editor.

4. Revision process

5. Poor-quality research: Why?

    a. Academic scientists need to publish.

    b. Poor training or investigators/writers

    c. Lack of reviewers with sufficient knowledge or time to review

    d. Least publishable unit: Several publications from same study

    e. Other influences

        i. Current political issues and hot topics

        ii. Industry

            (a) Design and funding of studies

            (b) Comments during publication stage

            (c) Ghost writers

            (d) Promotional activities

REFERENCES

1. Byerly WG. Working with the institutional review board. Am J Health Syst Pharm 2009;66:176-84.

2. Clauson KA, Polen HH, Marsh WA. Clinical decision support tools: performance of personal digital assistant versus online drug information databases. Pharmacotherapy 2007;27:1651-8.

3. Enfield KB, Truwit JD. The purpose, composition, and function of an institutional review board: balancing priorities. Respir Care 2008;53:1330-6.

4. Gim S, Vincent WR III. Contemporary approaches for evidence-based pharmacotherapy. J Pharm Pract 2013;26:95-102.

5. Grossman S, Zerilli T. Health and medication information resources on the World Wide Web. J Pharm Pract 2013;26:85-94.

6. Hamilton CW. How to write and publish scientific papers: scribing information for pharmacists. Am J Hosp Pharm 1992;49:2477-84.

7. Harvey E. Evidence-based pharmacotherapy. In: Shumock G, Brundage DM, Chapman MM, et al., eds. Pharmacotherapy Self-Assessment Program, 5th ed. Kansas City, MO: ACCP, 2005:115-30.

8. Kier KL, Goldwire M. Drug information resources and literature retrieval. In: Dunsworth TS, Richardson MM, Chant C, et al., eds. Pharmacotherapy Self-Assessment Program, 7th ed. Lenexa, KS: ACCP, 2013:41-64.

9. Malone PM, Kier KL, Stanovich JE. Drug Information: A Guide for Pharmacists, 4th ed. New York: McGraw-Hill, 2011.

10. Nathan JP. Drug information the systematic approach. J Pharm Pract 2013;26:78-84.

11. Ness RB; for the Joint Policy Committee, Societies of Epidemiology. Influence of the HIPAA privacy rule on health research. JAMA 2007;298:2164-70.

12. Pyon EY. Primer on clinical practice guidelines. J Pharm Pract 2013;26:103-11.

13. Sackett D. Evidence-based medicine: what it is and what it isn't. BMJ 1996;213:71-2.

14. Sackett DL, Straus SE, Richardson WS, et al. Evidence-Based Medicine: How to Practice and Teach EBM, 2nd ed. London: Churchill-Livingstone, 2000.

15. Tietze KJ. Clinical Skills for Pharmacists: A Patient-Focused Approach, 3rd ed. St. Louis: Elsevier, 2011.

16. Van Way CW III. Writing a scientific paper. Nutr Clin Pract 2002;22:636-40.

17. West PM. Literature evaluation. In: Shumock G, Brundage DM, Chapman MM, et al., eds. Pharmacotherapy Self-Assessment Program, 5th ed. Kansas City, MO: ACCP, 2005:93-114.

ANSWERS AND EXPLANATIONS TO SELF-ASSESSMENT QUESTIONS

1. Answer: C

Answers A and B, a review article in Pharmacotherapy and dosing information from Lexicomp, are examples of tertiary literature, one printed and one electronic. Answer D, a PubMed search using the key words fluticasone furoate, vilanterol, and COPD, is an example of secondary literature. Answer C, a study evaluating clopidogrel for the treatment of acute venous thromboembolism, is correct.

2. Answer: B

Although advertisements (Item A is correct) do not always indicate an unreliable Web site, each of the other distractors is a reasonable indicator that some attention is being paid to the content.

3. Answer: A

The responses in Answers B–D should all be viewed with skepticism when reviewing a website. The Health On the Net Foundation seal of approval (Answer A) is an external tool that is useful in assessing the quality of a website.

4. Answer: D

Answer A would provide the most up-to-date guideline and a tertiary source, but using it would likely take the longest time when incorporating the most recent studies. Answers B and C, UpToDate and Pharmacotherapy, respectively, are both tertiary sources, and although they would include studies, they would not provide the most recent new evidence for this condition because the chapter and review article would both have a time delay between writing and publication. Answer D, PubMed, would allow the searching of the primary literature to locate the most recent studies in this area.

5. Answer: D

The PICO format is associated with the ASK step of the five-step EBM process. Each of the other options is associated with one of the other steps in the process.

6. Answer: B

Federal law guidance for IRB membership simply states that membership must contain a chairperson, a scientific member, a nonscientific member (Item B is correct), a layperson unaffiliated with the institution, and a practitioner. There is no requirement for the others indicated.

7. Answer: B

Eighteen items are identified as PHI in federal law. A town (Item A) or state (Item D) of residence is not one of them and are incorrect. Similarly, the age of a patient (Item C) (unless > 90) is not PHI

Policy, Practice, and Regulatory Issues

Anna Legreid Dopp, Pharm.D.

Pharmacy Society of Wisconsin
Madison, Wisconsin

POLICY, PRACTICE, AND REGULATORY ISSUES

ANNA LEGREID DOPP, PHARM.D.

PHARMACY SOCIETY OF WISCONSIN
MADISON, WISCONSIN

Learning Objectives

1. List the congressional committees and government agencies that regulate health care in the United States.
2. Explain recent federal legislative and regulatory activity that affects the delivery of health care.
3. Describe the regulatory actions that govern the prescription drug approval process and the conduct of human subjects' research.
4. Identify the regulatory and oversight bodies with jurisdiction over health system delivery of care.
5. Describe national quality initiatives aimed at improving health care delivery and patient health outcomes.
6. Explain medication policy implications at an institutional level.

Self-Assessment Questions

Answers and explanations to these questions may be found at the end of this chapter.

1. With respect to reporting for adverse drug experiences, which is the best option to correctly describe the purpose of MedWatch Form FDA 3500A?
   A. Is for voluntary reporting by health care professionals of a serious adverse event, product quality problem, or product use error with a U.S. Food and Drug Administration (FDA)-regulated drug, biologic, medical device, or dietary supplement.
   B. Is for consumer reporting of adverse drug experiences.
   C. May contain patient identifiers and still comply with the Health Insurance Portability and Accountability Act (HIPAA) Privacy Rule.
   D. Is the mandatory form to be submitted by investigational new drug (IND) reporters, manufacturers, distributors, importers, and facility personnel.

2. When considering the generic drug approval process, which choice is best to correctly define a generic drug?
   A. Follows the Accelerated New Drug Application regulatory pathway for approval.
   B. Must be bioequivalent to the branded product.
   C. Must be therapeutically equivalent to the branded product.
   D. Will be rated "A" in the Orange Book if it is not therapeutically equivalent.

3. If a medication guide is part of a Risk Evaluation and Mitigation Strategies (REMS) program as an element to ensure safe use, which option best describes it?
   A. Must be provided when a drug is dispensed in an outpatient setting and will be used without direct supervision by a health care professional.
   B. Does not need to be provided to a hospital inpatient receiving that drug.
   C. Cannot be removed from that REMS program in the future.
   D. Does not need to be provided when a drug is dispensed to a health care professional for administering to a patient in an outpatient setting.

4. Which option is best to correctly state when an IND application should be submitted to the FDA?
   A. Before preclinical studies.
   B. After preclinical studies, before phase I clinical trials.
   C. During phase II studies.
   D. After phase III studies, before market approval.

5. Which is the best choice for correctly defining a phase II clinical trial?
   A. A study that tests a new drug or treatment on a few subjects for the first time.
   B. A preliminary study of the intervention's efficacy that compares it with an existing intervention or placebo.
   C. A study that evaluates a drug or intervention on a larger sample of subjects and assesses efficacy and adverse effects.
   D. A study consisting of postmarketing studies to obtain additional information about risks, benefits, and best use recommendations.

6. Which is the most accurate definition of an adverse drug reaction?

   A. Injury from a medication that did not result from a medication error and was not preventable.

   B. Injury caused by medication use.

   C. Injury caused by a medication error.

   D. Injury potential because of a medication error.

7. Which option is best to correctly name the legislative act that created an abbreviated FDA approval pathway for generic drugs?

   A. Kefauver-Harris Amendments of 1992.

   B. Hatch-Waxman Act of 1984.

   C. Durham-Humphrey Amendment of 1951.

   D. Biologics Price Competition and Innovation (BPCI) Act of 2009.

8. Which description best depicts FDA approval of a biosimilar?

   A. A biosimilar is approved through the abbreviated new drug application pathway.

   B. Clinical data are required.

   C. Interchangeability is granted with the initial FDA approval.

   D. Equivalence to the originator (reference) biologic will be listed in the Orange Book.

BPS Pharmacotherapy Specialty Examination Content Outline

This chapter covers the following sections of the Pharmacotherapy Specialty Examination
Content Outline:

1. Domain I: Patient-Centered Pharmacotherapy,
    a. Task 2: Disseminate pharmacotherapy plans to patients, caregivers, and interprofessional team members using appropriate forms of communication and patient education strategies in order to optimize outcomes: Knowledge of 6
2. Domain II: Drug Information and Evidence-Based Medicine
    a. Task 3: Conduct pharmacotherapy-related research using appropriate scientific principles in order to ensure optimal patient care: Knowledge of 3
3. Domain III: System-Based Standards and Population-Based Pharmacotherapy
    a. Task 1: Implement effective medication use systems in order to improve system- and population-based pharmacotherapy: Knowledge of 1, 2, 4, 6
    b. Task 2: Incorporate health information technology within patient care processes in order to ensure effective medication use: Knowledge of 1
    c. Task 3: Employ safety systems in accordance with established standards in order to promote a safe medication use process: Knowledge of 1, 2, 3
    d. Task 4: Implement public health initiatives that target recognized benchmarks in order to improve population health: Knowledge of 1

OVERVIEW

The purpose of this review of policy, practice, and regulatory issues is to highlight areas of importance for clinical pharmacists as they pertain to policies governing patient care delivery and clinical research activity. Specifically, this chapter addresses rules, regulations, and quality initiatives at the institutional and national levels.

I. INSTITUTIONAL MEDICATION USE POLICY CONSIDERATIONS

1. Formulary Management
   a. Basics
      i. Formulary management is an ongoing process for a health care organization to establish medication use policies on drugs, therapies, and drug-related products that are evidence based and cost-effective for certain patient populations.
      ii. The Joint Commission Medication Management Standard Chapter requires the hospital to develop and approve criteria for selecting medications that include indications for use, effectiveness, drug interactions, potential for errors and abuse, adverse drug events, sentinel event advisories, populations served, other risks, and costs.
      iii. The Centers for Medicare & Medicaid Services (CMS) Conditions of Participation (CoP) requires that medical staff establish a formulary system.
      iv. A pharmacy and therapeutics (P&T) committee develops consensus on medication use policies and formulary management.
      v. Evidence-based evaluation of medications for inclusion on a formulary includes a drug use review or drug use evaluation (DUE) (Box 1).

Box 1. Elements of a Drug Use Evaluation Monograph

Brand and nonproprietary names	Pregnancy category and use in breastfeeding mothers
FDA approval information, including date and FDA rating	Clinical trial analysis and critique
For biosimilars, interchangeability status	Comparison of efficacy, safety, and cost-effectiveness
Pharmacology and mechanism of action	Medication safety assessment and considerations
FDA-approved indications	Financial analysis based on use within a health system
Potential off-label uses	Recommendation for inclusion or exclusion
Dosage forms and strengths	
Pharmacokinetic considerations	
Use in special populations (e.g., pediatric, geriatric, hepatic, or renal insufficiency)	

FDA = Food and Drug Administration

   b. Definitions
      i. Formulary – A continually updated list of medications and related information, developed using the clinical judgment of pharmacists, physicians, and other experts in the diagnosis and treatment of disease and promotion of health
      ii. DUE – Process used to assess the appropriateness of drug therapy by evaluating data on drug use in a given health care environment compared with predetermined criteria and standards
      iii. Medication use evaluation (MUE) – Performance improvement method that focuses on evaluating and improving medication-use processes related to prescribing, medication preparation, dispensing, administering, and monitoring

    c. Formulary management strategies
       i. Preferential use of generic drugs
       ii. Formulary exclusions
       iii. Formulary restrictions: Restricting prescriptive authority to a particular service or disease state
       iv. Therapeutic interchange: Authorized exchange of therapeutic alternatives in accordance with previously established and approved written guidelines, policies, or protocols within a formulary system
       v. Guided-use requirements: Include use criteria, clinical practice guidelines, and operating procedures
       vi. MUE: MUEs differ from DUEs in that MUEs emphasize improving patient outcomes using a process that identifies, resolves, and prevents medication-related problems (actual or potential). Steps in conducting MUEs include:
          (a) Establishing and implementing criteria, guidelines, treatment protocols, and standards of care for medications and medication use policies
          (b) Selecting medications for MUE on the basis of adverse medication events or risk of events, signs of treatment failures, expense of medication, patient population or disease state
          (c) Identifying data points and collecting data
          (d) Evaluating adherence to criteria, guidelines, treatment protocols, and standards of care for medications and medication use policies
          (e) Interpreting and reporting MUE findings
          (f) Identifying and implementing improvement strategies in the medication-use process
2. Medication Safety Monitoring and Reporting
    a. Medication errors are the broadest category and have the highest frequency of occurrence, whereas adverse drug events are rare, occurring in 1% of medication errors.
       i. Grades of certainty criteria, including certainty, probable/likely, possible, and unlikely, determine whether an adverse event is caused by a medication.
       ii. Table 1 outlines the differences between medication errors, adverse drug events, and adverse drug reactions, or non-preventable adverse drug events.

Table 1. Differences Between Medication Errors, Adverse Drug Events, and Adverse Drug Reactions

Term	Definition	Example
Medication error	Any error occurring in the medication process (ordering, transcribing, dispensing, administering, and monitoring)	Order filled for the wrong patient
Adverse drug event	Injury resulting from medication use; may or may not result from a medication error	Hemorrhage from heparin
Adverse drug reaction	Injury not caused by medication error, non-preventable and caused by the drug at normal doses and with normal use	Allergic reaction in a person with no known allergies
Potential adverse drug event	Medication error with the potential for injury	Overdosage of a medication that was intercepted before patient administration
Preventable adverse drug event	Injury caused by medication error	Overdosage of a medication that resulted in a hospitalization

b. In 1999, the IOM released a report titled "To Err Is Human," which stated that medical errors claim as many as 98,000 lives a year. The 2004 IOM report titled "Patient Safety: Achieving a New Standard for Care" revealed the high incidence of adverse events occurring in hospitals.

c. The Patient Safety and Quality Improvement Act of 2005 (Patient Safety Act) and the Patient Safety and Quality Improvement Final Rule (Patient Safety Rule) were a congressional response to these reports.

    i. Encourages health care providers and organizations to voluntarily report and share patient safety information without fear of legal action

    ii. Authorized the creation of patient safety organizations (PSOs)

        (a) PSOs can be private or public entities, profit or not-for-profit entities, provider entities such as a health system, or other entities.

        (b) PSOs provide a secure mechanism for the collection, aggregation, and analysis of data to identify and reduce risks and hazards that may occur with patient care delivery.

        (c) The ACA charges PSOs to assist health systems with a high rate of risk-adjusted readmission rates to decrease readmission rates and improve transitions of care.

    iii. The Agency for Healthcare Research and Quality (AHRQ) created the Patient Safety Organization Privacy Protection Center to support the implementation of the Patient Safety Act. The Privacy Protection Center provides technical assistance to PSOs to ensure that data on patient safety events submitted to the Network of Patient Safety Databases are non-identifiable.

    iv. Data are submitted to PSOs through Common Formats, developed by AHRQ for acute care hospitals and skilled nursing facilities. Common Formats provide a systematic process for reporting adverse events, near misses, and unsafe conditions, and they allow a hospital to report harm from all causes.

        (a) In March 2013, CMS communicated that although the use of Common Formats is not required for CoP for Quality Assessment and Performance Improvement surveys, hospitals that use them will be in a better position to meet Quality Assessment and Performance Improvement requirements.

        (b) CMS surveyors were also encouraged to become familiar with Common Formats.

d. Adverse drug events should be reported to the U.S. Food and Drug Administration (FDA) Adverse Event Reporting System, a database with more than 400 million adverse event and medication error reports.

    i. MedWatch Form FDA 3500 for voluntary reporting is for health care professionals to report a serious adverse event, product quality problem, or product use error with an FDA-regulated drug, biologic, medical device, or dietary supplement. The Health Insurance Portability and Accountability Act (HIPAA) Privacy Rule specifically permits health care professionals to disclose protected health information (PHI) for public health purposes.

    ii. MedWatch Form FDA 3500A is for regulated industry following investigational new drug (IND) and biologic regulations and user facilities such as hospitals and nursing homes.

    iii. MedWatch Form FDA 3500B is available for consumer reporting.

    iv. Vaccine-related adverse effects, veterinary medicine product adverse events, and suspected unlawful Internet sales of medical products should not be reported to MedWatch.

    v. The Sentinel Initiative is being implemented in stages to complement existing reporting systems, and it will have functionality to query electronic medical records, administrative and insurance claims, and registries.

e. The Institute for Safe Medication Practices began in 1975 to promote medication error prevention and initiated a voluntary practitioner error-reporting program.

    i. The institute is a nonprofit PSO.

    ii. Publishes four medication safety alert newsletters for acute care settings, ambulatory care settings, nurses, and medications

f. The University HealthSystem Consortium (UHC) is an alliance of academic medical centers and affiliated hospitals.
    i. It is an AHRQ-listed PSO: the UHC Performance Improvement PSO.
    ii. Offers the UHC Patient Safety Net, a web-based inpatient and outpatient safety event–reporting system that consolidates and aggregates data for specific event types and offers best practices and policies to address common systemic areas for improvement
g. The Vaccine Adverse Event Reporting System is a national postmarketing vaccine safety surveillance program managed by the Centers for Disease Control and Prevention (CDC) and the FDA for vaccine-related adverse events to be reported, analyzed, and made available to the public. The National Childhood Vaccine Injury Act of 1986 requires health care professionals and vaccine manufacturers to report to the Department of Health and Human Services (DHHS) specific adverse events that occur after the administration of routinely recommended vaccines.
h. Occupational Safety and Health Administration
    i. Ensures safe and healthful working conditions for employees
    ii. Is part of the U.S. Department of Labor and was granted regulatory authority through the Occupational Safety and Health Act of 1970
i. The United States Pharmacopoeia (USP) develops standards, enforceable by the FDA, on the identity, strength, quality, and purity of medications and dietary supplements, including compounded products.
j. The General Chapters are as follows: Required (numbered below <1000>), Informational (numbered <1XXX>), or Specific for dietary supplements (numbered <2XXX>); the chapters pertaining to compounding include the following:
    i. USP 795: Pharmaceutical Compounding for Nonsterile Preparations
    ii. USP 797 (being revised): Pharmaceutical Compounding for Sterile Preparations (CSPs)
    iii. USP 800: Hazardous Drugs: Handling in Healthcare Settings
k. Pharmacies may be subject to inspection against these standards by boards of pharmacy, the FDA, the Joint Commission, and other entities. In October 2015, CMS issued a revision to its Pharmaceutical Services CoP State Operations Manual that aligned USP requirements with their standards of practice for drug compounding, particularly for CSPs.
l. USP 797 standards assign risk levels (low, medium, and high) according to requirements for the types of admixtures and preparation procedures.
m. CSPs have been under scrutiny because of deaths associated with microorganism contamination. An area of interest for organizations is beyond-use dating and sterility for CSPs. According to USP 797, if sterility testing has been performed, pharmacies can assign a beyond-use date based on the maximum chemical stability as listed in valid references. If sterility testing has not been performed, pharmacies must use beyond-use dating according to the level of risk and storage (Table 2).

Table 2. Beyond-Use Dating for Compounded Sterile Products

Risk Category	Room Temperature (20°C–25°C)	Refrigerator (2°C–8°C)	Freezer (≤ 10°C)
Immediate use	1 hr	1 hr	N/A
Low	48 hr	14 days	45 days
Low w/12-hr beyond-use date	≤ 12 hr	≤ 12 hr	N/A
Medium	30 hr	9 days	45 days
High	24 hr	3 days	45 days

3. Supporting Patient Access to Medications
   a. Options exist for supporting and supplementing patient access to medications. Pharmacists are a conduit for linking patients to medication discount and prescription assistance programs.
   b. The 340B Drug Pricing Program, authorized through the Medicaid Drug Rebate Program in 1990 and expanded by the ACA in 2010, allows specific categories of safety-net providers to become established entities and procure outpatient prescription drugs at discounted prices. The 16 categories of covered entities use the discounts to expand or develop new services.
      i. Eligibility is defined at the level of the health care facility and not the individual; however, the Health Resources and Services Administration's (HRSA's) Office of Pharmacy Affairs states that only patients with an established relationship with the covered entity are eligible to receive 340B purchased drugs.
      ii. Covered entities can procure drugs at 340B prices and distribute them in the following ways
         (a) Procurement by the covered entity and distribution by covered entities with in-house pharmacies or to an outpatient clinic for direct administration to patients
         (b) Procurement by the covered entity but distribution to the patient from a contracted pharmacy
   c. Patient and prescription assistance programs are operated by drug manufacturers to provide free medications to patients who cannot afford them.

II. CONGRESSIONAL OVERVIEW, COMMITTEES WITH JURISDICTION OVER HEALTH-RELATED POLICY, AND THE LEGISLATIVE PROCESS

1. Congress is bicameral, with two legislative chambers.
2. Laws and Regulations: Basics
3. The Senate is composed of 100 elected, voting members. Legislation and tasks are divided into 20 standing committees, 68 subcommittees, and 4 joint committees. The committees that have jurisdiction over health-related policy include the following:
   a. Appropriations Committee writes the legislation that allocates federal funds to the many government agencies, departments, and organizations on an annual basis and, in particular, funds discretionary programs.
   b. Finance Committee has jurisdiction over issues that pertain to taxation and health programs under the Social Security Act including Medicare, Medicaid, and the Children's Health Insurance Program.
   c. Health, Education, Labor and Pensions (HELP) Committee, as it pertains to health, authorizes agencies, institutes, and programs under DHHS, which includes the FDA, National Institutes of Health (NIH), and CDC.
   d. Committee on Veterans' Affairs oversees issues related to veterans' affairs (VA), including the VA health system.
   e. Aging Committee was initially established as a temporary committee but transitioned to a permanent, special committee without legislative authority for matters relating to older Americans.
   f. Legislation is reviewed by the committee with the most jurisdiction over the provisions in the bill. For example, the Pharmacy and Medically Underserved Areas Enhancement Act (S 314) was referred to the Committee on Finance because it amends the Medicare program.
4. The House of Representatives is composed of 435 elected, voting members and six delegates from the U.S. territories or from Washington, D.C., with nonvoting privileges. Legislation and tasks are divided into 20 standing committees, 4 joint committees, and 1 select committee. The committees with jurisdiction over health-related policy include the following:
   a. Appropriations has jurisdiction similar to that listed above.
   b. Ways and Means has jurisdiction over taxation and most programs authorized by the Social Security Act, similar to the Senate Finance Committee.

    c.   Energy and Commerce is the oldest standing committee of the House of Representatives. It has oversight of DHHS and is similar to the Senate HELP committee.

    d.   Veterans' Affairs oversees issues related to VA.

    e.   Legislation is sent to any committee that has jurisdiction over any of the provisions in the bill. For example, the Pharmacy and Medically Underserved Areas Enhancement Act (HR 592) was referred to the Energy and Commerce Subcommittee on Health and the Ways and Means Committee.

5.   Legislative Process (Figure 1)

    a.   Legislation is drafted by a member of Congress, a congressional committee, a constituent, a state legislature, or an executive communication from the president or an administrative agency.

    b.   Once introduced, the bill, joint resolution, concurrent resolution, or simple resolution is generally referred to the relevant committees for consideration, markup, and approval.

    c.   Action, debate, and voting on legislation, which are dictated by rules, differ greatly between the Senate and the House of Representatives.

Figure 1. Legislative process.

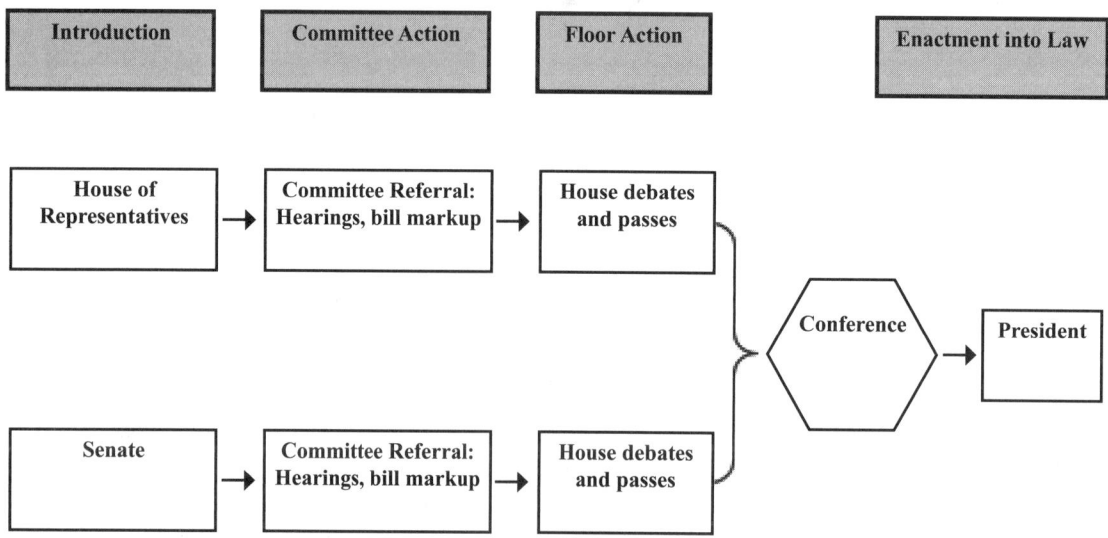

6.   Definitions

    a.   Authorization bills grant authority for a program or agency to exist or promulgate regulations. A program must still receive an appropriation in order to receive funding.

    b.   An appropriation is a sum of money designated for a particular purpose by an act or bill.

    c.   Entitlement spending for programs such as Medicare, Medicaid, and Social Security is automatically set according to eligible recipients. Levels of spending can be changed only by eligibility criteria changes.

    d.   Discretionary spending represents annual spending levels determined by Congress; such spending is optional.

    e.   Continuing resolution continues funding for a program if the congressional fiscal year, ending September 30, ends without a new appropriation in place.

7. Recent Legislative Activity with Regulatory Policy Implications
   a. The American Recovery and Reinvestment Act (ARRA) of 2009 provided a vehicle for passing the Health Information Technology for Economic and Clinical Health (HITECH) Act. The HITECH Act authorizes the U.S. DHHS to create programs to improve health care quality, safety, and efficiency through the promotion of health information technology, including electronic health records (EHRs) and health information exchanges (HIEs). The goal of HITECH is to facilitate and expand the secure, electronic movement and use of health information among organizations according to nationally recognized standards.
      i. Created the Office of the National Coordinator for Health Information Technology (ONC) to coordinate nationwide standards and implementation efforts
      ii. The Standards and Certification Criteria Final Rule is the initial approach to adopting standards, implementing specifications, and providing certification criteria to increase the interoperability, functionality, utility, and security of health information technology and to support its meaningful use.
      iii. The Electronic Health Records Incentive Programs was issued by CMS to provide a financial incentive to eligible professionals, eligible hospitals and critical access hospitals, and Medicare Advantage Organizations that are "meaningful users" of EHRs. ARRA 2009 specified three main components for "meaningful use":
         (a) Use of certified EHRs in a meaningful manner (e.g., e-Prescribing)
         (b) Use of certified EHR technology for electronic exchange of health information to improve the quality of health care
         (c) Use of certified EHR technology to submit clinical quality and other measures
      iv. Incentive payments began in fiscal year 2011 and will gradually decrease until fiscal year 2015, when penalties are to be put into effect.
      v. HITECH also affects research because it imposes new penalties for breaches in HIPAA and PHI; the Office for Civil Rights within DHHS will audit for compliance.
      vi. An HIE is defined as a process for exchanging health information, and an HIO (health information organization) is a model for exchanging information at local, regional (known as RHIO [regional health information organization]), or state levels. ONC's goal for HIE is for patient information to be accessible across organizational, vendor, and geographic boundaries. Regulations related to HIE are aimed at increasing interoperability, increasing consumer and provider trust to mobilize information, and decreasing the cost and complexity of the exchange. Three forms of HIE are defined:
         (a) Directed exchange – Ability to send and receive secure information electronically between care providers to support coordinated care
         (b) Query-based exchange – Ability for providers to find and/or request information on a patient from other providers
         (c) Consumer mediated exchange – Ability for patients to aggregate and control the use of their health information among providers
   b. The Patient Protection and Affordable Care Act of 2010 (ACA) contains several provisions, ranging from protecting consumers to improving health care quality and lowering costs to increasing access to care. As the law translates into regulation, unique opportunities exist for pharmacists to become engaged.
      i. Funding opportunities will be available for pharmacists to show their contributions as providers of medication therapy management.
      ii. The patient-centered medical home model emphasizes primary care as a central role in managing the chronic conditions of patients using a team-based care approach.

   iii. Accountable care organizations (ACOs) are a set of providers associated with a defined population of patients accountable for the quality and cost of care delivered to that population.

   iv. The Independence at Home Demonstration Program promotes the interdisciplinary collaboration of clinicians to provide home-based medical care for Medicare beneficiaries.

   v. The Biologics Price Competition and Innovation (BPCI) Act of 2009 is a provision in the ACA that creates an abbreviated approval pathway for follow-on biologic products, known as "biosimilars."

   vi. The Physician Payments Sunshine Act (i.e., Sunshine Act) requires manufactures of drugs, medical devices, and biologicals that participate in federal health care programs to report payments and items of value given to physicians and teaching hospitals. It also requires manufacturers and group purchasing organizations to report physician ownership or investments.

     (a) CMS authorized to implement the Sunshine Act as the Open Payments Program

     (b) Reports on 2013 data were released in September 2014.

c. The Safe and Secure Drug Disposal Act of 2010

   i. Authorized the Drug Enforcement Administration (DEA) to promulgate rules for patient disposal of unused controlled substances and controlled substance disposal by long-term care facilities

   ii. The Disposal of Controlled Substances Final Rule, enacted on October 9, 2014, allows the transfer of unwanted and unused controlled substances from an ultimate user (i.e., patient) to an authorized collector for safe, secure, and responsible disposal.

     (a) Authorized collectors include manufacturers, distributors, reverse distributors, narcotic treatment programs, hospitals and clinics with on-site pharmacies, and retail pharmacies, including long-term care facilities and specialty pharmacies.

     (b) Allows ultimate users to voluntarily dispose of controlled substances through take-back events, mail-back events, and collection receptacles

     (c) Regulates each element of the disposal process, including transfer, deliver, collection, return, and recall of controlled substances

d. The FDA Safety and Innovation Act of 2012 amends the federal Food, Drug, and Cosmetic (FD&C) Act to revise and extend the user fee programs for prescription drugs and medical devices to establish user fee programs for generic drugs, biosimilars, and other purposes.

   i. Addresses drug shortages and states that the manufacturer of a drug that is life supporting, life sustaining, or intended for use in the prevention or treatment of a debilitating disease or condition, including use in emergency medical care or during surgery, must notify the Secretary of DHHS of a permanent discontinuation in the manufacturing of the drug that may disrupt supply in the United States, together with the reasons for discontinuation, at least 6 months before the date of discontinuation

   ii. Additional provisions include responding to those failing to report a shortage, expediting manufacturer inspections, publishing a drug shortage list, authorizing hospitals to repackage drugs without registering as an establishment if distributing within a health system, and requiring the Comptroller General to conduct a study on the impact of medication shortages.

c. The Drug Quality and Security Act of 2013

   i. Establishes a new section (503B) in the FD&C Act to allow a compounding facility to voluntarily register as an outsourcing facility with the FDA. The outsourcing facility must give a licensed pharmacist direct oversight over compounded drugs. Other requirements include the following: only drugs with bulk ingredients listed as approved by the secretary can be compounded, the facility must report to the secretary every 6 months and undergo inspection by the FDA, the facility must report serious adverse events, and the facility must label products identifying them as a compounded drug.

    ii. Adds a new section to the FD&C Act with product-tracing requirements ("track-and-trace") for drug manufacturers, repackagers, wholesale distributors, and dispensers to provide trans-action details when pharmaceutical products change ownership. Entities will also need to respond promptly in the event of a recall or an illegitimate product suspicion or investigation. Implementation of these requirements has been delayed twice, extending the compliance deadline from July 1, 2015, to March 1, 2016.

    iii. Increases wholesale distributor licensure standards

  f. Medicare Access and CHIP Reauthorization Act (MACRA) of 2015

    i. Legislation repealed the sustainable growth rate (SGR) physician reimbursement methodology that threatened to reduce Medicare physician payments for more than a decade.

    ii. Represents a shift in reimbursement from fee-for-service to pay-for-performance or pay-for-value

      (a) Establishes the alternative payment model for physicians participating in patient-centered medical homes, ACOs, and Medicare shared-savings programs

      (b) Establishes the merit-based incentive payment system (MIPS) that reimburses on the basis of quality, resource use, clinical practice improvement activities, and meaningful use of EHR

    iii. Sunsets three existing value-based payment adjustments through the Physician Quality Reporting System, the Value-Based Payment Modifier, and the EHR incentive program and combines them into MIPS

    iv. Promises to revise and replace the EHR incentive program known as meaningful use

    v. Reauthorized the State Children's Health Insurance Program through fiscal year 2017

III. U.S. GOVERNMENT DEPARTMENTS AND AGENCIES WITH PRIMARY REGULATORY IMPACT ON THE PRACTICE OF PHARMACY

1. DHHS is the agency charged with protecting the health of Americans. Appropriations to DHHS represent the largest share of nondefense discretionary funding, at 32% of federal monies appropriated. The follow-ing agencies are located within DHHS:

  a. FDA is responsible for the safety of most foods (human and animal) and cosmetics, and it regulates both the safety and effectiveness of human drugs, biologics (e.g., vaccines, blood products, therapeutic proteins), medical devices, and animal drugs.

  b. CMS administers Medicare, Medicaid, and the State Children's Health Insurance Program. It is driving the Value-Based Purchasing Program, the Medicare Shared Savings Program, and the EHR Meaningful Use Incentive Program, and it develops CoP and Conditions for Coverage that health care organizations are required to meet in order to participate in Medicare and Medicaid programs.

  c. The Agency for Healthcare Research and Quality (AHRQ) supports research that helps people make better-informed decisions and improves the quality of health care services.

  d. CDC provides programs that reduce the health and economic consequences of the leading causes of death and disability. An example is Healthy People, which provides science-based national goals and objectives with 10-year targets designed to guide national health promotion and disease prevention efforts.

  e. HRSA improves access to health care through programs that strengthen the health care workforce, build healthy communities, and achieve health equity for people who are geographically isolated and/or economically or medically vulnerable. HRSA houses the National Center for Health Workforce Analysis charged with estimating the supply and demand for health care workers and designating shortage criteria in order to establish Health Professional Shortage Areas or Medically Underserved Areas or Populations.

2. U.S. Department of Justice (DOJ): Has jurisdiction over the DEA, which prevents, detects, and investigates the diversion of controlled substances and monitored chemicals.

3. U.S. Environmental Protection Agency seeks to protect human health and the environment.

    a. Through the Resource Conservation and Recovery Act of 1976, the U.S. Environmental Protection Agency has jurisdiction over rules governing the disposal of solid and hazardous waste.

    b. The Management Standards for Hazardous Waste Pharmaceuticals Rule proposes new regulations for health care facilities (including pharmacies) and reverse distributors in the handling of hazardous waste pharmaceuticals in order to improve environmental protection.

4. Departments and agencies of the U.S. government make rules and adjudicate (enforce) them within areas of delegated authority.

    a. The Administration Procedure Act of 1946 granted agencies of DHHS the power to promulgate rules and regulations that have the effect of substantive law.

    b. Codification of general and permanent rules is published in the Federal Register, and the public is allowed to provide feedback within a prespecified time limit.

        i. Example: DHHS CMS 42 Code of Federal Regulations (CFR) parts 424 and 431: Medicare and Medicaid Programs; Changes in Provider and Supplier Enrollment, Ordering and Referring, and Documentation Requirements; and Changes in Provider Agreements. This final rule expanded the definition of nonphysician practitioners on hospital staffs to include pharmacists.

        ii. Example: DOJ DEA 21 CFR Parts 1300, 1301, 1304, et al.: Disposal of Controlled Substances. This final rule governs the secure disposal of controlled substances by DEA registrants and ultimate users.

    c. Final rules are published in the CFR, which has 50 titles that are updated every year on a staggered basis.

        i. Title 21: Food and Drugs

            (a) Institutional Review Boards (21 CFR Part 56) contains standards for the composition, operation, and responsibility of an institutional review board (IRB) that reviews and approves of studies for products regulated by the FDA.

            (b) Differences exist between this regulation and that of the Common Rule for the definitions of research, human subjects, and IRB. Both need to be considered when conducting research.

            (c) IRB review is required for clinical investigations designed for submission to the FDA in support of an application or marketing permit. Exemptions from an IRB requirement are outlined in the text of this rule.

        ii. Title 42: Public Health

            (a) Contains rules related to HHS, CMS, and the Office of Inspector General-Healthcare

            (b) Federally qualified health centers, organizations that receive grants for enhanced reimbursement from Medicare and Medicaid for offering health care services to all patients regardless of their ability to pay, are regulated by rules outlined in Medicare CMS regulations in Title 42.

        iii. Title 45: Public Welfare

            (a) Common Rule (45 CFR Part 46): Federal Policy for the Protection of Human Subjects (revisions proposed in 2015 with finalization planned for 2016)

              • Defines research as a systematic investigation, including research, development, testing, and evaluation, designed to develop or contribute to generalizable knowledge

              • Defines a human subject as a living individual about whom an investigator obtains data through intervention or interaction with the individual or identifiable private information

              • Defines an IRB in the context of the rule and is different from that of 21 CFR 56. Typical exemptions from IRB requirements include research conducted in certain educational settings or involving educational tests or surveys.

(b) HIPAA (45 CFR Parts 160, 162, and 164)
- Enacted through HIPAA and enforced by the DHHS Office for Civil Rights
- The suite of HIPAA regulations for patient privacy and security is outlined in the Transactions and Code Set Standards, Identifier Standards, Privacy Rule, Security Rule, Enforcement Rule, and Breach Notification Rule.

IV. ACCREDITING ORGANIZATIONS AND QUALITY IMPROVEMENT EFFORTS

1. The Joint Commission is a not-for-profit, independent organization that sets standards for accrediting health care facilities through its mission "to continuously improve health care for the public, in collaboration with other stakeholders, by evaluating health care organizations and inspiring them to excel in providing safe and effective care of the highest quality and value."
    a. Accredits and certifies more than 20,500 health care organizations in the United States
    b. Standards address an organization's performance in functional areas of patient rights, patient treatment, medication safety, and infection control. Hospitals provide data from a selection of 57 inpatient measures.
    c. National Patient Safety Goals were established to help accredited organizations address specific areas of concern in patient safety in the areas of ambulatory health care, behavioral health care, critical access hospital, home care, hospital, laboratory, long-term care, Medicare or Medicaid long-term care, and office-based surgery.
    d. The ORYX is a Joint Commission performance measurement and improvement initiative implemented to integrate outcomes with accountability measures in the areas of acute myocardial infarction, heart failure, pneumonia, surgical care improvement project, children's asthma care, perinatal, hospital outpatient measures, venous thromboembolism, substance abuse, tobacco treatment, emergency department care, immunization, hospital-based inpatient psychiatric services, and stroke in its accreditation process.
        i. Common standardized measures between the Joint Commission and CMS are called National Hospital Quality Measures.
        ii. Accountability measures and processes that result in the greatest improvement in patient outcomes have been identified by the Joint Commission. These measures and processes must be of sound scientific evidence, be in proximity between process and outcome, accurately measure the process, and minimize adverse effects without inducing unintended consequences. Measures are updated semiannually and include areas such as acute myocardial infarction, heart failure, pneumonia, surgical care improvement project, children's asthma care, venous thromboembolism, and stroke.
    e. The Targeted Solutions Tool, created by the Joint Commission Center for Transforming Healthcare, provides a process for accredited hospitals to measure performance, identify barriers to excellent performance, and implement proven solutions.
    f. Tracer methodology is a process used by an on-site surveyor to evaluate a patient's medical record as a road map to move through a health care organization to assess and evaluate its compliance with standards and systems to provide care and services. First-generation tracers follow a patient through care areas, whereas second-generation tracers focus on major organizational areas, such as high-alert medications or medication shortages.
2. The National Committee for Quality Assurance (NCQA) is a private, not-for-profit organization with a mission to improve the quality of health care through measurement, transparency, and accountability.
    a. Accreditation programs, certification programs, physician recognition programs, and distinctions are directed at health plans, such as health maintenance organizations, preferred provider organizations, and consumer-directed health plans, physician networks, medical groups, and individual physicians.

b. Responsible for three key efforts to measure and improve health care quality: assessment of on-site clinical and administrative processes (around 54% of NCQA measures), through data collection for the Healthcare Effectiveness Data and Information Set (HEDIS) (around 33% of NCQA measures), and measuring member satisfaction through the Consumer Assessment of Healthcare Providers and Systems survey (around 13% of NCQA measures)

    c. Produces several public reports, including "The State of Health Care Quality," which is an overall assessment of the performance of the American health care system; "America's Best Health Plans" in collaboration with *U.S. News & World Report;* and the online Health Plan Report Card with a searchable database detailing health plans' accreditation and performance ratings

    d. NCQA will establish criteria for ACOs, created by the ACA. Principles of ACOs include the following:

        i. Strong foundation of primary care

        ii. Reliable reporting of measures to support quality improvement and to eliminate waste and inefficiencies to reduce cost

        iii. Commitment to improving quality and patient experience while reducing per capita costs

        iv. Collaboration with stakeholders in a community or region

        v. Creating and supporting a sustainable workforce.

    e. HEDIS is a tool that consists of more than 81 measures across five domains of care that health plans use to measure performance and focus improvement efforts.

        i. Measures are developed by identifying a clinical area to evaluate. The process includes conducting an extensive literature review, developing the measure, vetting it with various stakeholders, and performing a field test that evaluates feasibility, reliability, and validity.

        ii. Domains include effectiveness of care, access of care, experience of care, utilization and relative resource use, and health plan descriptive information.

    f. The Quality Compass is a comparison tool that allows users to view measure results and benchmark information that ranks health plans using the HEDIS measures.

3. The National Quality Forum is a nonprofit organization that aims to improve quality through a three-part mission. (1) Build consensus on national priorities and goals for performance improvement and work in partnership to achieve them. (2) Endorse national consensus standards for measuring and publicly reporting on performance. (3) Promote the attainment of national goals through education and outreach programs.

    a. Membership includes stakeholders from consumer organizations, public and private purchasers, physicians, nurses, accrediting and certifying bodies, supporting industries, and health care research and quality improvement organizations.

    b. Through the passage of the Medicare Improvements for Patients and Providers Act of 2008, DHHS entered into a contract with the National Quality Forum to establish a portfolio of quality and efficiency measures for use in reporting on and improving health care quality for the federal government to determine a return on investment in health care spending.

    c. Formulation of a national strategy and priorities for health care performance measurement to review and synthesize evidence related to 20 high-priority conditions identified by CMS that account for more than 95% of their costs

    d. Implementation of a consensus process for endorsement of health care quality measures

    e. Maintenance of consensus-endorsed measures

    f. Promotion of EHRs

    g. Focused measurement of the development, harmonization, and endorsement efforts to fill critical gaps in performance measurements

4. AHRQ
   a. The agency within DHHS that supports research that helps people make more informed decisions and improves the quality of health care services through its mission to improve the quality, safety, and effectiveness of health care for all Americans
   b. Health service research provides clinical, health care system, and public policy decision-makers evidence-based information on health outcomes, quality, cost, use, and access to improve the quality of health care services.
   c. Comparative effectiveness research (CER) is the conduct and synthesis of systematic research comparing different interventions and strategies to prevent, diagnose, treat, and monitor health conditions. The concept of CER was introduced in the Medicare Modernization Act of 2003, but it received more funding and attention in ARRA 2009 when the Federal Coordinating Council for Comparative Effectiveness Research was established. It is composed of members from DHHS agencies such as AHRQ, FDA, NIH, CMS, CDC, Office of Minority Health, ONC, HRSA, and Substance Abuse and Mental Health Services as well as from the Veterans Health Administration and the Department of Defense and Office of Management and Budget.
   d. The Consumer Assessment of Healthcare Providers and Systems assesses consumer experiences with health care. The Clinician and Group, Health Plan, and In-Center Hemodialysis surveys can be reviewed by patients and consumers, quality monitors and regulators, provider organizations, health plans, community collaboratives, and public and private purchasers of health care as a means to make informed decisions and improve health care services.
   e. The Effective Health Care Program funds individual researchers, research centers, and academic organizations to work together with AHRQ to produce effectiveness and CER for clinicians, consumers, and policy-makers.
5. The Pharmacy Quality Alliance
   a. The mission of the Pharmacy Quality Alliance is to improve the quality of medication use across health care settings through a collaborative process in which key stakeholders agree on a strategy for measuring and reporting performance information related to medications.
   b. Develops performance measures, including proportion of days covered, gap in medication therapy, diabetes medication dosing, suboptimal treatment of hypertension in patients with diabetes, use of high-risk medications in older adults, drug-drug interactions, and medication therapy for people with asthma
6. The American Society of Health-System Pharmacists (ASHP) is a national accrediting organization for pharmacy residency and pharmacy technician training programs.
7. The Accreditation Council for Pharmacy Education sets standards for education of pharmacists to prepare them for the delivery of pharmacist provided patient care.
8. The Center for Pharmacy Practice Accreditation, established by the American Pharmacists Association, the National Association of Boards of Pharmacy, and ASHP, offers accreditation for pharmacy practice sites on the basis of adherence to comprehensive and patient-centered medication use performance measures.
9. The Leapfrog Group is a voluntary program that works with employers to enable and direct purchasing power toward health care decisions focused on safety, quality, and value. It compares hospital performance on the metrics most important to consumers and purchasers of care. A Hospital Safety Score of A, B, C, D, or F has been applied to more than 2500 hospitals on the basis of prevention of errors, accidents, injuries, and infections.

V. THE U.S. FOOD AND DRUG ADMINISTRATION AND THE PRESCRIPTION DRUG APPROVAL PROCESS

1. The FDA and the Prescription Drug Approval Process
   a. Basics
      i. Most federal laws that authorize the FDA to promulgate rules are enacted by amendments to the FD&C Act, and they are organized in Title 21 of the CFR. The FDA is funded through discretionary spending every fall in Congress's appropriations bill written by the Senate and House appropriations committees, but the Senate HELP and the House Energy and Commerce committees have jurisdiction over its reauthorization.
      ii. Organized by the Office of the Commissioner, Medical Products and Tobacco, Foods and Veterinary Medicine, and Global Regulatory Operations and Policy. The following offices and centers affect medication use:
         1. Office of the Commissioner conducts overall agency coordination; the FDA's top official, the commissioner, requires Senate confirmation.
         2. Office of Regulatory Affairs, the largest office, regulates all inspection and enforcement activities.
         3. National Center for Toxicological Research supports the six product centers with scientific technology, training, and technical expertise.
         4. Center for Drug Evaluation and Research (CDER) regulates prescription and nonprescription drugs.
         5. Center for Biologics Evaluation and Research regulates biologic products, including vaccines, blood products, and gene therapy.
         6. Center for Devices and Radiological Health regulates medical devices.
         7. Center for Food Safety and Applied Nutrition regulates most foods, food additives, infant formulas, dietary supplements, and cosmetics.
         8. Center for Tobacco Products regulates tobacco-containing products.
         9. Center for Veterinary Medicine regulates feed, drugs, and devices used for pets, farm animals, and other animals.
   b. Definitions
      i. The Abbreviated New Drug Application (ANDA) contains data that, when submitted to the FDA's CDER, Office of Generic Drugs, allow the review and ultimate approval of a generic drug product.
      ii. An authorized generic drug is a listed drug that is marketed, sold, or distributed directly or indirectly to the retail class of trade. Its labeling, packaging (other than repackaging as the listed drug in blister packs, unit doses, or similar packaging for use in institutions), product code, labeler code, trade name, or trademark differs from that of the listed drug.
      iii. A biologics license application is a submission that contains specific information on the manufacturing processes, chemistry, pharmacology, clinical pharmacology, and medical effects of a biologic product (monoclonal antibodies, enzymes, immunomodulators, growth factors, and cytokines) seeking approval to market in the United States.
      iv. A clinical trial is a research study of humans conducted to answer specific questions about vaccines, new therapies, or new ways of using known treatments. Clinical trials are required by the FDA to determine whether new drugs or treatments are both safe and effective.
      v. The interchangeability of a biosimilar product allows it to be substituted for the legend (brand) biologic with an expectation that the same clinical outcome will occur and without the requirement of notification or intervention of a prescriber.

      vi. An Investigational New Drug Application (INDA) is used for a new drug, a new indication, or an off-label use that will be used in a clinical investigation's preclinical development for that new drug to be distributed across state lines before full FDA review.

     vii. A New Drug Application (NDA) is the vehicle through which drug sponsors formally propose that the FDA approve a new pharmaceutical for sale and marketing in the United States.

2. History of the Regulation of Drugs and Human Subjects' Research

   a. The Drug Importation Act of 1848: Prohibited the importation of unsafe or adulterated drugs at key ports of entry

   b. The Biologics Control Act of 1902

     i. Mandated annual licensing of establishments to manufacture and sell vaccines, sera, antitoxins, and similar products in interstate commerce

     ii. Authorized Hygienic Laboratory, precursor of the National NIH, to conduct regular inspections for purity and potency

   c. The Pure Food and Drug Act of 1906

     i. Prohibited interstate commerce of adulterated or misbranded drugs

     ii. Required labeling of selected dangerous and addictive substances

     iii. Identified the United States Pharmacopoeia and the National Formulary (USP/NF) as official standards for drugs

   d. The FD&C Act of 1938

     i. Required that firms prove evidence of safety to the FDA before marketing

     ii. Placed drug advertising under the jurisdiction of the Federal Trade Commission

     iii. Recognized the USP/NF as the official compendia of drug standards

   e. The Durham-Humphrey Amendment of 1951: Amended the FD&C Act of 1938 to statutorily differentiate prescription and nonprescription drugs

   f. The Kefauver-Harris Amendments of 1962

     i. Established the requirement for drug firms to demonstrate efficacy as well as safety

     ii. Statutory requirement to obtain informed consent for research subjects

     iii. Authorized the FDA to regulate advertising of prescription drugs and establish good manufacturing practices

   g. The Comprehensive Drug Abuse Prevention and Control Act of 1970 (i.e., Controlled Substance Act) authorized the DEA and FDA to regulate the manufacture, classification (schedule), importation, possession, use, and distribution of controlled substances.

   h. The Orphan Drug Act of 1983: Established grants, federal assistance for research, and tax incentives to develop drugs targeted for a patient population of less than 200,000

   i. The Drug Price Competition and Patent Term Restoration Act of 1984 (Hatch-Waxman Act): Authorized the FDA to create an abbreviated regulatory pathway through the ANDA for generic drugs

   j. The Food and Drug Administration Act of 1988: Officially established the FDA as an agency in DHHS

   k. The Prescription Drug User Fee Act of 1992 (PDUFA)

     i. Requires drug, biologics, and medical device (Medical Device User Fee Amendments) manufacturers to pay fees for product applications, supplements, and other services

     ii. Reauthorized every 5 years (1997, 2002, 2007, 2012, expected 2017)

   l. The Dietary Supplement Health and Education Act of 1994: Allows nutritional supplements and vitamins to be regulated

m. The FDA Modernization Act of 1997
   i. Streamlines clinical research on drugs and devices
   ii. Has exclusivity provisions for pediatric drugs
   iii. Authorizes the creation of a databank (ClinicalTrials.gov) to provide easy access to information on federally and privately supported clinical trials for a wide range of diseases and conditions
   iv. Provides abstracts of clinical study protocols that investigators are required to submit
       (a) Summary and purpose of study
       (b) Recruiting status
       (c) Criteria for patient participation
       (d) Location for trial and specific contact information
       (e) Research study design
       (f) Phase of trial
       (g) Disease or condition and drug or therapy under study
   v. More than 200,000 clinical trials have been listed with locations in all 50 states and in 191 countries.

n. The FDA Amendments Act of 2007
   i. Vehicle for reauthorizing PDUFA
   ii. Statutory authority to require Risk Evaluation and Mitigation Strategies (REMS)
   iii. Expanded the requirements for the types of drugs that must be registered on ClinicalTrials.gov; requires the submission of results for certain clinical trials
   iv. Reauthorized the Best Pharmaceuticals for Children Act and the Pediatric Research Equity Act. Both were designed to encourage more research into, and more development of, treatments for children

o. The Family Smoking Prevention and Tobacco Control Act of 2009: Gave the FDA authority to regulate tobacco products

p. The BPCI Act passed as a provision within the ACA.
   i. Established a regulatory approval pathway for biosimilars (or follow-on biologics)
   ii. Created FDA-administered periods of regulatory exclusivity for certain brand-name drugs and follow-on products
   iii. Created a patent dispute resolution procedure for use by brand-name and follow-on biologic manufacturers

q. The Reducing Prescription Drug Shortages Executive Order was signed by President Barack Obama on October 31, 2011. It requires the FDA to:
   i. Broaden the reporting of manufacturing discontinuances that may lead to shortages of drugs that are life supporting or life sustaining or that prevent debilitating disease
   ii. Expedite regulatory reviews to avoid or mitigate existing or potential drug shortages. Reviews may include new drug suppliers, manufacturing sites, and manufacturing changes.
   iii. Communicate to the DOJ any evidence of or behaviors by market participants that have contributed to stockpiling or exorbitant prices

r. The FDA Safety and Innovation Act of 2012 (reviewed earlier)
   i. Reauthorized PDUFA
   ii. Established the Biosimilar User Fee Act of 2012 to assess and collect fees for biosimilar biological products
   iii. Established the "breakthrough therapy" drug approval pathway
   iv. Increased stakeholder involvement in FDA processes by providing for the establishment of a patient-focused drug development initiative

s. The Drug Quality and Security Act of 2013 (reviewed earlier)

3. Prescription Drug Approval Path
   a. The 1962 amendments included a provision requiring manufacturers of drug products to establish a drug's effectiveness by "substantial evidence."
      i. It has been the FDA's position, based on the language of the statute and the legislative history of the 1962 amendments, that Congress generally intended to require at least two adequate and well-controlled trials, each convincing on its own, to establish effectiveness.
      ii. In 1997 under the FDA Modernization Act, section 505(d) was amended to make it clear that the agency may consider "data from one adequate and well-controlled clinical investigation and confirmatory evidence" to constitute substantial evidence if the FDA determines that such data and evidence are sufficient to establish effectiveness.
   b. Preclinical studies
      i. Laboratory and animal studies that assess safety and biologic activity in various model systems
         (a) ED_{50} is the amount of drug that produces a specific effect in 50% of animals tested.
         (b) LD_{50} is the amount of drug that causes death in 50% of animals tested.
      ii. Toxicologic studies completed
         (a) Effects on the fetus in pregnant mice, rats, rabbits, or baboons
         (b) May or may not translate into human fetal adverse effects
         (c) Fetal effects in humans may occur that were not observed in animal studies.
         (d) Basis for pregnancy categories B, C, and some D
      iii. An INDA is drafted and submitted to the FDA. It must contain a general plan of investigation, drug information (i.e., chemistry, pharmacology, toxicology, pharmacokinetics, biologic disposition, laboratory and animal testing data, and existing human data), protocol, manufacturing, and control of the drug.
   c. Phase I drug trial
      i. Initial introduction of an IND into humans, typically 20–80 healthy volunteers
      ii. Goal is to garner information on the pharmacokinetic and pharmacodynamic properties and safety profile of the investigational drug to design a well-controlled and robust phase II trial.
   d. Phase II drug trial
      i. Controlled clinical studies conducted in no more than several hundred subjects
      ii. Goal is to evaluate the drug's effectiveness for a particular indication in patients with the disease or condition under investigation and to determine the common short-term adverse effects and risks associated with the drug.
   e. Phase III drug trial
      i. Involves administering the investigational drug to a range of several hundred to several thousand patient subjects in different clinical settings to confirm its safety, efficacy, and appropriate dosage
      ii. Goal is to gather necessary additional information about effectiveness and safety for evaluating the overall benefit-risk relationship of the drug and to provide an adequate basis for physician labeling.
      iii. The step before the sponsor's submission of an NDA to the FDA for approval to market the drug (Box 2)
      iv. Once an NDA is submitted, it is classified with a code that reflects both the type of drug being submitted and its intended uses. The numbers 1–7 are used to describe the type of drug:
         (a) New molecular entity (1)
         (b) New salt of previously approved drug (2)
         (c) New formulation of previously approved drug (3)
         (d) New combination of two or more drugs (4)
         (e) Already marketed drug product (i.e., new manufacturer) (5)
         (f) New indication for currently marketed drug or switch from prescription to over the counter (6)
         (g) Already marketed drug product without a previously approved NDA (7)

    v. Letter code describes the review priority of the drug.
        (a) S = standard review for drug similar to currently available drugs.
        (b) P = priority review for drugs that represent significant advances over existing treatments.
    vi. Not all phase III drugs are approved, and the FDA can impose a clinical hold at any stage.

Box 2. Components of the New Drug Application

Index	Nonclinical pharmacology and toxicology
Summary	Human pharmacokinetics and bioavailability
Chemistry, manufacturing, and control	Microbiology (for antimicrobial drugs only)
Samples, methods, and labeling	Clinical data
Safety update report	Case report forms
Statistical analysis	Patent information
Case report tabulations	Patent certification
Other pertinent information	

    f. Phase IV drug trial
      i. Also called postmarketing studies
      ii. May be required by the FDA to identify additional information about the drug's risks, benefits, and optimal use
      iii. Verify effectiveness or focus treatment on special populations
    g. Generic drugs
      i. In 2014, more than 80% of all drugs dispensed were generic.
      ii. A generic drug product is identical to an innovator drug product in active ingredient, dosage form and strength, route of administration, quality, and intended use. It must also demonstrate bioequivalence, showing that there are no significant differences in the rate and extent of absorption of the therapeutic ingredient. The Drug Price Competition and Patent Term Restoration Act of 1984, also known as the Hatch-Waxman Act, defined bioequivalence statutorily as a means to approve a generic drug.
      iii. Once an ANDA is submitted to and approved by CDER's Office of Generic Drugs, the applicant can manufacture and market the generic drug as a safe, effective, and low-cost option to the public.
      iv. All approved multisource products are listed in the FDA's *Approved Drug Products with Therapeutic Equivalence Evaluations* (Orange Book). The therapeutic equivalence coding system, using A or B, helps health care providers determine whether the FDA evaluated a product to be therapeutically equivalent to other pharmaceutically equivalent products.
        (a) A code: An approved generic product considered therapeutically equivalent to other pharmaceutical equivalents
        (b) B code: An approved generic product that is not considered therapeutically equivalent to other pharmaceutical equivalents
      v. ANDAs generally do not require preclinical or clinical data; rather, they must demonstrate bioequivalence.
      vi. Pharmaceutical equivalents (Table 5)

Box 3. Criteria for Medications to Be Pharmaceutical Equivalents

Three criteria:
☐ Must contain the same active ingredient
☐ Must be the same dosage form and route of administration
☐ Must be of identical strength or concentration
Differences allowed:
☐ Shape
☐ Releasing mechanism
☐ Labeling (limited differences)
☐ Scoring
☐ Excipients (colors, flavors, preservatives)

    vii. Therapeutic equivalents can be substituted with the expectation that the substituted product will produce the same clinical effect and safety profile as the prescribed product.
        (a) Criteria
            (1) Pharmaceutical equivalent
            (2) Therapeutic equivalence codes rated "A" by the FDA
            (3) Designates a brand-name drug or a generic drug as the reference-listed drug
            (4) Demonstrates bioequivalence
        (b) Assigns therapeutic equivalence code according to data submitted in an ANDA to demonstrate bioequivalence
            (1) An ANDA contains adequate scientific evidence, established through in vivo or in vitro studies, of bioequivalence of the product to the reference-listed drug.
            (2) Products deemed by the FDA not therapeutically equivalent are rated "B."
    viii. An authorized generic is a drug that is produced by the brand company under the NDA but marketed as a generic, and a regular generic is produced under an ANDA. It is identical to the brand alternative in both active and inactive ingredients. The federal FD&C Act establishes a 180-day exclusivity period after approval of an ANDA. In this period, the FDA cannot approve other ANDAs for the same drug product.
    ix. At-risk launch of a generic occurs when a generic drug manufacturer challenges the validity of the existing patent of a brand drug.
    x. Follow-on biologics or biosimilars are drugs or vaccines that have been produced in living cells.
        (a) Biosimilars are approved new versions of an innovator biologic product after patent expiration. Although this is an area of controversy between the government, industry, and patient advocacy organizations, biosimilars offer a means to decrease the rapidly rising costs of biologic products.
        (b) Legislation has created a statutory pathway for the FDA to approve these products after 12 years of data exclusivity for the manufacturer of a new biologic product.

(c) In support of the implementation of the BPCI Act of 2009, the Biosimilar Implementation Committee, staffed by CDER, Center for Biologics Evaluation and Research, the Office of Chief Counsel, and the Office of the Commissioner, has developed several guidances for industry relating to quality and scientific considerations in demonstrating biosimilarity, clinical pharmacology data required to demonstrate biosimilarity, reference product exclusivity for biological products, and nonproprietary naming of biological products. As of this writing, final naming guidance and draft interchangeability guidances are awaited. These guidances do not establish legally enforceable responsibilities of the FDA; rather, they describe current thinking on a topic unless a specific regulatory or statutory requirement is cited.

(d) Table 3 compares the regulatory pathway differences between small molecules and biologics for FDA approval.

Table 3. Regulatory Approval Pathway Comparison for Small Molecule and Biologic Products

Product	Regulatory Pathway	Nonproprietary Name	Indications	Interchangeability	Clinical and Trial Data Requirement
Small Molecule (Food, Drug, and Cosmetic Act)	New Drug Application (505(b)1 and 2)	N/A; Legend (Brand) drug	N/A; Legend (Brand) drug	N/A; Legend (Brand) drug	Clinical data required; safety and efficacy data requirement
	Abbreviated New Drug Application (505(j))	Same as originator	Same as originator	Granted with initial approval (e.g., Orange Book rating)	Clinical data not required; bioequivalence data requirement
Biologic (Public Health Services Act)	Biologics License Application (351(a))	N/A; Innovator (Reference) drug	N/A; Legend (Brand) drug	N/A; Legend (Brand) drug	Clinical data required; purity, safety, and potency data requirement
	Biosimilar Application (351(k))	Uncertain, may be different	May or may not have all indications, extrapolation allowed	Not automatically granted at initial approval – Requires additional review (e.g., Purple Book rating)	Clinical data required; abbreviated data requirement with purity, safety, and potency (i.e., totality of the evidence)

xi. Medical devices
   (a) An instrument, apparatus, implement, machine, contrivance, implant, in vitro reagent, or other similar or related article, including a component part, or accessory that is:
   (1) Recognized in the official NF, or the USP, or any supplement to them
   (2) Intended for use in the diagnosis of disease or other conditions, or in the cure, mitigation, treatment, or prevention of disease, in humans or other animals
   (3) Intended to affect the structure or any function of the body of humans or other animals that does not achieve any of its primary intended purposes through chemical action within or on the body of human beings or other animals and that does not depend on being metabolized for the achievement of any of its primary intended purposes
   (b) Regulated by the Center for Devices and Radiological Health
   (1) To be approved, a medical device manufacturer must submit a premarket approval application ensuring the device's safety and efficacy.
   (2) If a medical device is essentially equivalent to an existing, legally marketed device, a 510(k) is submitted for premarket notification.
   (3) An investigational device exemption allows an investigational device to be used in a clinical study to collect the safety and effectiveness data required to support a premarket approval application or a premarket notification 510(k) submission to the FDA.

    (c) Classified according to the risks associated with the device:

        (1) Class I: Deemed low risk and therefore subject to the least regulatory control

        (2) Class II: Higher-risk devices than class I that require greater regulatory controls to ensure reasonable safety and efficacy

        (3) Class III: Highest-risk devices, subject to the greatest regulatory control; must be approved by the FDA before marketing

  xii. REMS

    (a) Is separate from the FDA's Risk Minimization Action Plans, which is a voluntary program for industry for drugs that have unusual risks but also unusual benefits

    (b) May be required by the FDA before or after approval if necessary to ensure that the benefits of a drug outweigh the risks

    (c) Requires that a drug be prescribed and dispensed with one of the following:

        (1) Medication guide or patient package inserts

        (2) Communication plan to health care providers (for NDAs or biologics license applications only, not ANDAs)

        (3) Elements To Assure Safe Use (ETASU) (Box 4)

        (4) Implementation system

Box 4. Risk Evaluation and Mitigation Strategies' Requirements of ETASU

ETASU may include one or more of the following:
☐ Health care providers who prescribe the drug have particular training or experience or are specially certified
☐ Pharmacies, practitioners, or health care settings that dispense the drug are specially certified
☐ Drug is dispensed only in certain health care settings
☐ Drug is dispensed to patients with evidence of safe use conditions such as laboratory test results
☐ Each patient using the drug is subject to monitoring
☐ Each patient using the drug is enrolled in a registry

ETASU = Elements To Assure Safe Use.

    (d) The FDA does not have the authority to impose penalties on pharmacies and pharmacists not in compliance with REMS requirements, but there may be legal implications such as mis-branding violations or civil liability issues.

    (e) Medication guides are not usually required as part of a REMS unless the REMS includes ETASU. If listed as an ETASU, a medication guide must be provided in all settings, including inpatient settings, outpatient settings but administered by a health care professional, and outpatient settings but dispensed to a patient.

  xii. Critical Path Initiative

    (a) Created in response to a significant decline in NDAs, biologics license applications, and medical device applications because of the widening gap between basic science discovery and the challenging, inefficient, and costly development of medical products

    (b) Prioritizes the most pressing developmental problems and identifies areas that provide the greatest opportunities for rapid improvement and public health benefit through three dimensions: safety assessment, evaluation of medical utility, and product industrialization

VI. INSTITUTIONAL REVIEW BOARD IMPLICATIONS FOR CLINICAL PRACTICE AND RESEARCH

1. By federal regulation, every institution that conducts or supports biomedical or behavioral research involving human participants must have an institutional review board (IRB) that initially approves and periodically reviews research protocols to protect the rights of human participants.

    a. Governed by FDA Title 21 Part 56 and DHHS Office for Human Research Protections regulations at Title 45 CFR Part 46; requires the IRB or ethics committee to protect the rights, safety, and well-being of all study subjects. Specifically, subpart A constitutes the Federal Policy (Common Rule) for the Protection of Human Subjects. In 2015, DHHS and 15 other federal agencies announced proposed changes to the Common Rule. The revisions are intended to better protect human subjects involved in research while facilitating valuable research and reducing burden, delay, and ambiguity for investigators. As of this writing, the final revised Common Rule has not been made public.

    b. An IRB is a committee of physicians, statisticians, researchers, community advocates, and others that ensures that a clinical trial is ethical and that the rights of study participants are protected. It is composed of at least five members with varying backgrounds to promote the complete and adequate review of research activities while adhering to institutional commitments and regulations, applicable law, and standards of professional conduct and practice.

        i. The committee must be sufficiently qualified through the experience, expertise, and diversity of its members, including race, gender, cultural background, and sensitivity to issues such as community attitudes, to promote respect for its advice and counsel.

        ii. At least one member whose primary concerns are in scientific areas

        iii. At least one member whose primary concerns are in nonscientific areas

        iv. At least one member who is not affiliated with the institution and who is not an immediate family member of a person affiliated with the institution

    c. IRB approval is required for interventional and observational studies, and applications must be reviewed annually.

2. A human subject is a living person about whom an investigator conducting research obtains (1) data through intervention or interaction with the individual or (2) identifiable private information.

3. Informed consent is the process of learning the key facts about a clinical trial before deciding whether to participate. An informed consent document describes the rights of the study participants and includes details about the study including purpose, duration, required procedures, risks, benefits, and key contacts.

4. Minimal risk means that the probability and magnitude of harm or discomfort anticipated in the research are no greater than those ordinarily encountered in daily life or during the performance of routine physical or psychological examinations or tests.

5. Research Exempt from IRB Requirements

    a. Research conducted in established or commonly accepted educational settings, involving normal educational practices such as:

        i. Research on regular or special education instructional strategies

        ii. Research on the effectiveness of the comparison between instructional techniques, curricula, or classroom management methods

    b. Research involving the use of educational tests (cognitive, diagnostic, aptitude, or achievement), survey procedures, interview procedures, or observation of public behavior, unless:

        i. Information obtained is recorded in such a manner that human subjects can be identified, directly or through identifiers linked to the subjects

        ii. Any disclosure of the human subjects' responses outside the research could reasonably place the subjects at risk of criminal or civil liability or be damaging to the subjects' financial standing, employability, or reputation

   c.   Research involving the collection or study of existing data, documents, records, pathologic specimens, or diagnostic specimens; if these sources are publicly available or if the information is recorded by the investigator in a manner such that subjects cannot be identified, directly or through identifiers linked to the subjects

   d.   Research involving no more than minimal risk, and minor changes made to approved research protocols, may be considered for expedited review.

6.   The HIPAA Privacy Rule: Supplements and expands the Common Rule regulation of human subjects' research

   a.   Protections for the confidentiality of PHI used in clinical practice, research, and the operation of health care facilities

   b.   PHI includes information that:

      i.   Is created or received by a covered entity, which includes health care providers, hospitals, insurance companies, and business associates

      ii.   Pertains to the past, present, or future physical or mental health, or condition of the individual

      iii.   Pertains to payment for the individual's health care

      iv.   Pertains to the provision of health care in the past, present, or future

      v.   Identifies an individual or could be used to identify an individual

      vi.   To use or disclose PHI for research purposes, one or more of the following must be obtained:

         (a)   Written authorization specifically for the use and disclosure of PHI for research purposes involving human subjects

         (b)   Waiver of authorization approved by an IRB: Use of de-identified information or limited data sets (limited data set [45 CFR §164.514(e)] defined for research, public health, and health care operations)

         (c)   Preparatory to research certifications

         (d)   Database registration

   c.   A provision within HIPAA also mandated adoption of a standard unique identifier for health care providers. The National Plan & Provider Enumeration System of CMS collects information from providers and assigns each a unique National Provider Identifier.

7.   Examples of typical documents submitted to the IRB for an initial review can be found at NIH's National Institute on Aging Clinical Study Investigator's Toolbox (Box 5).

Box 5. Documents That May Need to Be Submitted to an IRB for Initial Review

Cover sheet	Recruitment materials
Conflict of interest assessment	Surveys, questionnaires, other instruments
Application	Federal grant, if applicable
Formal protocol	Documentation of IRB approval from another institution
Informed consent forms	Data and safety monitoring plan
HIPAA authorization forms	Additional supportive documents as requested by IRB

HIPAA = Health Insurance Portability and Accountability Act; IRB = institutional review board.

8.   Informed Consent

   a.   A statement that the study involves research, an explanation of the purposes of the research, the expected duration of the subject's participation, a description of the procedures to be followed, and the identification of any procedures that are experimental

   b.   A description of any reasonably foreseeable risks or discomforts to the subject

   c.   A description of any benefits to the subject or to others that may reasonably be expected from the research

   d.   A disclosure of appropriate alternative procedures or courses of treatment that might be advantageous to the subject

e. A statement describing the extent to which confidentiality of records identifying the subject will be maintained

f. For research involving more than minimal risk, an explanation of whether there is any compensation and an explanation of whether any medical treatments are available if injury occurs and, if so, what they consist of, or where further information may be obtained

g. An explanation of whom to contact for answers to pertinent questions about the research and research subjects' rights and of whom to contact in the event of a research-related injury to the subject

h. A statement that participation is voluntary, that refusal to participate will involve no penalty or loss of benefits to which the subject is otherwise entitled, and that the subject may discontinue participation at any time without penalty or loss of benefits to which the subject is otherwise entitled

i. Waiver will be considered if
    i. Research involves no more than minimal risk to subjects
    ii. The waiver or alteration will not adversely affect the rights and welfare of subjects
    iii. The research could not practicably be carried out without the waiver or alteration

j. When appropriate, the subjects will be provided with additional pertinent information after participation.

VII. INVESTIGATIONAL DRUG SERVICE

1. Investigational Drug Service (IDS)

    a. The ASHP Policy on Institutional Review Boards and Investigational Use of Drugs (0711) strongly supports pharmacists' management of the control and distribution of drug products used in clinical research.

    b. The purpose of an IDS is to procure, manage, prepare, dispense, and dispose of investigational drugs according to protocol and in compliance with the state and federal requirements that govern investigational drug activities.

    c. Drugs, as defined by the FD&C Act, are "(A) articles intended for use in the diagnosis, cure, mitigation, treatment, or prevention of disease, and (B) articles (other than food) intended to affect the structure or any function of the body of man or other animals" (FD&C Act, sec. 201(g)(1)). An investigational drug is a chemical or biologic substance that has been tested in a laboratory and been approved by the FDA to be tested in human subjects. An investigational (also referred to as experimental) drug may be:
        i. A new chemical or compound that has not been approved by the FDA for general use
        ii. An approved drug undergoing further investigation for an approved or unapproved indication, dose, dosage form, or administration schedule or under an INDA in a controlled, randomized, or blinded clinical trial

    d. In addition to the regulations outlined by the Office for Human Research Protections (Common Rule) and the FDA to conduct research in accordance with the principles of good clinical practice and human subjects' protection, an IDS has federal and state requirements.
        i. The Joint Commission standards require policies for the use of investigational drugs that specifically address their storage, dispensing, labeling, and distribution.
        ii. The U.S. Environmental Protection Agency and the Occupational Safety and Health Administration regulate the disposal of investigational drugs.
        iii. ASHP provides practice standards.
        iv. The local IRB has its own requirements.
        v. State-specific laws may vary.

e. Study-specific notebook: The notebook is maintained where study drugs are stored. It contains the files and contents listed in Table 4.

Table 4. Example of Documents Stored in Study-Specific Notebooks Maintained by an Investigational Drug Service

File Section	Contents
Protocol	Copy of the research protocol
Drug information	Investigator's brochure, drug data sheet, package inserts (if commercially available)
Pharmacy procedures	Study-specific pharmacy procedure information
Logs, forms, and labels	Study-specific materials
Procurement details	Receipt and disposition records
Correspondence	Correspondence
Computer matters	Copies of order entry codes
Billing	Financial agreements with investigator
IRB	IRB submission application, approval, and consent forms
Miscellaneous	Miscellaneous documentation
Master patient log	Record of patients enrolled
Drug accountability records	Data accountability record for each drug, dosage form, package size, and strength

IRB = institutional review board.

2. An investigational drug pharmacist's duties may include the following:
   a. Participating on an IRB as a voting member
   b. Maintaining a working relationship with the IRB, P&T committee, principal investigators, and the pharmacy department
   c. Reviewing new and existing investigational drug study protocols
   d. Meeting with investigators, study monitors, and other study personnel responsible for coordinating the logistics of a clinical trial
   e. Receiving, organizing, and maintaining the contents of study notebooks
   f. Providing randomization, blinding, or control functions of a clinical trial
   g. Conducting the training of IDS staff and personnel regarding investigational protocols and study drug procedures

REFERENCES

Congressional Offices with Jurisdiction over Health-Related Policy and the Legislative Process

1. CMS Open Payments Program. Available at http://cms.gov/openpayments/. Accessed December 10, 2015.

2. C-SPAN Congressional Glossary. Available at http://legacy.c-span.org/guide/congress/glossary/alphalist.htm. Accessed December 10, 2015.

3. Lipton HL. Pharmacists and health reform: go for it. Pharmacotherapy 2010;30:967-72.

4. Office of the National Coordinator for Health Information Technology (ONC). Available at http://healthit.gov. Accessed December 10, 2015.

5. U.S. House of Representatives. Available at www.house.gov. Accessed December 10, 2015.

6. U.S. Senate. Available at www.senate.gov. Accessed December 10, 2015.

Agencies of DHHS with Primary Regulatory Impact on the Practice of Pharmacy

1. AHRQ.gov [homepage on the Internet]. Available at www.ahrq.gov. Accessed December 10, 2015.

2. CDC.gov [homepage on the Internet]. Available at www.cdc.gov. Accessed December 10, 2015.

3. CMS.gov [homepage on the Internet]. Available at www.cms.gov. Accessed December 10, 2015.

4. Code of Federal Regulations (CFR). Available at www.gpo.gov/fdsys/browse/collectionCfr.action?collectionCode=CFR. Accessed December 10, 2015.

5. FDA.gov [homepage on the Internet]. Available at www.fda.gov. Accessed December 10, 2015.

The FDA and the Prescription Drug Approval Process

1. Clinical Trials. Available at http://clinicaltrials.gov. Accessed December 10, 2015.

2. FDA.gov [homepage on the Internet]. Available at www.fda.gov. Accessed December 10, 2015.

3. Generic Pharmaceutical Association. Available at www.gphaonline.org/. Accessed December 10, 2015.

4. National Cancer Institute (NCI). Clinical Trial Information. Available at www.cancer.gov/clinicaltrials. Accessed December 10, 2015.

5. Past, Present, and Future of FDA Human Drug Regulation. Available at www.fda.gov/Training/ForHealthProfessionals/ucm209538.htm. Accessed December 10, 2015.

6. Presidential Actions, Executive Orders. Available at www.whitehouse.gov/briefing-room/presidential-actions/executive-orders. Accessed December 10, 2015.

7. U.S. Food and Drug Administration (FDA). How Is FDA Organized? Available at www.fda.gov/AboutFDA/Transparency/Basics/ucm194884.htm. Accessed December 10, 2015.

8. U.S. Food and Drug Administration (FDA). Approved Risk Evaluation and Mitigation Strategies (REMS). Available at www.accessdata.fda.gov/scripts/cder/rems/index.cfm. Accessed December 10, 2015.

9. U.S. Government Accountability Office. Drug Pricing: Research on Savings from Generic Drug Use. Available at www.gao.gov/assets/590/588064.pdf. Accessed December 10, 2015.

IRB Implications for Clinical Practice and Research

1. Code of Federal Regulations (CFR). Title 45 CFR Part 46. Available at www.hhs.gov/ohrp/humansubjects/guidance/45cfr46.html. Accessed December 10, 2015.

2. National Institute on Aging. Clinical Study Investigator's Toolbox. Available at www.nia.nih.gov/research/dgcg/clinical-research-study-investigators-toolbox. Accessed December 10, 2015.

Investigational Drug Services

1. American Society of Health-System Pharmacists (ASHP). Policy Position: On Institutional Review Boards and Investigational Use of Drugs. Available at www.ashp.org/DocLibrary/BestPractices/ResearchPositions.aspx. Accessed December 10, 2015.

2. Brigham and Women's Hospital. Investigational Drug Service. Available at www.brighamandwomens.org/research/CCI/IDS.aspx. Accessed December 10, 2015.

3. National Cancer Institute (NCI). Clinical Trial Information. Available at www.cancer.gov/clinicaltrials/. Accessed December 10, 2015.

4. Seattle Children's Hospital Investigational Drug Service. Available at www.seattlechildrens.org/research/cores/ids/. Accessed December 10, 2015.

5. U.S. Department of Veterans Affairs. Investigational Drugs and Supplies Handbook. Available at www.va.gov/vhapublications/ViewPublication.asp?pub_ID=2497. Accessed December 10, 2015.

6. University of Pittsburgh Cancer Institute. Investigational Drug Services. Available at www.upci.upmc.edu/ids/index.cfm. Accessed December 10, 2015.

The Joint Commission, National Committee for Quality Assurance, National Quality Forum, and Agency for Healthcare Research and Quality

1. Agency for Healthcare Research and Quality (AHRQ). Available at www.ahrq.gov. Accessed December 10, 2015.

2. American Society of Health-System Pharmacists (ASHP). Effective Health Care Program. Available at http://effectivehealthcare.ahrq.gov/. Accessed December 10, 2015.

3. Chassin MR, Loeb JM, Schmaltz SP, et al. Accountability measures: using measurement to promote quality improvement. N Engl J Med 2010;363:683-8.

4. Healthcare Effectiveness Data and Information Set (HEDIS). Available at www.ncqa.org/HEDISQualityMeasurement.aspx. Accessed December 10, 2015.

5. Joint Commission.org [homepage on the Internet]. Available at www.jointcommission.org/. Accessed December 10, 2015.

6. Joint Commission. Center for Transforming Healthcare Targeted Solutions Tool. Available at www.centerfortransforminghealthcare.org. Accessed December 10, 2015.

7. National Committee for Quality Assurance (NCQA). Available at www.ncqa.org/. Accessed December 10, 2015.

8. National Quality Forum (NQF). Available at www.qualityforum.org. Accessed December 10, 2015.

9. Pharmacy Quality Alliance (PQA). Available at www.PQAAlliance.org. Accessed December 10, 2015.

Institutional Medication Use Policy Considerations

1. Agency for Healthcare Research and Quality (AHRQ). Patient Safety Organizations. Available at www.pso.ahrq.gov. Accessed December 10, 2015.

2. Agency for Healthcare Research and Quality (AHRQ). Patient Safety Organizations Common Formats. Available at www.pso.ahrq.gov/formats/commonfmt.htm. Accessed December 10, 2015.

3. American Society of Health-System Pharmacists (ASHP). Discussion Guide for Compounding Sterile Preparations. Available at www.ashp.org/doclibrary/policy/compounding/discguide 797-2008.pdf. Accessed December 10, 2015.

4. American Society of Health-System Pharmacists (ASHP). Formulary Management Endorsed Document. Available at www.ashp.org/DocLibrary/BestPractices/FormEndPrinciples.aspx. Accessed December 10, 2015.

5. American Society of Health-System Pharmacists (ASHP). Formulary Management Guideline: Pharmacy and Therapeutics Committee and the Formulary System. Available at www.ashp.org/DocLibrary/BestPractices/FormGdlPTCommFormSyst.pdf. Accessed December 10, 2015.

6. American Society of Health-System Pharmacists (ASHP). Formulary Management Statement. Available at www.ashp.org/DocLibrary/BestPractices/FormStPTCommFormSyst.pdf. Accessed December 10, 2015.

7. American Society of Health-System Pharmacists (ASHP). Principles of a Sound drug formulary system [consensus statement]. In: Hawkins B, ed. Best Practices for Hospital & Health-System Pharmacy: Positions and Guidance Documents of ASHP. Bethesda, MD: ASHP, 2006:110-3.

8. American Society of Health-System Pharmacists (ASHP). Guidelines on Medication-Use Evaluation. Formulary Management – Guidelines. Available at https://www.ashp.org/DocLibrary/BestPractices/FormGdlMedUseEval.aspx. Accessed December 13, 2015.

9. Bates DW, Cullen DJ, Laird N, et al. Incidence of adverse drug events and potential adverse drug events. Implications for prevention. ADE Prevention Study Group. JAMA 1995;274:29.

10. Committee on Data Standards for Patient Safety, Board on Health Care Services. Patient Safety: Achieving a New Standard for Care. Washington, DC: National Academies Press, 2004.

11. Department of Health and Human Services (DHHS) Centers for Medicare & Medicaid Services (CMS). Letter on AHRQ Common Formats. Available at www.chpso.org/sites/main/files/file-attachments/survey-and-cert-letter-13-19.pdf. Accessed December 10, 2015.

12. Gandhi TK, Seger DL, Bates DW. Identifying drug safety issues: from research to practice. Int J Qual Health Care 2000;12:69-76.

13. Institute of Medicine (IOM). To Err Is Human: Building a Safer Health System. Available at www.iom.edu/Reports/1999/To-Err-is-Human-Building-A-Safer-Health-System.aspx. Accessed December 10, 2015.

14. Joint Commission. Medication Selection Criteria for Hospitals. Available at www.jointcommission.org/assets/1/6/Updated_med_sel_criteria_hospitals.pdf. Accessed December 10, 2015.

15. Patient Safety Organization (PSO) Privacy Protection Center. Available at https://www.psoppc.org/psoppc_web. Accessed December 10, 2015.

16. U.S. Food and Drug Administration (FDA). FDA MedWatch Program. Available at www.fda.gov/Safety/MedWatch/default.htm. Accessed December 10, 2015.

17. U.S. Pharmacopeial Convention. Available at www.usp.org/. Accessed December 10, 2015.

18. Vaccine Adverse Event Reporting System. Available at https://vaers.hhs.gov/index. Accessed December 13, 2015.

ANSWERS AND EXPLANATIONS TO SELF-ASSESSMENT QUESTIONS

1. Answer: D

The FDA requires manufacturers, packers, and distributors of marketed prescription drug products to establish and maintain records and to make reports to the FDA of all serious, unexpected adverse drug experiences associated with the use of their drug products. Form FDA 3500 is for voluntary reporting by health care professionals, consumers, and patients, whereas 3500A is the mandatory form to be submitted by IND reporters, manufacturers, distributors, importers, and facility personnel, making Answer D correct and Answer A incorrect. Manufacturers, packers, and distributors should not include the names and addresses of individual patients. However, health care providers can continue to make adverse event reports under the HIPAA Privacy Rule. The HIPAA Privacy Rule is not intended to disrupt or discourage adverse event reporting in any way. In fact, the Privacy Rule specifically permits covered entities (e.g., pharmacists, physicians, hospitals) to report adverse events and other information related to the quality, effectiveness, and safety of FDA-regulated products, both to the manufacturers and directly to the FDA. As an explanation, the following statement has been provided: "The HIPAA Privacy Rule recognizes the legitimate need for public health authorities and others responsible for ensuring public health and safety to have access to PHI to carry out their public health mission. The rule also recognizes that public health reports made by covered entities are an important means of identifying threats to the health and safety of the public at large, as well as individuals. Accordingly, the rule permits covered entities to disclose PHI without authorization for specified public health purposes." However, names of patients, individual reporters, health care professionals, hospitals, and geographic identifiers in adverse drug experience reports are not releasable to the public under the FDA's public information regulations, making Answer C incorrect. Answer B is incorrect because consumers and patients should complete Form 3500B.

2. Answer: B

A generic drug must prove bioequivalence to a branded product to gain approval, making Answer B correct. The regulatory pathway for a generic drug is through the ANDA, not through the Accelerated New Drug Application, making Answer A incorrect. Generic drugs need not be therapeutically equivalent to a branded product, making Answer C incorrect; however, if they are not therapeutically equivalent, they will be rated "B" in the Orange Book, making Answer D incorrect.

3. Answer: A

If a drug is subject to an ETASU REMS that requires the provision and review of a medication guide, it must be provided when a drug is dispensed in an outpatient setting and will be used without direct supervision by a health care professional, making Answer A correct. Moreover, it must be provided in all settings as specified in the REMS program, including inpatient settings and outpatient settings, making Answers B and D incorrect. Requirements of a REMS to provide a medication guide can be revised and removed after approval at a later point, making Answer C incorrect.

4. Answer: B

An IND application is used for a new drug, a new indication, or off-label use that will be used in a clinical investigation's preclinical development for that new drug to be distributed across state lines before undergoing full FDA review. An IND is drafted and submitted to the FDA after a preclinical study, before a phase I clinical trial, when the IND is first introduced into human subjects, making Answer B incorrect and Answers A, C, and D incorrect. The application must contain a general plan of investigation, drug information (i.e., chemistry, pharmacology, toxicology, pharmacokinetics, biologic disposition, laboratory and animal testing data, and existing human data), protocol, and manufacturing and control of the drug. An NDA is submitted after phase III studies, before market approval, making Answer D incorrect.

5. Answer: C

Answer C, a study that evaluates a drug or intervention on a larger sample of subjects and assesses efficacy and adverse effects, is correct. Answer A matches a phase I trial, Answer B matches a phase III trial, and Answer D matches a phase IV trial.

6. Answer: A

An adverse drug reaction is a non-preventable adverse drug event that is not the result of a medication error (Answer A is correct). Answer B is the definition of an adverse drug event, Answer C is the definition of a preventable adverse drug event, and Answer D is the definition of a potential adverse drug event.

7. Answer: B

Answer B is correct. The Drug Price Competition and Patent Term Restoration Act of 1984, commonly called the Hatch-Waxman Act, named after the two lead sponsors, Representative Henry Waxman and Senator Orrin Hatch, is the legislative act that created an abbreviated FDA approval pathway for generic drugs. The Kefauver-Harris Amendments pertain to the requirement of a drug to show efficacy in addition to safety, making Answer A incorrect. The Durham-Humphrey Amendment differentiated prescription drugs from nonprescription drugs, making Answer C incorrect. The BPCI Act of 2009 was a provision passed in the 2010 ACA, and it created an abbreviated approval pathway for follow-on biologic products, or biosimilars, making Answer D incorrect.

8. Answer: B

Biosimilars approved through a biosimilar 351(k) pathway have a clinical data submission requirement, making Answer B correct. Review of the application will consider the totality of evidence, which includes purity, safety, potency, and clinical trial data. This is different from the generic ANDA approval pathway, in which the only data submission requirement is for bioequivalence to be established between the generic drug and the legend (brand) drug, making Answer A incorrect. Interchangeability decisions have yet to be determined by the FDA; however, the FDA has indicated that interchangeability with an innovator product will not be granted on initial application, making Answer C incorrect. Designation of interchangeability will be denoted in the Purple Book, not the Orange Book, making Answer D incorrect.

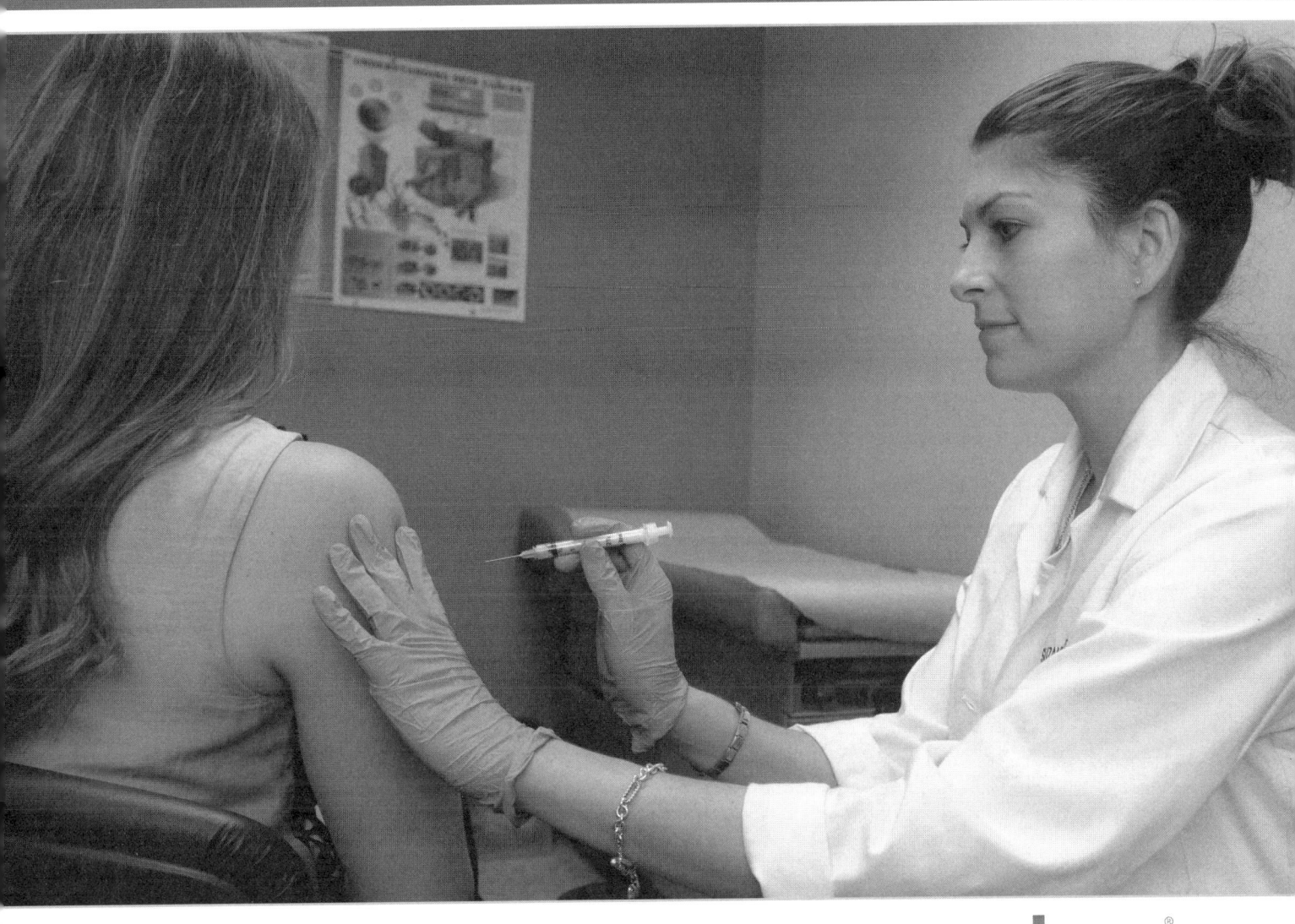

Board of Pharmacy Specialties bps®

2016 Recertification Guide

Specialty Certification in:
Ambulatory Care Pharmacy
Critical Care Pharmacy
Nuclear Pharmacy
Nutrition Support Pharmacy
Oncology Pharmacy
Pediatric Pharmacy
Pharmacotherapy
Psychiatric Pharmacy

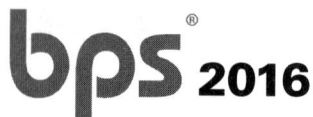

TABLE OF CONTENTS

RECERTIFICATION

This guide is intended for use by BPS-certified pharmacists who are interested in being recertified. It provides information on BPS recertification processes: eligibility requirements, application procedures and recertification examination administration.

This document is ONLY A GUIDE. The information, procedures and fees detailed in this publication may be amended, revised, or otherwise altered at any time and without advance notice by the Board of Pharmacy Specialties. The provision of this Guide does not confer any rights upon an applicant. The information contained in this Guide supersedes information contained in all previous editions of the BPS Recertification Guide.

Recertification assures the public and the profession that certified practitioners undergo periodic evaluation. Participating in continuing education opportunities or preparing for the recertification exam also offers the opportunity for certificants to increase knowledge in a specialty area and to stay up-to-date with current developments in the field. The Board of Pharmacy Specialties requires all board-certified specialists to recertify every seven years. If a BPS-certified specialist does not apply for recertification by the deadline date of August 1, 2016 the individual will be removed from the official roster of board certified specialists. If a certified pharmacist fails to successfully complete the recertification process, extension of certification may be granted for a one-year period, at the sole discretion of BPS, while the individual seeks to successfully complete the process.

Once a BPS-certified specialist has been deleted permanently from the roster, that individual may no longer use the designation or initials associated with that specialty (e.g., Board Certified Nuclear Pharmacist, BCNP) nor display the BPS certificate. Reinstatement can be achieved only by the successful completion of the entire certification process.

Please note, each specialty area has its own approved continuing education programs and requirements designed to assess a practitioner's knowledge in their particular subject area. **Continuing education credit earned through an approved professional development program will only be counted towards that specific specialty area. There is no overlap in continuing education programs between specialty areas unless noted by BPS and the provider.**

Board of Pharmacy Specialties
2215 Constitution Avenue, NW
Washington, DC 20037-2985
• Tel: (202) 429-7591 • Fax: (202) 429-6304
• info@bpsweb.org • www.bpsweb.org

BPS office hours are Monday through Friday, 8:30am to 5:00pm (Eastern Time). The BPS office is closed on all U.S. Federal holidays.

BPS RECERTIFICATION REQUIREMENTS

AMBULATORY CARE

Recertification Requirements

Pharmacists who earn the designation Board Certified Ambulatory Care Pharmacist (BCACP) will be required to maintain their certification over a seven-year period by completing one of the following professional development activities:

- Achieving a passing score on the 100-item, multiple choice objective recertification examination, based on the content outline for the Ambulatory Care Pharmacy Specialty
  OR
- Earning 100 hours of continuing education credit provided by a professional development program approved by BPS

A current, active license to practice pharmacy is required for recertification.

Board Certified Ambulatory Care Pharmacists are also required to pay the BPS Annual Certification Maintenance fee of $125 each year for years one through six and a $400 recertification fee in year seven.

Option One: Examination

Achieve a passing score on the 100-item, multiple choice objective recertification examination, based on the content outline of the certification examination (refer to the Ambulatory Care Content Outline for details).

Domain 1: Patient-Centered Care: Ambulatory Care Pharmacotherapy (37% of the examination).

Domain 2: Patient-Centered Care: Collaboration and Patient Advocacy (29% of the examination).

Domain 3: Translation of Evidence into Practice (14% of the examination)

Domain 4: Practice Models and Policy (14% of the examination).

Domain 5: Population and Public Health (6% of the examination).

Option Two: Continuing Education

Earn 100 hours of continuing education credit from the approved professional development programs offered by the American College of Clinical Pharmacy (ACCP) and/or the joint program offered by the American Society of Health-System Pharmacists (ASHP) and the American Pharmacists Association (APhA).

No more than 50 hours will be accepted by BPS during the first three years of the recertification cycle. Further,

Ambulatory Care Pharmacy Preparatory Review and Recertification Courses offered by either of the approved providers may only be completed for recertification credit up to two times, in nonconsecutive years, during the seven-year recertification cycle. To achieve the 100-hour requirement, the BCACP may participate in recertification offerings from both BPS-approved ambulatory care pharmacy providers.

For BCACPs who are also certified in Pharmacotherapy, ACCP and ASHP will provide opportunities for dual continuing education credits that overlap across both specialties with the Clinical Reasoning Series and Intensive Study programs. Please be advised that each year, candidates are only allowed to earn six (6) total hours towards their BCACP & BCPS certifications using these continuing education courses.

CRITICAL CARE PHARMACY
Recertification Requirements
Recertification for Board Certified Critical Care Pharmacists (BCCCP) requires assessment of a practitioner's knowledge and skill through one of the two methods:
- Achieving a passing score on the 100-item, multiple-choice objective recertification examination (administered by BPS), based on the content outline for the Critical Care Pharmacy Specialty in their seventh year following initial certification; OR
- Earning 100 hours of continuing education credit provided by professional development programs approved by BPS

A current, active license to practice pharmacy is required for recertification.

Board Certified Critical Care Pharmacists are also required to pay the BPS Annual Certification Maintenance fee of $125 each year for years one through six and a $400 recertification fee in year seven.

Option One: Examination
Achieve a passing score on the 100-item, multiple-choice recertification examination, which is based on the content outline of the certification examination (refer to the Critical Care Pharmacy Content Outline on the BPS website for details).
Domain 1: Clinical Skills and Therapeutic Management (66% of examination).
Domain 2: Practice Administration and Development (15% of examination).
Domain 3: Information Management and Education (19% of examination).

Option Two: Continuing Education
Earn 100 hours of continuing education credit provided by the joint program offered by the American College of Clinical Pharmacy and the Society of Critical Care Medicine and/or the American Society of Health-System Pharmacists (ASHP).

Critical Care Pharmacy Preparatory Review and Recertification Courses offered by any of the approved providers may only be completed for recertification credit up to two times, in nonconsecutive years, during the 7-year recertification cycle.

NUCLEAR PHARMACY
Recertification Requirements:
Recertification for Board Certified Nuclear Pharmacists (BCNP) will be accomplished through one of two methods:
- Achieving a passing score on the 100-item, multiple choice objective recertification examination, based on the content outline of the certification examination; OR
- Earning 100 hours of continuing education provided by the professional development program approved by BPS offered through the Purdue University College of Pharmacy.

At the time of recertification, the BCNP is also required to certify that (s)he is not currently under suspension by either the U.S. Nuclear Regulatory Commission or a State Radiation Control Organization.

Board Certified Nuclear Pharmacists are also required to pay the BPS Annual Certification Maintenance fee of $125 each year for years one through six and a $400 recertification fee in year seven.

All candidates for recertification must have a current active license to practice pharmacy.

Option One: Examination
Achieve a passing score on the 100-item, multiple choice objective recertification examination based on the content outline (refer to the Nuclear Pharmacy Content Outline on the BPS website for details).
Domain 1: Procurement, Storage, and Handling (16% of examination).
Domain 2: Preparation, Compounding, and Dispensing (38% of examination).
Domain 3: Quality Assurance (17% of examination).
Domain 4: Health and Safety (19% of examination).
Domain 5: Drug Information and Professional Consultation (10% of examination).

Option Two: Continuing Education
Beginning January 1, 2016, BPS has designated Purdue University College of Pharmacy as the new continuing education provider for professional development in nuclear pharmacy.

A BCNP recertifying via CE is required to earn 100 hours over the seven-year certification period. There are no restrictions as to which lessons in which years may be used to obtain the required number of hours.

NUTRITION SUPPORT PHARMACY

Recertification Requirements

Recertification for Board Certified Nutrition Support Pharmacists (BCNSP) is based on the following activities:

- Earning a minimum of 30 hours of continuing education in nutrition support with no less than 10 hours earned every two years. These hours must be from providers approved by the Accreditation Council for Pharmacy Education (ACPE).
- Achieving a passing score on the 100-item, multiple-choice recertification examination, based on the content outline of the certification examination.

A current, active license to practice pharmacy is required for recertification.

Board Certified Nutrition Support Pharmacists are also required to pay the BPS Annual Certification Maintenance fee of $125 each year for years one through six and a $400 recertification fee in year seven.

Examination

Achieve a passing score on the 100-item, multiple-choice recertification examination, which is based on the content outline of the certification examination (refer to the Nutrition Support Pharmacy Content Outline on the BPS website for details).

Domain 1: Clinical Practice: Provision of Patient-Centered Nutrition Support
- Subdomain A: Assessment (22% of examination).
- Subdomain B: Design and Initiation of a Therapeutic Plan of Care (27% of examination).
- Subdomain C: Monitoring and Management (14% of examination)

Domain 2: Nutrition Support Operations
- Subdomain A: Practice Management (7% of examination).
- Subdomain B: Policy and Protocol Management (7% of examination).
- Subdomain C: Compounding Operations (16% of examination).

Domain 3: Retrieval, Interpretation, Generation, and Communication of Knowledge in Nutrition Support (7% of examination).

ONCOLOGY PHARMACY

Recertification Requirements

Recertification for Board Certified Oncology Pharmacists (BCOP) requires assessment of a practitioner's knowledge and skills through one of two methods:

- Achieving a passing score on the 100-item, multiple-choice objective recertification examination, based on the content outline of the certification examination; OR
- Earning 100 hours of continuing education credit provided by a professional development program approved by BPS.

A current, active license to practice pharmacy is required for recertification.

Board Certified Oncology Pharmacists are also required to pay the BPS Annual Certification Maintenance fee of $125 each year for years one through six and a $400 recertification fee in year seven.

Option One: Examination

Achieve a passing score on the 100-item, multiple-choice objective recertification examination, based on the content outline of the certification examination (refer to the Oncology Pharmacy Content Outline for details).

Domain 1: Patient Management and Therapeutics. (57% of the examination).

Domain 2: Research and Education. (22% of the examination).

Domain 3: Practice Administration and Development. (17% of the examination).

Domain 4: Public Health and Advocacy. (4% of the examination).

Option Two: Continuing Education

Earn 100 hours of continuing education credit from the approved professional development program offered by the American College of Clinical Pharmacy (ACCP) in conjunction with the American Society of Health-System Pharmacists (ASHP), and/or the Hematology/Oncology Pharmacy Association (HOPA). Please note, BCOP must complete the review course at least once, but no more than three times during the seven-year recertification cycle.

PEDIATRIC PHARMACY

Recertification Requirements

Recertification for Board Certified Pediatric Pharmacy Specialists (BCPPS) requires an assessment of practitioner's knowledge and skills through one of two methods:

- Achieving a passing score on the 100-item, multiple-choice objective recertification examination (administered by BPS), based on the content outline for the Pediatric Pharmacy Specialty in their seventh year following initial certification; OR
- Earning 100 hours of continuing education credit provided by a professional development program approved by BPS.

A current, active license to practice pharmacy is required for recertification.

Board Certified Pediatric Pharmacy Specialists are also required to pay the BPS Annual Certification Maintenance fee of $125 each year for years one through six and a $400 recertification fee in year seven.

Option One: Examination

Achieve a passing score on the 100-item multiple choice recertification examination, based on the content outline of the certification examination (refer to the Pediatric Pharmacy Content Outline on the BPS website for details).

Domain 1: Patient Management (58% of the examination).

Domain 2: Practice Management (20% of the examination).

Domain 3: Information Management and Education (18% of the examination).

4: Public Health and Advocacy. (4% of the examination).

Option Two: Continuing Education

Earn 100 hours of continuing education credit provided by the professional development programs offered by the American College of Clinical Pharmacy (ACCP) and/or the American Society of Health-System Pharmacists (ASHP) and/or the Pediatric Pharmacy Advocacy Group. Pediatric Pharmacy Preparatory Review and Recertification Courses offered by any of the approved providers may only be completed for recertification credit up to two times, in nonconsecutive years, during the 7-year recertification cycle.

PHARMACOTHERAPY

Recertification Requirements

Recertification for Board Certified Pharmacotherapy Specialists (BCPS) is an assessment of a practitioner's knowledge and skills through one of two methods:

- Achieving a passing score on the 100-item, multiple-choice objective recertification examination, based on the content outline of the certification examination; OR
- Earning 120 hours of continuing education credit provided by professional development programs approved by BPS.

A current, active license to practice pharmacy is required for recertification.

Board Certified Pharmacotherapy Specialists are also required to pay the BPS Annual Certification Maintenance fee of $125 each year for years one through six and a $400 recertification fee in year seven.

Option One: Examination

Achieve a passing score on the 100-item, multiple-choice objective recertification examination, based on the content outline of the certification examination (refer to the Pharmacotherapy Content Outline on the BPS website for details). Please note, a new pharmacotherapy content outline will be used in Fall 2016. **Please check the BPS website for updates.**

Domain 1: Patient-specific Pharmacotherapy (60% of the examination).
Domain 2: Retrieval, generation, interpretation and dissemination of knowledge in pharmacotherapy (25% of the examination).
Domain 3: Systems and Population-based Pharmacotherapy (15% of the examination).

Option Two: Continuing Education

Earn 120 hours of continuing education credit from the approved professional development programs offered by the American College of Clinical Pharmacy (ACCP) and/or the American Society of Health-System Pharmacists (ASHP).

No more than 60 hours may be earned prior to the end of the fourth year of certification. However, all 120 hours may be earned during the last three years of certification. To achieve the 120 hour requirement, recertification candidates may participate in recertification offerings from both BPS approved pharmacotherapy continuing education providers.

The Pharmacotherapy Review & Recertification courses offered by either of the approved providers may only be completed for recertification credit up to two times, in nonconsecutive years. All other components may be completed every year throughout the seven-year recertification cycle to earn recertification credit.

For BCPS who are also certified in Ambulatory Care pharmacy, ACCP and ASHP will provide opportunities for dual continuing education credits that overlap across both specialties with the Clinical Reasoning Series and Intensive Study programs. Please be advised that each year, candidates are only allowed to earn six (6) total hours towards their BCPS & BCACP certifications using these continuing education courses.

PSYCHIATRIC PHARMACY

Recertification Requirements

Recertification of Board Certified Psychiatric Pharmacists (BCPP) requires an assessment of a practitioner's knowledge and skills through one of two methods:

- Achieving a passing score on the 100-item multiple choice recertification examination, based on the content outline of the certification examination; OR
- Earning 100 hours of continuing education credit provided by a professional development program approved by BPS.

A current, active license to practice pharmacy is required for recertification.

Board Certified Psychiatric Pharmacists are also required to pay the BPS Annual Certification Maintenance fee of $125 each year for years one through six and a $400 recertification fee in year seven.

Option One: Examination

Achieve a passing score on the 100-item multiple choice recertification examination, based on the content outline of the certification examination (refer to the Psychiatric Pharmacy Content Outline on the BPS website for details).

Domain 1: Patient Management (62% of the examination).
Domain 2: Information Management (25% of examination).
Domain 3: Health Policy and Practice Management (13% of examination).

Option Two: Continuing Education

The BPS-approved professional development program for Psychiatric Pharmacy is currently offered by the College of Psychiatric and Neurologic Pharmacists (CPNP).

The BCPP is required to earn 100 hours credit from this program.

Please note, BCPPs recertifying via continuing education are required to complete the Review Course a minimum of once, and a maximum of two times during their seven-year recertification cycle. The Review Course is revised and released every other year on the even year (2016, 2018, etc.). Given this revision cycle, individuals cannot repeat the current edition of the Review Course for BCPP Recertification or ACPE credit.

APPROVED BPS PROFESSIONAL DEVELOPMENT PROGRAMS FOR RECERTIFICATION

Please contact the following organizations for further information on approved CE programs.

For Ambulatory Care Pharmacy

American College of Clinical Pharmacy (ACCP)
(913) 492-3311 • FAX (913) 492-0088
(ACCP) - BPS Approved Ambulatory Care Pharmacy Recertification Program

American Pharmacists Association (APhA)
(202) 628-4410
www.pharmacist.com

American Society of Health-System Pharmacists (ASHP)
(301) 664-8700 • FAX (301) 652-8278
(ASHP) - BPS Approved Ambulatory Care Pharmacy Recertification Program

For Critical Care Pharmacy

American College of Clinical Pharmacy (ACCP)
(913) 492-3311 * FAX (913) 492-0088
(ACCP) - BPS Approved Critical Care Recertification Program

Society of Critical Care Medicine (SCCM)
(847) 827-6869 * FAX (847) 827-6886
(SCCM) - BPS Approved Critical Care Pharmacy Recertification Program

American Society of Health-System Pharmacists (ASHP)
(301) 664-8700 * FAX (301) 652-8278
(ASHP) - BPS Approved Critical Care Pharmacy Recertification Program

For Nuclear Pharmacy

Purdue University College of Pharmacy
Robert Heine Pharmacy Building
(765) 494-1361 * FAX (765) 494-7880
http://ce.pharmacy.purdue.edu

For Nutrition Support Pharmacy

Continuing education in Nutrition Support must be from providers approved by the Accreditation Council for Pharmacy Education (ACPE).

For Oncology Pharmacy

American College of Clinical Pharmacy (ACCP)
(913) 492-3311 • FAX (913) 492-0088
(ACCP) - BPS Approved Oncology Recertification Program

American Society of Health-System Pharmacists (ASHP)
(301) 664-8700 · FAX (301) 652-8278
(ASHP) - BPS Approved Oncology Recertification Program

Hematology Oncology Pharmacy Association (HOPA)
(877) 467-2791
HOPA- BCOP Recertification

For Pediatric Pharmacy

American College of Clinical Pharmacy (ACCP)
(913) 492-3311 • FAX (913) 492-0088
(ACCP) - BPS Approved Pediatric Pharmacy Recertification Program

American Society of Health-System Pharmacists (ASHP)
(301) 664-8700 • FAX (301) 652-8278
(ASHP) - BPS Approved Pediatric Pharmacy Recertification Program

Pediatric Pharmacy Advocacy Group (PPAG)
(901) 820-4434 • FAX (901) 767-0704
(PPAG) - BPS Approved Pediatric Pharmacy Recertification Program

For Pharmacotherapy

American College of Clinical Pharmacy (ACCP)
(913) 492-3311 • FAX (913) 492-0088
(ACCP) - BPS Approved Pharmacotherapy Recertification Program

American Society of Health-System Pharmacists (ASHP)
(301) 664-8700 • FAX (301) 652-8278
(ASHP) - BPS Approved Pharmacotherapy Recertification Program

For Psychiatric Pharmacy

College of Psychiatric & Neurologic Pharmacists (CPNP)
(402) 476-1677 • FAX (888)551-7617
https://cpnp.org/bcpp/recertification/products

RECERTIFICATION TIMELINE

Please view the chart below to determine your year of recertification. Remember, your certification becomes active December 31st of the year in which you sit for the initial certification exam or recertify, (July 1st for those initially certified during a Spring test window) and is active for a full seven years.

Initial Testing Year/ Year Last Recertified	Recertify by December 31 of
2009	2016
2010	2017
2011	2018
2012	2019
2013	2020
2014	2021
2015	2022

RECERTIFICATION APPLICATION PROCEDURES

It is the candidate's responsibility to submit an application that is completely and accurately filled out. Incomplete applications will not be processed. It is the candidate's responsibility to ensure the application is submitted by the deadline of August 1, 2016. Candidates who wish to recertify by testing in the Spring 2016 exam window must submit their application by March 11, 2016 (see Spring 2016 Candidate's Guide for a complete list of important deadlines). Those candidates wishing to test in the Fall 2016 exam window, or those using BPS-approved continuing education programs MUST submit their application by the August 1 deadline. Applications can be submitted through your MyBPS account.

CE hours for recertification may continue to be earned through the end of the calendar year for credit towards recertification.

Providers of BPS approved continuing education programs report all CE hours for recertification directly to BPS.

PROCESSING APPLICATIONS

All recertification applicants will be notified of their eligibility within 20 working days of BPS' receipt of their application and fee. Those candidates recertifying via examination will be contacted via email to schedule their exam after submitting a completed recertification application.

FEES AND PAYMENT METHODS

Recertification Fee
The fee for recertification is four hundred U.S. dollars ($400) and is due at the time the recertification application is submitted (no later than August 1, 2016).

The recertification fee helps cover the costs of the development and administration of recertification processes and the ongoing operations of the Board and its Specialty Councils. All fees are subject to change at the sole discretion of the Board.

Fee Payments
Payments are made in U.S. dollars by check, cashier's check, or money order made payable to Board of Pharmacy Specialties, or by credit card (VISA, MasterCard, American Express, Discover). Purchase orders are NOT accepted.

Declined Credit Cards and Returned Checks
When a credit card transaction is declined you may submit an alternate credit card for processing. When a check is returned for non-sufficient funds, payment must be sent by certified check or money order for the amount due. BPS reserves the right to charge fees incurred as a result of a check returned for insufficient funds.

Forfeiture of Fees/No Refunds
Candidates who fail to arrive at the Testing Centers on the date and time of the scheduled examination will forfeit their examination fees and must re-register by contacting BPS. Examination fees may NOT be transferred to another test window.

RECERTIFICATION VIA CE

Candidates who plan to recertify using BPS approved continuing education programs MUST submit their recertification application by the deadline date of **August 1, 2016** even if you have not completed your CE requirements.

The deadline to complete the required CE for recertification is **December 31, 2016.** If you believe you will not complete the CE requirement by the end of the year in which you are due to recertify, you may request an extension (see Request for Extension).

> **Important Dates for Candidates Recertifying Via CE**
> **Recertification Application Deadline**
> **August 1, 2016**
> **CE Requirement Deadline**
> **December 31, 2016**

EXAMINATION INFORMATION

Test Dates

BPS offers both a Spring and a Fall testing window for those candidates recertifying via exam. The Spring testing window will run between April 21, 2016 and May 7, 2016. The Fall window will run between September 21, 2016 and October 8, 2016. Recertification candidates licensed outside of the United States and Canada should view the section "Information for Foreign-licensed Candidates" beginning on page 10 for information on exam administration in their country. Candidates testing in Egypt and Saudi Arabia will take the paper-based exam on April 20, 2016 & April 21, 2016. In all other countries the BPS recertification exam will be administered via computer by Castle Worldwide (Castle), BPS's approved testing provider, through its affiliated test sites. Recertification candidates must schedule the date, time and location of their examination within the scheduled test administration window. Please see the Candidate's Guide for a complete list of deadlines and important dates.

Important Dates

Spring 2016 Application Deadline
March 11, 2016

Fall 2016 Application Deadline
August 1, 2016

Examination Dates

Spring 2016 Examination Window
April 21, 2016 - May 7, 2016

April 20 & 21, 2016 (Egypt and Saudi Arabia) (Paper-based Testing)

Fall 2016 Examination Window
September 22, 2016 - October 8, 2016 (Computer-based Testing)

September 21 & 22, 2016 (Egypt and Saudi Arabia) (Paper-based Testing)

Test Sites

BPS candidates can schedule their examinations at more than 450 test sites within the United States and more than 200 test sites outside of the United States through an arrangement with Castle. Test site locations can be found on the Castle website: http://www.castleworldwide.com/castleweb/clients/testing-services/testing-facilities.aspx.

Once an application is approved by BPS, applicants will be contacted by Castle to begin the scheduling process. Castle will contact you via email. It is recommended that applicants add ibt@castleworldwide.com to the list of acceptable addresses so that the emails to not get blocked by a spam filter.

Once a testing appointment is scheduled, the candidate will be notified of the exact test location, date, and time via email. The candidate must bring his/her printed confirmation to the test site. Please note that this confirmation will contain critical information, including the candidate's testing password.

The candidate also must bring current, government-issued photo identification with signature to the test site. Acceptable forms of identification include driver's licenses, passports, and government-issued identification cards. **The name on your identification must match the name on file with BPS.** If this is not the case, submit a Name Change Request through your MyBPS account. In order to help assure the greatest probability that candidates will receive their preferred test site and date, BPS recommends registering as early as possible once the schedule has been established.

Refer to the Candidate's Guide and/or www.bpsweb.org for a complete list of scheduling deadlines.

The testing network available to candidates has ample seats to meet demand for the BPS examinations. Castle will employ reasonable efforts to secure the test site and date requested by the candidate; however, BPS cannot guarantee availability of a testing session at a specific location within the designated testing period. Seats are filled on a first-come, first-served basis, based on test site availability.

Candidates may reschedule a testing session up to four (4) business days in advance of the schedule testing appointment through Castle's scheduling system. **BPS staff will not process change requests.** A $50 nonrefundable fee payable to Castle Worldwide will apply.

DANTES Program

Overseas U.S. military pharmacists may sit for BPS certification using the DANTES program through Military Education Centers. When candidates are sent a notice to schedule from Castle, they should contact Castle directly with the location and contact information from the DANTES site.

Scheduling

In order to help assure the greatest probability that certificants receive their preferred test site and date, BPS recommends registering as early as possible. Please view the Candidates Guide or visit www.bpsweb.org for a full list of priority deadlines.

Domestic Candidates must submit their scheduling request at least four (4) days prior to their preferred testing date during the scheduled test administration window. Non-U.S. candidates must submit their scheduling request at least ten (10) business days prior to their preferred testing date.

Castle will issue a Notice to Schedule (NTS) e-mail to approved certificants based upon the schedule noted. The NTS email will provide certificants with a unique username/password and the URL address to access Castle's online test scheduling system. Castle will issue a Notice to Schedule (NTS) e-mail to approved certificants based upon the schedule noted on the BPS website.

Castle will provide telephone and e-mail support to certificants on matters related to scheduling a testing appointment. Voicemail will accept certificants inquiries outside of normal U.S. business hours [Eastern time].

Once a testing appointment is scheduled, the certificant will be notified of the exact test location, date, and time via email. **The certificant must bring his/her printed confirmation to the test site.**

The certificant also must bring a current, government-issued photo identification with signature to the test site. Acceptable forms of identification include driver's licenses, passports, and government-issued identification cards. Unacceptable forms of identification include gym memberships, warehouse memberships, school identification cards, credit cards, and identification with signature only (no photo).

The certificant's name as it appears on the confirmation email must match the certificant's name as it appears on the government-issued photo identification. Certificant are responsible for contacting BPS with any name changes that occur after the submission of their application by submitting a name change request through their MyBPS account.

Rescheduling

Certificants may reschedule a testing session up to four (4) business days in advance of the scheduled testing appointment through Castle's scheduling system. BPS staff will not process change requests. A $50 nonrefundable fee, payable to Castle, will apply.

Day of Testing	Appointment: Must Reschedule/ Cancel By:
Monday	Tuesday of the previous week
Tuesday	Wednesday of the previous week
Wednesday	Thursday of the previous week
Thursday	Friday of the previous week
Friday	Monday of the current week
Saturday / Sunday	Tuesday of the current week

Special Circumstances

In the following situations and with appropriate documentation, certificants may change their testing session with fewer than four (4) days' notice. Certificants must contact Castle directly with documentation in order to reschedule. A $50 nonrefundable fee, payable to Castle, will apply.

(i) Serious illness (either the candidate or an immediate family member)

(ii) Death in the immediate family

(iii) Disabling accident

(iv) Court appearance

(v) Jury duty

(vi) Unexpected military call-up

Withdrawals

Candidates who withdraw from the exam recertification process after the application deadline (March 11, 2016 or August 1, 2016) will be charged a late withdrawal administrative fee of $200 ($250 if the exam has been

scheduled). Candidates who have withdrawn from the recertification process can maintain their credential and remain in good standing by immediately requesting an extension (see Request for Extension).

BPS will review requests for emergency withdrawals with decisions made on a case-by-case basis. Acceptable withdrawal requests, with appropriate documentation (e.g., physician's letter, police report, etc.) will be considered under the following situations:

(i) Serious illness (either the candidate or an immediate family member)

(ii) Death in the immediate family

(iii) Disabling accident

(iv) Court appearance

(v) Jury duty

(vi) Unexpected military call-up

Supporting documentation must be submitted to BPS within seven (7) days after the exam date. Candidates whose withdrawal request is not approved by BPS will forfeit all testing fees. Applications cannot be deferred from the Fall exam cycle into the next calendar year.

Checking In on Examination Day:

Recertification candidates should arrive at the test site at least 15 minutes in advance of the scheduled testing appointment time. If a candidate arrives at the test site 30 minutes after his/her scheduled testing appointment time and is refused admission, then the candidate will forfeit his/her appointment. **If an appointment is forfeited, there is no refund of the testing fee.**

The candidate must present <u>a valid government-issued photo identification with signature along with a printout of his/her testing appointment confirmation email.</u> Candidates will be required to sign in and will be instructed on where to store personal items and where to keep identification. The candidate's identity will be verified every time he/she enters or leaves the testing room.

Once the candidate has been checked-in, he/she will be escorted by testing staff to a workstation. The candidate must remain at the workstation unless authorized to leave by test site staff. Candidates may not leave the room without test site staff permission. If the candidate leaves the testing room without permission prior to completing his/her examination, he/she will forfeit the testing appointment and there will be no refund of testing fees.

Test site staff will provide the candidate with an erasable note board and pen, which may be replaced as needed during the test. The candidate may not remove the note boards or pens, and candidates are not allowed to use their own scratch paper or writing tools. Additionally, candidates will be provided with a calculator available on their computer screen for use during the exam.

Testing room temperature can be unpredictable; therefore, we suggest that you bring appropriate clothing with you (e.g., sweater, sweatshirt without hood) to help you adapt to a cooler or warmer climate in the examination room. Bring earplugs if you are sensitive to noise. If you choose to bring earplugs, they will be subject to examination by the testing center staff.

Prohibited Items

Candidates are expressly prohibited from bringing the following items to the test site:

- Cameras, cell phones or other mobile devices, optical readers, or other electronic devices that include the ability to photograph, photocopy, or otherwise copy test materials
- Notes, books, dictionaries, or language dictionaries
- Book bags or luggage
- iPods, MP3 players, headphones, or pagers
- Calculators, computers, PDAs, or other electronic devices with one or more memories
- Personal writing utensils (i.e., pencils, pens, and highlighters)
- Watches
- Food and beverage
- Hats, hoods, or other headgear, unless required for religious purposes

All items are subject to inspection by the proctor if suspicious behavior is detected. If Castle test site personnel determine that a candidate has brought any prohibited items to the test site, the candidate's item may be demanded and held for an indefinite period of time by Castle test site personnel. BPS and Castle reserve the right to review the memory of any electronic device that may be in the candidate's possession at the test site to determine whether any test materials have been photographed or otherwise copied.

If the review determines that any test materials are in the memory of any such device, BPS and Castle reserve the right to delete materials and/or retain them for subsequent disciplinary action. Upon completion of the review and any applicable deletions, BPS and Castle will return the device to the candidate, but will not be responsible for the deletion of any materials that may result from the review, whether or not such materials are test materials.

By bringing any such device into the test site in contravention of BPS and Castle policies, the candidate expressly waives any confidentiality or other similar rights with respect to the device, BPS and Castle review of the memory of the device, and/or the deletion of any materials. BPS, Castle, the examination site, and the test site staff are not liable for lost or damaged items brought to the examination site.

Inclement Weather and Cancellations

Castle will attempt to contact candidates in the event of a test site closure due to inclement weather to reschedule their appointment. As sites close, emails are issued to candidates

impacted notifying them of the closures, and Castle's website is also updated with this information. However, because closures can occur at any time during inclement weather, it is the responsibility of the candidate to contact Castle to receive the most up-to-date information regarding if a center is open or to reschedule the examination appointment. If a test site is officially closed, candidates will not be charged a rescheduling fee. If a test site is open and the candidate does not keep his or her appointment, the candidate forfeits all fees.

Retaking the Examination

If a recertification candidate fails to achieve a passing score on the examination, retaking the examination must take place within the following year. During this period, the individual's certification remains active; however, this period will be treated as a one-year extension on a one-time only basis, assuming the candidate has not already been granted an extension. No additional extension will be granted beyond this one-year period. The fee for retaking the examination is $200. Candidates who wish to retake the examination will be asked to submit an abbreviated application form through their MyBPS account. All recertification requirements must be completed by the end of the one-year extension, including passing the recertification exam, or that individual's certification will lapse and his/her name will be removed from the official roster of BPS-certified pharmacist specialists. Once removed permanently from the roster, reinstatement can be achieved only by the successful completion of the entire certification process.

For full information on the BPS examination process, please refer to the BPS website or the 2016 Candidate's Guide.

INFORMATION FOR FOREIGN LICENSED CANDIDATES

BPS certification is oriented primarily toward pharmacists licensed and practicing in the U.S. Recertification candidates who are not licensed to practice in the U.S. must submit a copy of their current, active, legal authorization to practice pharmacy in their country of origin or residence, along with their application form. If these documents are not in English, notarized English translations must be provided by the candidate, at the candidate's expense.

Throughout BPS specialty recertification examinations, all measures from laboratory test results are expressed in traditional units.

The Board is aware that examination questions dealing with procedures or regulatory issues in the U.S. are not necessarily pertinent to candidates who practice in foreign countries. However, all candidates are given the same examination and are held to the same standard of achievement, regardless of the country in which they practice and the regulations under which they practice.

Please note BPS certification does not confer the privilege to practice pharmacy in the U.S. or any other country.

Recertification candidates planning on testing in Egypt and Saudi Arabia should refer to the Spring or Fall 2016 Candidate's Guides for information regarding test administration in their country.

REQUEST FOR EXTENSION

Candidates seeking recertification who believe that they will not be able to sit for the recertification examination in their recertification year or who believe that they will not be able to complete all required CE by December 31 of the year in which they are to recertify may request an extension of their certification status. This request should be submitted via your MyBPS account. Certificants must upload a recertification application form and the $400 recertification fee must be submitted prior to this request for extension, plus any past fees including a $5 annual penalty. As part of the extension request, a candidate must submit a written request (in PDF or JPG format), providing specific reasons for not being able to sit for the examination or to meet the December 31 deadline for CE, as well as outline a plan for meeting all recertification requirements by December 31 of the following year. The request must be received by BPS by December 31 of the year in which the candidate is to recertify.

All requests will be reviewed on a case-by-case basis. **The Board may grant a one-year extension on a one-time only basis.** No additional extension will be granted beyond this one-year period. All recertification requirements must be completed by the end of the one-year extension or that individual's certification will lapse and his/her name will be removed from the official roster of BPS-certified pharmacist specialists.

When recertification is accomplished through a continuing professional development program for any specialty, all hours creditable to a specific seven-year recertification period must be earned within that period (plus an additional year, if granted an extension). Credit hours may not be carried over from one seven-year period to the next.

The "due date" of a professional development program which is established by its provider determines the year the program is creditable, regardless of when it is completed and submitted by the certificant.

If a certificant is recertifying via exam, they will only be granted one opportunity to test, and must pass the exam in their extension year. No additional extensions will be granted for examination retakes. If a candidate is granted an extension and successfully recertifies, it will result in resetting the certificants next certification date by one year to seven years from the end of the extension.

QUESTIONS

Board of Pharmacy Specialties®

2215 Constitution Avenue, NW
Washington, DC 20037-2985
202.429.7591 • FAX 202.429.6304
info@bpsweb.org • www.bpsweb.org